Sleep and Rehabilitation

A Guide for Health Professionals

Sleep and Rehabilitation
A Guide for Health Professionals

Julie M. Hereford, PT, DPT

President and Cofounder
CORE Services, Inc.
St. Louis, Missouri

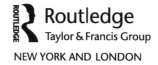

Routledge
Taylor & Francis Group

NEW YORK AND LONDON

First published 2014 by SLACK Incorporated

Published 2024 by Routledge
605 Third Avenue, New York, NY 10158

and by Routledge
4 Park Square, Milton Park, Abingdon, Oxon, OX14 4RN

Routledge is an imprint of the Taylor & Francis Group, an informa business

Library of Congress Cataloging-in-Publication Data

Hereford, Julie M., author.
Sleep and rehabilitation : a guide for health professionals / Julie M. Hereford.
        p. ; cm.
 Includes bibliographical references and index.
 ISBN 978-1-61711-033-7 (alk. paper)
 I. Title.
 [DNLM: 1. Sleep—physiology. 2. Rehabilitation—methods. 3. Sleep Disorders—physiopathology.
4. Sleep Disorders—therapy. WL 108]
RC547
616.8'498—dc23
                          2013025040

ISBN: 9781617110337 (pbk)
ISBN: 9781003526438 (ebk)

DOI: 10.4324/9781003526438

DEDICATION

For Henry

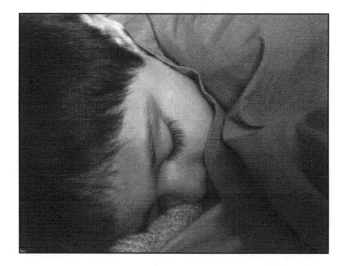

CONTENTS

Instructors: *Sleep and Rehabilitation: A Guide for Health Professionals Instructor's Manual* includes ancillary materials specifically available for faculty use. Included are PowerPoint slides. Please visit www.efacultylounge.com to obtain access.

ACKNOWLEDGMENTS

First and foremost I would like to acknowledge my parents for their unflagging support in life and particularly during this project. You taught me to wonder, you taught me to ask questions, you taught me to seek answers, and most importantly, you taught me to *do*. You offered me the space and the encouragement to write. I particularly want to thank my mother for helping me to stay on task.

I would like to thank Theresa Beach for her consistent and excellent care of my son, Henry. Knowing that you were there providing countless hours of care and support gave me the confidence, ability, and time I needed to read, research, and write. Thank you for your friendship and encouragement throughout this project. Thank you, too, for your assistance with research, syntax, grammar, and the ever present Oxford comma. I am grateful for your help with all the odds and ends, especially during the final push to complete the project and all the things I have forgotten to mention here.

I want to acknowledge the sacrifices that Henry has had to make during this project. He has been so patient with the time this has taken away from him.

To Molly Mebruer, Jessica Hoskins, and Amy Hereford: I cannot thank you enough for your unwavering dedication and commitment to this project. For fixing computer glitches, finding lost documents, clearing my space, guarding my office, finding time, dealing with my occasional unreasonable states, and celebrating milestones. Thank you for inspiring me and believing that I really could do this! I am lucky to have you.

To my business partner and friend, Mark Murray: For over 20 years, we have worked together and made our dream come true. Thank you for all you are, my friend. I can't imagine what my professional and personal life would be without you as such a major part of it.

To my friend and colleague J. Paul Rutledge, MD, for being the original inspiration for this work. You have helped me to understand patient care in a better and more complete way. And you were the first person who helped me to see how important sleep is in all aspects of patient care.

To Sarah Hereford for her outstanding and meticulous editing skills.

To Caren Schlossberg-Wood for her beautiful drawings and illustrations that helped bring this textbook to life.

To the rest of my family, friends, and colleagues who have helped and tolerated and encouraged me: Nancy, Lori, Lesley, Karen, Art, Karen Sue, Chris, Mary Lou, John, and Marian. You have each helped me in big and little ways and your help made this possible. I certainly have not mentioned everyone, but know that I hold you dear.

And, finally, to all of my patients who continue to inspire and teach me.

ABOUT THE AUTHOR

Julie M. Hereford, PT, DPT graduated from Saint Louis University with a BS in physical therapy and a master's of science in research from the Department of Anatomy and Neurobiology in 1989. As part of the graduate program in anatomy, Dr. Hereford performed original animal research comparing the effect of ultrasound, intra-articular injection, and phonophoresis on the morphology of articular cartilage and other joint structures that was presented at state, national, and international conferences. Dr. Hereford completed a doctorate in physical therapy and was named the Graduate with Distinction for her work in that program. In addition to national and state physical therapy organizations, Dr. Hereford is a member of Sigma Xi Research Society and served on the executive board of the Occupational Injury Prevention and Rehabilitation Society. She lectures frequently to colleagues and students and offers presentations to community groups. Course presentations include a variety of manual therapy technique courses, basic science review courses, and anatomical dissection courses. Dr. Hereford and Dr. J. Paul Rutledge have developed a course series for sleep science including "Sleep and Rehabilitation," "Sleep and Mental Health," and "Sleep and Learning." Dr. Hereford is the president and cofounder of CORE Services, Inc. in St. Louis, Missouri.

CONTRIBUTING AUTHORS

Michael D. Hoefs, DDS, DABCP (Chapter 22)
Craniofacial Pain Center of Nebraska
Lincoln, Nebraska

Duane C. Keller, DMD, FAGD, Dip. IBO (Chapter 25)
Keller Professional Group
St. Louis, Missouri

Bridget E. Lovett, OTR/L, CEAS (Chapter 23)
Clinic-Based Therapist
Lovett Family Wellness Center
Children's Hospital Colorado
Centennial, Colorado

Lauren E. Milton, OTD, OTR/L (Chapter 23)
Assistant Professor of Occupational Therapy
School of Health Professions
Maryville University
St. Louis, Missouri

Mark E. Murray, MS, BIAC, LPC (Chapter 26)
Partner, CORE Services, Inc.
St. Louis, Missouri

J. Paul Rutledge, MD (Foreword)
Diplomat of the American Board of Psychiatry and
    Neurology
St. Louis, Missouri

Catherine Siengsukon, PT, PhD (Chapter 21)
Assistant Professor
Physical Therapy and Rehabilitation Science
University of Kansas Medical Center
Kansas City, Kansas

PREFACE

The purpose of this book is to provide rehabilitation professionals with a source of information that will help them gain a better understanding of sleep and its impact on the rehabilitation process. It is widely accepted that sleep is an important factor in overall health and that it is necessary for the recovery of various physiologic, metabolic, and neurologic processes. It is less widely known that dysfunctional sleep may contribute to delayed recovery from injury due to disruption in connective tissue regeneration. Research has also shown that dysfunctional sleep can interfere with the consolidation of both experiential memory and motor learning. Disruption of these processes caused by disordered sleep can interfere with rehabilitation and delay physical performance improvement and the achievement of treatment goals.

This book will describe sleep and sleep disorders from a rehabilitation perspective. In order to have a thorough understanding of how sleep will impact rehabilitation, it is necessary to understand the role that sleep plays in overall health and the impact that dysfunctional sleep has on general health and well-being. Much of the current understanding of sleep has come from research studies in which sleep is manipulated experimentally in order to disrupt one or more stages of sleep or to prevent sleep completely, and then study the resultant alterations in brain activity and the impact on physiology, psychological processes, and metabolism. For example, when sleep is temporarily reduced in healthy subjects, they show increased cortisol levels, reduced glucose tolerance, and increased sympathetic nervous system activity. In addition, a number of studies have linked chronic pain conditions with dysfunctional sleep patterns. These studies suggest not only that pain may cause sleep dysfunction but also that dysfunctional sleep can aggravate pain by decreasing the pain threshold and pain tolerance and increasing tissue irritability; it may also disrupt the endogenous pain modulation system. Though the physiological mechanism underlying this relationship is not completely understood, it appears likely that the relationship between pain and sleep dysfunction involves aberrant processing of tactile-cutaneous sensory inputs at the mesoencephalic level and in the trigeminal nucleus during wakefulness and sleep.

Cardiovascular function is another important factor to consider as part of many rehabilitation programs; it is important for the rehabilitation professional to understand the impact sleep has on this system. A short sleep cycle impacts cardiovascular function and results in increased heart rate and blood pressure. It can also cause increased sympathetic nervous system tone, which may significantly magnify an individual's response to stressful stimuli.

Sympathetic nervous function modulates multiple systems and it should be considered as a part of any treatment program because increased sympathetic tone can have an adverse effect on the rehabilitation process. Sleep deprivation and dysfunctional sleep, especially obstructive sleep apnea, can cause sympathetic hyperactivity. The specific impact of increased sympathetic tone is not well understood, but it can have significant effects on overall health and physiologic function and can be an important risk factor in psychological disorders such as anxiety, depression, and mental illness.

Because of the multisystem repercussions of dysfunctional sleep, assessment of sleep habits is fundamental to rehabilitation and should be included as part of the clinical history of every patient seen for a rehabilitation evaluation. This book will provide the clinician with evidence-based practice guidelines for evaluating sleep quality and quantity in the rehabilitation setting and recommend a referral algorithm.

Once a clinician identifies a sleep dysfunction, the individual should be referred for a sleep study or polysomnogram. This book is not intended as a clinical guide to polysomnography, but will provide the rehabilitation professional with a basic understanding of the data gathered during a sleep study and will introduce common terminology utilized in the process. It will teach the reader to interpret the sleep study in order to effectively guide the patient and will define common sleep disorders that are likely to be found in the rehabilitation patient, giving a clinical picture of each. It will summarize the effects of sleep dysfunction on multiple physiological systems but will consider its implication specifically in the context of rehabilitation. It is designed to help the rehabilitation professional gain a better understanding of sleep and its dysfunction.

One of the most important parts of this book is an exploration of current research that deals with sleep and motor learning. Though it is important to understand the effects of sleep and sleep disorders on overall health, it is also important to understand the implications of disordered sleep on the rehabilitation process. In particular, recent research has shown that sleep is tied to consolidation of motor learning. It follows that dysfunctional sleep may interfere with the ability to incorporate particular restorative movement patterns that are learned and practiced during a rehabilitation session unless the appropriate stage of sleep is achieved within a specific time frame. This book will discuss ways in which sleep might be manipulated in order to enhance the rehabilitation process.

The last section of the book will provide the reader with material that can be used to meet the specific needs of particular patient populations. For instance, the sleep needs for a patient with a neurological injury are likely different from those of an endurance athlete. The ways in which sleep can be manipulated to enhance the rehabilitation process for various patient types will be discussed. This section will also explore the relationship between sleep dysfunction, sensory integration, sympathetic tone, and the mechanics of respiration. Evaluation of problems in these areas will be presented and treatment techniques designed to address these issues will be outlined.

The overall goal of this work is to assist the rehabilitation provider in working with a patient with sleep dysfunction to improve overall quality and quantity of sleep in order to improve the outcome of the rehabilitation intervention.

FOREWORD

Sleep and Rehabilitation: A Guide for Health Professionals represents an important contribution to the field of rehabilitation. As skilled clinicians, we are sometimes left in the dark when patients fail to make the progress we expect despite our skill and their hard work. We question this lack of progress and look for answers. This book makes clear that often the answers to that question lies in the darkness of sleep. While steadily unraveling and unlocking the mystery that is sleep, our authors equip health professionals with the knowledge and tools needed to recognize and effectively treat those obstacles that prevent patients from reaching their rehabilitative goals.

With a growing body of evidence documenting the problems associated with improper sleep, this book could not have come at a better time. A diminishment in productivity both at work and at home, fatal accidents at job sites and in the sky, and the rise in obesity rates have all been linked to insufficient or ineffective sleep. By possessing an understanding of the science of sleep and its mechanics and disorders, health professionals not only improve patients' lives but also put themselves at the forefront of those successfully combating the underlying cause of these problems. Unfortunately, in today's health care environment, there can be a tendency to treat the most obvious symptoms with the most common therapy rather than treating the underlying cause. The truth is that most physical problems requiring rehabilitation are issues that affect our bodies 24 hours a day, not just the hours one is awake and active. If sleep is not evaluated, health professionals may not simply be missing a piece of the picture but may be failing to recognize the part of the problem that is slowing or even defeating their therapeutic efforts.

Dr. Julie M. Hereford sets her presentation of sleep in this context. This book not only furnishes the reader with a thorough understanding of sleep itself but also examines the issues presented when sleep is dysfunctional or disordered due to structural abnormalities or other health-related issues. It provides the knowledge needed to recognize our sleep-disordered patients and apply some therapeutic techniques that may offer some relief of symptoms related to disordered sleep. Importantly, this volume provides a common language to assist the rehabilitation professional to engage in conversation with other health professionals about our patients' sleep and the problems associated with it in order to assist the patient in finding solutions to sleep problems which can improve overall health. This book also provides a framework for the clinical decisions we must make as rehabilitation professionals for and about our patients. For many patients, it is imperative that we have the knowledge about sleep and sleep disorders to make accurate diagnoses that will lead to accurate prognoses about our patients' ability to benefit from our interventions. The format of this text—first providing the reader with a solid grounding in the mechanisms of sleep and its many disorders and dysfunctions, the addition of information on evaluation and treatment of the sleep-disordered patient, and, finally, special implications for rehabilitation professionals—provides students and clinicians alike with the basis for clinical decision making.

This book has also given me the opportunity to see my many years of collaboration with Dr. Hereford come to fruition. Though I have had the great pleasure to meet and work with a variety of health professionals throughout my over 30 years as a psychiatrist, it was my meeting with Dr. Hereford that I count among my most fortuitous. It was because of my own need for physical therapy many years ago that I came to know Dr. Hereford and further came to appreciate her skill as a clinician and educator. Though her dedication to her field, her expansive knowledge of the intricacies of the human body, and her excellent clinical skills were soon apparent, it was my continued need for physical therapy that led to an opportunity that we as health professionals so often seek: a shared conversation about that which interests us as clinicians. Dr. Hereford was eager to hear my ideas about sleep and its impact on mental health concerns and to have a forum to discuss her interest in the same topic as it applied to her patients. Out of those meetings grew a shared desire to present to other health professionals the information we found so professionally fulfilling and so helpful to our patients. The resulting series of seminars was happily well received and was, in some measure, the impetus for this volume that addresses these issues in a comprehensive manner.

Although our work together may have been the stimulus for her to explore the importance of sleep in rehabilitation therapy, she has taken that exploration to a new level. Her thorough exposition of the nature and function of sleep across the life span clarifies how it influences the function and dysfunction of the body. She offers clear guidelines for any clinician to screen for possible sleep disorders and pursue collaboration with other professionals to have the disorders diagnosed and treated. The implications for rehabilitative therapy are made clear. Her work provides essential information for any rehabilitation therapist or other clinician who wants to make a real difference for the people he or she treats by a better understanding of the whole person. As new research continues to elucidate connections between the central nervous system and every other system in our bodies, anyone who does not appreciate the intricate effects of sleep in that picture will be left in the dark. Dr. Hereford's work is a cornerstone of the information that is essential to any clinician who does not want to become obsolete in the near future.

What *Sleep and Rehabilitation: A Guide for Health Professionals* ultimately gives us is one more opportunity to strengthen the quality of care we provide our patients. I am confident that readers will agree that this is a truly welcome contribution to our field. May this book be a source of insight and inspiration to our shared mission to provide the best treatment for those who entrust themselves to our care.

J. Paul Rutledge, MD
Diplomat of the American
Board of Psychiatry and Neurology
St. Louis, Missouri

Section I

Basic Science of Sleep

1

Introduction

Julie M. Hereford, PT, DPT

Why do rehabilitation professionals need to know about sleep? It is one of the primary functions in which every patient engages. As will be explored in this book, sleep is a biological imperative. It is even considered an "occupation" in some areas of rehabilitation. It is necessary for normal health and well-being and is a critical factor in recovering from illness and injury. Abnormal sleep patterns, or *disordered sleep*, can be an important contributing factor in the development of systemic disease. Sleep occupies nearly one third of a normal individual's life; therefore, it seems reasonable that every health care provider should have some understanding of the mechanisms involved in sleep, the processes that influence sleep, and those that are influenced by sleep.

It is not enough to know that a patient needs sleep in order to maintain a healthy life. It has been well established that sleep is essential for the survival and integrity of most living organisms. The exact function of sleep, however, continues to remain somewhat speculative despite a growing understanding of the processes that initiate and maintain sleep. It is clear that sleep is important for multiple physiological processes including brain function, thermoregulation, neuronal detoxification, and energy conservation.

Observation of human behavior appears to indicate that humans are relatively flexible in sleeping and waking behavior at any given time during the day or night. This suggests that an individual can wake up and perform simple and complex tasks at almost any time of the day or night at will. Although humans often attempt to override the biological need for sleep, this need actually has an awesome power over the lives of humans. If an individual goes without sleep or drastically reduces it, the desire or the need to sleep will quickly become more important than life itself (Figure 1-1). In fact, at some point, sleep is so preemptive that an individual cannot stay awake even to avoid death.

Examples of the extraordinary sleep drive that can overwhelm an individual, even in the face of death, can be seen in the number of automobile accidents that are linked to a driver falling asleep at the wheel. In fact, in a recent report the National Highway Traffic Safety Administration estimated that there are 56,000 sleep-related accidents annually in the United States, resulting in 40,000 injuries and 1550 fatalities[1] (Figure 1-2). A study undertaken by the National Transportation Safety Board estimates that as many as 30% of commercial road transport crashes are related to sleep and fatigue.[2]

Sleepiness has been known to impair the judgment of long-haul truck drivers so that they continue driving even though they risk falling asleep. Intense sleepiness or extreme difficulty maintaining wakefulness for more than 2 or 3 days can cause a need for sleep that is so compelling and powerful it cannot be avoided. An individual may in fact fall asleep while operating a vehicle, even though the risk of such behavior is obvious. This strongly suggests that the function of sleep is so important that it may supersede all other activities, if the debt is great enough.

There have been several industrial disasters and accidents linked to sleep deprivation, fatigue, and inattention that have made worldwide news. Investigators have ruled that sleep deprivation in critical workers was a significant causative factor in the nuclear accident at Three Mile Island in 1979 and in the core meltdown at Chernobyl in 1986[3] (Figure 1-3). Sleep deprivation was ruled a significant factor in the grounding of the *Exxon Valdez* oil tanker in Prince

Hereford JM. *Sleep and Rehabilitation:*
A Guide for Health Professionals (pp 3-5).
© 2014 Taylor & Francis Group.

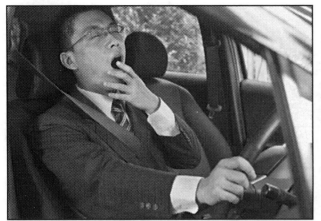

Figure 1-1. The drive for sleep can be so powerful that it can overwhelm basic survival instincts. (From Fotolia.com.)

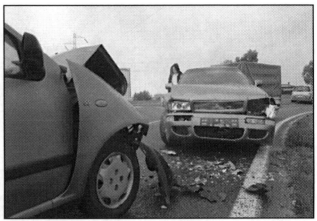

Figure 1-2. Drowsy driving can have deadly results and is on the rise. (From Fotolia.com.)

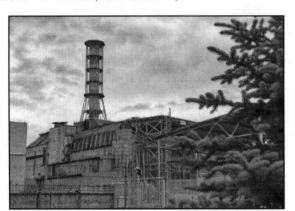

Figure 1-3. The nuclear meltdown at Chernobyl in 1986 was one of several major industrial disasters related to sleep deprivation of workers. (From Fotolia.com.)

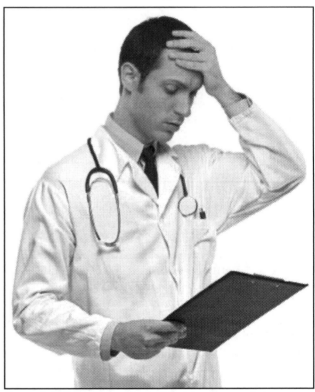

Figure 1-4. Sleep deprivation is linked to many workplace errors; in the medical field, these have sometimes resulted in death. (From Fotolia.com.)

William Sound, Alaska, in 1989[4] which cost millions of dollars and caused untold ecological and environmental damage. The explosion of the space shuttle *Challenger* was caused by extreme sleep deprivation in operation engineers who were trying to solve problems after the shuttle launch had been scrubbed several times.[5] This was a particularly high-profile launch because of the nature of that flight, which was carrying the first teacher in space, Christa McAuliffe. There was added pressure to make this launch because the subsequent mission, which would carry two exploratory probes, had a limited window for success. Repeated delays of the *Challenger* launch were a source of embarrassment for the program, increasing the stress and sleep deprivation of the launch crew. This was likely a contributing cause of the critical decision to launch despite problems with the vehicle that led to the explosion 73 seconds after lift-off.

The link between sleep deprivation and medical errors in hospitals is an increasingly recognized problem (Figure 1-4). The Institute of Medicine estimated that 50,000 to 100,000 deaths and over a million injuries were caused by preventable medical error, many of which are thought to be the result of sleep deprivation.[6]

Humans spend an significant amount of time sleeping, generally occupying up to one third of an individual's life. In fact, human society has been largely organized around the need for sleep. Caves, huts, houses, apartment buildings, and hotels are all clustered together so that humans can be safe and secure during sleep. Much of time, recreation and social activities are organized around the demand for sleep.

Understanding that sleep is a powerful and significant driver of life, it becomes important to understand *what* sleep is. Defining sleep is complicated because it consists of 2 very different stages that are so markedly different from one another that they must be described separately. Sleep is generally divided into rapid eye movement (REM) sleep and non-rapid eye movement (NREM) sleep. REM sleep involves a state of sleep in which there are binocularly synchronous rapid movements of the eye. In addition, there is a suppression of voluntary motor function resulting in nearly complete muscle atonia in all but a few select facial muscles and the muscles of the ossicles of the ear during REM sleep. Somatic reflexes are depressed. Activity of the autonomic nervous system is irregular and accelerated. The brain is clearly more active during REM sleep than during NREM sleep and, in some respects, even more active than it is during wakefulness. In fact, measurement of central nervous system activation strongly suggests that the brain reaches peak activity during REM sleep. There is unique metabolic activity, gene expression, and neurosecretion associated with sleep. In contrast, NREM sleep has an entirely different electroencephalogram pattern and lacks the visible ocular movements and twitches. Whereas REM sleep, also called *paradoxical sleep*, produces a distinctive rapid sawtooth pattern, NREM sleep produces a pattern that is more synchronized and slow. Autonomic function and general bodily physiology appear to present a more regular pattern of activity during NREM sleep compared to REM sleep.

What is essential to understand is that sleep is not a state in which the brain rests. In fact, it is no more conceivable that the brain needs to rest than that the liver needs to rest. On the contrary, certain cognitive and noncognitive processes are specifically associated with particular phases in the sleep cycle. Rather than being a time when the brain rests, it is a period of major and critical activity that does not occur during wakefulness. It appears that the essential difference between normal wakefulness and normal sleep is the degree of perception. During wakefulness, the individual is conscious of the external world. The individual can engage with and respond to stimuli within that environment. During wakefulness, humans foster survival, interact in the real world, find food, reproduce, and engage in a variety of meaningful activities. The fundamental essence of sleep, on the other hand, seems to be disengagement from the outer world and, to some extent, an engagement with an inner dream world (Figure 1-5). This disengagement is an active process in which sensory input is blocked or modified to a level that results in essential perceptual blindness and deafness.

Understanding what sleep is invites further investigation into how a clinician might use this powerful activity to the best benefit of a patient. In particular, one might ask whether there are ways in which sleep can be manipulated or used advantageously with regard to the rehabilitation process. This text will explore the basic science of sleep. The neurobiology of sleep will be discussed in some detail in order to understand how pathways and neurotransmitters that are influenced during rehabilitation are also influenced during sleep. Because of these interconnections,

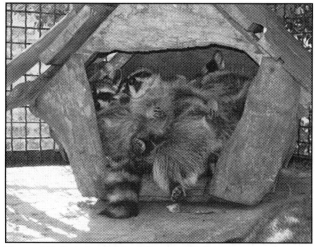

Figure 1-5. Sleep in all animals is a time of disengagement from the outer world. (From Fotolia.com.)

one might reasonably conclude that interference in sleep may complicate progress toward rehabilitation goals.

To that end, this text will discuss the impact that sleep has on motor learning and motor planning. The text will further suggest ways in which a rehabilitation professional can recognize an individual with a potential sleep disorder and recommend ways that the rehabilitation provider can intervene and refer the patient for appropriate testing. This text will assist the rehabilitation provider in being able to interpret findings from a standard sleep study and utilize that information in treatment planning. In addition, this text will suggest ways in which a rehabilitation provider may assist a patient to improve the quality of sleep.

REFERENCES

1. SmartMotorist.com. Driver fatigue is an important cause of road crashes. Available at: http://www.smartmotorist.com/traffic-and-safety-guideline/driver-fatigue-is-an-important-cause-of-road-crashes.html. Accessed December 20, 2011.
2. National Highway Transportation Safety Administration. Research on drowsy driving. Available at: http://www.nhtsa.gov/Driving+Safety/Distracted+Driving/Research+on+Drowsy+Driving. Accessed July 11, 2011.
3. ThirdAge.com. 6 Disasters caused by lack of sleep. Available at: http://www.thirdage.com/sleep/6-disasters-caused-by-lack-of-sleep. Accessed July 18, 2011.
4. *Exxon Valdez* Oil Spill Trustee Council. Details about the accident. Available at: http://www.evostc.state.ak.us/facts/details.cfm. Accessed July 17, 2011.
5. Space on NBCNews.com. Seven myths about the shuttle *Challenger* disaster. Available at: http://www.msnbc.msn.com/id/11031097/ns/technology_and_science-space/t/myths-about-challenger-shuttle-disaster/#.UFh9v66Djng. Accessed July 17, 2011.
6. Zhang J, Patel VL, Johnson TR. Medical error: is the solution medical or cognitive? *J Am Med Inform Assoc.* 2008;6(suppl):75-77.

What Is Sleep?

Julie M. Hereford, PT, DPT

Defining sleep is far more complicated than it appears to be on the surface. Sleep is not simply a single biological process, nor is it a single neurological process. Rather, it is a complex interaction between biology and neurology. In order to answer the question "What is sleep?" it is important to understand what happens to an organism when it sleeps, why an organism sleeps, and what mechanisms underlie sleep.

Sleep is definitely not a state during which the brain rests (Figure 2-1). In fact, nerve cells in the brain fire 5 to 10 times more frequently during certain stages of sleep than during wakefulness. The brain does not require rest any more than other organs in the human body do; it is not the case that engaging in more activity during wakefulness will reliably produce more sleep. It is also not the case that physical rest during wakefulness removes the urge to sleep. If anything, the opposite is true. For instance, if one simply sits around all day, perhaps just watching television or reading for pleasure, the urge for sleep seems to increase compared to a day in which one is relatively physically active. Surprisingly, the answer to the question of why organisms sleep—specifically, why humans sleep—is not completely clear.

Sleep is not a passive event in which one's brain "runs out of energy" and goes to sleep to rest. In fact, the mechanisms within the brain for sleep are remarkably complex and coordinate to actively induce and maintain sleep. Without normal, synchronous, and rather precise control, sleep may become disordered. Further, if certain parts of the brain are destroyed or inactivated by injury or disease thereby causing inhibition of certain neural activity, sleep mechanisms can be reduced or certain stages of sleep may be eliminated entirely. This book will explore normal neurological mechanisms that induce and maintain sleep and will discuss some of the systemic sequelae that may result due to disordered sleep when normal neurological processes are disrupted.

The complexity of this topic requires the definition of some terminology that is generally accepted in the literature regarding the science of sleep. To that end, this text will utilize 4 criteria to define sleep. First, sleep consists of very little movement. Generally, during normal sleep, the organism does not walk, talk, or write. Second, sleep usually entails adopting a stereotypic posture, usually lying down (Figure 2-2A and B). Stereotypic sleep posture is species specific. Most individuals adopt a particular posture in order to go to sleep, which may be considered that individual's *comfort posture*. This posture will also vary somewhat by individual within a species. In humans, this posture may be affected by the environment in which one sleeps but may also be affected by the condition of the body. For example, if an individual is suffering from an acute musculoskeletal injury, it may require alteration from a typical comfort posture during sleep. This is, in fact, an important consideration when obtaining subjective information during an initial evaluation of a patient. It is important to determine whether the typical posture in which the patient usually goes to sleep has been maintained or if circumstances such as pain or airway issues have caused a change in posture in order to be able to fall asleep.

A third criterion that is used to define sleep is that it involves a reduced response to stimulation. That is, the individual usually does not respond to low-intensity sounds, touches, or other sensory stimulation. Sensory threshold will vary with the stage of sleep and with age. For

Hereford JM. *Sleep and Rehabilitation:*
A Guide for Health Professionals (pp 7-18).
© 2014 Taylor & Francis Group.

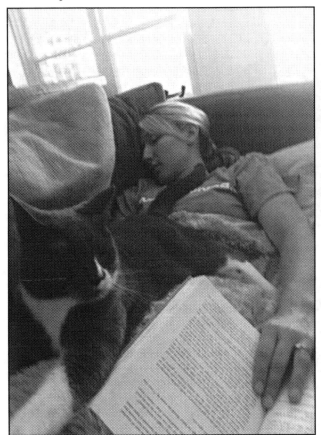

Figure 2-1. During sleep the brain is not at rest. Sleep is not a passive event. (Reprinted with permission from L. Callaham.)

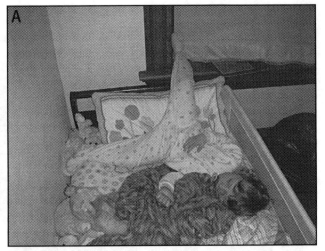

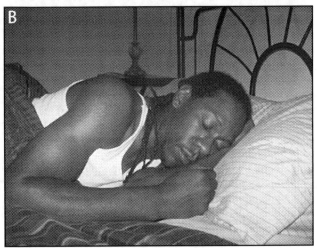

Figure 2-2. Sleep involves getting into a stereotypic posture. (Reprinted with permission from J. Hoskins and T. Hereford.)

example, the auditory threshold is relatively high in the very young sleeper but is often lower as the sleeper ages, which explains why a baby can sleep through a seemingly impossibly loud environment but an older adult may awaken at minimal auditory intrusion.

The fourth criterion of sleep is reversibility. One can readily be awakened from sleep, as distinguished from a coma or death, in which an individual is unable to reverse out of the state into normal wakefulness.

In addition to these 4 criteria that define sleep, certain physiological changes within the body and brain are also commonly utilized to identify sleep and describe its various stages. The sleeping brain produces particular electrical patterns that are typical of specific stages of sleep. For example, the brainwave pattern produced during rapid eye movement (REM) sleep differs substantially from that seen during non-rapid eye movement (NREM) sleep. In fact, electrophysiological changes are a common clinical method of describing sleep. Additionally, certain physiological changes including heart rate changes, body temperature changes, and changes in respiratory rate and rhythm are typical during sleep and can be used to define its various stages.

Clinically, sleep is studied by polysomnography (PSG), which uses multiple measurements of physiological function and brainwave activity during sleep. There are 3 primary measures that have been used to define sleep from a physiological perspective. The measures include electroencephalogram (EEG), electrooculogram (EOG), and electromyogram (EMG). These 3 measures are simultaneously recorded so that the relationships among the 3 can be seen immediately. These criteria have been chosen based on historical precedent, relative ease of measurement, and the discrimination power of each measure.

How Sleep Is Measured

An EEG records electrical activity or brainwaves produced by voltage fluctuations resulting from electrical activity of neurons within the brain (Figure 2-3). These brainwaves are recorded via electrodes that are placed at specifically described sites on the scalp. Billions of neurons in the brain produce its electrical charge by membrane potentials that pump ions across membranes. These

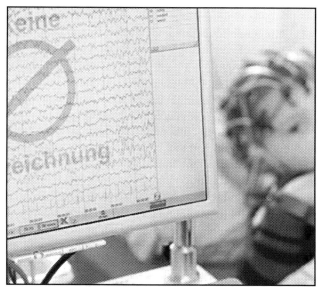

Figure 2-3. EEG records the electrical activity of the brain via electrodes adhered to the scalp with conductive gel. (From Fotolia.com)

propagate action potentials across neurons in a process known as volume conduction. When the electrical wave reaches the electrode on the scalp, it pushes or pulls electrons on the metal of the electrode resulting in a positive or negative charge. This is then measured by a voltmeter and recorded as part of the EEG.[1] The electrical activity of a single neuron is far too small to record; therefore, the recorded EEG wave reflects the summation of the synchronous activity of thousands or millions of neurons that have similar spatial orientation.

Scalp EEG activity shows oscillations at a variety of frequencies. Several of these oscillations have characteristic frequency ranges and spatial distributions and are associated with different states of brain functioning that are of particular interest when studying sleep (eg, waking and the various sleep stages). These oscillations represent synchronized activity over a network of neurons. The neuronal networks underlying some of these oscillations are understood (eg, the thalamocortical resonance underlying sleep spindles), though many others are not (eg, the system that generates the posterior basal rhythm). Research that measures both EEG and neuron spiking has shown that the relationship between the two is complex, with the power of surface EEG in only 2 bands (gamma and delta) relating to neuron spike activity.[2]

A clinical EEG is used to measure electrical activity over a 20- to 40-minute period and often includes administration of various sensory stimuli in order to provoke neuronal irritability and to help to determine neurological disorders such as epilepsy. EEG is also utilized as part of a sleep study or PSG, although the electrode placement is different from that of a full clinical EEG evaluation and recordings are taken across a full night's sleep rather than for a short period of time (Figures 2-4, 2-5, and 2-6).

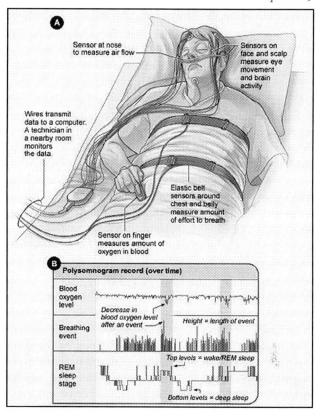

Figure 2-4. The polysomnography uses EEG, electrooculogram, and EMG to record brain and muscle activity while the subject sleeps. (Reprinted with permission from the National Heart, Lung, and Blood Institute Health Information Center.)

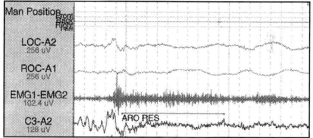

Figure 2-5. Three bipotentials, the EEG, EOG, and EMG, are the primary measures that have been used historically to define physiological sleep. They are recorded simultaneously so that the relationships among the 3 can be seen immediately. These criteria were chosen based on historical precedent, relative ease of measurement, and discriminating power. (Reprinted with permission from American Sleep Medicine of St. Louis.)

The stages of sleep as seen on EEG were first described by Dr. Alfred Loomis in 1937. Loomis utilized electroencephalography when he and his coworkers separated sleep EEG into 5 different levels from wakefulness through deep sleep.[3] In a paper published in 1957, Drs. William Dement and Nathaniel Kleitman identified REM and reclassified sleep into REM sleep and 4 stages of NREM sleep.[4] In 1968, Drs. Allan Rechtschaffen and Anthony Kales developed standardized criteria for defining sleep stages in a method known as the R&K Sleep Scoring Manual, or R&K System, which divided NREM sleep into 4 stages. This method

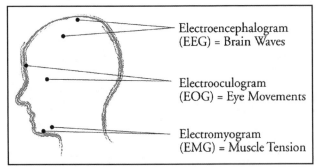

Figure 2-6. Normal site for placement of EEG, EOG, and EMG electrodes during a polysomnography study.

further defined stages 3 and 4 sleep as slow-wave sleep (SWS), in which delta waves are produced. Specifically, stage 3 sleep is defined as that in which delta wave sleep composes less than 50% of sleep and stage 4 sleep is sleep in which delta sleep composes more than 50% of the sleep EEG pattern.[5] The R&K system had been the system utilized to evaluate sleep until the American Academy of Sleep Medicine (AASM) revised it in 2007. The revised sleep scoring system also includes arousal and respiratory events, cardiac activity, and limb movement information. The scoring system revisions were published as The AASM Manual for the Scoring of Sleep and Associated Events.[6] EEG is one of the 3 primary physiological measures used to define and study sleep. The other 2 are EOG and EMG.

An EOG is a recording of the differences in electrical potential between surface electrodes placed on either side of the head near the side of the eye. The electrodes record eye movements and eye position (Figure 2-7).

Electrooculography is not, however, a measurement of the EMG activity of the extraocular muscles. Instead, it measures the movement of the eyeball itself. Although the precise mechanism is not completely understood, the most likely theory, the cornea–retinal dipole theory, states that an electric dipole is formed through the eye because the cornea is positively charged and the retina is negatively charged. A dipole is measured as the difference in this electrical field. As the eye changes direction, so does the dipole, and this can be detected and recorded as an electrical signal (see Figure 2-5). EMG signals from facial muscles may create artifacts in the tracing of EEG of the brain during PSG.[7]

Sleep studies utilize EOG as one of the bipotentials that are recorded to help determine the stage of sleep, particularly REM sleep. During this phase of sleep, as the name implies, there may be very rapid and random eye movements. These REM sleep bouts usually occur every 90 to 120 minutes and may last from 5 to 30 minutes. This is the type of sleep that is usually associated with active dreaming and is accompanied by profound muscle atonia, changes in respiratory and cardiac function, and markedly increased brain activity. It is often during this phase of sleep that there is less precise control of physiological activity, which may lead to disordered sleep (see Chapters 11 and 12).

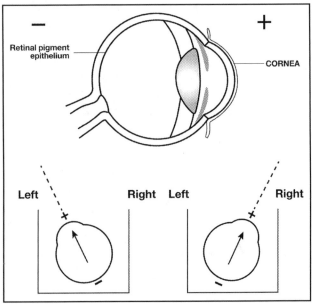

Figure 2-7. EOG. The eye acts as a dipole. The cornea is positively charged and the retina is negatively charged, which creates a dipole with an electrical field that can be measured. When the eye moves, electrodes placed in a lateral position to the eye record changes in the electrical potential which give the characteristic EOG tracings during polysomnography.

EMG is the last of the 3 commonly utilized bipotentials that are measured during a sleep study. An EMG measures the electrical activity of skeletal muscles recorded with the placement of small electrodes applied to the skin's surface. Electrode placement is usually under the chin and over the shin area. An electrode is placed over both of these areas to pick up increased muscle activity in the jaw, which may indicate the presence of bruxism, and over the shin to detect abnormal limb movement during sleep. The EMG records muscular activity that is a result of an action potential stimulated by a message within motor centers in the brain that eventually finds its way to a neuromuscular junction propagating down the alpha motor neuron and releasing acetylcholine (Ach). Ach travels across the neuromuscular junction and causes Ach-gated receptors to open, allowing sodium ions to flow into the cell, causing it to depolarize. The potential change activates voltage-dependent sodium channels, which results in action potential that propagates throughout the muscle fiber. The current creates potentials in the extracellular space that may be recorded by electromyography. This potential can occur 60 to 100 times per second and a single action potential may last 1 to 3 ms, although the time of muscle contraction may last 10 to 100 ms. The contraction of the muscle as a result of a single action potential is called a *muscle twitch*. If the action potentials continue at a successive rate, the muscle does not have time to relax and the twitches are additive and observed as muscular contractions. If this occurs at a high enough frequency, the force output of the muscle will plateau as a tetanus response. With temporal

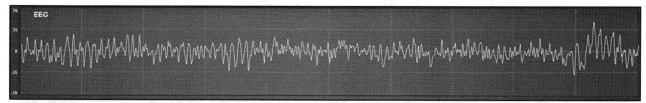

Figure 2-8. EEG of awake drowsy state. Alpha and theta wave activity. EEG activity shows low-voltage, random, fast waves. (Reprinted with permission from CORE Services, Inc.)

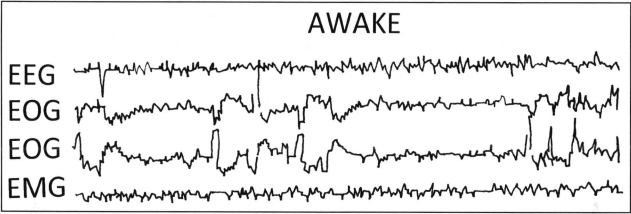

Figure 2-9. EEG, left EOG is listed first and right EOG is listed next, followed by an EMG of the awake state. (Reprinted with permission from CORE Services, Inc.)

or spatial summation of action potentials, musculature is recruited for the desired muscle activity. The force output of the muscle can be related to the amplitude of the EMG signal. That is, the fewer muscle fibers that are recruited, the smaller the EMG signal. With a stronger muscle contraction resulting from higher-frequency muscle recruitment, the greater the amplitude of the EMG signal. The overall amplitude of an EMG signal is related to the number, size, and frequency of recruited motor units, measured in millivolts. EMG monitoring during the course of a sleep study provides information regarding nerve and muscle function and may be useful in diagnosing neurological disorders and conditions that present in characteristic ways during sleep. Restless leg/legs syndrome and periodic limb movement are examples of these. Measuring EMG activity is also useful in distinguishing between REM and NREM sleep, because there is postsynaptic inhibition that occurs during REM sleep and will be characterized as a relative quiescence of motor activity during REM sleep.

STAGES OF WAKEFULNESS AND SLEEP

Wakefulness

Although the differences between wakefulness and sleep seem readily apparent, closer examination reveals some surprising differences between the 2 states. Typical

and obvious components of wakefulness are consciousness and awareness of the external environment. Wakefulness can also be described in the context of PSG recording. For example, wakefulness as described by EEG findings in a wakened, neurologically intact human subject usually alternates between 2 major patterns. First is a low-voltage (~10 to 30 µV), fast activity (16 to 25 Hz) pattern that is often called an activation or desynchronized pattern. The activation pattern is most prominent when subjects are alert with their eyes open and are scanning the visual environment (Figure 2-8). REMs may be abundant or scarce depending on the amount of visual scanning. Muscle activity may be high or moderate depending on the degree of muscle tension and general activity of the subject. This EEG activity may be considered beta activity in which the individual is very alert and active.

The EEG pattern seen in Figure 2-9 was recorded from an individual who was awake with eyes closed. These potentials are generally recorded from the parietal and occipital lobes and posterior parts of the temporal lobes. The EEG pattern in an individual who is awake with eyes closed is a sinusoidal pattern at 8 to 12 Hz of about 20 to 40 mV. This is called alpha activity and is typically most abundant in the subject who is relaxed, non-attentive, and perhaps drowsy and with the eyes closed. Alpha wave activity usually occurs in a synchronized fashion, connecting both hemispheres of the brain (Figure 2-10). This alpha activity may immediately precede descent into a sleeping state.

Wakefulness and EEG desynchronization are precisely controlled events in the brain and require coordinated excitatory innervation of the forebrain. Several parallel

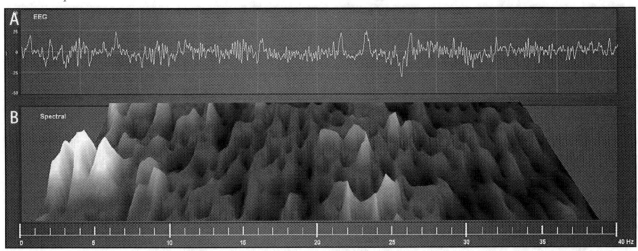

Figure 2-10. Alpha waves. (A) Drowsy wakefulness (B) with spectral analysis. EEG waves oscillate at 8 to 12 cycles per second. (Reprinted with permission from CORE Services, Inc.)

ascending tracts including glutamate, acetylcholine, and serotonin and norepinephrine neurotransmitter pathways appear to contribute to the state of wakefulness.[8] Studies indicate that activation of the cortex is accomplished by several major pathways from the brain stem through the thalamus, through the basal forebrain and hypothalamus, and by way of 2 pathways directly projecting from the locus coeruleus and dorsal raphe.[8] When first described, this system was known as the ascending reticular activating system, but further study has revealed that cells of this system lie outside the reticular formation and so the term ascending activating system is now more commonly used. The ascending activating system describes several components throughout the brain stem and midbrain whose discharge rates increase before the first sign of the change to the EEG desynchronized state. Cells that project to the thalamus are cholinergic and localized to the laterodorsal tegmentum/pedunculopontine (LDT/PPT) region. These remain active when the EEG is desynchronized during wakefulness and REM sleep. Discharge rates decline during NREM sleep. Glutamatergic projections from reticular formation, monosminergic projections from the locus coeruleus, and serotonergic projections from the dorsal raphe demonstrate a significant state-related change in discharge rate, with the highest rate occurring during wakefulness, decreased during NREM sleep, and completely silent during REM sleep.[9] These data show that sleep is actively regulated and specific stages of sleep are induced and maintained by particular neurotransmitters.

Another neuropeptide called *orexin* or *hyocretin* has been identified as a neurotransmitter that contributes to wakefulness (Figure 2-11). This neurotransmitter sends excitatory projections to components of the ascending activating system and appears to enhance general arousal and EEG desynchronization. It is thought to help control the transition between sleep and wakefulness.[10,11]

What follows will describe specific sleep stages from stage 1 to stage 4 sleep. It should be noted that sleep

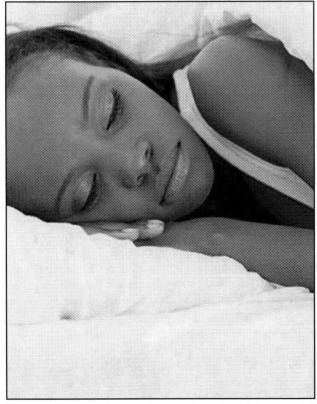

Figure 2-11. Orexin or hyocretin is a neurotransmitter that may control the transition between sleep and wakefulness. (From Fotolia.com)

architecture, or the manner in which sleep progresses across a night's sleep, does not follow a 1 to 4 pattern. Rather, sleep architecture varies according to brain activity and certain environmental conditions. For simplicity of discussion, however, these stages will be described in numeric order.

Onset of Sleep

Normal adult human sleep is initiated through NREM sleep. Infants may enter sleep through REM sleep, but if

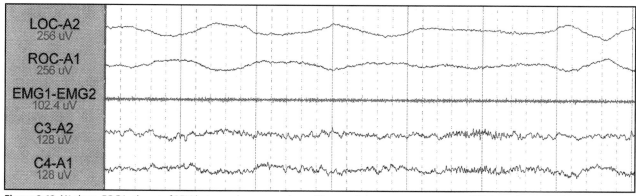

Figure 2-12. N1 sleep. EOG is absent of REM but may show some slow rolling synchronous eye movements. EEG shows 3- to 7-Hz theta waves. EMG shows a marked decrease in activity. (Reprinted with permission from American Sleep Medicine of St. Louis.)

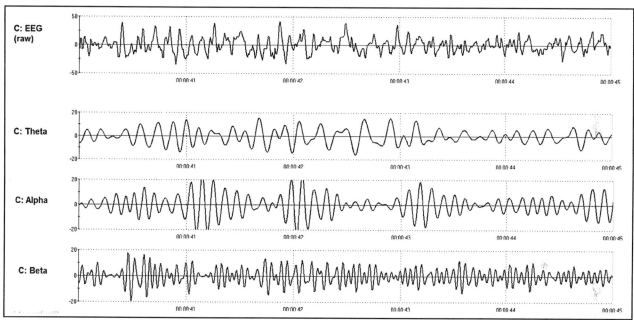

Figure 2-13. This illustration shows a raw EEG with theta, alpha, and beta waves imbedded in a single tracing. The top tracing is the raw wave. The second segment shows only the theta wave that has been pulled out of the raw wave form. The third tracing is only the alpha wave and the last segment is only the beta wave form. (Reprinted with permission from CORE Services, Inc.)

an adult enters a sleeping state through REM sleep, it may be considered a pathological event as is sometimes seen in narcolepsy.

"Falling asleep" does not appear to be a singular event, as sensory awareness, self-consciousness, memory, and logical thought processes and response to external stimuli recede. Rather, it appears to be actively controlled by specific brain centers. Generally, normal adult sleep is initiated with stage 1 (N1) sleep; however, N1 can sometimes be difficult to identify clearly from drowsy, relaxed wakefulness. Muscle activity is usually considerably decreased, but EMG findings cannot specifically identify the moment of onset of sleep. Electrooculography may show some changes as sleep approaches with the slowing of eye movements and the onset of asynchronous, slow rolling movements. EEG tracings, however, show a more clear change from the rhythmic alpha wave activity.

Stage 1 Sleep

As an individual begins to become drowsy and adopts a sleep posture, closes the eyes, and begins to generate alpha waves, he may easily drift into sleep. Stage 1 sleep is difficult to distinguish from wakefulness based solely on observation. EEG activity can make this distinction, however (Figure 2-12). In fact, if an individual is awakened from stage 1 sleep, he or she may likely report that he or she was not asleep, indicating that the perception of sleep is variable at this stage. This is frequently seen in the classroom or in the evening in front of the television. When a companion awakens the individual, he or she may well deny having been asleep at all. EEG readings would likely show alpha wave activity decreased from the high alpha that is seen during non-attentive relaxation with the eyes closed (Figure 2-13). The EEG will consist mostly of low-voltage,

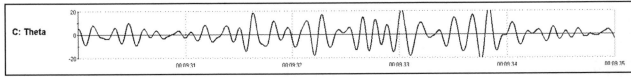

Figure 2-14. Theta waves characteristic of N1 sleep. (Reprinted with permission from CORE Services, Inc.)

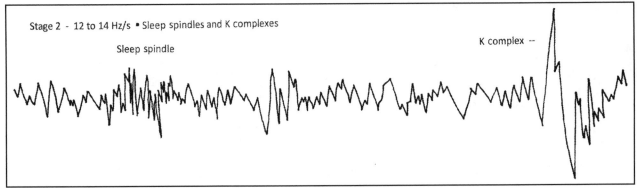

Figure 2-15. Sleep spindles and K-complexes characteristic of N2 sleep. (Reprinted with permission from CORE Services, Inc.)

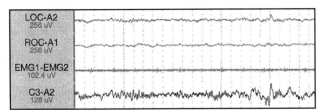

Figure 2-16. Stage N2 sleep. (Reprinted with permission from American Sleep Medicine of St. Louis.)

mixed-frequency activity with scarce alpha wave activity. Brain wave activity is at the 3- to 7-Hz range (Figure 2-14). Rapid asynchronous eye movement is absent, but slow, rolling, and asynchronous movement may appear.

Behavioral factors also change as an individual enters stage 1 sleep. Though simple automatic motor activity may be possible, generally there is a cessation of physical activity. The exception to this is the continuation of "automatic" activity such as an individual continuing to operate a vehicle after having fallen asleep. The individual cannot, however, respond appropriately to external stimuli with the same immediacy that he or she would be able to while awake, explaining the frequency of sleep-related traffic injuries and deaths.

Individuals who have entered into stage 1 sleep experience a perceptual disengagement in which they show decreased responsiveness to visual and auditory stimulus. Interestingly, particular olfactory stimuli are maintained during the initial phase of sleep. Sensing of strong pleasant or unpleasant odors appears to be maintained in stage 1 sleep but not beyond.[12] Though responsiveness to stimuli is generally decreased at the onset of sleep, it is not the case that an individual becomes unable to respond to meaningful stimuli. For example, an individual has a lower arousal threshold for his or her own name as opposed to someone else's. Likewise, a mother has a significantly lower arousal

threshold for the cry of her own child over an unrelated child. That is, an individual has a lower arousal threshold for meaningful versus non-meaningful auditory stimuli. According to one study, this remaining responsiveness seems to indicate that part of the brain maintains some awareness and can become activated in the presence of meaningful stimuli.[13]

Stage 1 sleep may be accompanied by sudden twitches and hypnic myoclonus, which are the sudden, substantial body or limb jerks that some individuals occasionally experience as they drop off to sleep. These are not pathologic but appear to be associated with increased stress and periods of disrupted sleep schedule and fatigue. Stage 1 sleep is essentially a transitional stage between wakefulness and sleep.

Stage 2 Sleep

Stage 2 (N2) sleep has a distinctive EEG pattern and specific brain activity. Against a continuing background of low-voltage, mixed-frequency EEG activity, bursts of distinctive rapid rhythmic 12- to 14-Hz sinusoidal waves called sleep spindles that last at least 0.5 seconds appear in the EEG. K-complexes often accompany sleep spindles and occur approximately 1 to 2 minutes apart during stage 2 sleep (Figure 2-15). Sleep spindles follow interaction between the thalamus and the cortex and have been correlated with maintenance of sleep in the presence of external noise. Sleep spindles occur immediately following muscle twitching and are related to motor learning, especially in the very young. They are associated with integration of new information into existing knowledge, memory consolidation, and remembering and forgetting.

K-complexes are the largest event that occurs in a normal human EEG (Figure 2-16). They consist of a brief high-voltage (75+ µV) peak followed by a slower positive complex at

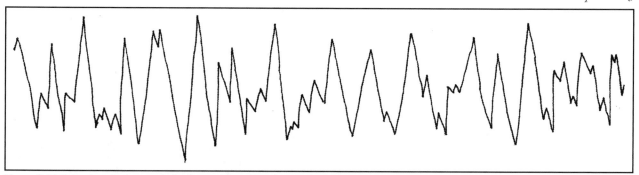

Figure 2-17. Delta sleep is characteristic of stage N3 and N4 sleep. EEG of delta waves oscillates at 0.5 to 2 cycles per second greater than 75 μV. (Reprinted with permission from CORE Services, Inc.)

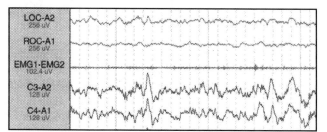

Figure 2-18. Stage N3 sleep. (Reprinted with permission from American Sleep Medicine of St. Louis.)

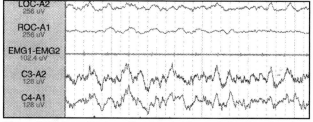

Figure 2-19. Stage N4 sleep. (Reprinted with permission from American Sleep Medicine of St. Louis.)

350 to 550 ms and another negative peak at approximately 900 ms. They occur every 1 to 2 minutes and are often followed by bursts of sleep spindles. K-complexes are thought to preserve sleep and are involved in information processing homeostasis of synapses and memory consolidation.[14]

Eye movements are rare and EMG activity is low to moderate during stage 2 sleep. Body temperature begins to decrease and the heart rate starts to slow. The sleeper loses complete conscious awareness of the environment, and muscular activity as measured by EMG is significantly decreased. Stage 2 sleep occupies 45% to 55% of total sleep time in the normal adult. It is associated with memory consolidation and is of particular interest when studying motor learning and memory and will be discussed in considerable depth in Chapter 21.

Stage 3 Sleep

Stage 3 sleep is characterized by high (>75 μV), slow (0.5 to 2 Hz) waves called delta waves (Figure 2-17). Although the 2007 American Academy of Sleep Medicine guidelines[6] have combined stage 3 and stage 4 sleep, many texts continue to describe stage 3 sleep as delta sleep or SWS with 20% to 50% delta waves (Figure 2-18) and stage 4 sleep as having greater than 50% SWS (Figure 2-19). Dividing SWS into stage 3 and stage 4 sleep in the sleep lab can prove daunting when striving for pure accuracy, and because the physiological function of SWS is very similar in N3 and N4, combining the data seems a reasonable method. Because the clinician utilizing this text to incorporate principles of sleep medicine into rehabilitation clinical practice is most likely to use sleep studies generated under the 2007 American Academy of Sleep Medicine guidelines,[6] this text

will generally combine stage 3 and stage 4 sleep and will refer to such sleep as N3 sleep, delta sleep, or SWS. These terms will be used interchangeably. However, in a detailed discussion of SWS, certain distinctions regarding the physiological and hormonal events that occur will be more specifically discussed, and it will be useful to divide SWS into N3 and N4. It should be kept in mind that the predominant difference between the two is the density of delta waves within the sleep stage.

Rapid Eye Movement Sleep

REM sleep is characterized by changes in the EEG pattern and significant physiological changes compared to NREM sleep and wakefulness. At the onset of REM sleep, the EEG reverts to a low-voltage, mixed-frequency pattern similar to that of stage 1 sleep (Figure 2-20). As REM sleep progresses, its brain activity is similar to the activity seen during wakefulness, and thus REM sleep has sometimes been called *paradoxical sleep*. Bursts of prominent REM are measured on electrooculography. The background EMG activity is virtually absent, but many small muscle twitches may occur against this low background activity (Figure 2-21).

For the most part, the major differences among N1, N2, and N3 sleep are found in the EEG patterns, and although there are some exceptions, the general physiology of these stages is fairly similar. The physiology of REM sleep, however, is dramatically different from NREM sleep or wakefulness. Heart rate and blood pressure can become erratic and irregular during REM sleep. Respiration can be similarly irregular and may be a contributing factor to sleep-related breathing disorders, which have a propensity

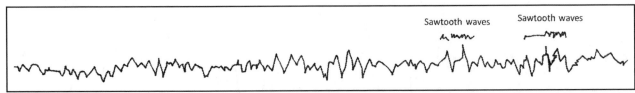

Figure 2-20. REM sleep characterized by low voltage, random, fast with sawtooth waves. (Reprinted with permission from CORE Services, Inc.)

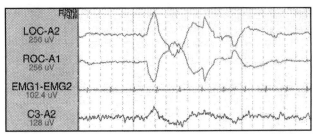

Figure 2-21. REM sleep. (Reprinted with permission from American Sleep Medicine of St. Louis.)

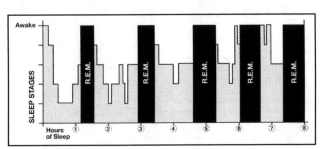

Figure 2-22. Normal sleep architecture histogram.

to occur during REM sleep compared to other stages of sleep. Body temperature regulation is also erratic during REM sleep and is marked by the loss of ability to regulate body temperature, causing it to migrate to the ambient temperature of the environment. This can be especially precarious in infants because of the prodigious amount of REM sleep that an infant usually has. The adult sleeping in an extreme temperature (such as in extreme cold during winter camping), will simply forgo REM sleep in order to maintain body temperature regulation. However, when the individual returns to a normal temperature environment in which to sleep he or she appears to "catch up" on REM sleep. This seems to indicate the important role of REM sleep in human function.

Normally, REM sleep occurs cyclically with NREM sleep with the average NREM–REM cycle lasting approximately 90 to 110 minutes. As the night progresses, REM sleep takes up more of the cycle and N3 and N4 take up less.

DISTRIBUTION OF SLEEP ACROSS A TYPICAL NIGHT

The distribution of the various sleep stages across one typical night's sleep is commonly illustrated in the form of a histogram and is referred to as the sleep architecture. The sleep histogram depicted in Figure 2-22 plots NREM and REM sleep over the course of one night. NREM is lightly shaded and REM sleep is depicted in black. In the neurologically intact normal adult, sleep is entered through NREM sleep at the beginning of the night. This is usually preceded by a period of drowsy wakefulness in which there is a significant amount of alpha wave activity. During this period of wakefulness, which occurs immediately prior to the onset of sleep, the individual may experience vivid visual hallucination-like images. This transition into sleep may

be accompanied by small muscle twitching or even hypnic myoclonia, which consists of significant group muscle jerking and is usually experienced by the individual as a sense of falling. This is normal activity but does tend to occur more frequently when the individual is under increased stress or has experienced disruption of the normal sleep cycle and is somewhat sleep deprived.

Sleep onset is an active neurological process and, as such, normally requires some time to move from drowsy wakefulness to stage 1 sleep. This process would normally require 10 to 20 minutes to "fall asleep." In fact, the individual who goes to sleep immediately upon going to bed may in fact be sleep deprived and thus not able to attain sleep by a normal physiological process. This may interfere with normal maintenance of sleep or may be an indication of poor sleep hygiene or another abnormality of sleep such as obstructive sleep apnea that interferes with the quality and quantity of normal restorative sleep. The manifestations and consequences of sleep deprivation can be substantial and may interfere with quality of life and may contribute to significant systemic pathology (see Section II).

A normal adult, upon sleep onset, will descend fairly quickly through N1 and N2 to deeper SWS, which consists of N3 and N4 sleep (Figure 2-23). In a typical night, the sleeper will experience two or three 15- to 20-minute bouts of SWS, or *restorative sleep,* during the early part of the total sleep cycle. From the onset of sleep to the end of the first REM period is the first sleep cycle and usually lasts from 90 to 110 minutes from sleep onset. There is a cyclic alternation between NREM and REM sleep that constitutes the basic sleep cycle. The average periodicity of this cycle is 90 to 110 minutes, although later cycles tend to be shorter than the earlier ones. SWS dominate NREM periods in the first part of the night but are completely absent during the later cycles. Toward the end of the night, very brief periods of wakefulness may interrupt sleep even in the normal sleeper (see Figure 2-23).

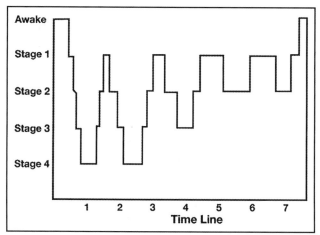

Figure 2-23. Sequences of states and stages of sleep on a typical night.

NREM sleep is often considered lighter sleep than REM sleep for a number of reasons. When subjects are awakened from NREM sleep, they report that they have been in lighter sleep than when they are awakened from REM sleep. Galvanic skin activity, which is sometimes used as an indicator of emotional arousal, is more frequent during NREM than during REM sleep. Muscle tone and spinal reflexes are maintained during NREM but are significantly inhibited during REM sleep. In some brain areas such as the raphe nuclei and the locus coeruleus, neuronal activity is maintained during NREM but is completely quiescent during REM.

In contrast, REM sleep is characterized by increased neural activity in some brain areas, such as the occipital cortex, compared to NREM sleep. These increases are sometimes greater even than during wakefulness. Brain temperature is usually decreased during NREM but is dramatically increased during REM sleep. Cerebral blood flow increases dramatically as the sleeper transitions from NREM to REM sleep. Heart rate, respiration rate, and blood pressure are much more variable during REM sleep than during NREM. The EEG of REM sleep resembles the EEG of wakefulness much more than does the EEG of NREM sleep. In fact, in most animals, the EEGs of REM sleep and wakefulness are almost indistinguishable. Muscle twitches are more frequent during REM sleep than during NREM sleep. Although dreaming occurs in all stages of sleep, dreaming is reported more frequently upon awakening from REM sleep than upon awakening from NREM sleep.

It is clear that NREM sleep and REM sleep are dramatically different entities in terms of brain wave activity, arousal threshold, and general physiology, so much so that they can be considered to be separate forms of sleep.

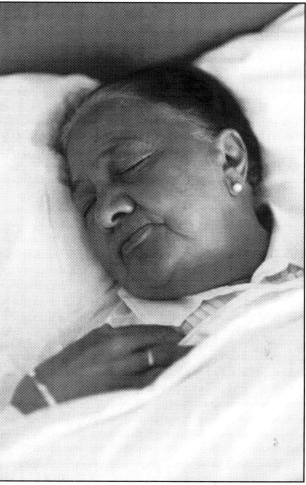

Figure 2-24. Sleep requirements change across the life span. (From Fotolia.com)

SLEEP REQUIREMENTS

Sleep requirements vary with age (Figure 2-24). Normal adults require 7 to 9 hours of sleep in a 24-hour period. The sleep requirements for infants, children, and young adults vary, with infants requiring a great deal of sleep and children requiring less as they get older. Pubescent young adults actually require slightly more sleep than children due to the significant demands of puberty. Contrary to popular belief, older adults do not have a decreased requirement for sleep. Instead, sleep in older adults is much more likely to be fragmented, and they are more likely to nap during the day to meet their sleep needs.

The greatest determinant of an individual's sleep requirement on any given night is the quality and quantity of sleep during the preceding night. Apart from that, volitional determinants such as staying up late or getting up early are superimposed on the genetic sleep need. Though there are those who reportedly do not require much sleep, sleep is a biological imperative and cannot be cheated without biological consequences. These consequences may manifest themselves in a variety of physiological and/or psychological ways. In addition to sleep deprivation, it is also possible to sleep too much. That is, the consequences of chronic excessive sleep, as may occur in some psychological disorders, can be as substantial as chronic sleep deprivation. This, of course, does not extend to the occasional sleep excess or deprivation. It is the chronicity of either that creates problems (see Chapters 11 and 12).

SUMMARY

It is clear that sleep is a complex and vital function that is necessary for the general health and neurocognitive function of the individual. Four criteria have been identified that constitute behavioral sleep. First, the sleeper produces very little movement. Second, the sleeper generally assumes a stereotypic posture; however, the drive for sleep can be so overwhelming that sleep is unavoidable and individuals will fall asleep anywhere in any posture if the sleep drive is strong enough. Third, the sleeper disengages from most external stimuli and appears to engage with an inner world. Finally, sleep is readily reversible and tends to occur in a cyclic fashion across a 24-hour day.

Sleep is able to be measured in a laboratory with PSG, which allows for measurement of several different physiological functions. These parameters help to describe different stages of sleep and are used diagnostically to determine the existence of disordered sleep. These measures include EOG to measure eye movement, EEG to measure brainwave activity, and EMG to measure muscle activity.

Sleep is divided into 2 distinct phases, NREM and REM sleep. It has been shown that these 2 phases are physiologically very different. NREM sleep is further subdivided into NREM stages 1 to 4, although most sleep labs now combine stage 3 and 4 sleep. The normal sleeper cycles between NREM and REM sleep throughout the night about every 90 to 110 minutes. This cycling can be measured and is known as *sleep architecture*. NREM stage 3 and 4 sleep, also known as SWS, usually occurs in the early part of the night, whereas NREM stage 2 sleep and REM sleep activity increases in density in the latter part of a normal night's sleep.

Sleep architecture varies across the life span, with infants experiencing an increased percentage of REM sleep and older individuals experiencing decreased percentages of NREM stage 3 and 4 sleep. Sleep requirements are greater in infancy, childhood, and during puberty but remain the same throughout adult life. Contrary to some beliefs, older adults require the same amount of sleep but may experience increased sleep fragmentation and thus have a loss in the quality of sleep. Daytime napping sometimes makes up for some of this sleep debt.

REFERENCES

1. Tatum WO, Husain AM, Benbadis SR. *Handbook of EEG Interpretation.* New York, NY: Demos Medical Publishing; 2008.
2. Whittingstall K, Logothetis NK. Frequency-band coupling in surface EEG reflects spiking activity in monkey visual cortex. *Neuron.* 2009;64:281–289.
3. Loomis AL, Harvey EN, Hobart GA. Cerebral states during sleep, as studied by human brain potentials. *J Exp Psychol.* 1937;21(2):127–144.
4. Dement W, Kleitman N. Cyclic variations in EEG during sleep and their relation to eye movements, body motility and dreaming. *Electroencephalogr Clin Neurophysiol.* 1957;9:673–690.
5. Rechtschaffen A, Kales A, eds. *A Manual of Standardized Terminology, Techniques and Scoring System for Sleep Stages of Human Subjects.* Washington, DC: Public Health Service, United States Government Printing Office; 1968.
6. Iber C, Ancoli-Israel S, Chesson A, Quan SF. *The AASM Manual for the Scoring of Sleep and Associated Events: Rules, Terminology and Technical Specifications.* Westchester, IL: American Academy of Sleep Medicine; 2007.
7. Croft RJ, Barry RJ. Removal of ocular artifact from the EEG: a review. *Neurophysiol Clin.* 2000;30:5–19.
8. Jones BE. From waking to sleeping: neuronal and chemical substrates. *Trends Pharmacol Sci.* 2005;26:578–586.
9. Steridae M, Datta S, Pare D, et al. Neuronal activities in brainstem cholinergic nuclei related to tonic activation processes in thalamocortical systems. *J Neurosci.* 1990;10:2541–2559.
10. Lu MG, Hassani OK, Alonso A, Jones BE. Cholinergic basal forebrain neurons burst with theta during waking and paradoxical sleep. *J Neurosci.* 2005;25:4365–4369.
11. Saper CB, Chou TC, Scammell TE. The sleep switch: hypothalamic control of sleep and wakefulness. *Trends Neurosci.* 2001;24:726–731.
12. Carskadon MA, Dement WC. Normal sleep and its variations. In: Kryger MH, Roth T, Dement WC. *Principles and Practice of Sleep Medicine.* 5th ed. St Louis, MO: Elsevier Saunders; 2011.
13. Portas CM, Krakow K, Allen P, et al. Auditory processing across the sleep–wake cycle: simultaneous EEG and fMRI monitoring in humans. *Neuron.* 2000;28:991–999.
14. Tononi G, Cirelli C. Sleep function and synaptic homeostasis. *Sleep Med Rev.* 2006;10:49–62.

3

Phylogeny of Sleep and Sleep Apnea

Julie M. Hereford, PT, DPT

Much of what has been learned about the nature and characteristics of sleep has been learned by studying the animal kingdom (Figure 3-1). Correlating sleep with other characteristics of a species can provide clues to the adaptive functions of sleep. Sleep has been studied in over 90 different animal species in different taxonomic groups, including mammals, birds, fish, reptiles, amphibians, and insects.

Sleep habits, sleep places, and sleep postures vary greatly among species. For example, moles and rabbits sleep in burrows, and zebras sleep out in the open. Cattle can sleep with their eyes open. Seals and hippopotamuses spend part of their sleep under the water. Gorillas settle into nests to sleep.

Sleep duration varies with the size of the animal. For example, giraffes sleep an average of 1.9 hours per 24-hour period (Figure 3-2), and elephants only sleep 2 to 3 hours per 24-hour period. The little brown mouse, on the other hand, sleeps more than 20 hours per 24-hour period.

Sleep has adapted and evolved over time to meet species specific needs for survival. For example, dolphins and porpoises sleep while swimming and can sleep with one half of their brain at a time while the other half is awake so as to permit these air-breathing mammals to come to the surface to breathe periodically (Figure 3-3). Horses and zebras spend the majority portion of every 24-hour period standing, part of the time in rapid eye movement (REM) sleep, by utilizing a passive locking mechanism in their limbs. Because both horses and zebras sleep out in the open, sleeping while standing allows them to move quickly if confronted by a predator.

The universality of sleep in mammals, despite all of the variations in duration and place, is evidence that sleep is indispensable. Not only do all mammals sleep but, as a rule, they experience cyclical alteration between non-rapid eye movement (NREM) and REM sleep. An outstanding exception to this pattern is the echidna, a spiny Australian ant-eater, a monotreme, which has no REM sleep, only NREM sleep (Figure 3-4). The reason for this is unclear.

Birds also sleep. Like mammals, birds have cycles of NREM and REM sleep but with some differences. One of the most striking differences is that both NREM and REM sleep episodes are quite short in birds. Their NREM sleep episodes average only about 2.5 minutes and REM sleep episodes only 9 seconds. Birds do not lose muscle tone during REM sleep as consistently as mammals do (Figure 3-5). There is also speculation that some birds sleep aloft during long transoceanic flights.

Species that are at greater risk of predation at their sleep sites tend to sleep less. In fact, one prominent theory proposes that how much an animal sleeps is largely determined by its status as a prey animal or as a predatory animal. This theory suggests that prey animals sleep less because sleep makes them vulnerable. This predation theory seems unlikely because the victims of predators are generally the very young, the sick, and the old even when they are wide awake. In addition, prey animals often sleep 12 hours or more per 24-hour period, which is as much or more than many predators (Figure 3-6).

There is also a well-established but modest relationship between daily sleep and body size in mammals (ie, small mammals tend to sleep more than large ones). The reasons for the relationship between sleep and size are thought to have something to do with energy conservation, which is a much greater problem for smaller mammals

Hereford JM. *Sleep and Rehabilitation:
A Guide for Health Professionals* (pp 19-23).
© 2014 Taylor & Francis Group.

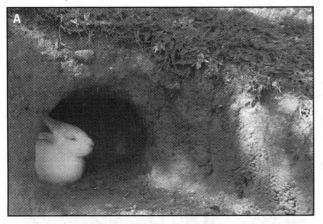

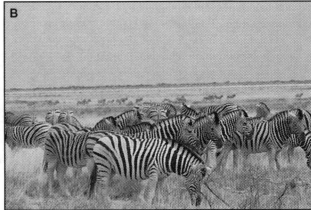

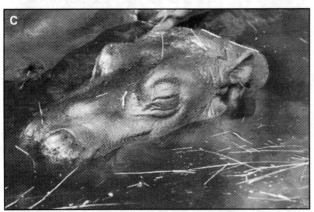

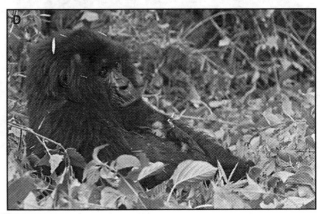

Figure 3-1. Animals vary greatly in the places and postures in which they sleep. (From Fotolia.com)

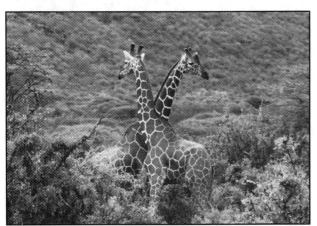

Figure 3-2. Sleep duration varies greatly from animal to animal, with the giraffe sleeping the least and the little brown mouse sleeping the most. (From Fotolia.com)

than for larger ones. For example, the energy expense for locomotion is much greater in smaller mammals. Because a smaller proportion of the body weight of a smaller mammal is composed of fat, smaller mammals have a more limited capacity for energy storage. Smaller mammals lose heat energy at a greater rate than larger mammals because of surface area in proportion to mass. In addition, larger mammals generally have more fat insulation and thicker fur than smaller mammals. Therefore, they

are better protected against heat loss. Sleep might help conserve energy especially in smaller mammals that are in almost constant danger of depleting their energy resources by providing long periods of lowered metabolic activity, resulting in a decrease in energy expenditure. However, the metabolic rate during sleep is only about 10% lower than during quiet wakefulness; therefore, the evolution of sleep is not explained by the energy conservation theory, when the animal could conserve this much energy with quiet rest as opposed to sleep. Additionally, if the animal simply rested rather than slept, it would be able to maintain the vigilance that is absent during sleep.

On the other hand, lowered vigilance may be an essential feature of sleep because it limits an animal's reactivity to the environment and therefore keeps it from being perpetually active, with resultant high cost to its energy reserves. It has also been proposed that sleep helps to regulate energy expenditure by maintaining specific temperatures that conserve energy resources.

Sleep appears to have some role in the length of the life span in various species. For example, there is a tendency for species of mammals that sleep the most to have shorter life spans. Long-lived mammals may have some characteristic that enables them to get by with less sleep. Species that are born relatively immature, such as the rat or cat, tend to have

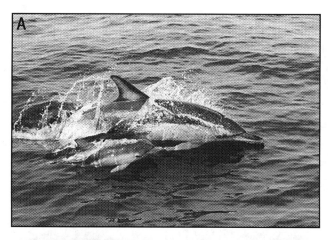

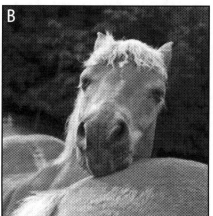

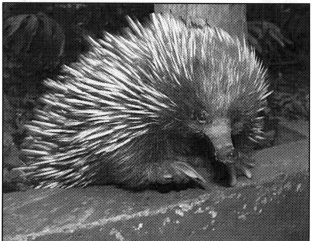

Figure 3-4. In keeping with the unique nature of Australian fauna, the Australian echidna is the only mammal that has no REM sleep. (From Fotolia.com)

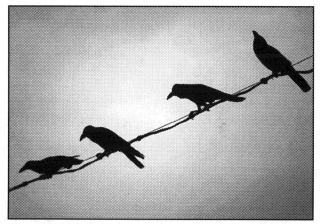

Figure 3-5. Birds do not lose muscle tone during sleep. (From Fotolia.com)

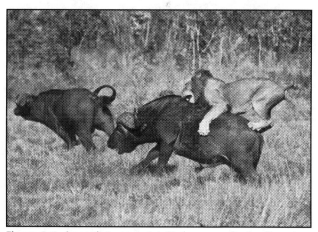

Figure 3-6. Somewhat counterintuitively, prey animals often sleep more than predators. (From Fotolia.com)

more REM sleep than species born with fairly mature regulatory systems, such as the guinea pig or the horse.

Sleep has evolved over time to meet the particular survival needs of each species. In humans and other mammals, sleep likely evolved from rest to become NREM sleep and REM sleep evolved from NREM sleep. The particular evolution of the neurobiology in humans accompanied this development and progressed further as the human mammal developed the capacity for speech. This evolution developed to meet the particular needs of the evolving brain in humans. Much later in the evolutionary cycle, the human began to adapt the structure of the upper airway as a natural selection pressure for the development of speech and language. In fact, some anthropologists believe that speech developed a mere 40,000 years ago.[1-3] Spoken language and the ability to communicate separated the human mammal from the rest of the animal kingdom. It is the ability to communicate in this manner that conferred an increased survival advantage on human species that could speak over those that could only grunt. Prior to the development of speech, the human mammal was evolving slowly over tens of thousands of years. Following the development of speech, evolution progressed relatively rapidly.

Communication about tribal defense, building a tool, or the acquisition of food provided an improved capacity for survival. For example, if an early human being was able to communicate a plan to trap an animal so that another could more easily strike it with a spear or arrow, chances for acquiring food improved. As gathering of food became less labor intensive, nutrition and survival rates improved and evolution moved forward. With the advent of speech, the early human being developed small communities that worked cooperatively to hunt, gather, and store food rather than to simply compete with one another for food. The ability to communicate led to the development of social groups and allowed one generation to communicate what it had learned to successive generations. Evolution of speech and language was followed by the development of written language. Prior to the written word, communication was immediate and vital. Once written communication was established, it separated the language from the individual speaker and the society and allowed it to become general knowledge available to the masses, even those existing great distances apart. This has allowed the human being to progress at a significantly faster pace than the rest of the animal kingdom. It also led to substantial evolution of the human brain to support the capacity for speech, language, memory, and learning. These developments likely necessitated the need for the evolution of sleep to support advancing brain processes.

Though the development of speech afforded very significant advantages to survival and advancements seen in modern society, it also carries with it some substantial disadvantages. The changes to the upper airway that were necessary to allow for the development of speech also led to the undesired consequence of predisposing the human being to obstructive sleep apnea. Humans and possibly some flat-faced dogs, such as the English bulldog, are the only mammals that can suffer from aspiration and acute airway obstruction (choking) as well as obstructive sleep apnea and sleep-disordered breathing.[4,5]

The evolution of the supralaryngeal vocal tract is unique in humans compared to that of close ancestors and other members of the animal kingdom. This evolution has involved migration of the foramen magnum anteriorly, creating an acute oral cavity–skull base angle. Shortening of the face, or splanchnocranium, which is made up of the mandible, palate, ethmoid, maxilla, and sphenoid, was necessary to reduce compression of the pharynx. The mandible moved posteriorly and rotated downward and created the obtuse gonial angle. This has also caused crowding of the teeth, which can be seen in humans with impacted third molars. Only humans, who have a shortened, laterally expanded dental arch that has allowed for speech, suffer from this crowding.[6] These developments resulted in decreases in the length of the oral cavity and contributed to the narrowing of the pharynx.[2]

The supralaryngeal tract narrowed and elongated, and the larynx descended. This descent shortened the palate and resulted in a loss of the epiglottis–soft palate lock-up mechanism, in which the epiglottis overlaps the soft palate. This allows food to be diverted laterally around the epiglottis such that alimentation and respiration can occur concurrently. With the loss of this mechanism, food is supposed to be channeled around the larynx, but there is a constant risk of aspiration. Charles Darwin noted this in *The Origin of Species* in which he wrote "… every particle of food and drink which we swallow has to pass over the orifice of the trachea, with some risk of falling into the lungs, notwithstanding the beautiful contrivance by which the glottis is closed. (p. 191)"[7]

The descent of the larynx contributed to the repositioning of the tongue into the oropharynx. Humans are the only mammals to have an oropharyngeal tongue.

The descent of the larynx and the migration of the foramen magnum created a right angle bend in the human vocal tract. The vocal tract then extends from the vocal chords through the oropharynx and oral cavity to the lips. It consists of a vertical segment that extends from the vocal chords to the top of the oropharynx and a horizontal segment that extends from the lips to the posterior wall of the pharynx. There exists an approximately 1:1 ratio between the vertical and horizontal segments of the vocal tract connected at a right angle bend. The closer this ratio is to exactly 1:1, the greater the vocal clarity is.[8] This angulation, though allowing for speech, reduces the respiratory efficiency of the upper airway. It also increases the chance of immediate death by asphyxiation, increases the risk of infection and impaction of the third molars, restricts breathing to some degree, and contributes to sleep-disordered breathing such as obstructive sleep apnea.

Sleep-disordered breathing is a risk factor for hypertension and is linked to early death by stroke and heart attack. It complicates cardiovascular disease and predisposes an individual toward accidents. It causes excessive daytime sleepiness, loss of productivity, and decreased quality of life. The onset of these consequences of sleep-disordered breathing is generally 40 to 50 years of age, which is generally beyond the life expectancy of early humans in which the anatomic changes occurred to allow for the production of speech. The only benefit to this evolutionary change in anatomic arrangement appears to be the production of speech. Natural selection pressure for speech and language was so powerful that it developed despite the substantial negative consequences. But it was also a likely catalyst for significant progress in the development of humans.

The concurrent series of events that developed in the central nervous system to support speech also likely contributed to the evolution of sleep. Sleep has evolved from resting of the organism into the complex behavior that is the focus of this text. As knowledge and understanding of sleep increase, the clinician will be able to use this information to the advantage of the patient undergoing a rehabilitation program.

REFERENCES

1. Diamond J. *The Third Chimpanzee: The Evolution and Future of the Human Animal.* New York, NY: Harper Collins; 1992.
2. Lieberman DE, McCarthy RC, Hilemae KM, Palmer JB. Ontongeny of postnatal hyoid and larynx descent in humans. *Arch Oral Biol.* 2001;46:117–128.
3. Lieberman DL. *The Evolution of the Human Head.* Boston, MA: President and Fellows of Harvard College; 2011.
4. Barsh LI. The origin of pharyngeal obstruction during sleep. *Sleep Breath.* 1999;3:17–21.
5. Hendricks JC, Kline LR, Kovalski RJ, O'Brien JA, Morrison AR, Pack AI. The English bulldog: a natural model of sleep-disordered breathing. *Am Physiol Soc.* 1987;63:1344–1350.
6. Miles AEW. The evolution of dentitions in the more recent ancestors of man. *Proc R Soc Med.* 1972;65:396–399.
7. Darwin C. *The Origin of Species: By Means of Natural Selection of the Preservation of Favoured Races in the Struggle for Life. 150 Anniversary Edition.* New York, NY: Signet Classics; 2003.
8. Lieberman P. *Eve Spoke.* New York, NY: Norton Press; 1988.

How Sleep Develops and Changes Throughout the Life Span

Julie M. Hereford, PT, DPT

Sleep changes significantly across infancy and childhood into young adulthood. In fact, age is probably the single most crucial factor that determines how humans typically sleep. Age impacts sleep more than gender, although males seem to be more susceptible to age-related changes than females.[1] Age affects sleep more than psychiatric illness, genetics, and to a large extent, even more than most physical illnesses. The only factor that can influence sleep in a specific incident more than age is the amount of time since the last episode of sleep.

Sleep undergoes a wide variety of modifications across the human life span that have a significant impact on the growth and development of humans. These modifications may be the result of disorders such as upper airway resistance, dysautonomia, or the modifications may simply be a function of aging.

Sleep has been shown to begin in a rudimentary form beginning around the seventh month of fetal life (Figure 4-1). Studies show that rapid eye movement (REM) sleep may be present as early as 26 to 28 weeks of gestation.[2,3] Direct electroencephalogram (EEG) measurement of the human fetus in utero is not technically reasonable; therefore, knowledge about early sleep habits is gleaned from observation of eye movements and from various animal models. It appears that the developing fetus spends most of its time asleep, cycling every 20 to 40 minutes between REM sleep and non-rapid eye movement (NREM) sleep.[2] It is not clear from current research exactly how sleep develops in the fetus, whether it simply appears or develops over time. Some research has been attempted on premature infants, but it is technically very difficult and rife with errors. Instead, researchers have turned to animal models, specifically sheep models, because fetus size and course of brain development in sheep are analogous to those of humans. Schwab et al[3] have hypothesized that there is cyclic patterning in the immature fetal brain that occurs every 5 to 10 minutes and changes slowly as the fetus grows. Schwab et al[3] concluded that sleep does not suddenly evolve from a resting brain in utero. Instead, these authors postulated that sleep changes including sleep stages and transitions are an actively regulated process. Schwab et al further suggested that the neurons that generate sleep mature before there is sufficient brain development for it to generate REM sleep. This sort of cyclic change in neuronal activity may stimulate other nerve cells to propagate into complex neural pathways.[3] This in utero cyclical neural activity may also represent a method by which the somatosensory system proliferates, targets, and refines neuronal networks. Some research has linked the cyclical nature of early fetal sleep and the development of REM sleep to the development of particular modalities of the somatosensory system.[2,3] Schwab et al continue to study this area and are investigating the impact of environmental stimuli including noise, light, or stress on the developing fetus. It is possible that aberrations in environmental stimuli at a vulnerable period in fetal or neonatal brain development may impact the more mature brain's tolerance to sensory input and may indeed be a significant factor in childhood and adult presentations of sensory integration deficits.[1-4] Continued research in this area will lead to a better understanding of the phases of fetal and neonatal growth and development that may be particularly vulnerable to injury or damage.

Hereford JM. *Sleep and Rehabilitation: A Guide for Health Professionals* (pp 25-34). © 2014 Taylor & Francis Group.

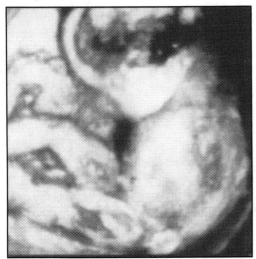

Figure 4-1. Sleep begins as early as the seventh month of fetal life. (Reprinted with permission from V. Mebruer.)

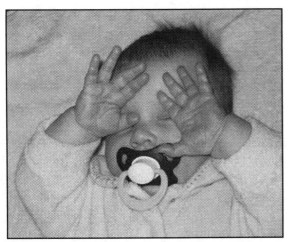

Figure 4-3. Infants tend to move directly from wakefulness to REM sleep. (Reprinted with permission from J. Hoskins.)

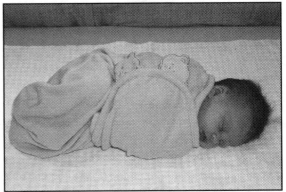

Figure 4-2. Newborns sleep 16 to 20 hours a day. (Reprinted with permission from J. Hoskins.)

What is known is how sleep manifests across the life span. Understanding normal sleep habits helps to identify deviation from the norm and the potential consequences of such deviation.

The premature neonate generally displays 2 stages of sleep: active sleep and quiet sleep. Active sleep, which resembles REM sleep, develops first and may inhabit as much as 75% to 80% of the total sleep time (TST) in this group. The amount of REM sleep in the premature infant is prodigious and can be substantially more than their full-term counterparts.

Full-term newborn infants sleep about 16 to 20 hours per 24-hour period, and sleep bouts are widely distributed across that time period (Figure 4-2). This sleep requirement is thought to be related to the brain development demands associated with the dramatic growth that occurs during this time frame.

Quiet sleep occupies approximately 50% of TST in neonates and gradually increases as the infant matures.

Quiet sleep does not usually occur at sleep onset until the infant is at least 3 months old. Instead, in the neonate, sleep onset is marked by active sleep resembling REM sleep until the infant is approximately 3 months of age. Active sleep occupies nearly 50% of TST, and this amount gradually decreases in amount as the infant matures. The relatively greater percentage of active or REM sleep in the neonate is presumed to be activation of central motor programs (Figure 4-3). In addition, immature versions of NREM and slow-wave sleep (SWS) begin to appear.

By 16 weeks of age, the total amount of sleep time that an infant requires decreases to approximately 14 to 15 hours per day and a clear diurnal pattern of sleep emerges. The percentage of time spent in specific sleep stages has shifted by 6 months of age to be approximately 30% REM sleep and 70% NREM sleep. TST remains roughly the same during the remainder of the first year of life. At birth the infant sleeps a great deal, mostly in active sleep but with occasional bursts of quiet sleep. Sleep is seemingly randomly interspersed with brief bouts of wakefulness. As the infant matures, there is a gradual consolidation of wakefulness into longer periods and a gradual consolidation of sleep into several periods of time; that is, the infant will generally establish a longer nocturnal sleep period with several long naps throughout the day. This is known as a *polycyclic sleep pattern.*

During the first year of life there is a gradual maturation of the sleep EEG patterns and the emergence of SWS or delta sleep. Sleep spindles are found during this period. Over the first year, there is also a gradual decline in the amount of active/REM sleep and a gradual decrease in TST.

It is during this time that the infant's parent or caregiver can work to manipulate sleep to better fit the family schedule, but it is very important that the parent or caregiver realize the critical importance of sleep in the infant and young child's overall growth and development, most particularly the development of neuronal pathways and overall brain development. Apart from proper nutrition, it is likely the single most important factor in brain development during the early years of life. There is a growing body of research

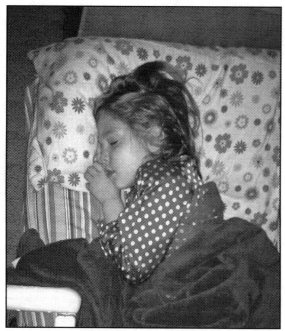

Figure 4-4. In children, sleep decreases to 10 to 12 hours per day, with naps disappearing around age 5. (Reprinted with permission from V. Mebruer.)

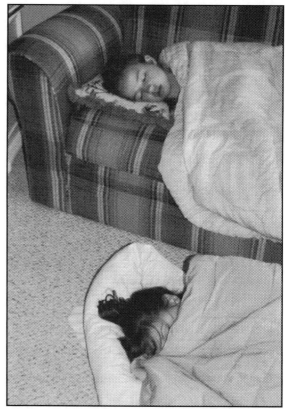

Figure 4-5. Hormonal changes make quality and quantity of sleep even more important in the adolescent. (Reprinted with permission from T. Mebruer.)

that links early sleep disorders including sleep apnea to various developmental and behavioral problems in children such as attention deficit disorders, sensory integration problems, and some learning disorders. It is very important that parents and caregivers understand this critically important issue and safeguard sleep as much as possible. It is vital that infants and children develop and maintain a sleep routine in order to achieve maximum brain growth and development. Occasional alterations in sleep schedule may be tolerated better by some infants and children than others. A frequently repeated complaint from the primary caregiver of a child is difficulty getting the child to initiate sleep. Often the parent will decide to keep the child up later in an attempt to get him or her tired enough to fall asleep. In reality, the overly tired child has an irritated brain that makes the active processes required to transition into sleep much more difficult. The infant will act out with restlessness, crying, or pleas for the parent's presence. Although a detailed discussion of development of sleep habits in the infant and child is outside the scope of this chapter, issues of establishing and maintaining a good sleep schedule early in life have been shown to lead to better health, behavior, and habits later in life.[4] Preservation of sleep routine, quantity, and quality are of significant importance. Providing guidance in sleep habits is one of the most important but underrecognized duties of parenthood.

In children up to approximately 5 years of age, TST has usually decreased to 10 to 12 hours per 24-hour period (Figure 4-4). By 2 years of age, sleep is usually consolidated into nocturnal sleep plus one afternoon nap. The afternoon nap usually disappears by the time the child reaches 5 to

6 years of age. Full EEG sleep staging is present by age 5. Boys have a mean average of 611 minutes of sleep, and girls have a mean average of 576 minutes of sleep per 24-hour period. The division of sleep architecture, or the breakdown of sleep stages, is generally 2% N1, 46% N2, 20% N3, and 32% REM sleep.[5,6] The arousal threshold in children under the age of 5 is nearly impervious in N3, particularly the auditory arousal threshold. One study reported that children in N3 sleep would not arouse even when subjected to 140 decibels, which is equivalent to the noise a jet plane engine makes upon take off at 100 yards.[7]

Parasomnias, or abnormal movements during sleep such as sleepwalking, sleep talking, or night terrors are more prevalent in this age. Nocturnal enuresis or bed-wetting is also common.

Sleep in pre-pubescent adolescents, considered to be between the ages of 5 to 12 years of age, usually declines in quantity. At 6 years of age, TST is usually between 9 and 12 hours confined to nighttime as afternoon naps disappear completely. On average boys sleep slightly less than girls (boys = 573 minutes, girls = 589 minutes) and sleep architecture changes slightly, with 2% N1, 48% N2, 20% N3, and 30% REM sleep.[5,8] Parasomnias are still a relatively frequent occurrence during this period of growth and development; however, nocturnal enuresis generally disappears

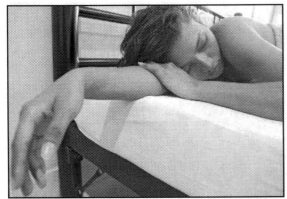

Figure 4-6. The young adult is often sleep deprived while learning to balance new responsibilities and social pressures. (From Fotolia.com)

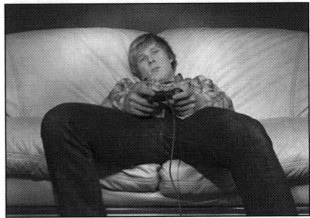

Figure 4-7. Adolescents have notoriously poor sleep habits. (From Fotolia.com)

in normal children, although it may last until an older age, up to age 10 in boys.[9]

The metabolic and hormonal demands of the body are substantial during puberty (between 12 to 18 years of age), and sleep plays an important role in the pubescent individual. Generally speaking, the adolescent may well require more sleep than the prepubescent individual because of the tremendous hormonal and metabolic demands. During this period, there is a gradual increase in the production of human growth hormone in N3 to N4 sleep, particularly in the most dense SWS or N4 sleep (Figure 4-5). The average TST for the adolescent appears to be 8.5 to 9 hours per 24-hour period. The total sleep requirement for the adolescent might be close to 9 to 10 hours per 24-hour period. At this age, human growth hormone and sex hormones begin to be secreted during N3 sleep and are only secreted during sleep (Figure 4-6). Sleep stages begin to approximate the adult pattern of sleep. There is a decrease in the frequency of REM periods but orgasm and ejaculation begin to occur during REM sleep. Sleep hygiene is notoriously poor, and this can become problematic in terms of behavior, learning ability, and even metabolic tolerances (Figure 4-7). The pubescent adolescent often develops a shift in circadian control of sleep and essentially develops a delayed sleep phase disorder. This explains why the average teenager, if left to his or her own devices, prefers to stay up late and sleep late into the morning. Paralleling this decrease in sleep quantity throughout adolescence is an increase in the tendency to fall asleep during the day, usually in class. These behaviors, if not properly understood as a part of development and/or a potential sign of sleep deprivation, may become a source of tension in family and academic life. They are, however, more likely than not a reflection of the increased metabolic and hormonal demands placed on the teenager going through puberty. It is difficult for the parent and child to resolve these issues because societal pressures do not align with normal biological changes that a teenager experiences. This mismatch between sleep requirement and actual sleep obtained may be the beginning of chronic

sleep deprivation. Some relatively easy steps can be taken to ease this burden. For instance, changing the time that adolescents start school has been shown to ameliorate a number of typical problems of teenagers in school.[8,10] In fact, a school district in Rhode Island shifted the start of its school day to try to accommodate for this issue. The school found that not only were the students better rested by self-report, but there was also a significant decrease in truancy and an improvement in multiple academic performance measures.[6]

As the individual continues to mature into early adulthood, considered to be age 18 to 30, TST is usually established at a level that best fits the habits and biological requirements of the individual. Sleep requirement in the adult is generally 7 to 9 hours per 24-hour period, and this requirement may have a strong genetic component. Although very rare, there are reports of individuals who are considered "short sleepers" who may require significantly less sleep without experiencing cognitive or physiological consequences of sleep deprivation. This is a very rare condition, and it is much more likely that individuals who boast that they require very little sleep have, in fact, a substantial sleep debt. These individuals may be suffering from long-term consequences of chronic sleep deprivation such as early onset of cardiovascular disease, insulin resistance and diabetes, and pain conditions.

Sleep in early adulthood is generally 7 to 9 hours, with sleep efficiency—defined as the TST divided by the total amount of time spent in bed—declining somewhat. Sleep efficiency in males is 91% to 99% and in females it is 94% to 98%. Sleep architecture takes on its characteristic adult form in the normal adult sleeper with N1 sleep occupying 2% to 6% of TST, N2 41% to 51% in males and 46% to 58% in females, and N3 6% to 26% in males and 11% to 25% in females. REM sleep occupies 22% to 34% in males and 21% to 29% in females.[8] Due to the pressures of college and perhaps professional education and stresses of early careers and usually very active social lives, young adults may

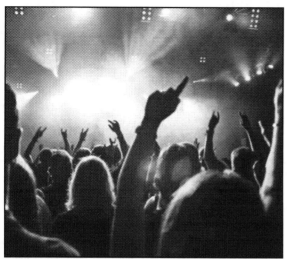

Figure 4-8. Sleep in early adulthood is often sacrificed voluntarily to the career and social pressures. (From Fotolia.com)

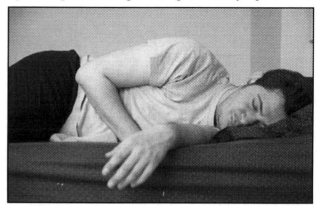

Figure 4-9. Sleep patterns shift into adulthood around age 30. (From Fotolia.com)

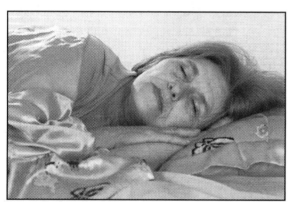

Figure 4-10. Though older adults are assumed to sleep longer than adults, they actually have less total sleep and lower-quality sleep. (From Fotolia.com)

"burn the candle at both ends" and wind up in a chronically sleep deprived state (Figures 4-6 and 4-8). Though the young adult has more resilience than the middle-aged or older adult, this may be the period of time in which the foundation is set for the long-term systemic consequences of chronic sleep deprivation, including things such as metabolic syndrome, insulin resistance, diabetes, and cardiovascular disease.

Sleep in early middle age, defined here as 30 to 45 years of age, may begin to show increased incidences of arousal and awakenings, which are considered a normal part of sleep at this stage of life (Figure 4-9). TST for males averages 419 minutes per night and for females TST averages 421 minutes per night. Sleep efficiency tends to begin to decline because of the increase in nocturnal arousals and awakenings and sometimes the increase in sleep latency. Sleep latency is defined as the length of time between getting into bed with the intention of sleeping and the onset of sleep. Sleep efficiency in males is usually 85% to 99% and for females it is 90% to 99%. Sleep architecture also shows gender differences as follows: N1 for males is 3% to 11%, for females 2% to 8%; N2 for males is 45% to 66%, for females 45% to 63%; N3 for males is 2% to 18%, for females 21% to 31%; and REM sleep for males is 19% to 27% and for females 31% to 31%.[8] Parasomnias are rare in this age group, but there is an increasing incidence of sleep disorders including obstructive sleep apnea, periodic limb movement disorder (PLMD), snoring, and insomnias.

In later middle age, defined here as age 45 to 65, TST changes slightly, with males getting an average of 390 minutes of sleep per night and females an average of 431 minutes of sleep per night. Sleep efficiency may show a further decline, with both male and female sleepers showing an average of 93% sleep efficiency. Awakenings and arousals tend to increase to 5.5 times per night for the average male and 5 times per night for the average female. Sleep architecture shows a general decrease in N3 sleep as a percentage of TST, and there continues to be a bit of a gender difference. N1 sleep is 4% to 12% in males and 3% to 7% in females; N2 is 52% to 72% in males and 51% to 65% in females; N3 is 0% to 12% in males and 5% to 17% in females; and REM sleep is 17% to 25% in males and 19% to 25% in females.[8]

Most evidence indicates that as an individual approaches old age, the amount of nocturnal sleep decreases (Figure 4-10). *Old age* or *elderly*, as described in sleep literature, varies somewhat by publication and seems to be an imprecise and somewhat arbitrary term to which it is impossible to assign an accurate age. For example, some older individuals are of such hale and hardy constitution that they do not seem old even in their early 80s. Others who have a less sturdy genetic substrate that has manifested as illness and disease, who have not attended to their health, or who have experienced substantial psychological and mental distress may seem to age much more rapidly and can be said to have entered old age in their 60s. For the purposes of this text—aware that it may be an arbitrary distinction that cannot be generally or universally applied—the "aging individual" will be defined as 65 years of age and older. Generally speaking, this age is the beginning of some of the changes in sleep that are a hallmark of old age.

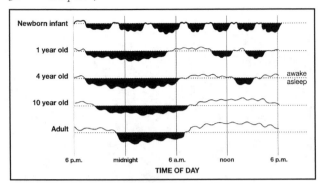

Figure 4-11. Cyliclic nature of sleep across the life span.

At this age, TST may decline slightly, although the sleep requirement is basically the same throughout adulthood. The older individual may experience a return to polycyclic sleep habits in which nocturnal sleep decreases to 5 to 6 hours but is enhanced with a 1- to 1.5-hour nap in the afternoon, making the TST 6 to 7.5 hours per 24-hour period. Rather than indicating a decreased need for TST, this decline is likely evidence of developing problems in the brain sleep mechanism. It is not at all uncommon for the older adult to lose the ability to consolidate sleep at night, making daytime napping a reasonable attempt to attain the TST necessary. Sleep efficiency declines significantly as the individual moves through old age because of the significant increase in sleep fragmentation. Increased numbers of arousals and awakenings may be due to medical problems or increased depression that sometimes accompanies the aging process. As mentioned previously, it may also be an indication of malfunctioning of the sleep mechanism either due to damage, such as from a stroke, or due to degeneration as may be seen in dementia or depletion of neurotransmitters. Sleep efficiency for males can be 57% to 97% and for females it can be 73% to 96%. Sleep architecture continues to show differences in gender as follows: N1 males 4% to 16%, females 4% to 12%; N2 males 38% to 72%, females 44% to 64%; N3 males 0% to 3%, females 0% to 18%; and REM sleep males 11% to 27% and females 15% to 25%.[11] An increased number of awakenings tends to be part of the aging process as well, with males ages 60 to 69 experiencing an average of 7.5 and females 4.5 awakenings. Awakenings actually decrease slightly for males to 5 per night but increase for females to 8.5 per night.

The other common feature of sleep and aging is an apparent disorder in circadian rhythm. This is perhaps related to loss of cells in the substantia nigra resulting in what is called *advanced-phase sleep disorder*. In this disorder, the individual desires sleep onset in the early evening and tends to awaken for the day in the very early hours of the morning. Sleep is more fragmented by wakefulness and is much more susceptible to disruption by noise. In fact, the auditory threshold is markedly diminished by the seventh or eighth decade of life.

It has been shown, however, that increased amounts of daily exercise and increased duration of daylight exposure tend to improve the reported quality of sleep in the aging individual.

HOW RAPID EYE MOVEMENT SLEEP DEVELOPS OVER THE LIFE SPAN

As previously noted, the quantity of active or REM sleep is exceedingly high in the premature infant and usually occupies at least 50% of TST in the newborn infant. The increased concentration of REM sleep in fetal life and in early infancy has led sleep researchers to speculate that this active sleep, which has not yet taken on the full characteristics of adult REM sleep, may be important for the maturation of the cerebral cortex and oculomotor system.[12] It may also be involved in the programming of the developing neuronal circuits and be associated with neuronal targeting and retraction.[13,14]

NREM and REM sleep have a cyclic nature beginning in fetal life, showing a rapid cycle that lengthens as the brain continues to grow and develop. These cycles occur approximately every 50 to 60 minutes in the infant and occur at approximately 90- to 110-minute intervals in the adult (Figure 4-11).

By the age of 2, REM sleep has taken on the EEG characteristics familiar to normal adult sleep. It occupies approximately 20% to 25% of TST, and this amount of REM remains fairly constant throughout childhood, adolescence, and adulthood.

Unlike normal neurologically intact adults, infants may pass directly from wakefulness to REM sleep, bypassing the normal first NREM cycle that initiates sleep in the adult. Despite the difference in the presentation of REM sleep, the percentage of TST of REM sleep does not vary appreciably, although, given the increase in TST in the infant and child, the total amount of time spent in REM is significantly higher in youth. This is thought by some to be related to memory consolidation and the rapid rate of learning that occurs in youth compared to adulthood.

There is some speculation that certain conditions of pathological aging such as Alzheimer's disease may result in a reduction of REM sleep, which is a reflection of the decrease in cholinergic function that is a hallmark of dementia (Figure 4-12).

Although the total percentage change of REM sleep does not occur in a situation of normal aging, the amount of NREM sleep does decrease with age (Figure 4-13). This decrease, in conjunction with the increased frequency of arousal and awakenings, may cause the older individual to experience a corresponding reduction in TST, although this may be somewhat offset by daytime napping.

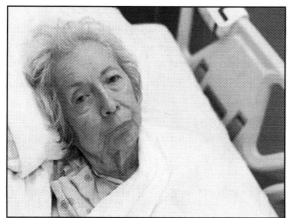

Figure 4-12. Alzheimer's patients show a decline in REM. (From Fotolia.com)

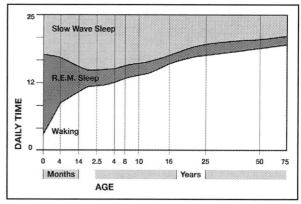

Figure 4-13. REM and NREM sleep distribution over 24-hour period.

HOW NON-RAPID EYE MOVEMENT SLEEP DEVELOPS

In contrast to REM sleep, SWS, or synchronized delta wave sleep, shows a gradual but relatively steady decline across the life span. A rudimentary version of NREM sleep, called *quiet sleep*, is evident in fetal life and infancy. This begins to develop and take on a more mature appearance during early childhood and is usually fully developed by the age of 5 years old. At this age, children typically have abundant high-amplitude SWS or delta wave sleep, which is relatively impervious to external disruption. Specifically, SWS in children displays a remarkably high auditory threshold. This threshold remains relatively high during SWS in adolescence into adulthood but begins to show a significant decline as a function of aging.

Beginning in early adolescence, there is a gradual decrease in SWS or N3 sleep that continues throughout adulthood. The decrease in N3 sleep is generally replaced by NREM N1 and N2 sleep.

By the time an average human being reaches the eighth decade of life, the highest density delta waves that occur during SWS, previously known as stage 4 sleep or N4, may be virtually absent, especially in males. The functional significance of the changes in SWS in a normal healthy individual is not precisely known, although speculation is that these changes may be related to the loss of neural plasticity and may be the harbinger of aging of the central nervous system.

SLEEP PATHOLOGIES

Pathological aspects of sleep tend to manifest at particular ages. Sleep pathologies may be related to deficits or pathologies during neurological development that accompanies the developmental course of sleep over the life span (see Section II).

Sleep parasomnias are usually diagnosed by analyzing an overnight sleep study called a *polysomnogram*. During this study, 25 or more sensors are attached to the study subject's head, thorax, abdomen, and leg in order to obtain EEG, electrooculogram (EOG), and electromyogram (EMG) data simultaneously in order to gather data during sleep. Analysis of these data can help define an individual's sleep architecture and is the standard test used to identify sleep parasomnias (see Chapter 16).

Night Terrors

A night terror, or *pavor nocturnus*, is a parasomnia disorder that is found in 6% of children, usually between the ages of 4 and 12, and in approximately 1% of adults.[15] Night terrors may develop suddenly, and episodes may occur for several weeks and then disappear without explanation for either the onset or cessation of the episodes. Different from a nightmare, which usually has more of a narrative story feel, a night terror generally consists of an overwhelming feeling of terror or dread. It usually consists of very strong emotional content without an identifiable story. It often involves a fear of being chased or trapped or suffocated. Night terrors usually occur within the first few hours of the night and occur during N3 or N4 sleep. Children who are experiencing a night terror may suddenly sit up in bed and scream and look extremely fearful or panicked. They often have multiple autonomic signs of significant emotional stress, including sweating, labored breathing, and rapid heart rate. They may appear to be awake but are not. They are generally inconsolable, confused, and do not respond to efforts to comfort them. The child usually cannot be awoken from this state and will likely have no recollection of the episode when he or she does awaken. There appears to be a genetic link to night terrors, but they appear to be related to other parasomnias as well.

Night terrors in adults, on the other hand, occur with much less frequency and seem to be related to poor

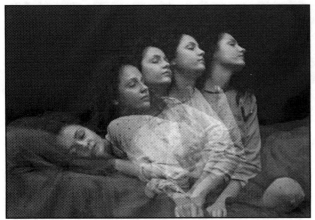

Figure 4-14. Sleepwalking occurs in 1% to 15% of the population. (From Fotolia.com)

quality or quantity of sleep or improper diet, particularly in an individual who also suffers from hypoglycemia.[16] Interestingly, the incidence of night terrors does not correlate with known mental illness.

Somnambulism

Somnambulism, more commonly known as sleepwalking, is a parasomnia that is most prevalent in children and usually disappears during adolescence (Figure 4-14). It occurs in 1% to 15% of the population, according to the National Sleep Foundation.[17] Although much more uncommon in adults, when it does occur the episodes tend to be 3 times more frequent and episodes may continue for years. Sleepwalking in old age, especially if it is a new onset, is usually indicative of another disorder such as dementia, drug toxicity, or seizure disorder.[18]

A sleepwalking episode may last for less than a minute up to 30 minutes. Sleepwalking nearly always consists of simple repetitive movement behaviors that occur during SWS. The sleepwalker's eyes are usually open and the individual may seem dimly aware of his or her surroundings. Although these episodes usually consist of simple tasks, there have been verified reports of more complex activities occurring during sleep including cleaning, driving, having sex, or even violent acts such as murder.[17,19–21]

There is some evidence that sleepwalking is an inherited autosomal-dominant disorder.[22] Sleepwalking generally occurs in the earlier part of the night during SWS and there is usually only one episode per night. The cause of sleepwalking is open to some degree of debate. Some have theorized that it occurs in childhood, resulting from an increased amount of SWS and the relative immaturity of the central nervous system.[18] Incidences of sleepwalking can be aggravated by sleep deprivation, fever, and excessive fatigue. Use of hypnotics or neuroleptics can lead to increased episodes of sleepwalking in susceptible individuals. In addition to practicing good sleep hygiene and avoiding sleep deprivation, treatment for sleepwalking usually consists of removing dangerous objects from the area or locking doors and windows to keep the potential sleepwalker from harm during an episode. Medication can be prescribed if necessary and can include low-dose benzodiazepines or tricyclic antidepressants.[23]

Nocturnal Enuresis

Nocturnal enuresis, more commonly known as bed-wetting, is defined as involuntary urination while asleep after the age at which bladder control has been attained. Though this is one of the most common complaints to the pediatrician, it is commonly an incidence of developmental delay rather than emotional issues or physical problems. Only 5% to 10% of bed-wetting is related to a specific medical problem. It is a more common problem in young boys, occurring in nearly 3% of boys as opposed to 1% of young girls. Because it is primarily a developmental issue, it usually resolves by the age of 10. Most treatment is behaviorally based and is directed at protecting or improving the child's self-esteem because it is unlikely there is a physical problem.

Trouble Sleeping Through the Night

Trouble sleeping through the night is a very common occurrence in toddlers and young children. In fact, approximately 30% of 1- to 4-year-olds have difficulty sleeping through the night, though this percentage decreases by the age of 8 to approximately 1% to 3%. The prevalence of poor sleep, especially awakening during the night, is relatively low during adolescence; instead, difficulty sleeping during adolescence is usually characterized by difficultly falling asleep. This may be related to caffeine intake or overstimulation immediately prior to bedtime (eg, watching scary, action-packed, or exciting television shows or playing interactive computer games). Excessive fearfulness can also become a problem during adolescence and may interfere with sleep onset.

Narcolepsy

Narcolepsy is a serious parasomnia that is characterized by excessive sleepiness and the sudden, involuntary onset of sleep at inappropriate times, known as *sleep attacks*. Narcolepsy is a relatively rare neurological disorder that affects 1 in 10,000 individuals and usually develops in adolescence. There appears to be a genetic component to narcolepsy that results in hypocretin-orexin deficiency, but there may also be environmental triggers during brain development such as viral infection that may contribute to the development of the disorder.[24]

Insomnia

Insomnia is by far the most prevalent sleep disorder in adulthood. Insomnia is characterized by difficulty falling asleep and/or staying asleep or a self-report of poor sleep quality or nonrestorative sleep. It is also usually accompanied by reports of functional impairment while awake. Episodes of sleep disruption occur several times per week and symptoms persist for more than 1 month. Insomnia is either primary (ie, not associated with any medical, psychiatric, or environmental cause, or secondary (ie, related to another condition). Approximately 1 in 4 individuals in their 30s suffer from insomnia. The incidence of insomnia rises to nearly 50% by the age of 70, with individuals reporting some degree of sleeplessness (see Chapter 26).

Periodic Limb Movement Disorder

Periodic limb movement disorder (PLMD) is a parasomnia that is characterized by involuntary movement, usually of the lower extremities during sleep. This disorder is not the same as restless leg/legs syndrome, in which symptoms may occur during wakefulness. The prevalence of PLMD is approximately 4%. PLMD may result in arousals that disrupt sleep and then lead to excessive daytime sleepiness. PLMD occurs during NREM sleep, so it tends to occur most frequently during the first half of the night.

Sleep Apnea

Sleep apnea is a sleep disorder characterized by periodic pauses in breathing that may result in decreased oxygen saturation. These respiratory pauses or *apneic events,* may last for a few seconds to 1 minute and may occur multiple times per hour. According to a study by the National Sleep Foundation, up to 25% of the United States population is at significant risk for sleep apnea.[25] Sleep apnea tends to occur more frequently at opposite ends of the life span. Sleep apnea may be classified as central sleep apnea, obstructive sleep apnea, or mixed sleep apnea, which has elements of both central and obstructive. Sleep apnea is commonly recognized by a sleep partner when an individual with the disorder snores heavily but then seems to stop breathing, followed by a gasp of air and resumption of normal respiration. These events may occur occasionally, but when the frequency increases to multiple times per hour or if the events result in multiple arousals from normal sleep architecture, the individual may be diagnosed with sleep apnea. The cause of sleep apnea may be centrally mediated in which the individual ceases to breathe and does not have a respiratory effort or it may be obstructive, in which there continues to be a respiratory effort but it is insufficient to overcome the collapse of the airway. When a sleep apneic event occurs, there is an increase in CO_2 concentration and a drop in O_2 saturation. This elevated CO_2 level eventually acts to drive restoration of normal respiration. Central sleep apnea occurring alone is relatively rare and accounts for only 0.4% of sleep apnea diagnoses.[26]

Obstructive sleep apnea is by far the most common form of sleep apnea, accounting for nearly 84% of cases.[25] This occurs when there is a physical obstruction to the airway and the normal respiratory effort available during sleep is insufficient to overcome the resistance in the system. This type of sleep apnea generally leads to arousal and may be accompanied by the characteristic snort or gasp for breath that some sleepers exhibit. Mixed sleep apnea accounts for approximately 15% of sleep apnea diagnoses and is a combination of obstructive and central sleep apnea events.

Regardless of the type of sleep apnea, the sleeper is usually unaware of these respiratory or arousal events. However, an individual who has repeated and persistent sleep apnea, regardless of its pathophysiology, may report symptoms of poor sleep habits including fatigue and excessive daytime sleepiness. Additionally, when arousals and apneic events disrupt the sleep architecture and affect the quality and quantity of sleep by diminishing sleep efficiency, the individual with sleep apnea will begin to develop sequelae associated with chronic sleep apnea.

Sudden Infant Death Syndrome

It has been postulated that sudden infant death syndrome (SIDS) is related to a deficiency in respiratory control during sleep and/or deficiency in the arousal mechanisms[27] and therefore may be considered a parasomnia. SIDS is characterized by a sudden death of an infant who is not predicted to die by medical history and usually leaves no obvious clues on postmortem exam as to the cause of death. Further research regarding causation in SIDS continues and understanding of this tragic syndrome has increased as knowledge of the science of sleep grows.

SUMMARY

Sleep is essential for normal growth and development as well as for normal restorative mechanisms to function across the life span. Sleep requirements change as people age; infants generally require the most sleep at 16 to 20 hours per day, and adults need the least at 7 to 9 hours per day (Figure 4-15). Different phases of life also display some variation in sleep architecture. Whereas infants spend the most time in REM sleep, this gradually changes and the amount of time spent in REM sleep remains fairly constant from age 2 through adulthood. The percentage of time spent in the various sleep stages also changes during life. Various pathologies of sleep tend to manifest themselves at characteristic times during a life span. Night terrors are common in young children, and insomnia is the most common sleep pathology seen in adults. Understanding these variations in sleep architecture and pathology allows the rehabilitation professional to more accurately assess sleep issues in a particular patient population.

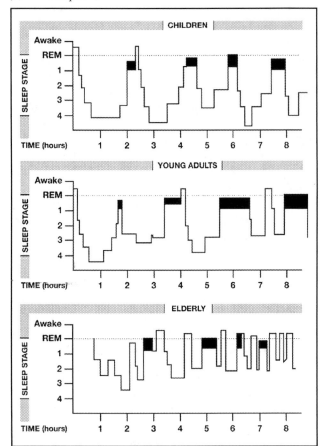

Figure 4-15. Sleep architecture histograms during particular age ranges.

REFERENCES

1. Bilwise DL. Normal aging. In: Kryger MH, Roth T, Dement WC, eds. *Principles and Practice of Sleep Medicine*. 5th ed. St Louis, MO: Elsevier Saunders; 2011.

2. American Institute of Physics. Baby's first dreams: sleep cycles of the fetus. Available at: http://www.sciencedaily.com/releases/2009/04/090413185734.htm. Accessed March 23, 2012.

3. Schwab K, Groh T, Schwab M, Witte H. Nonlinear analysis and modeling of cortical activation and deactivation patterns in the immature fetal electrocorticogram. *Chaos*. 2009;19:1–8.

4. Weissbluth M. *Healthy Sleep Habits, Happy Child*. New York, NY: Random House Publishing Group; 2003.

5. Kahn A, Dan B, Groswasser J, Franco P, Sottiaux M. Normal sleep architecture in infants and children. *J Clin Neurophysiol*. 1996;13(3):184–197.

6. Rettner R. Delaying school start times benefits teens. Available at: http://www.livescience.com/6684-delaying-school-start-times-benefits-teens.html. Accessed March 23, 2012.

7. Owens JA. Sleep in children: cross-cultural perspectives. *Sleep Biol Rhythms*. 2004;2(3):165–173.

8. College of Education and Human Development. Later start times for high school students. Available at: http://www.cehd.umn.edu/research/highlights/Sleep. Accessed March 23, 2012.

9. Mahowald MW, Rosen GM. Parasomnias in children. *Pediatrician*. 1990;17:21–31.

10. National Sleep Foundation. Backgrounder: later school start times. Available at: http://www.sleepfoundation.org/article/hot-topics/backgrounder-later-school-start-times. Accessed March 23, 2012.

11. White M. Development of sleep architecture and sleep across the lifespan. Available at: http://psych.fullerton.edu/mwhite/473pdf/473%20Sleep%20Across%20Lifespan.pdf. Accessed March 23, 2012.

12. Mirmiran M, Someren EV. The importance of REM sleep for brain maturation. *J Sleep Res*. 1993;2(4):188–192.

13. Kavanau JL. Memory, sleep and the evolution of mechanisms of synaptic efficacy maintenance. *Neuroscience*. 1997;79:7–44.

14. Bottjer S. Neural strategies for learning during sensitive periods of development. *J Comp Physiol A Neuroethol Sens Neural Behav Physiol*. 2002;188:917–928.

15. American Psychiatric Association. *Diagnostic and Statistical Manual of Mental Disorders*. 4th ed, text rev. Washington, DC: American Psychiatric Association; 2000.

16. Carranza CR, Dill JR. *Banishing Night Terrors and Nightmares: A Breakthrough Program to Heal the Traumas That Shatter Peaceful Sleep*. New York, NY: Kensington Publishing Corp; 2004.

17. Mahowald M. Sleepwalking. Available at: http://www.sleepfoundation.org/article/sleep-related-problems/sleepwalking. Accessed March 23, 2012.

18. Swanson J, ed. Sleepwalking. *Sleep Disorders Sourcebook*. Detroit, MI: Omnigraphics; 1999.

19. Smith M. SLEEP: sex while sleeping is real, and may be no joke. Available at: http://www.medpagetoday.com/primarycare/sleepdisorders/3568?np=1&xid=ob_pcp. Accessed August 11, 2011.

20. Martin L. Can sleepwalking be a murder defense? Available at: http://www.lakesidepress.com/pulmonary/Sleep/sleep-murder.htm. Accessed April 3, 2012.

21. Nowak R. Sleepwalking woman had sex with strangers. *New Scientist*. 2004. Available at: http://www.newscientist.com/article/dn6540. Accessed April 30, 2007.

22. Dogu O, Pressman MR. Identification of sleepwalking gene(s): not yet, but soon? *Neurology*. 2011;76:12–13.

23. Lavie P, Malhotra A, Pillar G. *Sleep Disorders: Diagnosis, Management and Treatment: A Handbook for Clinicians*. London, UK: Martin Dunitz; 2002.

24. Maret S, Tafti M. Genetics of narcolepsy and other major sleep disorders. *Swiss Med Wkly*. 2005;135:662–665.

25. Hiestand DM, Britz P, Goldman M, et al. Prevalence of symptoms and risk of sleep apnea in the US population—Results from the National Sleep Foundation Sleep in America 2005 Poll. *Chest*. 2006;130:780–786.

26. Morgenthaler TI, Kagramanov V, Hanak V, Decker PA. Complex sleep apnea syndrome: is it a unique clinical syndrome? *Sleep*. 2006;29:1203–1209.

27. Harper RM, Kinney HC. Potential mechanisms of failure in the sudden infant death syndrome. *Curr Pediatr Rev*. 2010;6:39–47. Available at: http://www.ncbi.nlm.nih.gov/pmc/articles/PMC3392684. Accessed April 10, 2012.

5

Non-rapid Eye Movement and Rapid Eye Movement Sleep

Julie M. Hereford, PT, DPT

Sleep is a naturally reoccurring state in which there is an absence of conscious awareness, a marked reduction in response to sensory stimuli, and a substantial change in voluntary muscular activity ranging from decreased activity to the marked atonia that characterizes rapid eye movement (REM) sleep. Sleep is distinguished from hibernation, coma, or death, in that it is cyclic and easily reversible. During sleep there is increased anabolic activity, the purpose of which seems to be to promote growth and regeneration of the immune system, nervous system, and musculoskeletal system. Sleep has been observed in all mammals, birds, some reptiles, amphibians, and fish and has even been studied in invertebrates (Figures 5-1 and 5-2). In fact, much of the current understanding of sleep has come from study of sleep in the animal kingdom (Figure 5-3). The function of sleep is not completely clear and continues to be an area of significant research. Current theories regarding the function of sleep will be discussed, but in order to understand the potential purpose of sleep, it is important to study the mechanisms by which sleep occurs.

Sleep is a cyclical event and consists of non-rapid eye movement (NREM) and REM sleep phases. In a normal sleeper, these phases proceed in a relatively orderly and predictable fashion throughout the night. The normal order of sleep stages is wakefulness → N1 → N2 → N3 → N2 → REM → natural awakening (see Figure 2-23).

In normal sleep architecture, there is greater slow-wave sleep (SWS; N3) earlier in the night and proportionately greater amounts of REM sleep later in the night. The cycling of NREM and REM takes on a characteristic appearance. As the understanding of normal sleep architecture increases, it sheds light upon disordered sleep. The study of the impact of disordered sleep has helped to clarify some of the functions of normal sleep. It is increasingly clear that the normal cycling of sleep between NREM and REM is important for normal physiological functioning. It is therefore important to understand the differences between NREM and REM sleep.

ONSET OF SLEEP

The hallmark of the onset of sleep is a behavioral disengagement from the environment and a substantial reduction in responsiveness to sensory stimuli compared to that of wakefulness. Normally sleep onset occurs when the individual enters NREM stage 1 sleep from wakefulness. It is most common to experience an increase in alpha wave activity, which occurs during drowsy wakefulness with eyes closed prior to sleep. It can be difficult to pinpoint the moment of transition into sleep unless one is attached to an electroencephalogram (EEG). Sleep is initiated as N1 sleep and transitions fairly rapidly to descending stages of sleep until one reaches N3 (consisting of N3 and N4 SWS). Infants may enter sleep going directly into REM sleep, but a normal adult sleeper never does this. In fact, if one finds onset of REM sleep immediately from wakefulness in an adult, one must consider the possibility of a narcolepsy diagnosis.

Constantin von Economo first postulated an ascending arousal system in the 1920s as a result of studies he carried out during an outbreak of encephalitis.[1] The ascending arousal system is located between the brain stem and basal forebrain that regulates sleep. von Economo established

Hereford JM. *Sleep and Rehabilitation: A Guide for Health Professionals* (pp 35-51).
© 2014 Taylor & Francis Group.

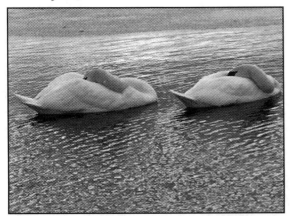

Figure 5-1. Sleep has been observed in birds, amphibians, and even invertebrates. (From Fotolia.com)

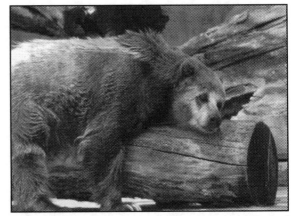

Figure 5-2. Sleep has been observed in mammals, reptiles, and fish. (From Fotolia.com)

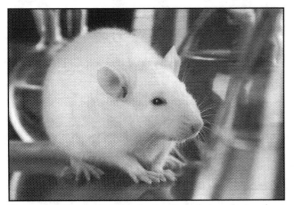

Figure 5-3. Much of our understanding of sleep comes from studies of animals. (From Fotolia.com)

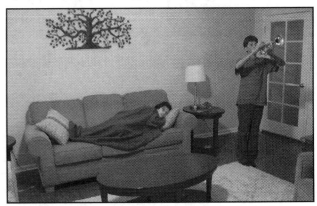

Figure 5-4. Sleep is accompanied by a profound reduction in responsiveness to outside stimuli. (Reprinted with permission from J. Hereford.)

that lesions between the midbrain and diencephalons caused prolonged sleepiness.[2]

As the body of knowledge on neurobiology has increased within the last several decades, two ascending arousal pathways have been identified. The first pathway is acetylcholinergic and has cell bodies located in the pedunculopontine and laterodorsal tegmental nucleus. This pathway ascends to the thalamus and activates relays within it. Neurons from this nucleus play an important role in transferring information between the thalamus and the cerebral cortex. These neurons are highly active during wakefulness and REM sleep and are minimally active during NREM sleep. The second pathway is monoaminergic and has neurons that originate in the locus coeruleus (norepinephrine), dorsal and median raphe nuclei (serotonin), ventral periaqueductal gray matter (dopamine), and tuberomammillary nucleus (histamine), and project to the lateral aspect of the hypothalamus and basal forebrain and then project throughout the cerebral cortex. The hypothalamic neurons contain orexin, and the basal forebrain neurons contain gamma-aminobutyric acid (GABA) and acetylcholine. Experimentally induced lesions of these pathways can cause profound sleep or may produce coma.[3,4]

Sleep-promoting neurons located in the ventrolateral preoptic nucleus are activated at sleep onset. These neurons project inhibitory neurons GABA type A and galanin to arousal-promoting neurons that contain histamine, serotonin, orexin, norepinephrine, and acetylcholine. Sleep is induced by activation of sleep-promoting neurons that produce inhibition of arousal-promoting neurons. These sets of neurons have shown reciprocal discharges. GABA also increases arousal-promoting neurons during NREM sleep, which acts as a mechanism to preserve sleep. Additionally, sleep-promoting neurons receive input from neurons that they inhibit, which suggests that the sleep–wake circuitry is a feedback loop that can process in either direction.[5,6]

Sleep onset is also accompanied by a profound reduction in responsiveness to sensory stimuli compared to wakefulness (Figure 5-4). This is exemplified when subjects are asked to respond to a flash of light in front of their eyes. They are able to do so accurately during wakefulness but fail to do so at the moment of onset of sleep. This failure to respond is not evidence of an inability to generate a response but rather a failure to see the stimulus; humans are essentially functionally blind during sleep.

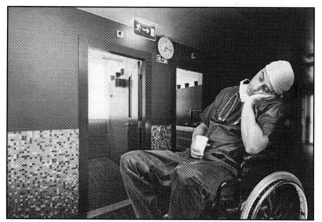

Figure 5-5. Hypnic myoclonia is linked to sleep deprivation, changes in sleep schedule, or psychological stress. (From Fotolia.com)

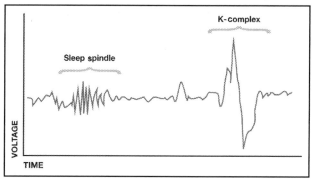

Figure 5-6. Sleep spindles and K-complexes characterize NREM sleep.

There is also a failure to respond to most auditory stimuli. Auditory arousal threshold increases across stages of sleep and is the highest during NREM stage 4 sleep. The auditory arousal threshold during sleep declines with increasing age and is far greater in children. In fact, a maximal auditory stimulus of nearly 140 decibels, which is the equivalent of the noise produced by a jet engine 100 yards overhead, did not cause any arousal in a group of children during the early part of a night's sleep. Auditory discrimination in a sleeping adult, however, is increased. That is, a person can be aroused more easily by the sound of his or her own name rather than someone else's name. In addition, a sleeping mother is more likely to awaken to the sound of the cry of her own baby, but is less likely to awaken to the cry of an unrelated infant. Auditory threshold can be manipulated by linking a stimulus to reward or punishment.

NON-RAPID EYE MOVEMENT SLEEP

According to the 2007 American Academy of Sleep Medicine (AASM) standards,[7] NREM sleep now consists of 3 stages, because N3 and N4 have been combined into N3 since the distinction between the 2 in polysomnography is the density of the delta wave activity.

Stage N1 sleep is that which the normal adult sleeper enters into from drowsy wakefulness (8 to 12 Hz) in which the brain is producing alpha waves with a frequency of 3 to 7 Hz. At the onset of sleep, the brain begins to produce theta waves, which have a frequency of 3 to 7 Hz. Sudden muscle twitches and hypnic myoclonia (the major muscle jerk that often arouses one out of sleep and is often accompanied by a report of the feeling of falling) may occur at the onset of N1 sleep. Hypnic myoclonia is more likely to occur when an individual is sleep deprived, is experiencing changes in sleep schedule, or is under increased psychological stress (Figure 5-5). This is seen with increasing frequency in graduate students, interns and residents, and shift workers.

Hypnagogic hallucinations, a mental phenomenon that occurs during threshold consciousness, may include lucid dreaming, hallucinations, out-of-body experiences, and sleep paralysis. This phenomenon occurs at the transition points between wakefulness and sleep or sleep and wakefulness. These phenomena are usually brief but can be extended in disordered sleep or in deliberate induction, as may occur during meditation.

In addition to increased arousal threshold to most sensory stimuli, normal sleepers usually lose some muscle tone and most conscious awareness of the external environment.

Stage 2 sleep, or N2, is characterized by 2 particular waveforms called *sleep spindles* and K-complexes (Figure 5-6).

A sleep spindle, sometimes called a *sigma band*, is a burst of oscillatory EEG activity that consists of 12 to 14 Hz waves that last at least 0.5 seconds. Sleep spindles are thought to represent an inhibitory response within the brain, which preserves the tranquil state of sleep. They are usually recorded over the frontal and central head regions. They may be synchronous or asynchronous, but they should be symmetrical and bilateral. They are generated in the thalamus and are a result of interactions between cells in the thalamus and the cerebral cortex. They have been shown to have a preservative effect on sleep, especially in the presence of external noise. Muscle twitching may be seen immediately following a burst of sleep spindle activity and this is thought to represent a part of motor learning.[8–11] Sleep spindles are also associated with the integration of new information into existing knowledge.[12] Fast sleep spindles are associated with directed remembering and forgetting.[13] Abnormalities in patterns of slow and fast sleep spindles have been associated with certain mental disorders such as schizophrenia.[14]

K-complexes are the other waveform that indicates the onset of N2 sleep. They are the largest event in a human EEG and are seen more frequently in the first sleep cycles. They consist of a brief negative high-voltage wave greater than 75 μV followed by a slower positive complex that lasts 350 to 550 ms ending in a negative peak. In normal N2 sleep, a K-complex occurs every 1.0 to 1.7 minutes and is often followed by bursts of sleep spindles. They occur spontaneously but also occur in response to external stimuli such as touch or sound or to internal stimuli such as respiratory disruptions. They are generated primarily in the frontal brain but can occur in widespread areas of the cortex.[15-17] K-complexes are sleep protective, in that they appear to suppress cortical arousal in response to external stimuli that the sleeping brain decides is not a signal of danger. They are also involved in information processing and memory consolidation. The K-complex aids in the activation of homeostasis of synapses by reducing the strength of synaptic connections that occur when they are activated during wakefulness. This then allows a kind of cortical rebooting in a systematic order so that memory engrams encoded during neuronal firing can be repeatedly practiced and consolidated.[18,19] K-complexes develop in infancy at approximately 5 to 6 months of age. During childhood there is a faster negative component that continues to become faster until adolescence. In the normal young adult sleeper, the frequency and amplitude of the K-complex is higher than in the normal sleeper as he ages. This decrease is consistent with the decrease in sleep spindle density and the power of delta wave sleep.[20]

A change in K-complex presentation is associated with several conditions, including obstructive sleep apnea (OSA), restless leg/legs syndrome, and epilepsy.

K-complexes are decreased during N2 in individuals with OSA, which seems to suggest a link between OSA and a blunting of cortical response to respiratory interruptions.[21-23]

Individuals who suffer from restless leg/legs syndrome tend to have increased numbers of K-complexes associated with abnormal leg movements. Though dopamine-enhancing medications can reduce leg movements, they do not reduce the density of K-complexes or reduce the complaint of non-restorative sleep, suggesting that leg movements are a symptom of the increased K-complex production. Drugs that inhibit REM sleep by increasing GABA such as benzodiazepines also reduce the density of K-complexes, and users report improvement in restorative sleep.

In some types of epilepsy, K-complex synchronization can trigger spike wave discharges, usually during transition phases of sleep. In nocturnal frontal lobe epilepsy, K-complexes are usually present at the start of the seizure.[24]

During N2 sleep, muscular activity decreases and conscious awareness of the external environment is completely inhibited. N2 sleep normally amounts to 45% to 55% of total sleep in adults.

N3 sleep, also known as delta sleep or SWS, is characterized by the presence of at least 20% of delta waves, which range from 0.5 to 2 Hz with an amplitude of >75 μV. This stage of sleep is sometimes called *restorative sleep* because production of some hormones, which are involved in cellular and neural regeneration, occurs almost exclusively during this stage of sleep. This is also the stage in which several common parasomnias occur, including night

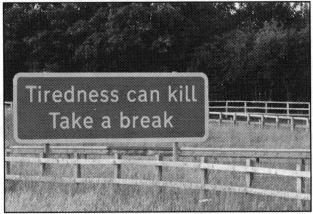

Figure 5-7. Drowsy driving is a deadly problem on roads. (From Fotolia.com)

terrors, nocturnal enuresis, and somnambulism. Although the AASM criteria now combine N3 and N4 sleep, there is reason to divide them out during a discussion of the physiological activities that occur during deep sleep. For these purposes, N3 sleep is defined as sleep that contains 20% to 50% delta waves and N4 sleep is sleep that contains greater than 50% delta waves during sleep.

In general, during NREM sleep simple automatic behaviors may occur. A very sleepy individual experiencing waxing and waning sleep may still be able to carry out fairly complex behavior such as driving a car. However, the competence with which the individual can accomplish this task is severely diminished and may result in tragic consequences. In fact, it is estimated by the National Highway Traffic Safety Administration that over 100,000 police-reported crashes result from drowsy drivers. There are approximately 1550 deaths and over 71,000 injuries from drivers who have actually fallen asleep at the wheel[25] (Figure 5-7).

SOME UNIQUE CHARACTERISTICS OF RAPID EYE MOVEMENT SLEEP

First identified in the early 1950s by Dement and Kleitman,[26] REM, as its name connotes, is characterized by random rapid eye movements but is also characterized by low muscle tone and a rapid, low-voltage EEG. It has since been divided into tonic REM and phasic REM. REM sleep typically occupies 20% to 25% of total sleep time and, generally, bouts of REM sleep occur with increasing duration during the latter half of the night. REM sleep generally produces the most memorable dreams, although dreaming occurs in every stage of sleep. The first bout of REM sleep usually begins approximately 90 to 110 minutes into a normal night's sleep. A normal adult sleeper will experience 4 to 5 bouts of REM sleep during a night's sleep. REM bouts are often followed by a brief period of very light

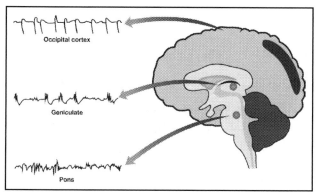

Figure 5-8. PGO waves.

sleep and some individuals may even awaken briefly after a REM bout. The relative amount of time one spends in REM sleep decreases from infancy throughout childhood. It can be composed of up to 80% of total sleep time in a newborn, and that percentage can be even higher in a premature infant. Percentage of REM sleep to total sleep time gradually decreases through childhood and usually reaches a steady point in early adolescence and remains relatively constant during normal adult sleep until old age. There can be disruption in the architecture of REM sleep as one reaches the seventh or eighth decade of life and there may be some decline in the total amount as a function of the aging brain.

REM sleep has been further divided into distinguishable tonic and phasic aspects. Phasic REM sleep is characterized by intermittent REM bouts with muscle twitches. Tonic REM sleep shows more persistent desynchronized sleep with an activated EEG tracing. One of the most characteristic aspects of tonic REM sleep is postsynaptic inhibition of voluntary skeletal musculature with the exception of external ocular musculature and musculature controlling the bones of the inner ear.

The onset of REM sleep is heralded by the generation of ponto-geniculo-occipital (PGO) waves (Figure 5-8). These are spiky waves that begin while the cortical EEG still shows signs of NREM sleep. This waveform is named according to the sites where they are most easily recorded but, due to technical difficulties, most of the research on PGO waves has been done in animal models. The PGO waves originate in the pons, travel to the lateral geniculate nucleus in the hypothalamus, and end in the occipital primary visual cortex. PGO waves occur most frequently during REM sleep and typically appear in clusters. The areas of activation of the PGO waves are areas that are responsible for eye movements, receipt of visual information, and processing of that visual information or creating or filling in visual information in a scene. These waves are initiated immediately prior to cortical EEG evidence of the onset of REM sleep and indicate that profound changes in neural activity are beginning to take place within the brain. One hypothesis suggests that PGO waves produce dreaming

and that the bursts of eye movement during REM sleep, which increase in intensity and duration as a night's sleep progresses, represent scanning of the hallucinated dream scene. PGO waves are representative of the powerful influence that activity in the pons of the brain stem has on other brain regions especially during sleep. It is also interesting that individuals who have been deprived of REM sleep can exhibit PGO waves in other stages of sleep, indicating an as-yet not understood physiological function of the PGO wave.

Another significant difference between NREM and REM sleep is the amount of somatic motor activity seen during the different stages of sleep. Although there are few motor events during NREM sleep, body repositioning and some other motor activities are possible during NREM. However, during normal REM sleep there is a postsynaptic inhibition of virtually all voluntary skeletal musculature, producing a nonreciprocal flaccid paralysis of major muscle groups during REM. A process of membrane hyperpolarization also decreases motor activity (Figure 5-9). The release of certain neurotransmitters—particularly the monoamines norepinephrine, serotonin, and histamine—ceases during REM sleep, and this is partially responsible for the muscle atonia characteristic of REM sleep.[27–29]

At intervals during phasic REM sleep that usually coincide with REM, there may be brief muscle twitches that occur primarily in peripheral musculature of the fingers and toes and in muscles of facial expression or muscles of mastication, particularly the masseter and temporalis. Twitching of the latter 2 muscles may be responsible for the production of bruxing of the teeth (see Chapter 22 and Chapter 25).

There is some evidence that the motor inhibition that is characteristic of REM sleep may be protective against the acting out of dreams. In fact, if the brain stem mechanisms subserving this state-dependent atonia become damaged or if there is dysfunction in certain neurotransmitters, a phenomenon in which the affected sleeper may engage in truly bizarre behavior may occur because of the loss of muscular inhibition. This disorder is known as *REM behavior disorder*. This may present itself as benignly as substantial muscular twitching or as significantly as complex integrated movement like kicking, grabbing, jumping out of bed, or screaming. There are a number of significant cases of REM behavior disorder in which an individual may even commit acts of violence. This disorder may have an acute onset that results from adverse reaction to certain medications or may occur during drug withdrawal. It may be more chronic and has been associated with certain neurodegenerative disorders such as Parkinson's disease[30] or neurological disorders such as narcolepsy.

The mechanisms that produce the atonia characteristic of REM sleep can also erupt during wakefulness, resulting in the characteristic "dropsy attacks" that occur in cataplexy, in which the individual experiences a sudden loss of motor function.

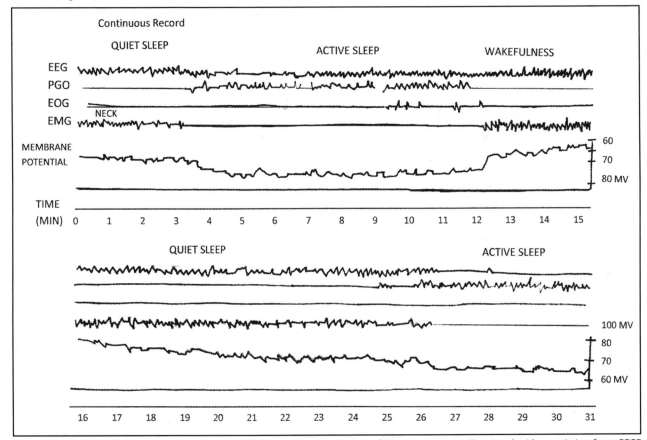

Figure 5-9. Hyperpolarization that causes motor inhibition that is characteristic of REM sleep atonia. (Reprinted with permission from CORE Services, Inc.)

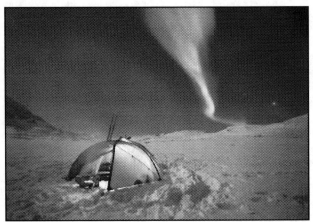

Figure 5-10. REM sleep is associated with the inability to regulate one's body temperature. (From Fotolia.com)

Various physiological functions become erratic and unstable during REM sleep. For example, heart rate and respiration become irregular during REM and body thermoregulation is disrupted. In fact, the loss of ability to regulate one's body temperature causes the body temperature to migrate toward the ambient temperature. This is particularly important when sleeping in extreme cold as one might do during fall or winter camping (Figure 5-10). Because of the inability to regulate body temperature during REM sleep, the normal sleeper will simply forgo REM sleep during the period of exposure to extreme cold. Interestingly, when allowed to return to a normal sleep environment, the sleeper will "catch up" on REM sleep by producing prodigious amounts of REM sleep to recover from the previous loss. Another important consideration in the thermoregulation disruption characteristic of REM sleep occurs with infants. Because of the marked increased in time that a newborn or infant spends in REM sleep, up to 80% of total sleep time, the infant is far less tolerant of spending time in temperature extremes.

Nocturnal penile tumescence normally occurs during REM sleep. In fact, an individual who experiences erectile dysfunction while awake but displays normal nocturnal penile tumescence may have a psychological component to the dysfunction rather than a physiological cause. Females may experience nocturnal clitoral tumescence and increased vaginal blood flow and transudation during normal REM sleep. During a normal night's sleep, genital tumescence commonly occurs for a total of 1 to 3 hours.

Changes in Physiological Processes Related to Different Sleep Stages

	Relaxed Waking	NREM Sleep	Tonic REM	Phasic REM
Sympathetic	P	P	S	S
Parasympathetic	P	P	P	P
Heart rate	70+	65+	60+	80+
Pupil diameter	O	0	0	O

Figure 5-11. Sympathetic and parasympathetic activity that occurs during wakefulness, NREM, and tonic and phasic episodes of REM sleep.

Central Nervous System Activity During Sleep

During NREM sleep, there is an overall reduction in the mean discharge rate of many neurons within the central nervous system. The metabolism of the brain also decreases during NREM sleep compared to wakefulness or REM sleep. During tonic REM sleep, the mean firing rate in many regions of the brain is significantly increased compared to NREM sleep, and some areas may even have a higher firing rate than during wakefulness. In short, the brain in REM sleep is extremely active, more active even than during some aspects of alert wakefulness. The visual system in particular exhibits a significant increase in neuronal discharge during REM sleep.

Autonomic Nervous System Function During Sleep

During NREM sleep, sympathetic activity stays at about the same level as during relaxed wakefulness. Parasympathetic activity increases during NREM sleep, resulting in a slight predominance of parasympathetic activity over sympathetic activity.

During tonic REM sleep, the imbalance between parasympathetic and sympathetic activity increases in favor of parasympathetic activity as a result of decreased sympathetic input compared to that in NREM sleep (Figure 5-11). During phasic REM sleep, both sympathetic and parasympathetic inputs increase and can be likened to putting one's foot on the brake and the accelerator at the same time.

The transient imbalance in autonomic drives during NREM and REM sleep generally favors a slight preponderance of sympathetic activation.

Autonomic nervous system function changes in the individual who has sleep apnea. Sympathetic neural activity during sleep and wakefulness is increased overall. This may be a factor in the greater risk of cardiovascular events observed in patients with OSA. Increased blood pressure is also associated with OSA and may result from sodium retention due to activation of the renin–angiotensin system.

Mechanisms responsible for the elevated autonomic tone seen in individuals with OSA include repetitive arousals, hypoxemia, and hypercapnia, which occur particularly in REM sleep. Effective positive airway pressure therapy used to treat OSA is extremely effective in reducing the elevation in autonomic tone. It is also possible that changes in the

mechanics of respiration associated with attempts to maintain an airway during sleep can cause mechanical changes in the autonomic system. This is an area that is of interest to the rehabilitation professional. It is possible that work to correct deficiencies in the mechanics of respiration and establish more homeostatic breathing patterns may translate to improved airway function during sleep. This is an important area in which the rehabilitation professional may be able to positively affect sleep-related breathing disorders.

Symptoms of respiratory disease can be affected by changes in autonomic tone. Stimulation of the sympathetic nervous system, particularly the adrenergic beta-2 receptors, produces bronchodilation. Increased parasympathetic tone leads to bronchoconstriction and increased mucus production. The nocturnal decrease in sympathetic activity and enhanced parasympathetic tone can give rise to worsening of lung function and asthma symptoms in the early morning hours.

Cardiovascular System Activity During Sleep

With the transition from relaxed wakefulness to NREM sleep, systemic blood pressure tends to decrease slightly and exhibits reduced variability. During tonic REM sleep, blood pressure remains about the same as during NREM sleep. However, during phasic REM sleep, blood pressure becomes unstable and may increase as much as 40 mm Hg, or approximately 30% over resting levels. Cardiac output is reduced during NREM sleep compared to wakefulness and continues at about the same level during REM sleep. Active vasodilatation occurs during NREM sleep and leads to decreased resistance in the circulatory system. Most vessels remain dilated during tonic REM sleep except for those in skeletal muscles, which undergo vasoconstriction. During phasic REM sleep, however, vasoconstriction is generalized and may be a mechanism by which blood pressure rises during phasic REM sleep.

Brain circulation varies according to the stage of sleep. Only a few brain areas show minimal increased blood flow during NREM sleep compared to relaxed wakefulness. In general, there is a slight decrease in overall brain circulation and temperature during NREM sleep. Changes occur during REM sleep. For instance, during tonic REM sleep most brain areas show an almost 50% increase in blood flow compared to that seen during wakefulness. However, during some parts of tonic REM sleep, the increase in brain blood flow in specific areas has been shown to be as high as 200%. During phasic REM sleep blood flow in most regions of the brain is further increased transiently. The exact quantification of this increase is difficult because these phasic REM episodes are usually brief.

As brain blood flow changes, so does brain temperature. Overall, brain temperature is decreased during NREM sleep when compared to alert wakefulness. Brain temperature does increase above waking levels during REM sleep as cerebral blood flow increases.

Renal System Function During Sleep

The renal system alters its function during normal sleep, mostly affecting the production of urine. Although not specifically confined to a particular stage of sleep, glomerular filtration rate, renal plasma flow, filtration fraction, and excretion of sodium, chloride, potassium, and calcium are all reduced during sleep. These changes in renal function act to produce less, more concentrated urine during sleep. These changes occur in both NREM and REM sleep but are more pronounced during REM sleep. This action occurs in conjunction with the body's release of a minute burst of antidiuretic hormone, known as *arginine vasopressin*. This hormone burst reduces kidney output well into the night so that the bladder does not get full until morning. This hormone cycle is not present at birth but usually develops in children between the ages of 2 and 6; these diurnal changes in antidiuretic hormone production may not occur until the age of 10. The ability to awaken when the bladder is full is a developmentally related function that develops at the same age but is separate from the hormone cycle. Conscious awareness of bladder filling occurs as a result of sympathetic neuronal pathways. As the bladder continues to fill, stretch receptors in the wall of the bladder in the detrusor muscle are activated, coupled with the desire to void. This information is relayed back to the cerebral cortex via S1 to S4 parasympathetic pelvic nerve fibers. Generally, the bladder pressure remains low due to the bladder's compliance as urine volume changes. Bladder compliance, or its ability to expand or contract, is due to the smooth muscle lining the bladder and collagen deposits within the wall together with neuronal mechanisms that inhibit the detrusor muscle from contracting, specifically adrenergic receptors that mediate relaxation. To maintain adequate kidney filtration rates, bladder pressure during filling must remain low. When the bladder reaches 150 to 200 mL of urine, the sensation of bladder fullness is transmitted to the central nervous system and the first desire to void occurs. Three hundred to 500 mL of urine is normal functional capacity, and the desire to void and discomfort is strong. Inhibition of the neurological function of bladder fullness and desire to void occurs during sleep so that an individual should not waken at the early stages of bladder filling. In fact, individuals who report that they have a "small bladder" because they have to get up multiple times a night to urinate should be evaluated for the presence of another factor, such as benign prostate hyperplasia. Disordered sleep often leads to this report, and the individual will assume that the sense of bladder fullness is what has awakened them. In reality, it is likely that disordered sleep is what awakened them and then they became aware of a normal conscious sense of bladder fullness. In normal individuals, bladder fullness will not cause awakening until the bladder reaches capacity at 300 to 500 mL.

Related to renal function, there is also a sleep-related increase in plasma aldosterone levels and increase in prolactin secretion, which is considered to potentiate the action of aldosterone. There is also an increase in parathyroid hormone release during sleep, which may affect calcium excretion.

Gastrointestinal Activity During Sleep

In individuals with a normal digestive tract, gastric acid secretion decreases during sleep and displays circadian rhythmicity; that is, its function varies according to the workings of the internal clock. Swallowing and salivary production decrease during sleep, and esophageal motility is reduced compared to production during wakefulness. These changes delay esophageal acid clearance and prolong mucosal acid contact in patients with gastroesophageal reflux disease. There is evidence that disordered sleep contributes to respiratory complications associated with gastroesophageal reflux disease. There is also evidence that although the sensory threshold is decreased during sleep, this may not be true in the upper gastrointestinal tract; some visceral sensation is actually increased during sleep. This mechanism seems to protect the tracheobronchial tree from aspiration of gastric contents that reflux during sleep. Positional changes of the system tend to favor reflux; the horizontal orientation of the esophagus and tracheobronchial tree in the supine or prone position during sleep tends to encourage reflux.

Patients with functional bowel disorders report more sleep complaints compared to normal subjects, which may be related to changes in autonomic function during sleep, particularly during REM sleep. This is especially true in patients with irritable bowel syndrome.[31] In addition, in individuals suffering from duodenal ulcers, there is a substantial increase in gastric acid secretion up to 3 to 20 times as great during sleep.

Respiratory Physiology During Sleep

Sleep removes the behavioral activity subserved by the respiratory apparatus and the cortical state-related

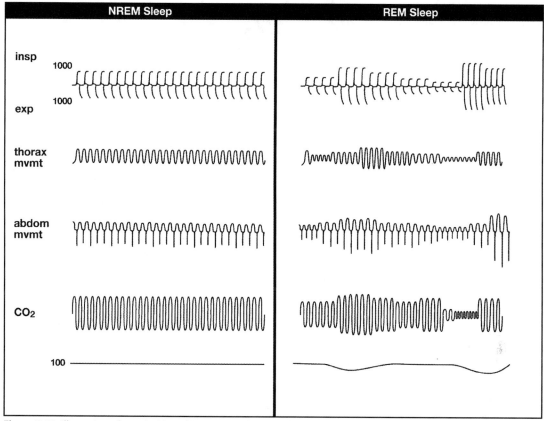

Figure 5-12. Illustration of a typical breathing pattern during NREM and REM sleep. This figure shows changes in ventilator effort as evidenced by a decrease and cessation of thoracic and abdominal movement. Note that this leads to immediate loss of CO_2 concentration in the face mask, but that SaO_2 saturation trails ventilator effort change. V = ventilatory volumes (mL) obtained from a pneumotachograph attached to a face mask; insp = inspiration; exp = expiration; thor mvt = thoracic movements; abd mvt = abdominal movements; SaO_2 = oxygen saturation (%).

non-metabolic drive that tonically stimulates breathing during wakefulness. This results in a loss of the normal respiratory drive that occurs during wakefulness, and these 2 phenomena result in a decrease in ventilation during sleep. The net result is that during NREM sleep there is a 13% to 15% fall in minute ventilation and a corresponding fall in alveolar ventilation so that the arterial partial pressure carbon dioxide (PCO_2) increases and arterial partial pressure oxygen (PO_2) decreases (Figure 5-12).

Control of Acid–Base Balance

Respiration changes substantially during different stages of sleep. One of the functions of respiration is to assist in maintaining homeostasis with the acid–base balance. Arterial blood gases measure this acid–base balance, and certain bodily enzymes cannot function outside the normal acid–base balance. Normal pH is between 7.35 to 7.45, and normal partial pressure arterial carbon dioxide ($PaCO_2$) is 35 to 45 mm Hg. Normal partial pressure arterial oxygen (PaO_2) is 80 to 100 mm Hg, and a person is considered hypoxemic when this number falls below 80 mm Hg. PaO_2 assesses perfusion or blood gas exchange. $PaCO_2$ assesses the adequacy of ventilation. An increase in respiratory rate or hyperventilation allows CO_2 (acid) to be blown off, thereby decreasing the $PaCO_2$. If this becomes excessive, respiratory alkalosis may occur. If the respiratory rate is decreased, as happens in sleep apnea or upper airway resistance syndromes in disordered sleep, hypoventilation causes the individual to retain CO_2 which increases $PaCO_2$, resulting in respiratory acidosis. The renal system also attempts to control this acid–base balance because the kidneys rid the body of hydrogen ions (H^+) and nonvolatile acids and maintain a constant bicarbonate level (HCO_3). Bicarbonate is the body's base.

Acidosis occurs when excessive H^+ and decreased HCO_3 cause a decrease in body pH. The renal system tries to adjust for this by excreting H^+ and retaining HCO_3. The respiratory system will try to compensate by increasing ventilation to blow off CO_2 and therefore decrease the acidosis.

Alkalosis occurs when H^+ decreases and HCO_3 increases. To compensate for this condition, the kidneys excrete HCO_3 and retain H^+. The respiratory system tries to compensate with hypoventilation to retain CO_2. The respiratory system can effect change in the acid–base balance in 15 to 30 minutes; the renal system, on the other

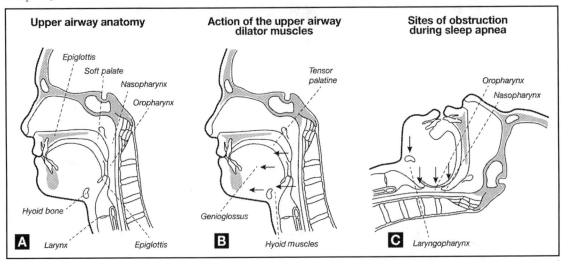

Figure 5-13. Anatomy of the airway and action of upper airway dilator muscles. Decreased tone in musculature during normal sleep, particularly during REM sleep, can cause momentary closure of the upper airway particularly if the genioglossus (tongue) muscle drops backwards into the airway.

hand, may take several hours or days to exert an effect on the acid–base balance.

During sleep, because of normal decreases in muscle tone and neural drive, there can be a minimal drop in oxyhemoglobin saturation and consequently a slight increase in carbon dioxide level. This is known as a *hypoxic* and *hypercapnic* ventilatory response, and it may occur to a minimal degree during normal sleep compared to wakefulness. Because of this hypoxic and hypercapnic ventilatory response, the respiratory drive is not as responsive to changes in acid–base balance. There is a greater change in hypoxemia and hypercapnea during REM sleep than during NREM. In fact, respiration can become somewhat unstable during REM sleep. PaO_2 may decrease 2 to 12 mm Hg and $PaCO_2$ may increase 2 to 8 mm Hg during sleep compared to wakefulness. SaO_2 may drop approximately 2% in a normal sleeper.

Upper airway muscle tone is diminished during sleep due to decreased respiratory neuron excitatory activity to the pharyngeal motor neurons. This decreases airway diameter and increases its vulnerability to collapse. Sleep also blunts the ventilatory response to the added inspiratory resistance because of the loss of muscular tone in the upper airway. There are gender differences in respiratory control. Hypoxic ventilatory responses may be similar during both wakefulness and NREM sleep in women. In men, there is a greater drop in hypoxic drive during sleep compared to wakefulness.

Though there are chemical and neuronal factors that change respiratory drive and capacity in sleep compared to wakefulness, there are also structural factors that impact this process (Figure 5-13). The upper airway can be considered to be a collapsible cylinder. Air flow within the upper airway is driven by changes in the nasal pressure, downstream pressure, and airway resistance. The patency of the

upper airway is influenced by length, caliber (Bernoulli effect), the pressure gradient against its wall, and its inherent collapsibility. The collapsibility of the upper airway is mediated by activation of the upper airway dilator muscles, increasing its resistance to collapse and increasing air flow. The muscles of the upper airway consist of the alai nasi in the nose; the levator veli palatini, palatoglosus, and tensor veli palatini in the palate; the genioglossus, geniohyoid, sternohyoid, and sternohyoid in the oropharanyx; and the circothyroid and posterior cricoarytenoid in the larynx.

Activation of these muscles can be diminished by sleep, alcohol, and muscle relaxants. This is why it is particularly important to warn patients against use of these agents in the presence of known untreated or undertreated upper airway resistance disorder. During wakefulness, reflex upper airway dilator muscle activation is triggered by negative subatmospheric intraluminal pressure. This reflex is diminished as sleep progresses through NREM sleep and transitions into REM sleep. Upper airway dilator response to hypoxia and hypercapnea is suppressed during NREM and especially during the transition into REM, where it may be completely abolished. There can be normal instability in respiratory drive along its pathway during REM sleep, so disordered sleep can result in significant respiratory events.

The activity of the genioglossus muscle, the primary muscle of the tongue, is inhibited by increased blood pressure that accompanies obstructive respiratory events and the subsequent arousals that follow them. Upper airway patency depends on activation of the upper airway dilator musculature that is sufficient to counteract the forces that cause airway collapse. Upper airway patency requires that these dilator muscles are properly synchronized to specific segments of the respiratory cycle; that is, activation of the upper airway muscles should precede activation of the diaphragm. This is an important concept and requires that there is normal length–tension ratio and motor firing patterns in these muscles. In Chapter 27, these concepts will be discussed at length. This is a way that the rehabilitation professional can have a direct impact on respiratory mechanics and therefore sleep. This is an important but largely ambiguous area of rehabilitation. Because patients normally spend one third of their lives asleep, it is important for the rehabilitation practitioner to understand the process of sleep and the direct influence it can have on the mechanics of the body system. It is important for the practitioner to learn how he or she can manipulate sleep and the rehabilitation process to achieve the best, most efficient outcomes for the patient.

A decrease in skeletal muscle tone is a normal feature of NREM sleep and relaxes the upper airway dilator muscles so that resistance to inspiratory air flow increases. During sleep, there is a decrease in the activity of muscles responsible for maintaining pharyngeal patency during inspiration. For normal patients in NREM sleep, breathing is automatic and regular because it is under chemical and mechanical feedback control. Breathing appears to be most dependent on the levels of CO_2 in the arterial blood, so much so that below a certain level of CO_2, called the *apneic threshold*, breathing efforts cease. During the transition between wakefulness and sleep, breathing can be periodic with regular fluctuations in amplitude. This is because fluctuations in the level of alertness and the changes between CO_2 set points for wakefulness and sleep. These oscillations dampen out as sleep becomes established. During REM sleep, breathing appears to be relatively free of chemical feedback control. It appears to depend on a higher cortical drive; as a result, breathing during REM sleep can be quite irregular. The greatest degree of irregular breathing occurs during phasic periods of REM sleep. Sleep alters not only respiratory patterns but also the respiratory response to both external and internal stimuli. There are some gender differences in this. In men, the hypoxic ventilatory response during sleep is lower during NREM sleep than during wakefulness, and this response decreases a bit more during REM sleep. In women, there is a slight change from wakefulness to NREM sleep. This might just reflect ventilatory hypoxic response that is present during wakefulness in women.[32] Hypercapnea during sleep normally triggers a reflexive increase in breathing and access to oxygen, such as may occur with a momentary arousal and turning the head during sleep. Failure of this reflex can be fatal and has been postulated to be a factor in sudden infant death syndrome (SIDS). The hypercapnic ventilatory response generally falls during normal sleep in adults and may drop as much as 50% during NREM compared to wakefulness. With loss of muscle tone that occurs in REM sleep, there is an increase in upper airway resistance that is generally up to twice the normal wakefulness value. In those who snore presumably due to altered upper airway anatomy, which can occur for a variety of reasons (see Chapter 27), the airway resistance

can increase to 10 times normal values during wakefulness. In certain individuals, the resistance during sleep becomes infinite and ventilation ceases altogether despite continued respiratory efforts. This is what happens in OSA. With the exception of certain flat-faced dogs, like the bulldog or pug, humans are the only mammals that have any significant OSA. This is thought to be due to the development of complex speech and language skills, which could only occur when the human larynx dropped below the tongue into the neck area.

There are 3 anatomic concepts and theories that should be considered when studying the mechanics of breathing, especially breathing during sleep. First is the property of the downwardly bent face, or *klinorhynchy*. This evolutionary concept looks at the migration of the facial skeleton as it moves forward and rotates under the brain cavity. This leads to a narrowing of the breathing passageways and a shortening of the facial bones, which causes airway narrowing. This is seen in primates and is most pronounced in humans who have relatively flat faces and short facial bones. There is even speculation that because of this skeletal compression, the human sinus passageways are more narrow to begin with, which leads to a predisposition toward sinus infection.

The descent of the larynx and the loss of the epiglottis soft palate lock-up results in the tongue and soft palate tissues becoming more pliable (Figure 5-14). In all other animals and in human infants, the epiglottis touches and overlaps behind the soft palate. But as the larynx descends, a space is created between the soft palate and the epiglottis called the *oropharanyx*, which is only present in humans. Human infants are born with a natural suck–swallow–breathing cycle, and the elevated epiglottis found in human infants helps to reduce the risk of aspiration of breast milk. As the epiglottis descends to its normal lower position in the later months of infancy as the face elongates, the risk of aspiration increases. Usually by this time the normal infant has perfected the act of swallowing so this is not an issue. This can, however, become an issue of critical importance in a child who is developmentally delayed and has swallowing dysfunction.

Migration of the foramen magnum is the final anatomical concept that affects humans in particular. This opening in the human skull is relatively forward compared to that of the chimpanzee and results in further crowding of the already narrowed airway, which occurs because of the shortening of the facial bones in humans (see Figure 5-14).

These anatomical considerations imply that all humans are susceptible to airway collapse to varying degrees. Because the upper airway has to simultaneously accommodate speech, breathing, and swallowing, it is logical that overdevelopment of any one of the components of the upper airway occurs at the expense of the others. There is speculation that speech and language development has ultimately been detrimental to the evolution of humans, evidenced

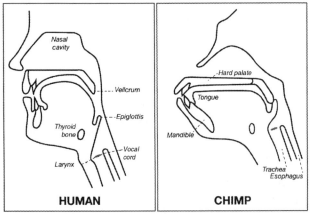

Figure 5-14. Illustration of migration of foramen magnum and larynx. Note differences in position of foramen magnum into a position closer to the oropharynx and the larynx under the tongue in humans. This relatively rapid evolution allowed for the development of speech to the detriment of the airway, especially during sleep. The only species who are able to choke to death and who develop OSA are humans and some flat-faced dogs.

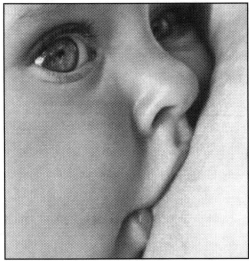

Figure 5-16. Breastfeeding was the only source of sustenance for babies until about 200 years ago. (From Fotolia. com)

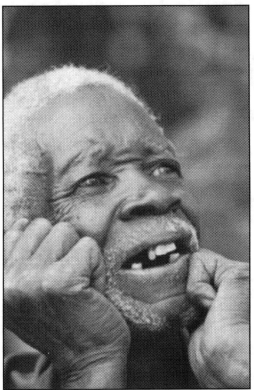

Figure 5-15. Tribal cultures introduced to a Western diet show declines in dental health within 1 to 2 generations. (From Fotolia.com)

relatively soft and highly refined and processed foods, the dental health and facial and jaw structures of these groups began to change. He noted that within 1 or 2 generations, the aboriginal people he was studying began to suffer from severe dental caries and misaligned teeth. In addition, those eating a Western diet had significant jaw structure narrowing, which caused major crowding of the teeth and increased dental caries and loss of teeth (Figure 5-15). In contrast, people living off the land with no Western influence in their diet remained healthy, vibrant, and cavity-free and with straight teeth. Their jaws were wide with broad arches and no teeth crowding. He found these phenomena repeatedly during his travels throughout the world investigating native and tribal cultures.

Another dentist, Dr. Brian Palmer,[34] has proposed that with the advent of bottle-feeding that began about 200 years ago and move away from breastfeeding, there has been a dramatic rise in the incidence of sleep-related breathing disorders (Figures 5-16 and 5-17). He postulated that the abnormal tongue position that is required to suckle on an artificial nipple somehow affects jaw development. He also suggested that the artificially elevated sucking forces needed to suckle from a bottle prevent proper widening of the infant's delicate jaw.

Regardless of the underlying mechanisms that have altered anatomy and increased upper airway resistance, there are a number of other ventilatory responses that are

by the fact that only humans can choke on a foreign object and die. Not being able to breathe well when sleeping supine may be another consequence of this anatomical evolution that has allowed human speech.

There are other theories that attempt to explain why there are so many sleep-related breathing problems in humans, which seem to be becoming more prevalent.

One theory that is widely discussed was put forth by Dr. Weston Price,[33] a dentist and amateur anthropologist who studied isolated cultures that lived and ate off the land. Dr. Price noticed that the aboriginal people of certain tribal cultures displayed normal teeth, without dental caries, and that the wide, well-developed midface and jaw structure was maintained. Over time, with the introduction of the Western diet, which contains significant amounts of altered by sleep. Sleep suppresses the arousal response to bronchial irritation. Coughing in patients with lung disease is suppressed by sleep, and an individual must arouse in order to cough. The arousal response to hypoxia alone is poor, although hypercapnea is a strong arousal stimulus that results in the waking of most individuals before a 15 mm Hg rise in $PaCO_2$ occurs.

Upper airway function in OSA and snoring is altered as well. Compared to control subjects, individuals with OSA often have anatomically narrower retropalatal and retroglossal air spaces that narrow further during sleep. Increase in activity of the upper airway dilators is often present during wakefulness to compensate for the narrow airway. Some of the causes for the narrowing of the airway may include adenoidal and tonsillar hypertrophy. This is especially important in children and has been shown to be related to development of behavioral conditions. Disordered sleep in children due to hypertrophic tonsils and adenoids can, and often does, result in increased upper airway resistance and can have substantial impact on behavioral aspects of childhood including symptoms of attention-deficit/hyperactivity disorder (see Chapter 15).

Other causes of narrowing of the upper airway may include macroglossia, which can be evidenced by the scalloping on the lateral borders of the tongue caused by indentation of the teeth onto a tongue that is larger than the space available for it. Micrognathia or retrognathia, both involving abnormal growth of the midface, can narrow the upper airway and may also be contributing factors to temporomandibular disorders related to disordered sleep (see Chapter 22 and Chapter 25).

Pharyngeal fat deposits in overweight or obese individuals will also narrow that upper airway and may be corrected by weight loss.

Sleep position can have an effect on the upper airway. For instance, the supine position will have an effect on the mandible and tongue because of the change in gravity in this position.

A reduction in lung volume caused by pulmonary disorders such as chronic obstructive pulmonary disease or restrictive diseases such as asthma can change the lower airway and result in sleep-related breathing disorders.

Endocrine Activity and Sleep

The production from the endocrine system serves to maintain the homeostatic balance of an organism. Endocrine activity promotes tissue growth, sexual development, absorption of sodium, and response to stress. Secretions of some hormones are directly related to the sleep process, whereas secretion patterns of other hormones are linked to circadian factors and not necessarily directly to a particular stage of sleep. To gain a better understanding of the relationship between the endocrine system and sleep, it is necessary to describe the specific hormones and their

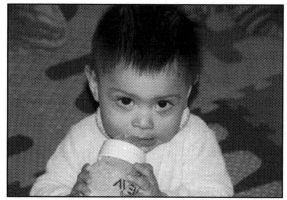

Figure 5-17. It has been proposed that the introduction of bottle feeding was accompanied by a dramatic increase in sleep-related breathing disorders. (Reprinted with permission from J. Hereford.)

relationship to sleep. Only the hormones that are related to sleep or disordered sleep will be discussed in the following section.

Human Growth Hormone

Human growth hormone (HGH) secretion, which stimulates growth and cellular reproduction and regeneration, is directly tied to sleep. The effects of HGH are generally anabolic. HGH acts by interacting with a specific receptor on the surface of cells. Increased height during childhood is the most commonly known function of HGH. It is also responsible for a number of other processes in normal physiological function including increased calcium retention, which strengthens and increases bone mineralization. It is also important in increasing muscle mass through sarcomere hyperplasia, which is why it is sometimes abused in competitive arenas. It promotes lipolysis, increases protein synthesis, and stimulates the growth of all internal organs except the brain. It plays a role in homeostasis and is involved in glucose metabolism by reducing its uptake by the liver. It also promotes gluconeogenesis in the liver, contributes to the maintenance and function of pancreatic islet cells, and stimulates the immune system. Clearly, this hormone has significant and variable functions. Because its secretion occurs during SWS, it is extremely important for an individual to have adequate SWS, otherwise known as *restorative sleep*.

If sleep is either advanced or delayed from its normal time, the peak episode of HGH secretion is advanced or delayed to coincide with the early part of sleep, regardless of its onset (Figure 5-18). Sleep-related HGH secretion is not present in infants younger than 3 months of age. In older children approaching puberty, virtually all HGH secretion occurs during the early part of sleep. With the advent of puberty, there is a great increase in sleep-related HGH, but there may also be several minor episodes of HGH secretion during wakefulness. In older sleepers, the relationship between sleep and HGH release declines, and it may cease altogether in the seventh or eighth decade of life.

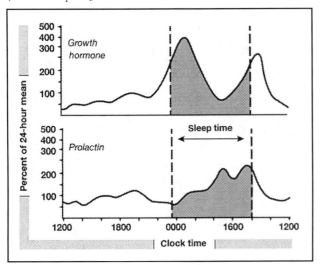

Figure 5-18. HGH and prolactin secretion during sleep.

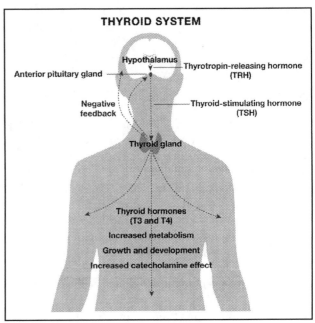

Figure 5-19. Function of thyroid hormones.

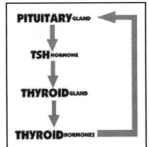

Figure 5-20. Schematic of thyroid production.

HGH-releasing hormone actually promotes sleep in men but may inhibit sleep in women. HGH-releasing hormone production is also increased in N3 and N4. Somatostatin, an HGH inhibitor, antagonizes HGH-releasing hormone, thus inhibiting HGH production. Decreased HGH production can interfere with sleep. Administration of actreotide, a somatostatin analogue, reduces NREM SWS. Gamma hydroxybutyrate and ritanserin increase NREM SWS and may increase HGH secretion.

Prolactin

Prolactin is a hormone produced in the anterior pituitary. Its levels increase during sleep, beginning about 30 to 90 minutes after the onset of sleep with maximum levels reached in the early morning (see Figure 5-18). Prolactin has many effects, including regulating lactation and orgasms. It is important for regeneration and repair of the central nervous system; it stimulates the proliferation of oligodendrocyte precursor cells, which then differentiate into oligodendrocytes, the cells responsible for formation of myelin coatings on axons in the central nervous system. Prolactin release is linked to sleep, so that as sleep is advanced or delayed, prolactin release corresponds with those changes. It is linked to sleep from puberty until old age. Prolactin secretion, however, is suppressed by sleep fragmentation. Administration of benzodiazepines can increase prolactin secretion during sleep.

Thyroid-Stimulating Hormone

Thyroid-stimulating hormone (TSH), or thyrotropin, is a peptide hormone that is secreted by thyrotrope cells in the anterior pituitary gland (Figures 5-19 and 5-20). TSH regulates endocrine function of the thyroid gland by stimulating the thyroid to secrete thyroxine (T_4) and triiodothyronine (T_3). TSH production is controlled by a thyrotropin-releasing hormone produced in the hypothalamus. This thyroid hormone feedback system is eventually responsible for the production of calcitonin, which acts to decrease serum calcium concentration. TSH release reaches its peak each day in the evening and then declines across the sleep period.

Parathyroid Hormone

Parathyroid hormone, also known as *parathormone*, is secreted by the chief cells of the parathyroid gland. It acts to increase the concentration of calcium in the blood. Unlike TSH, parathyroid hormone levels increase during sleep. Since TSH reaches its peak in the evening and declines during sleep, and parathormone is produced during sleep, the control of circulating calcium has a significantly sleep-related component.

Gonadotropins, Luteinizing Hormone, Follicle-Stimulating Hormone, and Testosterone

Gonadotropins, luteinizing hormone (LH), and follicle-stimulating hormone release herald the onset of puberty. LH release triggers ovulation and corpus luteum development in females. Its analogue, interstitial cell-stimulating hormone in males, stimulates Leydig cell production of testosterone. The release of these sex hormones occurs at sleep onset and is inhibited during wakefulness. The sleep-related release of LH is the first sign of puberty and is thought to be the event that initiates puberty in females. After puberty, the sleep-related release of LH no longer occurs. Release of follicle-stimulating hormone, which regulates the development, growth, pubertal maturation, and reproductive processes, also occurs during sleep and is inhibited by wakefulness.

Testosterone levels in males continue to be highest during sleep until old age, when the sleep-related pattern of testosterone release is no longer present.

Cortisol

Cortisol is involved in response to stress and anxiety and has a primary function to increase blood sugar and store sugar in the liver as glycogen. It also acts to suppress the immune system. The release of corticotropin-releasing hormone (CRH) from the hypothalamus stimulates secretion of adrenocorticotropic hormone by the anterior pituitary, which in turn increases cortisol release from the adrenal cortex in a pulsatile fashion. The highest levels of plasma cortisol occur toward the end of sleep or just after awakening. Sleep onset, regardless of its time, has an inhibitory effect on cortisol release; thus, sleep can modulate the ongoing pattern of cortisol release. Normally, secretion of cortisol appears to be more closely linked to circadian rhythm than it does to sleep; however, sleep fragmentation and awakenings increase cortisol secretion. CRH increases vigilance and inhibits sleep. Administration of CRH, adrenocorticotropic hormone, or cortisol decreases REM sleep. CRH decreases NREM stage 3 and 4 sleep, whereas cortisol enhances NREM stage 3 and 4 sleep.

Melatonin

Melatonin, which is a pervasive and powerful antioxidant with a particular role in protection of nuclear and mitochondrial DNA, is released from the pineal gland and follows a circadian rhythm that is influenced by light, not by sleep. Sleep does not potentiate melatonin release in the daytime, and wakefulness does not inhibit it at night. Nocturnal melatonin release is inhibited by light. Its patterns of release adjust slowly, taking 10 to 12 days to reverse to a change in a light–dark cycle. This should be a consideration in jet lag and in shift work. Receptors for melatonin have been localized to the suprachiasmatic nucleus of the hypothalamus, which is strongly implicated as the mammalian circadian pacemaker. Melatonin functions in part as a hormonal transducer of light–dark signals. Seasonal information provided by this system has significant interactions with reproductive activity in many mammals.

Leptin

Leptin is a hormone that plays a key role in regulating energy intake and energy expenditure, including appetite and metabolism. There is some controversy regarding the

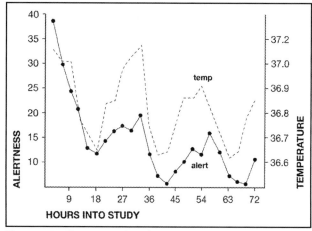

Figure 5-21. This is a graphic of sham data showing the relationship between body temperature and alertness. In this example, average subjective alertness and body temperature of 15 subjects experiencing 72 hours of sleep deprivation under temporal isolation.

regulation of leptin by melatonin during the night. One research group suggested that increased levels of melatonin caused a downregulation of leptin.[35] However, in 2004, Brazilian researchers[36] found that when insulin is readily available, it allows melatonin to interact with insulin and upregulate insulin-stimulated leptin expression, therefore causing a decrease in appetite while sleeping.

Ghrelin

Ghrelin is a hormone produced mainly by P/D1 cells lining the fundus of the human stomach and epsilon cells of the pancreas that stimulates hunger. Ghrelin levels increase before meals and decrease after meals. It is considered the counterpart of the hormone leptin. Ghrelin plays a significant role in neurotrophy, particularly in the hippocampus, and is essential for cognitive adaptation to changing environments and the process of learning. Studies suggest that sleep deprivation may be associated with high levels of ghrelin and obesity. There appears to be an inverse relationship between hours of sleep and blood plasma concentration of ghrelin; that is, as the hours of sleep increase, ghrelin concentrations are considerably lower, thereby potentially reducing appetite and decreasing the risk of obesity.[37]

Insulin

Blood levels of glucose and insulin may decline during sleep. Insulin resistance may develop and levels of insulin may decrease during sleep deprivation. Because there are a number of hormones that have an impact on glucose metabolism, it is a reasonable conclusion that sleep deprivation or disordered sleep may have a negative impact on metabolism and may be a contributing factor to insulin resistance.

THERMOREGULATION

Body temperature regulation is an important aspect of homeostasis and is important to keep internal organs at a relatively constant temperature (Figure 5-21). Overall, body temperature remains at a lower level during sleep than during wakefulness. Body temperature fluctuates somewhat throughout the day. The daily temperature pattern persists even in the absence of sleep, but it does correlate with cycles of alertness (see Figure 5-21). The preoptic area of the anterior hypothalamus normally controls body temperature. Homeostatic control of body temperature is apart from the sensation of the temperature. Strategies to control body temperature vary according to the situation, and small fluctuations are accomplished by internal mechanisms. It is true, however, that during NREM sleep body temperature is at a lower set point than during wakefulness.

State-dependent regulation of temperature involves control mechanisms independent of those responsible for the circadian pattern of sleep. Body temperature is regulated during NREM at a lower set point than during wakefulness. Shivering is initiated at a lower temperature and sweating will occur during NREM sleep when the ambient temperature is high or even when it is at what would be considered a normally neutral temperature if the individual were awake. This explains why a person may go to sleep in a comfortably climate-controlled room but wake sweating, because the set point of the temperature is lower during NREM sleep.

Thermoregulation ceases as the sleeper transitions into REM sleep. Shivering and sweating in response to temperature changes stops altogether. For as long as REM sleep persists, body temperature will drift toward the ambient temperature. In extremes of environmental temperature, sleep will become disrupted. REM sleep is reduced much more than NREM sleep so that body temperature usually continues to be actively regulated. Newborn human infants may be at particular risk, however, for catastrophic thermal events during sleep because they have such a large amount of REM sleep and because the drive to maintain REM sleep is very great.

IMMUNE FUNCTION AND SLEEP STAGES

During systemic infection, people often experience increased lassitude or sleepiness. Sleepiness associated with hepatic failure can be relieved in seconds by administration of a benzodiazepine receptor antagonist. This leads one to the conclusion that sleep plays a role in immune function.

Acute infections and inflammatory processes can give rise to sleepiness mediated in part by central nervous system cytokines, particularly interleukin (IL)-1 and tumor necrosis factor-alpha (TNF-α). Sleep deprivation can impair antibody response to vaccination and alter specific immune parameters.

Cytokines affect sleep by either enhancing or inhibiting it. For example, fibroblast growth factor, IL-1, IL-2, IL-6, IL-8, IL-15, and IL-18, nerve growth factor, and TNF-α all enhance sleep. Conversely, the cytokines' insulin-like growth factor and IL-4, IL-10, and IL-13 inhibit sleep.

The effects of sleep deprivation on immune parameters include an increase in IL-1, interferon, and TNF-α. There is also a change in the number of T-lymphocytes and natural killer cells, a change in lymphocyte mitogenesis and phagocytosis, and a change in circulating immunoglobulins and immune complexes as a consequence of sleep deprivation.

In animal studies there is a very large change in sleep patterns during infection. In fact, sleep changes in an animal are a major sign of infectious disease. These sleep changes are adaptive and play a role in nonspecific host defenses. The general pattern after bacterial or fungal infection is an initial period of enhancement of NREM sleep followed 1 to 2 days later by a period of suppressed NREM. REM sleep is inhibited throughout the course of a bacterial or fungal infection.

SUMMARY

Sleep is divided into 2 broad categories, NREM and REM sleep. Each sleep stage is associated with physiological, neurological, and psychological activity. NREM sleep is further divided into NREM stages 1, 2, and 3. Stage 3 sleep was previously divided into stage 3 and stage 4 sleep depending upon the density of delta wave activity, but the AASM[7] has combined these 2 stages into NREM stage 3 for scoring purposes. NREM stage 3 sleep is also known as *slow-wave sleep*.

Much of what is known about the physiological, neurological, and psychological functions of sleep has been learned from sleep deprivation studies and observational studies of animals. It is clear that significant hormonal, immune, and reparative activities occur primarily during sleep. Acute and chronic sleep deprivation caused by short sleep or disordered sleep has been shown to contribute to illnesses and diseases related to these changes in physiological function.

This chapter suggests that the rehabilitation provider may be able to influence sleep in patient populations by evaluating the mechanics of respiration and improving function, thereby maximizing respiratory function during wakefulness and decreasing the potential for airway collapse during sleep.

REFERENCES

1. Reid AH, McCall S. Henry JM, Taubenberger JK. Experimenting on the past: The enigma of von Economo's encephalitis lethargica. *J Neuropathol Exp Neurol.* 2001;60(7):663-670.

2. Pearce JM. Baron Constantine von Economo and encephalitis lethargica. *J Neurol Neurosurg Psychiatry.* 1996;60(2):167.

3. Saper CB, Scammell TE, Lu J. Hypothalamic regulation of sleep and circadian rhythms. *Nature.* 2005;437:1257-1264.

4. Haung ZL, Urade Y, Hayaishi O. Prostanglan and adenosine in the regulation of sleep and wakefulness. *J Physiol.* 2009;437(7):33-38.

5. McGinty D, Szymusiak R. Hypothalamic regulation of sleep and arousal. *Front Biosci.* 2008;8:1257-1264.

6. Gallopin T, Luppi PH, Cauli B, et al. The endogenous somnogen adenosine excites a subset of sleep-promoting neurons via A2A receptors in the ventrolateral preoptic nucleus. *Neuroscience.* 2005;134:1377-1390.

7. Iber C, Ancoli-Israel S, Chesson A, Quan SF. *The AASM Manual for the Scoring of Sleep and Associated Events: Rules, Terminology and Technical Specifications.* Westchester, IL: American Academy of Sleep Medicine; 2007.

8. Blumberg MS, Lucas DE. Dual mechanisms of twitching during sleep in neonatal rats. *Behav Neurosci.* 1994;108:1196-1202.

9. Khazipov R, Sirota A, Leinekugel X, Holmes GL, Ben-Ari Y, Buzsaki G. Early motor activity drives spindle bursts in the developing somatosensory cortex. *Nature.* 2004;432:758-761.

10. Petersson P, Waldenstrom A, Fahraeus C, Schouenborg J. Spontaneous muscle twitches during sleep guide spinal self-organization. *Nature.* 2003;424:72-75.

11. Seelke AH, Karlsson KA, Gall AJ, Blumberg MS. Extraocular muscle activity, rapid eye movements, and the development of active and quiet sleep. *Eur J Neurosci.* 2005;22:911-920.

12. Tamminen J, Payne JD, Stickgold R, Wamsley EJ, Gaskell MG. Sleep spindle activity is associated with the integration of new memories and existing knowledge. *J Neurosci.* 2010;30:14356-14360.

13. Saletin JM, Goldstein AN, Walker MP. The role of sleep in directed forgetting and remembering of human memories. *Cereb Cortex.* 2011;21:2534-2541.

14. Ferrarelli F, Huber R, Peterson MJ, et al. Reduced sleep spindle activity in schizophrenia patients. *Am J Psychiatry.* 2007;164(3):A62.

15. Roth M, Shaw J, Green J. The form, voltage distribution and physiological significance of the K-complex. *Electroenceph Clin Neurophysiol.* 1956;8:385-402.

16. Webster KE, Colrain IM. Multichannel EEG analysis of respiratory evoked-potential components during wakefulness and NREM sleep. *J Appl Physiol.* 1998;85:1727-1735.

17. McCormick L, Nielsen T, Nicolas A, Ptito M, Montplaisir J. Topographical distribution of spindles and K-complexes in normal subjects. *Sleep.* 1997;20:939-941.

18. Tononi G, Cirelli C. Sleep function and synaptic homeostasis. *Sleep Med Rev.* 2006;10:49-62.

19. Cash SS, Halgren E, Dehghani N, et al. Human K-complex represents an isolated cortical down-state. *Science.* 2009;324:1084-1087.

20. Wauquier A. Aging and changes in phasic events during sleep. *Physiol Behav.* 1993;54:803-806.

21. Huang J, Colrain IM, Melendres MC, et al. Cortical processing of respiratory afferent stimuli during sleep in children with the obstructive sleep apnea syndrome. *Sleep.* 2008;31:403-410.

22. Gora J, Trinder J, Pierce R, Colrain IM. Evidence of a sleep-specific blunted cortical response to inspiratory occlusions in mild obstructive sleep apnea syndrome. *Am J Respir Crit Care Med.* 2002;166:1225-1234.

23. Afifi L, Guilleminault C, Colrain IM. Sleep and respiratory stimulus specific dampening of cortical responsiveness in OSAS. *Respir Physiol Neurobiol.* 2003;136:221-234.

24. El Helou J, Navarro V, Depienne C, et al. K-complex-induced seizures in autosomal dominant nocturnal frontal lobe epilepsy. *Clin Neurophysiol.* 2008;119:2201-2204.

25. National Sleep Foundation. Drowsy drivers: facts and stats. Available at: http://drowsydriving.org/about/facts-and-stats/ Accessed April 19, 2012.

26. Dement W, Kleitman N. Cyclic variations in EEG during sleep and their relation to eye movements, body motility and dreaming. *Electroencephalogr Clin Neurophysiol.* 1957;9:673-690.

27. Hobson JA. REM sleep and dreaming: towards a theory of proto-consciousness. *Nat Rev.* 2009;10:803-813.

28. Aston-Jones G, Gonzalez M, Doran S. Role of the locus coeruleus–norepinephrine system in arousal and circadian regulation of the sleep–wake cycle. In: Ordway MA, Schwartz MA, Frazer A, eds. *Brain Norepinephrine: Neurobiology and Therapeutics.* New York, NY: Cambridge University Press; 2007:157-195.

29. Siegel JM. REM sleep. In: Kryger MH, Roth T, Dement WC, eds. *Principles and Practice of Sleep Medicine.* 4th ed. St Louis, MO: Elsevier; 2005:120-135.

30. Gugger JJ, Wagner ML. Rapid eye movement sleep behaviour disorder. *Ann Pharmacother.* 2007;41:1833-1841.

31. Orr WC, Chen CL. Sleep and the gastrointestinal tract. *Neurol Clin.* 2005;23:1007-1024.

32. Berthon-Jones M, Sullivan CE. Ventilatory and arousal responses to hypoxia in sleeping humans. *Am Rev Respir Dis.* 1982;125:632-639.

33. Price WA. *Nutrition and Physical Degeneration.* 8th ed. Cleveland, OH: Price Pottenger Nutrition Foundation; 2008.

34. Palmer B. *Breastfeeding and Frenulums.* Available at: www.brianpalmerdds.com/pdf/Bfing_Frenum03.pdf. Accessed July 1, 2013.

35. Kus I, Sarsilmaz M, Colakoglu N, Kukne A, Ozen OA, Yilmaz B, Kelestirmur H. Pinealectomy increases and exogenous melatonin decreases leptin production in rat anterior pituitary cells: an immunohistochemical study. *Physiol Res.* 2004;53(4):403-408.

36. Patel SR, Hu FB. Short sleep duration and weight gain: a systemic review. *Obesity.* 2008;16(3): 643-653.

37. Taheri S, Lin L, Austin D, Young T, Mignot E. Short sleep duration is associated with reduced leptin, elevated ghrelin, and increased body mass index. *PLoS Med.* 2004;1(3):e62.

6

Brain Mechanisms of Sleep and Wakefulness

Julie M. Hereford, PT, DPT

Waking and consciousness depend on the activity of neurons within the brain stem reticular formation. The reticular formation is a network of nerve pathways and nuclei that are located within the brain stem and connect motor and sensory neurons to and from the spinal cord, the cerebellum, and the cerebrum (Figure 6-1). It is estimated that a single neuron in this network may synapse with as many as 25,000 other neurons. The reticular formation is involved in the sleep–wakefulness cycle. It also acts to filter incoming stimuli to discriminate irrelevant background sensory information. It is essential in governing some basic functions including respiration and cardiovascular function. Other basic functions that require an intact reticular formation include somatic motor control involved in maintaining tone, balance, and posture, especially during movement. The reticular formation relays visual and auditory signals to the cerebellum for integration and provides pathways that dictate motor coordination. The reticular formation also includes other motor nuclei that allow the eyes to track and fixate and nuclei that produce rhythmic signals to the musculature of breathing and swallowing.

The reticular formation contains centers for cardiovascular control. It has relay pathways for pain and is the origin of cells that generate descending pain modulation. It is involved in habituation, the process by which the brain learns to ignore repetitive, meaningless stimuli in favor of other stimuli that are deemed important. Finally, the reticular formation is important in modulating states of sleep and wakefulness. It has projections to the thalamus and cerebral cortex that allow it to exert some control over which sensory signals reach the cerebrum and come to conscious attention. It plays a central role in states of consciousness. Damage to the reticular formation can lead to irreversible coma.

Neurons in the reticular formation form the ascending reticular activating system. They project into the thalamus and excite cells that project to widespread areas of the cerebral cortex to produce the cortical activation that occurs during wakefulness. Brain stem reticular neurons project into the hypothalamus and basal forebrain where neurons that also project to the cerebral cortex and participate in the maintenance of an alert cortex are located.

LOCALIZATION OF BRAIN MECHANISMS SUBSERVING WAKEFULNESS

Wakefulness and the electroencephalogram (EEG) desynchronization that characterizes it require excitatory input from the forebrain. Several apparently redundant ascending pathways are active in this state, but experimental work has concluded that no single pathway is responsible; rather, they combine to contribute to the state of wakefulness (Figure 6-2). Neurotransmitters for these pathways include the monoamines, serotonin, and norepinephrine as well as glutamate and acetylcholine.[1] Cell bodies for these pathways are located in the brain stem.

The ascending activating system (AAS), which includes the reticular formation, has cells located at the pons–midbrain junction that project to the thalamus. These

Hereford JM. *Sleep and Rehabilitation: A Guide for Health Professionals* (pp 53-60). © 2014 Taylor & Francis Group.

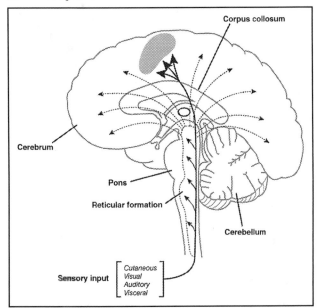

Figure 6-1. The reticular activating system of the human brain. Various sensory inputs send nonspecific impulses into the reticular formation via collaterals (dark arrowed lines) as well as to specific sensory areas of the cerebral cortex (shaded). In turn, the reticular formation sends nonspecific impulses throughout the cortex (curved, dashed lines) to "awaken" the entire brain.

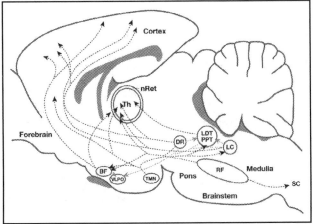

Figure 6-2. The principal activating systems that support wakefulness are displayed in this schematic of a sagittal section of the midbrain. Excitatory influences are shown in dark lines and inhibitory in lighter lines. Th = thalamus; TMC = tuberomammillary nucleus; DR = dorsal raphe; BF = basal forebrain; VLPO = ventrolateral preoptic area; LC = locus coeruleus; LDT/PPT = laterodorsal tegmentum/pedunculo-pontine region; RF = reticular formation.

neurons show increased rate of discharge prior to the first changes seen in EEG that indicate desynchronization typifying wakefulness. These neurons that project to the thalamus are cholinergic and are located in the laterodorsal tegmentum/pedunculopontine region (LDT/PPT). Neurons remain active during wakefulness and during rapid eye movement (REM) sleep, whenever the EEG shows a characteristic desynchronized pattern. These neurons show decreased discharge during non-rapid eye movement (NREM) sleep.[2,3]

In addition to the LDT/PPT, there are other projections from the reticular formation to the thalamus including norepinephrine projections from the locus coeruleus and serotonergic projections from the dorsal raphe.[4]

The locus coeruleus is a norepinephrine system located in the dorsolateral pons and is the major source of norepinephrine in the brain. Norepinephrine-producing neurons from the locus coeruleus project to the spinal cord, brain stem, midbrain, cerebellum, hippocampus, thalamus, and cerebral cortex. It receives projections from a wide spectrum of neurons with various neurotransmitters including opiate, glutamate, gamma-aminobutyric acid (GABA), serotonin, and epinephrine.[5] It is significantly involved in generating and maintaining the state of wakefulness. The suprachiasmatic nucleus, which is responsible for circadian rhythms that regulate cyclic sleep and wakefulness, activates the locus coeruleus through the dorsomedial hypothalamus. Activity of the locus coeruleus is greatest during wakefulness, decreases during NREM sleep, and is completely absent during REM sleep.

Corticotropin-releasing factor, produced by cells in the periventricular nucleus of the hypothalamus, initiates the production of adrenocorticotropin from the anterior pituitary during stress and also stimulates the locus coeruleus. Therefore, the locus coeruleus plays a role in regulation of the sleep–wake cycle and in stress-related behavior.

Neurons from the raphe nuclei project from the brain stem to almost every area of the brain. One of these nuclei, the dorsal raphe nucleus, contains the largest pool of serotonergic neurons in the brain. It projects inhibitory neurons containing serotonin to the dentate gyrus and the hippocampus. Microinjection studies have shown that the dorsal raphe has a major inhibitory projection to the dorsolateral pons that promotes sleep.[6]

The monoamine pathway containing histamine also shows increased discharge during wakefulness. Cells for this pathway are located in the tuberomammillary nucleus of the caudolateral hypothalamus. Another ascending cholinergic pathway originating in the basal forebrain sends widespread projections to the thalamus. These pathways relay excitatory projections to the cortex from the brain stem through the thalamus and basal forebrain and hypothalamus and send direct excitatory projections to the cortex from the locus coeruleus and dorsal raphe nucleus.

GABA modulates input to the raphe nuclei. Serotonergic neurons in the dorsal raphe nucleus decrease activity as a sleeper moves from wakefulness to slow-wave sleep (SWS) to REM sleep while GABA activity increases. It is unclear whether the GABAergic neurons decrease ascending serotonergic output by direct inhibition of serotonergic neurons in the raphe nuclei or by inhibition of GABA interneurons. Studies show that blocking the GABA receptors activates the glutamatergic pathway and promotes sleep.[7] Morphine increases the release of serotonin in the dorsal raphe nuclei by inhibiting GABAergic projections. The dorsal raphe and raphe magnus are also components of the descending pain modulation system.

In addition to these pathways, a neuropeptide called *hypocretin/orexin* plays an important role in sleep regulation and wakefulness.[8,9] Hypocretin/orexin-producing cells located in the dorsolateral hypothalamus send excitatory projections to the cholinergic pontine reticular formation, spinal cord, locus coeruleus, dorsal raphe nuclei, amygdala, and basal forebrain. These cells play a role in the regulation of sleep and wakefulness and also play an important role in attention, learning, memory, feeding-energy regulation, and pain modulation.[9] These neurons stimulate noradrenergic, serotonergic, and histaminergic pathways that promote wakefulness. Hypocretin/orexin also appears to be important in controlling the gate from one state to another in order to ensure a coordinated transition between states of sleep and wakefulness and is responsible for rapid switching during these transitions.[10,11] Studies of narcolepsy and cataplexy have shown that, in these disorders, there can be an 85% to 95% decrease in hypocretin/orexin neurons.[8]

SLEEPINESS

Several factors lead to a state of sleepiness. The first and perhaps greatest driving force for sleepiness and the desire to sleep is the amount of time that has passed since the last sleep episode. The homeostatic drive for sleep increases as the time since the last sleep bout increases. It appears that accumulation of extracellular adenosine may be a factor in this drive. Adenosine can inhibit cholinergic and non-cholinergic neurons in the basal forebrain of the AAS.

Another important factor in the development of sleepiness and the increased drive for sleep is the circadian system. This system follows a 24-hour periodicity and is influenced by light rather than the length of time since the last sleep or the length of wakefulness. It is modulated through the suprachiasmatic nucleus with inhibitory projections to components of the AAS.

THE ONSET OF SLEEP

A group of cells that contain GABA and galanin are located in the vertrolateral preoptic (VLPO) area of the basal forebrain and have been shown to be active during sleep. These cells show first signs of activity during drowsy wakefulness and continue to be active throughout NREM sleep[12] (Figure 6-3). Neurons from the VLPO are inhibited by neurotransmitters of the AAS and send inhibitory projections throughout all components of the system. Thus,

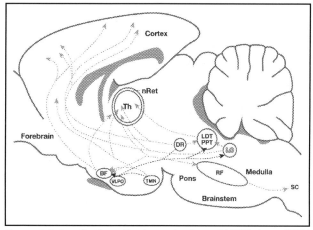

Figure 6-3. Localization of brain mechanisms of NREM sleep. NREM sleep is marked by a reduced discharge rate in the AAS (light arrows) as the inhibitory influence (dark arrows) from cells in the ventrolateral preoptic region increases. Th = thalamus; DR = dorsal raphe; BF = basal forebrain; VLPO = ventrolateral preoptic area; LDT/PPT = laterodorsal tegmentum/pedunculopontine region; nRet = nucleus reticularis; RF = reticular formation; SC = spinal cord.

neurons from the VLPO and AAS are self-reinforcing in that they disinhibit their own influence on the system. In this way, these pathways help stabilize wakefulness or NREM sleep and ensure the rapid transition between sleep and wakefulness states once the system is altered by temporal or circadian influences. This system is also influenced by orexin to help coordinate these changes in the AAS.

The thalamus plays a major role in orchestrating changes in cortical neuron discharge patterns from wakefulness to NREM sleep because of its ability to alter the discharge rate according to varying levels of AAS neurotransmitters allowing for rapid and smooth transitions between states of wakefulness and NREM sleep.

LOCALIZATION OF BRAIN MECHANISMS SUBSERVING NON-RAPID EYE MOVEMENT SLEEP

Much of what is understood about the function of the reticular formation and the entire AAS has come from lesion studies, electrical and chemical stimulation studies, and transection studies. The following is a summary of a number of these studies.

Lesion studies of the anterior hypothalamus and the adjacent forebrain or basal forebrain have been shown to produce long-lasting insomnia.[13] There is consistent damage to this area in individuals with Alzheimer's disease. This is thought to contribute to the characteristic insomnia that accompanies the disorder.

Electrical and chemical stimulation studies have shown that there is a unique electrical discharge pattern in the basal forebrain. Studies have shown that stimulation of this area of the brain produces NREM sleep. These cells discharge maximally during NREM sleep but show relatively little activation during REM sleep and wakefulness. Stimulation, recording, and lesion studies all implicate the basal forebrain in the control of NREM sleep.[14–17]

The nucleus of the solitary tract (NTS) is a solitary area of myelinated axons within the gray matter located along the length of the medulla oblongata in the dorsal respiratory group[18] (Figure 6-4).

The NTS is divided into the rostral gustatory nucleus and the caudal neurons. It carries visceral sensation and taste from cranial primary afferents and is related to cardiovascular, respiratory, and gastrointestinal functions. Injection studies have shown that the NTS is involved in the generation of sleep.[19] The NTS can also be powerfully stimulated by distention of the carotid sinus and produces behavioral sleep. Low-frequency stimulation of the vago-aortic nerve or stimulation to the NTS also produces SWS on EEG. Inactivation of the lower brain stem regions, including the NTS, produces a profound arousal. There is some evidence that certain NTS neurons increase discharge during NREM sleep. These neurons are reciprocally interconnected with cells in the midbrain EEG arousal region. These data suggest that the NTS region may constitute a second center for the regulation of NREM sleep.[20] It is likely that several widely separated brain regions are sufficient to generate NREM sleep and that these regions interact in order to trigger the onset and maintenance of NREM sleep. Rapid oscillations between nuclei that generate sleep and those that cause arousal are responsible for alternating states of wakefulness and NREM sleep. This rapid cycling has been linked to the occurrence of night terrors and sleepwalking.[21] Another study shows that endogenous opioids may be involved in controlling activity generated by the NTS, which enhance EEG synchronization usually associated with behavioral SWS.[22]

As sleep progresses to stage 2, GABAergic neurons gradually depolarize as the influence of the AAS decreases. Sleep spindles, caused by network interactions between GABAergic thalamic nucleus reticularis neurons and thalamocortical neurons, begin to appear.[23] As sleep transitions into deeper levels, the influence of the AAS is completely inhibited and sleep is maintained. EEG tracings show increasing density of high-voltage, SWS, also called *delta wave activity*. Thalamocortical neurons are maintained in a hyperpolarized state by the absence of depolarizing influence. There are bursts of SWS that are synchronized and inhibit internal and external sensory inputs through the thalamus to the cortex, thereby maintaining SWS.

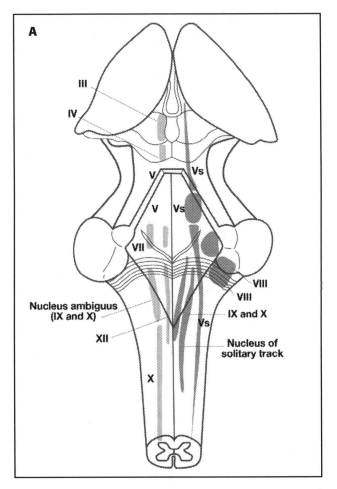

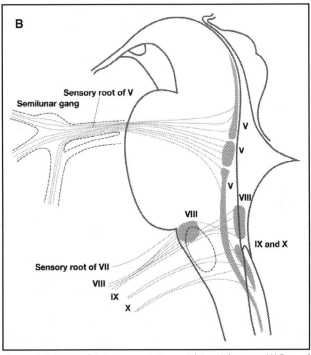

Figure 6-4. NTS and its interconnections with cranial nerves. (A) Frontal view and (B) sagittal view.

LOCALIZATION OF BRAIN MECHANISMS OF RAPID EYE MOVEMENT SLEEP

REM sleep is controlled by a different area of the brain than NREM sleep. Neuropsychological, radiological, and pharmacological findings and lesion and transection studies suggest that REM sleep is controlled by brain stem mechanisms that are cholinergic[24] (Figure 6-5). REM sleep should not be mistakenly identified as *dream sleep* because REM sleep is controlled by completely different brain mechanisms than dreaming. REM sleep is a function of brain stem activity. Dreaming may occur in any stage of sleep, and studies indicate that it is controlled by forebrain mechanisms. The neurobiology of dreaming will be discussed in Chapter 9.

Early ablation, stimulation, and recording studies by Jouvet[25] concluded that REM sleep is controlled by brain stem mechanisms in the pons (Figure 6-6). This conclusion has been proven in subsequent studies. In fact, REM sleep generator mechanisms have been shown to be able to survive disconnection from over 95% of the rest of the central nervous system.[26] On the other hand, destruction of only a very small region of the brain stem can permanently prevent REM sleep even if the rest of the brain remains intact and functional. This further supports the notion of a pontine REM generator mechanism.

Areas in the brain stem, particularly in the pontine tegmentum as well as adjacent areas of the midbrain and areas in the hypothalamus, contain neurons known as REM-on cells that are active during REM sleep and REM-off cells that are minimally active during REM sleep. The REM-on cells are likely involved in the initiation of REM sleep. These cells utilize neurotransmitters GABA, acetylcholine, glutamate, or glycine. REM-on cell activity is also responsible for the muscular atonia that is characteristic of REM sleep.[30-32] During REM sleep, certain monoamines including norepinephrine, serotonin, and histamine are completely inhibited. These are the neurotransmitters used by the REM-off cells. Loss of this function can lead to loss of muscle atonia and result in REM behavior phenomenon, in which certain automatic actions can be carried out, as if the individual were acting out a dream.

In a review article, Solms reported on a number of transection, lesion and microinjection studies that have helped to localize REM sleep generators. The conclusion of these studies is that the pons is both necessary and sufficient to generate the basic phenomena of REM sleep.[24] Transection studies localized REM sleep generation to the pons. In order to further localize the pontine neurons responsible for generating REM sleep, lesion studies were undertaken.[24] These studies showed that a lesion occupying the lateral portion of the pontine tegmentum, an area that includes the nucleus

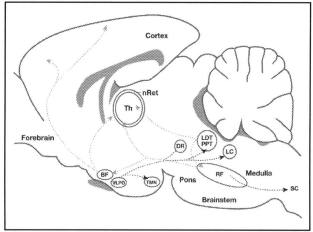

Figure 6-5. Localization of brain mechanisms of REM sleep. REM sleep is characterized by inhibition (dark arrows) of the monoaminergic (locus coeruleus and dorsal raphe) activating systems from the ventrolateral preoptic area. REM-on cells of the LDT/PPT project caudally to the reticular formation and are disinhibited. Forebrain activation is supported by cholinergic systems (LDT/PPT and basal forebrain) during REM sleep. Th = thalamus; DR = dorsal raphe; BF = basal forebrain; VLPO = ventrolateral preoptic area; LDT/PPT = laterodorsal tegmentum/pedunculo-pontine region; RF = reticular formation.

reticularis pontis oralis and the site ventral to the locus coeruleus, appears to be critical in the control of REM sleep. This small area recruits the massive change in brain neuronal activity that characterizes REM sleep. Lesions in this area block both the atonia of REM sleep and the expression of motor activity during REM sleep. Lesions limited to noradrenergic neurons of the locus coeruleus, which is adjacent to the reticularis pontis oralis, do not block REM sleep. Studies that induce chemical depletion of norepinephrine also fail to block REM sleep.[24]

The lateral pontine and medial medullary reticular area contains cells that discharge at a high rate throughout REM sleep. These cells have little or no activity during NREM sleep. During waking, these cells are generally silent, even during vigorous movement. It should be noted that some of these cells are active during head lowering and related postural changes, which involve reduction of tone in extensor musculature.

The pontine REM sleep-activating cells, also known as REM-on cells, are distributed throughout the lateral pontine region. The medullary REM-activating cell population is thought to mediate suppression of muscle tone that characterizes REM sleep via excitatory projections to the lower brain stem (Figure 6-7). REM muscle atonia is also mediated by inhibitory projections to spinal motor neurons. The subsequent suppression of muscle tone is produced by postsynaptic inhibition of the motor neurons.

Some neurons within the pons fire bursts of action potentials during REM sleep. These neurons excite other neurons in the thalamus, which excite neurons in the cortex. The phasic excitation that results is called *ponto-geniculo-occipital* (PGO) waves.

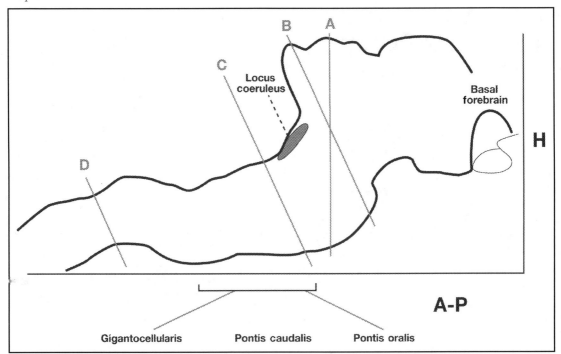

Figure 6-6. Figure of transection studies of the pons and midbrain.

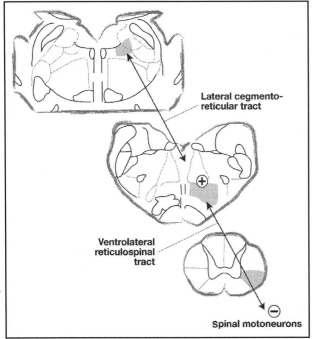

Figure 6-7. Schematic of the theoretical mechanism subserving muscle atonia characteristic of REM sleep. Neurons of the nucleus reticularis pontis oralis of the midbrain (shaded area, top section) exert an excitatory influence via lateral tegmentoreticular tract on neurons in the medulla (shaded area, middle section), which in turn exert a generalized inhibition on spinal motor neurons via ventrolateral reticulospinal tract.

Noradrenergic cells of the locus coeruleus and serotonergic cells of the raphe have similar discharge patterns during the sleep–wake cycle (Figure 6-8).

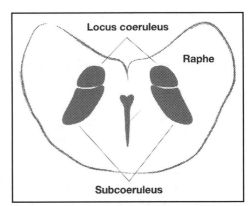

Figure 6-8. A cross section of the brain stem at the pons level shows the raphe, or serotonergic neurons, right in the midline of the brain stem. The locus coeruleus cells are more lateral.

During wakefulness, the discharge of these sets of cells is very regular and tonic in contrast to the burst–pause discharge pattern seen in most reticular neurons. During the initial stages of NREM sleep, discharge in both serotonergic and noradrenergic cells slows dramatically. During REM sleep, these cells have their lowest discharge rates, and many are completely silent.

REM sleep can be elicited by microinjection of acetylcholine into the pons. Most of the mechanisms that drive the very complex behavioral state of REM sleep are localized to a very small area of the brain stem. In an intact animal, many brain regions distant from the pons actively participate in the control of the REM sleep state.

Transection studies have determined that the pons is sufficient to generate much of the phenomenology of REM sleep. Lesion studies have identified a small region in the lateral pontine tegmentum corresponding to lateral areas of the nucleus reticularis pontis oralis and the region immediately ventral to the locus coeruleus, which is required to form normal REM sleep, primarily the motor inhibitory component. Unit recording studies have revealed a population of cells within this region that are selectively active during REM sleep.

Experimental manipulations and pathological states allow further localization of the mechanism that generates REM sleep. Lesion studies have demonstrated that atonia and EEG desynchrony can be individually dissociated from the REM sleep state. REM sleep can exist without muscle atonia and with a synchronized EEG. Cholinergic stimulation of different regions within the pons can induce either of these abnormal presentations of REM sleep.

Two medullary and one pontine region are able to produce the complete suppression of muscle tone seen in REM sleep.[31] This was shown clinically and experimentally. Pontine and medullary lesions can produce REM sleep without atonia, a condition known clinically as *REM behavior disorder.* Conversely, atonia can occur without REM sleep and can be evoked by injection of the cholinergic agonist carachol or the cholinesterase inhibitor physotigmine into the dorsal pons. This results in a loss of muscle tone during wakefulness, a condition that is clinically known as *cataplexy.* It can be triggered by strong emotion or physical activity, among other variables. Physiologically, it is similar to the atonia in REM sleep state. A stimulus, which would produce arousal in an intact individual, produces cataplexy in narcoleptics. Hypersensitivity of cholinergic cells in the pons and/or medial medulla produces the atonia seen during attacks of cataplexy.

SUMMARY

Cortical activation originates in the basal forebrain. This area is important for homeostatic control of sleep and wakefulness. Inhibition of these neurons leads to increased SWS or delta sleep. Increased bursts of activity in the cholinergic basal forebrain activate the cortex, which begins to produce gamma and theta waves characteristic of wakefulness. During wakefulness, the AAS maintains a depolarized state of the thalamocortical and cortical cells; this prevents the appearance of delta sleep. These neuronal pathways also include cholinergic neurons in the basal forebrain and LDT/PPT, norepinephrine, serotonin, and glutamate containing neurons in the brain stem. Single spike discharge from the thalamocortical relay cells allows transmission of sensory information to the cortex and the individual is thus able to interact with the environment. This transmission of sensory input is increasingly inhibited as one progresses through the stages of NREM sleep. Postsynaptic inhibition of spinal motor neurons disallows response to sensory input during REM sleep.

REFERENCES

1. Jones BE. From waking to sleeping: neuronal and chemical substrates. *Trends Pharmacol Sci.* 2005;26:578–586.
2. McCormick DA, Bal T. Sleep and arousal: thalamocortical mechanisms. *Annu Rev Neurosci.* 1997;20:185–215.
3. Steriade M, McCormick DA, Sejnowski TJ. Thalamocortical oscillations in the sleeping and aroused brain. *Science.* 1993;262:679–685.
4. Aston-Jones G, Gonzalez M, Doran S. Role of the locus coeruleus-norepinephrine system in arousal and circadian regulation of the sleep–wake cycle. In: Ordway GA, Schwartz MA, Frazer A, eds. *Brain Norepinephrine: Neurobiology and Therapeutics.* New York, NY: Cambridge University Press; 2007;275-297.
5. Aston-Jones G, Shiekhattar R, Akaoka H, et al. Afferent regulation of locus coeruleus neurons: anatomy, physiology and pharmacology. *Prog Brain Res.* 1991;88:47–75.
6. Nitz DA, McNaughton BL. Hippocampal EEG and unit activity responses to modulation of serotonergic median raphe neurons in the freely behaving rat. *Learn Mem.* 1999;6(2):153–167.
7. Li S, Varga V, Sik A, Kocsis B. GABAergic control of the ascending input from the median raphe nuclei to the limbic system. *J Neurophysiol.* 2005;94:2561–2574.
8. Kiyashchenko LI, Mileykovskiy BY, Maidment N, et al. Release of hypocretin (orexin) during waking and sleep states. *J Neurosci.* 2002;22:5282–5286.
9. Ebrahim IO, Howard RS, Kopelman MD, Sharief MK, Williams AJ. The hypocretin/orexin system. *J R Soc Med.* 2002;95:227–230.
10. Lu J, Sherman D, Devor M, Saper CB. A putative flip-flop switch for control of REM sleep. *Nature.* 2006;441:589–594.
11. Saper CB, Chou TC, Scammell TE. The sleep switch: hypothalamic control of sleep and wakefulness. *Trends Neurosci.* 2001;24:726–731.
12. Szymusiak R. Magnocellular nuclei of the basal forebrain: substrates of sleep and arousal regulation. *Sleep.* 1995;18:478–500.
13. Basics of sleep behavior. *Brain mechanisms of sleep and wakefulness.* Available at: http://www.sleepsources.org/uploads/sleepsyllabus/fr-e.html. Accessed April 9, 2012.
14. Steininger TL, Alam MN, Gong H, Szymusiak R, McGinty D. Sleep–waking discharge of neurons in the posterior lateral hypothalamus of the albino rat. *Brain Res.* 1999;840:138–147.
15. Kumar VM, Datta S, Chihina GS, Gandhi N, Singh B. Sleep-awake responses elicited from medial preoptic area on application of norepinephrine and phenoxybenzamine in free moving rats. *Brain Res.* 1994;322(2):322–325.
16. Kodama T, Takahashi Y, Honda Y. Enhancement of acetylcholine release during paradoxical sleep in the dorsal tegmental field of the cat brain stem. *Neurosci Lett.* 1990;114:277–282.
17. Hammond EJ, Uthman BM, Reid SA, Wilder BJ. Electrophysiological studies of cervical vagus nerve stimulation in humans: I. EEG effects. *Epilepsia.* 1992;33:1013–1020.
18. King MS. Anatomy of the rostral nucleus of the solitary tract. In: King MS, ed. *The Role of the Nucleus of the Solitary Tract in Gustatory Processing.* Boca Raton, FL: CRC Press; 2007;17-38.
19. Chou TC, Bjorkum AA, Gaus S, Lu J, Scammell TE, Saper CB. Afferents to the ventrolateral preoptic nucleus. *J Neurosci.* 2002;22:977–990.
20. Gottesmann C. The neurophysiology of sleep and waking: intracerebral connections, functioning and ascending influences of the medulla oblongata. *Prog Neurobiol.* 1999;59:1–54.
21. Brown RE, Basheer R, McKenna JT, Strecker RE, McCarley RW. Control of sleep and wakefulness. *Physiol Rev.* 2012;92:1087–1187.
22. Reinoso BF, de Andres I. Effects of opioid microinjections in the nucleus of the solitary tract on the sleep-wakefulness cycle states in cats. *Anesthesiology.* 1995;82:144–152.
23. Steriade M, McCarley RW. *Brain Control of Wakefulness and Sleep.* New York, NY: Kluwer Academic/Plenum; 2005.

24. Solms M. Dreaming and REM sleep are controlled by different brain mechanisms. *Behav Brain Sci.* 2000;23(6):843-850.

25. Jouvet M. Paradoxical sleep—a study of its nature and mechanisms. *Prog Brain Res.* 1965;18:20–62.

26. Shiromani PJ, Fishbein W. Continuous pontine cholinergic microinfusion via mini-pump induces sustained alteration in rapid eye movement (REM) sleep. *Pharmacol Biochem Behav.* 1986;25(6):1253-1261.

27. Hobson JA. Sleep and dreaming: induction and mediation of REM sleep by cholinergic mechanism. *Current Opinion Neurobiol.* 1992;2(6):759-763.

28. Datta S Mavanji V, Ullor J Patterson EH. Activation of phasic pontine-wave generator prevents rapid-eye-movement sleep deprivation-induced learning impairment in the rat: A mechanism for sleep-dependent plasticity. *J Neurosci.* 2004;24(6):1416-1427.

29. Hobson JA. REM sleep and dreaming: towards a theory of proto-consciousness. *Nat Rev.* 2009;10:803–813.

30. Aston-Jones G, Gonzalez M, Doran S. Role of the locus coeruleus-norepinephrine system in arousal and circadian regulation of the sleep–wake cycle. In: Ordway GA, Schwartz MA, Frazer A, eds. *Brain Norepinephrine: Neurobiology and Therapeutics.* New York, NY: Cambridge University Press; 2007:157–195.

31. Siegel JM. REM sleep. In: Kryger MH, Roth T, Dement WC, eds. *Principles and Practice of Sleep Medicine.* 4th ed. St Louis, MO: Elsevier; 2005:120–135.

32. Schenck CH, Mahowald MW. REM sleep behavior disorder: clinical, developmental and neuroscience. Perspectives 16 years after its formal identification in SLEEP. *Sleep.* 2002;25(2):120-138.

7

Chemical and Neuronal Mechanisms of Sleep

Julie M. Hereford, PT, DPT

Chemical and neuronal mechanisms that control and regulate sleep occur via a variety of neurotransmitters. Neurotransmitters are endogenous chemicals that transmit a signal from a neuron across a synapse to a target cell in order to communicate between the nerve cells (Figure 7-1). Neurotransmitters are packed into synaptic vesicles that are clustered beneath the membrane in the nerve terminal on the presynaptic side of the synapse. They are released into the synaptic cleft and diffuse across where they bind with receptor sites on the postsynaptic side of the cleft. The release of the neurotransmitter is stimulated by an action potential or a gradated electrical potential. Low-level release can occur without electrical stimulation. Once the neurotransmitter crosses the gap and excites or inhibits the connecting neuron it diffuses away, it is actively denatured by enzymes or reabsorbed by protein complexes called *transporters* on the surface of the originating neuron. Neurotransmitters are synthesized from precursors such as amino acids, which are plentiful in a normal healthy diet. Biosynthesis generally requires only a few steps to convert an amino acid into a neurotransmitter.

There are many different neurotransmitters, but the discussion here will be limited to those that are directly or indirectly involved in the sleep–wake cycle. Some of these neurotransmitters have multiple functions, which will be noted for the reader to consider possible related functions within the system.

REVIEW OF NEUROTRANSMITTERS OF SLEEP

Norepinephrine

Also known as *noradrenaline*, norephinephrine is a catecholamine that functions as a hormone and a neurotransmitter. Areas that produce or are affected by norepinephrine are known as *noradrenergic*. The terms *norepinephrine* and *noradrenaline* are used interchangeably, one derived from Greek and the other from Latin. For the purpose of clarity, the term *norepinephrine* will be used.

Norepinephrine is a crucial factor in sleep neurochemistry. It is found in the ascending activating system and is involved in regulation of sleep and wakefulness. Certain medications such as amphetamine and modafinil increase extracellular norepinephrine and therefore enhance the wakefulness promotion pathways. The neurotransmitter gamma-aminobutyric acid (GABA) inhibits norepinephrine. Norepinephrine influences the synthesis of melatonin. It shares reciprocal signaling with histamine. A number of currently available antidepressants affect the signaling of norepinephrine and can be used for their effects on sleep promotion. Adrenergic antagonists, which block norepinephrine, are also known to have considerable sedative side effects.

Hereford JM. *Sleep and Rehabilitation: A Guide for Health Professionals* (pp 61-68). © 2014 Taylor & Francis Group.

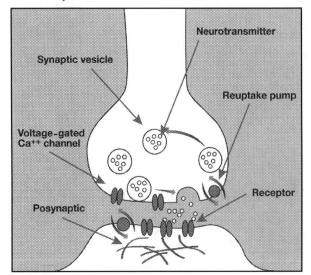

Figure 7-1. Structure of a typical neuronal synapse.

In addition to its actions as a neurotransmitter in the brain, norepinephrine is used in the sympathetic nervous system and affects cardiac function. Because norepinephrine release increases in sympathetic neurons, the heart rate increases. Norepinephrine is part of the fight-or-flight response in that it triggers the release of glucose, increases blood flow to skeletal musculature, and increases the brain's oxygen supply. It increases vascular tone and therefore increases blood pressure.

Norepinephrine is synthesized from dopamine and is released from the adrenal medulla into the blood as a hormone. It is also released from noradrenergic neurons in the locus coeruleus.

Noradrenergic neurons in the brain have widespread areas of influence. They affect alertness, arousal, and have an influence on the reward/pleasure system. These neurons originate from the locus coeruleus and act on adrenergic receptors in the amygdala, cingulate gyrus, cingulum, hippocampus, hypothalamus, neocortex, spinal cord, striatum, and thalamus. Projections from the lateral tegmental field act on adrenergic sites in the hypothalamus.

Dopamine

Dopamine is a catecholamine that functions as a neurotransmitter in the brain. In humans, there are 5 different types of dopamine receptors (D_1, D_2, D_3, D_4, and D_5). Dopamine is produced in the substantia nigra of the basal ganglia and in the ventral tegmental area. It plays an important role in reward-driven learning; certain addictive stimulant drugs such as cocaine and methamphetamine act on the dopaminergic system. There is even evidence that people with extraverted personality traits tend to have a higher level of dopamine than introverts.[1]

Several diseases are associated with irregularities of the dopaminergic system. Parkinson's disease is caused by a loss of dopamine-secreting neurons in the substantia nigra. There also appears to be an association with dopamine deficiency and the symptom of periodic limb movement disorder, which occurs during sleep.

Elevated levels of dopamine activity in the mesolimbic pathway and decreased levels in the prefrontal cortex are associated with schizophrenia. One theory of attention-deficit hyperactivity disorder (ADHD) is that it involves a decreased level of dopamine activity.

The level of activity in dopamine-dependent neurons varies only slightly over a 24-hour period, leading to questions regarding whether it has a role in sleep regulation. However, clinical findings in individuals with Parkinson's disease and abusers of methamphetamine reveal consistent sleep-related symptoms. Methamphetamine is known to be a potent stimulant that blocks the transporter complexes for dopamine, serotonin, and norepinephrine. Modafinil binds to the dopamine transporter, but the actual mechanism by which the resulting compound promotes wakefulness remains unclear.[2]

Caffeine is the most widely used stimulant in the world, and it acts by blocking adenosine. Adenosine accumulates in the brain during waking time. It has been postulated that when adenosine accumulation has reached a critical level, adenosine receptors are triggered and brain activity begins to slow as sleep approaches.[3] Caffeine works by blocking adenosine receptors, thereby preventing the neurotransmission of the "sleep signal." Dopamine signaling works to keep the brain awake until adenosine levels rise to a threshold that overwhelms the effects of dopamine. Caffeine blocks adenosine to maintain wakefulness. Adenosine receptors and dopamine receptors can be found in some of the same areas of the brain. It appears that dopamine fights the tendency of adenosine to promote sleep.

Dopamine remains active during rapid eye movement (REM) sleep when neurons containing norepinephrine and serotonin become silent. These dopamine neurons produce the psychotic-like mental activity of dreaming.[4] If there is a reduction in the dopaminergic neuron activity in the substantia nigra during REM sleep, there can be a loss of the skeletal muscle atonia that usually characterizes REM sleep in a disorder called *REM behavior disorder*. Patients with this condition may perform simple automatic actions or complex activities in which they appear to act out their dreams, with sometimes catastrophic results.[5] The dopamine neuron loss increases the activity of the globus pallidum, which inhibits midbrain structures. These structures inhibit spinal motor neurons, and their inhibition prevents the development of skeletal muscle atonia during REM sleep.[6]

Acetylcholine

Acetylcholine is a neurotransmitter that operates in the peripheral nervous system by activating muscles and in the central nervous system, where it acts as a neuromodulator in that the cholinergic system tends to inhibit excitatory actions. It is also a major neurotransmitter in the autonomic nervous system.

In the peripheral nervous system, acetylcholine binds to receptors on skeletal muscle fibers and opens sodium channels, initiating the sequence of steps that result in muscle contraction. In cardiac musculature, it acts via a muscarinic receptor to inhibit contraction.

In the autonomic nervous system, acetylcholine is released in all preganglionic and postganglionic neurons in the parasympathetic system and all preganglionic neurons in the sympathetic system.

In the central nervous system, acetylcholine exerts a variety of neuromodulator effects. It has an important role in the enhancement of sensory perceptions upon awakening and acts to help sustain attention.[7,8] Cholinergic neurons—that is, those neurons that utilize acetylcholine as a neurotransmitter—play a critical role in arousal and cognitive function, neural plasticity, and reward. Its release is greater during REM sleep than during wakefulness or non-rapid eye movement (NREM) sleep.[9]

Damage to the cholinergic system is associated with memory deficits that are characteristic of Alzheimer's disease. Because acetylcholine promotes REM sleep, it is plausible that the loss of REM sleep that characterizes Alzheimer's disease may have a cause–effect relationship. Anticholinergic drugs are also known to interfere with memory and learning processes.

Histamine

Histamine is an organic nitrogen compound produced by basophils and mast cells as part of the inflammatory response. Histamine acts to increase capillary permeability and is released as a neurotransmitter from cells in the posterior hypothalamus and in various tuberomammillary nuclei. These histaminergic neurons project to the cortex through the medial forebrain bundle and are known to modulate sleep. H1 histamine receptor antagonists, or antihistamines, produce sleep. Destruction of histamine-releasing neurons or inhibition of histamine synthesis causes an inability to remain awake. H3 receptor antagonists increase wakefulness. Histaminergic neurons have the most wakefulness-related firing patterns. They are active during wakefulness, decrease activity level during relaxation, and are completely silent during REM and NREM sleep. Histaminergic neurons have been shown to become active before there are physical signs of awakening. Histamine has an inhibitory effect that protects against susceptibility to convulsion, drug sensitization, denervation supersensitivity, ischemic lesions, and stress. It has been suggested that histamine controls the mechanisms by which memories and learning are forgotten.[10,11]

Histaminergic neurons play an important role in memory and learning by direct influence on memory or by modulating release of acetylcholine.[12] These neurons are located in the tuberomammillary nucleus of the hypothalamus and send projections indirectly via the raphe nuclei and directly to the cortex to promote wakefulness and process emotional memory. Descending histaminergic neurons activate cholinergic neurons in the mesopontine tegmentum, which activates the neocortex via the thalamus and hypothalamus. Histaminergic neurons regulate acetylcholine release in the amygdala, which is associated with processing emotional memory. Experimental microinjection models of histamine into the bilateral amygdala resulted in learning impairments.[13] Microinjections of histamine into the neocortex decrease cholinergic tone through H3 receptors, and systemic administration of H3 receptor agonist also impairs performance of learning.[14]

One study showed that nitric oxide synapses exist on the cholinergic neurons of the laterodorsal and pedunculopontine tegmental nuclei, which send projections to the medial pontine reticular formation.[15] Stimulation of the medial pontine reticular formation evokes a REM sleep-like state and causes hypotonia of the upper airway musculature. Microinjections of Ng-nitro-l-arginine inhibits nitric oxide synapses in the medial pontine reticular formation and significantly decreases the duration of REM sleep. Research findings suggest that nitric oxide increases the release of acetylcholine in the medial pontine reticular formation and promotes REM sleep.[16]

Glutamate and Aspartate

Glutamate and aspartate are excitatory amino acids that function in the sleep–wake cycle. Studies have shown that aspartate levels are highest during slow-wave sleep (SWS) and decrease during REM sleep. They decrease even further during awakening. Concentration of glutamate increases during SWS and in individuals receiving narcotics. Glutamate also decreases production during REM sleep and while awake.[17,18]

Glutamate and aspartate concentrations depend on brain metabolism and can be affected by changes in microcirculation which can occur during states of hypoxemia, ischemia, hypoglycemia, and oxidative stress.[19] A decrease in concentration impacts glutamate, especially N-methyl-D-aspartate (NMDA) receptor activity, which acts as a molecular device for controlling synaptic plasticity and memory consolidation.[20] Glutamate NMDA receptors in the rostral pons also regulate inspiration. NMDA receptor antagonists decrease REM duration but do not affect SWS or the duration of wakefulness.[21]

Changes in microcirculation are known to occur during certain stages of normal sleep, and these changes may be more pronounced in disordered sleep.[22] During REM sleep,

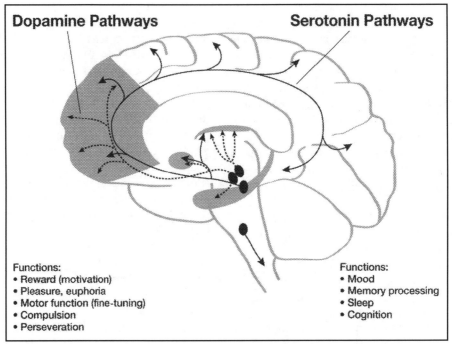

Figure 7-2. This figure shows the general location and function of the dopamine and serotonin pathways within the brain.

production of nitric oxide, which is a vasodilatory agent, increases, but it decreases during SWS. This correlates with the cholinergic neuron activity and PGO wave frequency.[23] Deprivation of nitric oxide biosynthesis elicits decreased sleep duration and increased slow-wave sleep.[24] Nitric oxide inhibitors in the pontine reticular formation cause a significant decrease in the release of acetylcholine.[25] These data indicate that cerebral blood flow and metabolism fluctuate during different stages of sleep and may cause changes in concentration of important excitatory neurotransmitters such as glutamate and aspartate. These fluctuations, in turn, may alter the duration and depth of sleep stages.

NEUROPEPTIDES

Corticotropin-Releasing Hormone

Corticotropin-releasing hormone (CRH), also known as *corticotropin-releasing factor*, is a neuropeptide that has a variety of physiological effects, including the expression of stress and anxiety reaction, vasoregulation, thermoregulation, growth and metabolism, metamorphosis, and reproduction. CRH is released as a prohormone, a committed intraglandular precursor of a hormone that has little hormonal effect by itself. Instead, it acts to enhance the strength of a hormone that already exists. CRH is found mainly in the paraventricular nucleus of the hypothalamus that regulates the release of adrenocorticotrophic hormone from the pituitary, thereby activating the

hypothalamic–pituitary–adrenal axis and thus causing the release of glucocorticoids, cortisol, mineralcorticoids, and dehydroepiandrosterone (DHEA). Marked reduction of CRH is seen in patients with Alzheimer's disease.[26] Studies have shown that sleep recovery following a period of forced wakefulness activates the hypothalamic–pituitary–adrenal axis and increases the release of CRH, which then impairs sleep.[27–30] Another study showed that experimental manipulation of the CRH system activates the hypothalamic–pituitary–adrenal axis and disrupts homeostasis of sleep and decreases normal sleep rebound that usually follows sleep deprivation.[31] In particular, there was a decrease in the length of REM sleep and a decrease in NREM and REM sleep, and an increase in episodes of wakefulness.

Serotonin

Serotonin, or 5-hydroxytryptamine, is a monoamine neurotransmitter that is derived from tryptophan (Figure 7-2). Most serotonin is found in the gastrointestinal system, where it regulates intestinal motility. The remaining 5-hydroxytryptamine is synthesized in serotonergic neurons in the central nervous system and regulates mood, appetite, and sleep. It also is involved in memory processing and learning.

At the onset of sleep, serotonin is secreted and promotes NREM sleep. On the other hand, secretion of norepinephrine occurs at the onset of REM sleep and promotes its continuationF. According to research, depression can be alleviated by awakening the patient at the onset of REM sleep, thus regulating the imbalance of norepinephrine and serotonin, but REM deprivation may increase aggression, which lasts after REM deprivation returns to normal.[32,33]

Serotonin is one of the most important neurotransmitters for regulating the sleep–wake cycle. When serotonin levels are low, sleep disturbance, depression, and chronic fatigue can occur. High levels of serotonin are associated with wakefulness and lower levels are associated with increased sleep. Though serotonin levels decrease during sleep compared to wakefulness, levels are lowest during REM sleep. When serotonin levels drop, acetylcholine rises and, conversely, rising serotonin levels inhibit the rise of acetylcholine.

Low serotonin levels result in sleep disruption and sleep disorders such as insomnia. Psychological and emotional stressors are common causes of decreased serotonin levels and cause disrupted sleep, depression, anxiety, and fatigue during the day.

Gamma-Aminobutyric Acid

GABA is the primary inhibitory neurotransmitter of the central nervous system. Activation of GABA produces sleep. It plays a role in regulating the state of excitability throughout the nervous system. It also regulates muscle tone. This can be seen in spastic paralysis, in which GABA absorption is impaired by nerve damage in an upper motor neuron lesion. GABA acts at inhibitory synapses by binding to receptors of both presynaptic and postsynaptic neuronal processes. This opens ion channels in which negatively charged chloride ions flow into the cell or positively charged potassium ions flow out of the cell. This decreases the membrane potential and causes hyperpolarization.

GABA stabilizes the brain by preventing excitability and stimulating relaxation and sleep. Human growth hormone from the anterior pituitary levels is significantly increased by GABA administration. This helps to preserve sleep cycles, thermoregulation, and pituitary function. Human growth hormone levels decrease with age and are thought to cause changes in sleep architecture and sleep disruptions that occur with increasing age. Diet, prolonged stress, and genetics have much to do with GABA deficiencies. GABA promotes tranquil rest and also has some influence over motor control, vision, and anxiety. Individuals who suffer from panic attacks, anxiety, depression, alcoholism, and bipolar disorders appear to have lower GABA levels.[34]

Adenosine

Adenosine is a purine nucleoside that plays an important role in energy transfer as part of adenosine triphosphate and adenosine diphosphate. It also plays an important role in signal transduction as cyclic adenosine monophosphate. Adenosine acts as an inhibitory neurotransmitter and plays a role in sleep promotion and suppression of arousal. It appears that adenosine concentration rises in relationship

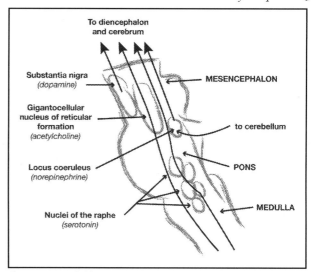

Figure 7-3. Multiple centers in the brain stem that release different neurotransmitters. These neurons send control signals upward into the diencephalon and cerebrum and downward into the spinal cord.

to increasing wakefulness time. Adenosine has an inhibitory effect in the central nervous system. Caffeine acts as a stimulant of the central nervous system by blocking adenosine binding at the receptor site, and thus adenosine, which normally slows the central nervous system, is inhibited, therefore allowing CNS arousal. A decrease in adenosine activity also causes increased activity of dopamine and glutamate.

ACTIVITY OF KEY NEUROTRANSMITTERS IN THE BRAIN DURING THE SLEEP–WAKE CYCLE

Norepinephrine is contained in neurons of the locus coeruleus, which project diffusely to the entire forebrain and cerebral cortex. These act to maintain and enhance cortical activation.

Dopamine is contained in neurons of the substantia nigra and ventral tegmental area. Dopaminergic neurons project to the striatum and frontal cortex and play an important role in behavioral arousal, movement, responsiveness, and cortical activation. Drugs such as amphetamine and cocaine enhance the release or synaptic concentration of dopamine and dramatically enhance and prolong wakefulness. Drugs that deplete dopamine produce a decrease in activity and cortical activation, which may have the effect of increasing sleep.

Acetylcholine has been localized to neurons within the reticular formation and basal forebrain. These neurons project to the forebrain and cerebral cortex and form an important component of the ascending activation system (Figure 7-3). Acetylcholine is released in highest concentrations from nerve terminals in the thalamus and cortex. This release is associated with cortical activation that occurs naturally during wakefulness and REM sleep. Nicotine, a cholinergic agonist, is a stimulant that produces prolonged and enhanced cortical activation. Nicotinergic antagonists and muscarinic cholinergic antagonists decrease cortical activation and cortical vigilance.

Histaminergic neurons are located within the caudal hypothalamus. These neurons project to the cerebral cortex. Drugs containing antihistamine produce drowsiness and decreased cortical activation, although this may not be solely because of the antihistamine.

Glutamate and aspartate are excitatory amino acids contained in many neurons that project to the cerebral cortex, forebrain, and brain stem. Glutamate and aspartate are released in the greatest amounts during wakefulness and make up an important component of the ascending activating system. Glutamate agonists produce a prolonged central excitation and cortical activation.

There are many peptides such as CRH, thyrotropin-releasing factor, and vasoactive intestinal peptide found in the central nervous system that are involved in the maintenance of cortical activation and wakefulness by either synaptic release or release into the cerebral spinal fluid.

Epinephrine, histamine, thyroid-stimulating hormone, or ACTH released into the blood can elicit or reinforce arousal and wakefulness by acting on brain areas outside the blood–brain barrier.

NEUROTRANSMITTER ACTIVITY DURING NON-RAPID EYE MOVEMENT SLEEP

NREM sleep is initiated by actively inhibiting the ascending activating system. Neurons that are particularly important for this inhibition are located within the lower brain stem and in the anterior hypothalamus. Serotonin, which is contained in the nucleus raphe and neurons in the brain stem, may also help to promote sleep, although the precise mechanism is still the subject of substantial research. Some pharmacological studies suggest that diffusely projecting serotoninergic neurons may facilitate the onset of sleep by dampening the response to sensory input. This may be the mechanism by which the serotonin precursor tryptophan may facilitate sleep. Cells of the nucleus raphe begin to slow and then cease discharge during NREM sleep. Because of this, they do not appear likely to be involved in actively generating NREM or REM sleep.

GABA is the chief inhibitory neurotransmitter in the central nervous system. It plays a role in regulating neuronal excitability throughout the nervous system. In humans, GABA is also directly responsible for the regulation of muscle tone. GABA is known to play a role in sleep, as is evidenced by the sedative effects of benzodiazepines, which are known to enhance the postsynaptic action of GABA. Similarly, barbiturates—which produce sedation or, in a higher dose, anesthesia—bind at or near the chloride ionophore of the benzodiazepine receptor complex and therefore indirectly enhance the effectiveness of GABA.

GABAergic neurons are located throughout the brain in the brain stem, thalamus, hypothalamus, basal forebrain, and cerebral cortex. They may shut off neurons within the ascending reticular activating system and may also inhibit transmission and activity in neurons that project to the thalamus and cortex. GABA is released from the cerebral cortex in the highest concentration during NREM sleep.

Adenosine may act to promote sleep, as suggested by the stimulant caffeine which blocks adenosine receptors. It is not known whether adenosine is released by specific neurons utilizing adenosine as a neurotransmitter or by all neurons as a metabolite of adenosine triphosphate where they are active. The latter mechanism would provide an explanation for fatigue as well as sleep onset.

There is some evidence to suggest the presence of a "sleep substance" peptide that accumulates in the brain and cerebrospinal fluid that promotes the onset of sleep. These peptides include the opiate peptides of a-acetyl melanocyte-stimulating hormone and somatostatin. Substances released into the blood such as insulin, cholecystokinin, prostaglandins, interleukins, growth hormone, and prolactin have been shown to have sleep-promoting actions (Figure 7-4). Many substances can induce, modify, and, to varying degrees, influence NREM sleep as well as REM sleep.

NEUROTRANSMITTER ACTIVITY DURING RAPID EYE MOVEMENT SLEEP

Many of the components of REM sleep are generated by neurons within the pontine tegmentum. Acetylcholine, which is contained within neurons in the pons, is critically involved in the generation of REM sleep. Experimentally increasing acetylcholine levels in the brain by administering physotigmine, an inhibitor of the catabolic enzyme, precipitates REM sleep during an ongoing period of NREM sleep and enhances the phasic periods of REM sleep. Blocking muscarinic receptors—which are acetylcholine receptors stimulated by its release from postganglionic fibers in the parasympathetic nervous system—can retard the appearance of REM sleep and reduce its phasic periodicity. Direct injection of the cholinergic agonist carbachol into the pontine tegmentum produces a full-blown state of REM sleep in cat models. These research findings suggest

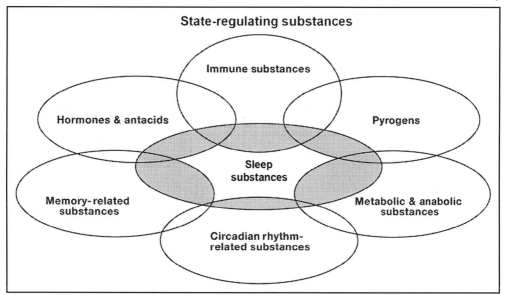

Figure 7-4. Schematic representation of the involvement of multiple hormonal factors in the regulation of sleep and wakefulness.

that pontine cholinoceptive neurons act upon other reticular neurons to excite ascending circuits and inhibit sensory and motor transmission.

Norepinephrine neurons of the locus coeruleus appear to act in a reciprocal manner to the cholinergic neurons that are selectively active during wakefulness. These are some of the chemical and neuronal systems that participate in the cyclic generation and maintenance of sleep and waking.

SUMMARY

Sleep is an active process that is generated and maintained in the brain by various neurotransmitters and neuropeptides. Key among these neurotransmitters are norepinephrine, which is involved in sleep regulation; acetylcholine, released in greater amounts during REM sleep as compared to wakefulness; and serotonin, one of the most important neurotransmitters in regulation of the sleep–wake cycle. Important neuropeptides include glutamate and aspartate, of which fluctuations in the concentration alter the duration and depth of sleep stages, and CRH, a regulatory hormone impacting the quantities of REM and NREM sleep. Various sleep stages are also mediated by neurotransmitters. REM sleep is turned on and off primarily by neurotransmitters in the pons.

REFERENCES

1. Rammsayer TH. Extraversion and dopamine: individual differences in response to changes in dopaminergic activity as a possible biological basis of extraversion. *Eur Psychol.* 1998;3:37–50.
2. Shelton J, Nishino S, Vaught J, Dement WC, Mignot E. Comparative effects of modafinil and amphetamine on daytime sleepiness and cataplexy of narcoleptic dogs. *Sleep.* 1995;18:817–826.
3. UT Southwestern Researchers. Release adenosine to slow cells, trigger sleep, UT Southwestern Researchers find. *ScienceDaily.* Available at: http://www.sciencedaily.com/releases/2005/04/050421213511.htm. Accessed September 28, 2013.
4. Gottesmann C. The neurochemistry of waking and sleeping mental activity: the disinhibition–dopamine hypothesis. *Psychiatry Clin Neurosci.* 2002;56:345–354.
5. Schenck CH, Mahowalf MW. REM sleep behavior disorder: clinical, developmental, and neuroscience perspectives 16 years after its formal identification in SLEEP. *Sleep.* 2002;25(2):120–138.
6. Eisensehr I, Linke, R, Noachtar S, Schwarz J, Gildehaus FJ, Tatsch K. Reduced striatal dopamine transporters in idiopathic rapid eye movement sleep behaviour disorder. Comparison with Parkinson's disease and controls. *Brain.* 2002;123(pt 6):1155–1160.
7. Jones BE. From waking to sleeping: neuronal and chemical substrates. *Trends Pharmacol Sci.* 2005;26:578–586.
8. Platt B, Riedel G. The cholinergic system, EEG and sleep. *Behav Brain Res.* 2011;221:499–504.
9. Vazquez J, Baghdoyan HA. Basal forebrain acetylcholine release during REM sleep is significantly greater that during waking. *Am J Physiol Regul Integr Comp Physiol.* 2001;280:R598–R601.
10. Yanai K, Tashiro M. The physiological and pathophysiological roles of neuronal histamine: an insight from human positron emission tomography studies. *Pharmacol Ther.* 2007;113:1–15.
11. Alvarez EO. The role of histamine on cognition. *Behav Brain Res.* 2009;199:183–189.
12. Blandina P, Efoudebe M, Cenni G, et al. Acetylcholine, histamine, and cognition: two sides of the same coin. *Learn Mem.* 2004;11:1–8.

13. Alvarez EO, Banzan AM. Effects of localized histamine micro-injections into the hippocampal formation on the retrieval of a one-way active avoidance response in rats. *J Neural Trans.* 1995;101(1-3):201-211.

14. Parmentier R, Ohtsu H, Djebbara-Hannas Z, Valatx JL, Watnabe T, Lin JS. Anatomical, physiological, and pharmacological characteristics of histidine decarboxylase knock-out mice: evidence for the role of brain histamine in behavioral and sleep–wake control. *J Neurosci.* 2002;22:7695-7711.

15. Leonard TO, Lydic R. Pontine nitric oxide modulates acetylcholine release, rapid eye movement sleep generation, and respiratory rate. J Neurosci. 17(2):774-785.

16. Leonard TO, Lydic R. Pontine nitric oxide modulates acetylcholine release, rapid eye movement sleep generation, and respiratory rate. *J Neurosci.* 1997;17:774-785.

17. McCormick DA, Bal T. Sleep and arousal: thalamocortical mechanisms. *Annu Rev Neurosci.* 1997;20:185-215.

18. Fillenz M. Physiological release of excitatory amino acids. *Behav Brain Res.* 1995;71:51-67.

19. Coyle JT, Puttfarcken P. Oxidative stress, glutamate, and neurodegenerative disorders. *Science.* 1993;262:689-695.

20. Li F, Tsien JZ. Clinical implications of basic research: memory and the NMDA receptors. *N Engl J Med.* 2009;361:302-303.

21. Prospéro-García O, Criado JR, Henriksen SJ. Pharmacology of ethanol and glutamate antagonists on rodent sleep: a comparative study. *Pharmacol Biochem Behav.* 1994;49:413-416.

22. Nikolaishvili L, Mitagvaria NP. In: Oniani T, ed. *Neurobiology of Sleep–Wakefulness Cycle.* Tbilisi, Georgia, Metsniereba; 1988:315-322.

23. Vincent SR, Williams JA, Reiner PB, el-Husseini A. Monitoring neuronal NO release in vivo in cerebellum, thalamus and hippocampus. *Prog Brain Res.* 1998;118:27-35.

24. Dzoljic MR, de Vries R, van Leeuwen R. Sleep and nitric oxide: effects of 7-nitro indazole, inhibitor of brain nitric oxide synthase. *Brain Res.* 1996;718:145-150.

25. Leonard TO, Lydic R. Pontine nitric oxide modulates acetylcholine release, rapid eye movement sleep generation, and respiratory rate. *J Neurosci.* 1997;17:774-785.

26. Hatzinger M, Z'Brun A, Hemmeter U, Seifritz E, Baumann F, Holsboer-Trachsler E, Heuser IJ. Hypothalamic-pituitary-adrenal system function in patients with Alzheimer's disease. *Neruobiol Aging.* 1995;16(2):205-209.

27. Machado RB, Tufik S, Suchecki D. Modulation of sleep homeostasis by corticotropin releasing hormone in REM sleep-deprived rats. *Int J Endocrinol.* 2010;2010:326151. doi: 10.1155/2010/326151.

28. Suchecki D, Lobo LL, Hipolide DC, Tufik S. Increased ACTH and corticosterone secretion induced by different methods of paradoxical sleep deprivation. *J Sleep Res.* 1998;7:276-281.

29. Koban M, Wei WL, Hoffman GE. Changes in hypothalamic corticotropin-releasing hormone, neuropeptide Y, and proopiomelanocortin gene expression during chronic rapid eye movement sleep deprivation of rats. *Endocrinology.* 2006;147:421-431.

30. Machado RB, Tufik S, Suchecki D. Chronic stress during paradoxical sleep deprivation increases paradoxical sleep rebound: association with prolactin plasma levels and brain serotonin content. *Psychoneuroendocrinology.* 2008;33:1211-1224.

31. Machado RB, Tufik S, Suchecki D. Modulation of sleep homeostasis by corticotropin releasing hormone in REM sleep-deprived rats. *Internat J Endocrinol.* 2010:1-12.

32. Carlson NR. *Physiology of Behavior.* 4th ed. Concord, MA: Simon & Schuster; 1991.

33. Ellman SJ, Antrobus JS, eds. *The Mind in Sleep.* 2nd ed. New York, NY: John Wiley & Sons; 1991.

34. Baetz M, Bowen RC. Efficacy of divalproex sodium in patients with panic disorder and mood instability who have not responded to conventional therapy. *Can J Psychiatry.* 1998;42:72-77.

Temporal Regulation of Sleep and Wakefulness

Julie M. Hereford, PT, DPT

In preceding chapters, the brain mechanisms and neurochemistry of sleep have been discussed at length. Another mechanism, a temporal system, influences and regulates sleep and is also known as the *circadian clock* (Figure 8-1). The term *circadian* takes its origin from the Latin *circa*, meaning approximately, and *dies*, meaning day.

A circadian rhythm is an internal biological process that is regulated by the circadian clock and has an entrainable oscillation of not exactly, but close to, 24 hours (Figure 8-2). Therefore, in order to synchronize with the precise 24-hour day that occurs due to the Earth's rotation, the circadian clock must reset daily by using external cues. Circadian rhythms have been observed in cyanobacteria, fungi, plants, and animals. They are endogenous but can adjust to external cues in the local environment known as *zeitgebers*. The most common zeitgeber is daylight. As early as the fourth century B.C., experimental observation of natural processes in plants and animals showed that, even in the absence of external cues, many plants and animals seemed to maintain a 24-hour periodicity to their behavior.[1] Later, scientists observed that even during periods of prolonged sleep deprivation, objective and subjective reports of sleepiness appeared to increase and decrease at relatively predictable times throughout a 24-hour period, in the absence of external cues such as light and temperature changes.[2,3] The genetic underpinnings for the concept of the circadian clock were suggested in the 1970s by Konopka and Benzer[4] when they were able to isolate the first gene of the circadian clock in a fruit fly. It was not until 1994 that Vitatema et al[3] discovered the first mammalian gene of the circadian clock. Therefore, although the concept of an internal clock has been around for a very long time, research to uncover the mechanisms of the circadian clock is relatively recent.

Circadian rhythms are said to be endogenous, which means that they are internally controlled and persist even in the absence of external cues. A circadian rhythm is also entrainable, which means that it can be reset by exposure to external stimuli such as light or temperature changes. The experience of jet lag is an example of an entrainment problem, in which one crosses one or more time zones and has a period of time before adjusting to local time. Another hallmark of circadian rhythms is their ability to maintain periodicity over a range of physiological temperatures. Differences in temperature may affect the kinetics of molecular processes, but the circadian rhythm helps to maintain a 24-hour periodicity despite changing cellular kinetics. This is known as *temperature compensation*. Circadian rhythms allow for anticipation of environmental changes and allow the organism to coordinate internal metabolic processes with its environment.[5] An animal is able to predict seasonal changes of weather conditions, food availability, or predator activity, thus improving its likelihood of survival. Circadian rhythm is also an important factor in governing various behaviors such as migration, hibernation, and reproduction.[6]

In recent years, there has been a great deal of research into the genetic components of the circadian clock. Though much is now known, there is much still to be learned. Current research suggests that there is an interlocked feedback loop of genetic products resulting in periodic fluctuations that the cells of the body interpret as a specific time of the day.[7] Cells communicate with one another to produce a synchronized output, which influences periodic release of hormones and results in characteristic rhythmic physiological activity. For instance, information regarding the time of day is relayed by the visual system to the brain

Hereford JM. *Sleep and Rehabilitation: A Guide for Health Professionals* (pp 69-76).
© 2014 Taylor & Francis Group.

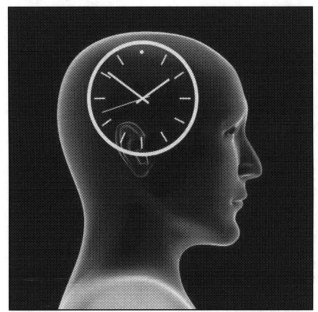

Figure 8-1. A circadian rhythm is an internal biological process. The circadian clock refers to the biological mechanism that regulates circadian rhythms. These terms are sometimes used interchangeably. (From Fotolia.com)

to the circadian clock to synchronize activity throughout the body including the timing of the sleep–wake cycle and fluctuations in body temperature, thirst, and appetite.

The light–dark cycle that occurs every 24 hours is one of the primary zeitgebers that influences circadian rhythm. A number of studies have examined the influence of this cycle on the circadian clock including several that kept animals and even humans in a completely light or completely dark controlled environment for an extended period.[8-11] It is consistently found that the organism tends to migrate to a so-called free-running cycle according to endogenous rhythms that may be shorter or longer than 24 hours. In the absence of light–dark zeitgebers, the environmental cues become out of phase with the circadian rhythm or other ultradian rhythms, which are predictable periods that repeat throughout a 24-hour circadian rhythm.[12,13] Other evidence of the importance of light–dark cycles to help maintain circadian rhythms can be seen on the International Space Station[14] in which light–dark transitions occur every 45 minutes, which results in changes in the thermal properties of the spacecraft and in the power generated from the solar arrays. This has been a source of circadian dyssynchrony that has led to disordered sleep. The current design of the spacecraft now takes this into consideration and mimics a light–dark cycle closer to the normal circadian rhythms of the astronauts.[14]

The primary circadian clock in humans is located in the suprachiasmatic nucleus of the hypothalamus. Destruction of the suprachiasmatic nucleus causes irreversible absence of a normal sleep–wake cycle. This nucleus receives input through the visual system in specialized ganglionic photosensitive cells. These cells contain melanopsin, a photopigment, and project via the retinohypothalamic tract to the suprachiasmatic nucleus, where entrainment to the local environment occurs.

Information received from the retina regarding the light–dark cycle is sent to the suprachiasmatic nucleus to be processed and then is passed on to the pineal gland located on the epithalamus. The pineal gland secretes melatonin in response to the light–dark cycle, peaking at night and decreasing to an undetectable level during the daytime. The pineal melatonin appears to feed back to the suprachiasmatic nucleus to modulate the circadian rhythm.[15]

Indoor lighting does not appear to affect circadian rhythms, and most humans achieve their best quality sleep during their individual chronotypical sleep period. That is, most humans have a particular time of day in which their physical functions including sleep, cognitive function, and hormonal levels are at an optimal level. Markers for measuring the timing to circadian rhythm include core body temperature, melatonin secretion by the pineal gland, and plasma level of cortisol[16,17] (Figure 8-3). These studies have shown that the average adult human temperature reaches its minimum approximately 2 hours prior to habitual awakening time. This timing can vary widely according to individual chronotypes.[17] Melatonin is undetectable during the daytime, but at the onset of decreasing light, it can be measured in blood or saliva (Figure 8-4).

Another marker of the activity of the circadian clock is the timing of the maximum plasma cortisol level. Cortisol levels present in the blood have diurnal variation, peaking in the early morning and reaching the lowest point between midnight and 4 AM, which is generally 3 to 5 hours after the onset of sleep.[18]

Light can advance or delay the circadian rhythm, depending on the timing of its application. In fact, light therapy has been prescribed for some time as a treatment for a number of disorders of circadian rhythm. Therapeutic lighting is a higher-intensity light than normal artificial home lighting. The illumination intensity needed to affect the circadian system needs to reach 1000 lux.[19] Melanopsin is most efficiently stimulated by light in the blue spectrum (470 to 485 nm).[20] The direction of the light is also an important factor in circadian rhythmicity in that light projected from above eye level is more effective than light projected from below eye level.[19]

Timing of medical treatment in coordination with circadian rhythm may increase efficacy and reduce drug toxicity or adverse reactions. This is particularly true in the timing of certain antineoplastic agents for the treatment of cancer.[21] Long-term disruption of circadian rhythms has been shown to have significant consequences on general health, particularly in cardiovascular disease.[22] Suppression of the production of melatonin caused by disturbances in circadian rhythm has been associated with increased risk of developing cancer.[23]

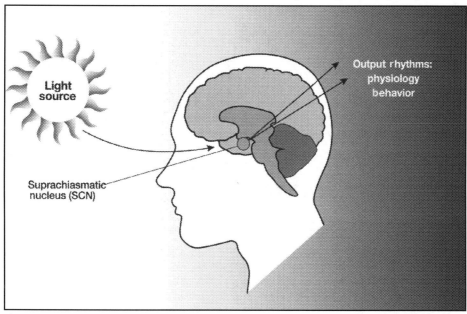

Figure 8-2. Biological clock in humans. Light and darkness influence circadian rhythms and related physiology and behavior through the suprachiasmatic nucleus.

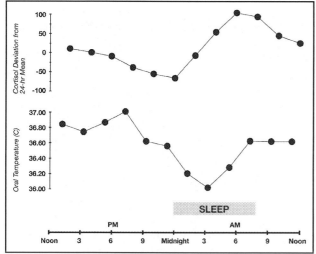

Figure 8-3. Twenty-four–hour fluctuation of cortisol levels and oral temperature.

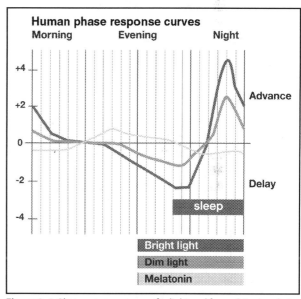

Figure 8-4. Phase response curves for light and for melatonin administration.

Some individuals engage in a short period of sleep during the day. Short daytime napping does not affect normal circadian rhythms, but daytime napping has been shown to decrease stress and improve productivity.[24,25]

Disturbances in circadian rhythms have been associated with health problems and psychiatric disorders. Generally, affected individuals get a normal quality and sufficient quantity of sleep if allowed to sleep according to their individual circadian clock. However, the dyssynchrony of circadian rhythm may interfere with the ability to engage in normal work, school, and social activities. Light therapy may be an effective treatment for a number of disorders of circadian timing.[26,27]

OTHER THOUGHTS ABOUT CIRCADIAN RHYTHM

Peaks of activity of various physiological systems vary according to the time of day. For example, core body temperature in humans is not a fixed value but, rather, varies across a 24-hour period. It is generally highest in mid-afternoon at near 100°F and is at its lowest point in the early morning hours before awakening, at as low as 96°F.

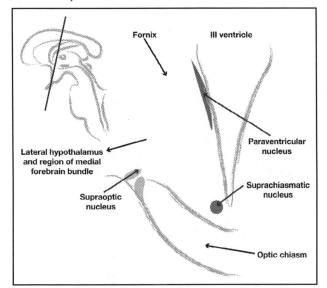

Figure 8-5. Schematic of the location of the suprachiasmatic nucleus.

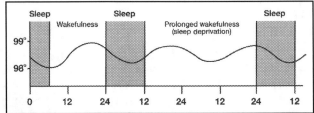

Figure 8-6. Fluctuation of an individual body temperature over 36 hours. Maximum temperature occurs during the day and minimum temperature at night. This figure shows that the daily temperature cycle continues even if one does not sleep. The intrinsic circadian rhythms of bodily functions are not dependent upon the daily alternation of sleep–wakefulness. Rather, the circadian fluctuations influence the tendency to sleep or remain awake.

Another example can be seen in plasma levels of hormones such as cortisol, human growth hormone, and prolactin. Urine production, heart rate, and blood pressure also follow patterns. This consistent presence of a diurnal rhythmicity appears to confer an adaptive advantage by optimizing energy expenditure and behavior in relationship to a changing external environment.

The circadian clock consists of a rhythmic organization of activity that persists even in the absence of environmental cues or zeitgebers. In the absence of periodic time cues, the circadian rhythm can drift to a longer or shorter time span than the typical 24-hour time period. Resetting to a 24-hour environmental cycle based on zeitgebers is known as *entrainment*.

Control of circadian rhythm resides in the suprachiasmatic nucleus of the hypothalamus (Figure 8-5). If the suprachiasmatic nucleus is destroyed, the amount of sleep and wakefulness will not necessarily change, but the normal 24-hour rhythmicity is no longer present. Time isolation experiments have shown that, in subjects who have lived for up to 6 months in special apartments without windows, telephones, television, radio, or any contact with the outside world, the sleep–wake cycle migrated to a free-running period that appeared to be greater than 24 hours. However, this famous study did not control for individuals turning lights off during sleep, which will change levels of melatonin and alter the sleep–wake cycle.[28] This is thought to be because of a feedback mechanism between the melatonin-producing pineal gland and the suprachiasmatic nuclei. In humans, it appears that the circadian period is fairly narrowly defined to 24 hours, 11 minutes. The clock appears to reset itself daily according to the Earth's rotation.[29] Alternating sunlight and darkness, warmth and cold, and noise and quiet along with other factors in the environment change rhythmically because of the Earth's rotation, which entrains the endogenous circadian oscillation to a period of 24 hours.

On the mornings after a later bedtime than usual, it is difficult to continue sleeping until 8 hours of sleep have been accumulated because of the entrained circadian oscillation that continues without interruption. This situation requires the individual to sleep when the cycle is on the upswing. Generally, this is only possible if there are other contributing factors such as an accumulated sleep debt or ingestion of drugs or alcohol that artificially alter the sleep–wake cycle.

Circadian rhythm is innate and internal, built into an organism, and does not, in fact, need to be driven from the outside. Cells removed from the suprachiasmatic nucleus and placed in culture maintain their own rhythm in the absence of external cues.[30] In experimental models in which an individual is placed in an isolated environment, the individual circadian rhythm begins to free-run. When free-running, body temperature changes its phase relationship to the sleep–wake cycle (Figure 8-6). Instead of reaching its lowest point toward the end of sleep, the low point occurred at the beginning of sleep. This change in the phase relationship between sleep and body temperature suggests that these 2 processes have 2 distinct timing mechanisms.[31]

Changes in physiological function are more precisely characterized as a secondary response to the rhythmic changes in sleep and wakefulness, rather than as a direct response to the circadian clock. There is speculation that the principal function of sleepiness is to rhythmically drive the organism to seek safety. For instance, the organism retreats to inactivity deep in a burrow, nest, or bed when the external environment is most hostile or least accommodating. Sleep and wakefulness are inextricably linked to the circadian clock, which strongly modulates their expression. For example, the circadian influence on human sleep in sleep deprivation experiments shows that alertness increases in the morning after subjects have been up all night, having not slept at all.

Neither the basal condition nor the free-running condition establishes that the circadian clock as directly controlling sleep and wakefulness. Rather, though circadian rhythms are extremely important in defining a sleep–wake cycle, there is a complex interaction among circadian and non-circadian influences. The circadian clock controls a homeostatic mechanism in which sleepiness increases in proportion to the time awake and eventually results in sleep onset. The reverse homeostatic mechanism, in which alertness increases with the amount of time spent asleep, may account for the timing of the onset of wakefulness. Despite severe sleep deprivation accumulating over several days, subjects were still unable to sleep during hours in the afternoon and evening that coincided with the peak of the circadian cycle when they would normally be awake. If a lesion occurs in the suprachiasmatic nuclei, however, sleep and wakefulness are no longer rhythmic. Instead, alternating episodes of sleep and wakefulness of varying length occur randomly throughout the day and night. However, if an animal in this experimental model is kept awake for a significant period of time and then allowed to fall asleep, the duration of the recovery sleep is increased above the normal baseline duration. This supports study supports circadian rhythm as a homeostatic regulator of sleep and wakefulness. The internal desynchronization seen in humans during free-running conditions is a complex interaction between homeostatic and circadian influences in timing of sleep.

Circadian rhythm modulates sleep states. Sleepiness is modulated by the circadian clock as well as by the homeostatic sleep drive and behavioral imperatives. Sleep tendency shows a nocturnal increase coincident with the trough in body temperature, but there is also a consistent peak sleep tendency and a minimum in sleep latency in the early afternoon, known as the *PM slump*. This trough in circadian rhythm persists independent of the timing of meals or other exogenous factors that are thought to augment sleepiness.

In addition to the relationship with sleep onset, circadian rhythm appears to have a relationship to rapid eye movement (REM) propensity with its peak near the minimum of body temperature. REM sleep that occurs coincident to the circadian peak appears to be prolonged compared to that which occurs at other points along the circadian pattern. If sleep onset occurs near the REM peak, then latency from sleep onset to REM onset will be very short. In contrast, sleep that occurs in the late afternoon or evening, when REM propensity is at its minimum, will exhibit brief REM periods and very long REM latencies. REM periods increase in length across the night's sleep and REM occupies an increasing percentage of the total sleep time later in the night.

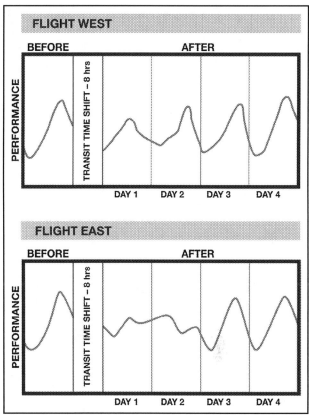

Figure 8-7. The effects of time displacement on the phase of the circadian rhythm of air pilots' performance in a simulator after simulated travel between destinations in the west and east. Restoration of baseline performance rhythms takes longer after eastward displacement.

DYSSYNCHRONY OF CIRCADIAN RHYTHMS

Individuals who suffer from insomnia and other sleep disorders may have a defect in the entrainment mechanism or in the innate oscillation mechanism such that these individuals may not have the ability to oscillate in synchrony with their environment.

Jet lag is a circadian dyssynchrony that results from changing time zones and zeitgeber orientation faster than the circadian clock can adjust. Jet lag is more severe, persistent, and annoying after eastward travel than it is after westward travel. Westward travel is in accord with the 24-hour circadian clock's tendency to drift to later hours. In contrast, eastward travel causes an advance to earlier hours, which runs against the clock's natural tendency.

The workload of an airline pilot is such that he or she may cross multiple time zones, experience multiple episodes of sunlight and darkness in one day, and spend many hours awake during the day and night. Pilots are often unable to maintain a normal sleep pattern coincident with their circadian rhythms (Figure 8-7). This situation can easily lead to fatigue and may be a significant contributing factor in pilot error and accidents. The National Transportation Safety Board continues to research methods of combating pilot fatigue.[32–34]

The second common circadian dyssynchrony is the "Monday morning blues." In this situation, an individual who normally goes to bed at a consistent time and awakens at a consistent time during the week decides to sleep an hour later on a Saturday morning. The individual therefore misses the normal early morning zeitgebers signal and, as a consequence, the 24-hour clock drifts approximately 1 hour later. The process repeats on Sunday morning. When the alarm clock rings at 6 AM on Monday morning, the body's clock is 2 hours behind and the individual struggles to get out of bed because, according to the individual's circadian clock, it is only 4 AM.

DISORDERS OF CIRCADIAN TIMING

Delayed Sleep Phase Syndrome

Delayed sleep phase syndrome (DSPS) usually occurs in adults. In this disorder, the circadian system is shifted to a position markedly later than normal (Figure 8-8). Sleep propensity rhythm shifts with it so that the individual with DSPS cannot fall asleep before 3 or 4 AM and they cannot awaken before noon without extraordinary effort. An apparent defect in the circadian entrainment mechanism prevents normal corrective shifts to earlier hours while allowing stable entrainment to the 24-hour cycle. This locks the individual into quasi-permanent jet lag and his or her functioning in a normal diurnal world is difficult. DSPS occurs to a lesser degree in young adults around puberty. This helps to explain the propensity of the pubescent child to prefer to go to sleep later and sleep later, a schedule that is often in conflict with academic and athletic pursuits and sometimes with family life.

Shift Work Syndrome

Shift work syndrome is a significant problem in the 24-hour modern world. In this condition, many shift workers cannot adapt to the dyssynchrony between circadian rhythms and work and sleep demands. The conflict is between the work schedule and circadian orientation. This often produces insomnia during the day when the individual tries to sleep and excessive sleepiness at night when the individual tries to work. Over time, the resultant chronic sleep deprivation produces general stress and a host of secondary medical disorders. As noted earlier, light therapy may offer some help for these workers as they try to adapt to this dyssynchrony.

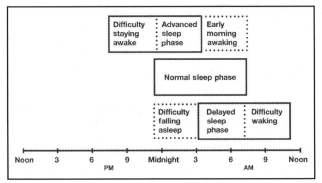

Figure 8-8. Schematic of conventional sleep–wake cycle and the sleep–wake cycle of DSPS and advanced sleep phase syndrome. The timing of the preferred sleep period in each syndrome is designated in bold lines. Dashed lines indicate sleep problems when a conventional schedule is attempted.

Entrainment Failure Syndrome

Entrainment failure syndrome is a persistence of a free-running sleep–wake rhythm despite the presence of adequate zeitgeber signals in the environment. This disorder can produce cyclic insomnia. It occurs much more commonly among the blind than among normally sighted individuals.

Clock Failure Syndrome

Clock failure syndrome is a rare condition that is a manifestation of a neurological disease. In individuals with clock failure syndrome, the anterior hypothalamus is affected and results in episodes of sleep and wakefulness that are scattered throughout the 24-hour period in a random fashion analogous to experimental models of suprachiasmatic lesions.

Changes in Circadian Rhythms With Age

Changes in circadian rhythms with age involve changes in circadian organization with advancing age. There is a decrease in the free-running period and, most notably, a shift of phase to earlier hours. There is also a decrease in the amplitude of the circadian variation, as well as a loss of neurons in the suprachiasmatic nuclei with increasing age.

The advance of the sleep–wake cycle to earlier in the evening is known as *advanced sleep phase syndrome*. In this syndrome, older adults may report overwhelming sleepiness at 7 or 8 PM that makes it impossible to remain awake. Then, by 3 or 4 AM the individual with advanced sleep phase syndrome is unable to continue sleeping. Older adults are often significantly distressed by this but, as with all disorders of circadian rhythm, quality and quantity of sleep are usually preserved. Rather, the timing of sleep onset and offset is dyssynchronous.

SUMMARY

In addition to neurochemical regulation of sleep, sleep is regulated by circadian rhythm. Circadian rhythm is an internally controlled oscillation of approximately 24 hours which has the capacity to be brought into a specific rhythm by external stimuli. This 24-hour internal clock is governed by the suprachiasmatic nucleus in the brain. Destruction of this structure causes irreversible loss of a normal sleep–wake cycle. Circadian timing, one's "circadian clock," is dependent upon melatonin secretion by the pineal gland, core body temperature, and plasma level of cortisol. This clock also plays an important role in thermal regulation.

Although circadian rhythms are endogenous, they adjust to external cues in the environment such as the light–dark cycle of the sun and social cues that are time specific, such as meals and social gatherings. Physiological systems are affected by the circadian clock and vary across a 24-hour period in relation to this clock. Core body temperature and specific hormone levels are driven by circadian rhythm, as are urine production, heart rate, and blood pressure. Though the physiologic systems are directly affected by circadian rhythm, physiologic functions or manifestations, such as sleepiness, exhibit a secondary response to the rhythmic changes in sleep and wakefulness. There is no evidence that the circadian clock directly controls the sleep–wake cycle, though it is extremely important in this cycle, as it plays a role in modulating sleep states and affecting the REM sleep propensity.

Disorders of circadian rhythm can disrupt sleep and be a source of chronic sleep deprivation as well as various psychological and physical disorders. Depression, Monday morning blues, jet lag, shift work syndrome, and clock failure syndrome affect sleep and are indirectly or directly related to difficulties or disorders of circadian rhythm.

REFERENCES

1. Gardner MJ, Hubbard KE, Hotta CT, Dodd AN, Webb AA. How plants tell the time. *Biochem J.* 2006;397:15–24.
2. Dijk D-J, von Schantz M. Timing and consolidation of human sleep, wakefulness, and performance by a symphony of oscillators. *J Biol Rhythms.* 2005;20:279–290.
3. Vitaterna MH, King DP, Chang AM, et al. Mutagenesis and mapping of a mouse gene, clock, essential for circadian behavior. *Science.* 1994;264:719–725.
4. Konopka R, Benzer S. Clock mutants of *Drosophila melanogaster. Proc Natl Acad Sci USA.* 1971;68:2112–2116.
5. Sharma VK. Adaptive significance of circadian clocks. *Chronobiol Int.* 2003;20:901–919.
6. McNamara P, Barton RA, Nunn CL. *Evolution of Sleep: Phylogenetic and Functional Perspectives.* New York, NY: Cambridge University Press; 2009.
7. Salk Institute. 'Alarm clock' gene explains wake-up function of biological clock. *ScienceDaily.* October 3, 2011. Available at: http://www.sciencedaily.com/releases/2011/09/110929161343. htm. Accessed September 28, 2013.
8. Aschoff J. Exogenous and endogenous components in circadian rhythms. *Cold Spring Harb Symp Quant Biol.* 1960;25:11-28.
9. Aschoff J. Circadian rhythms: influences of internal and external factors on the period measured in constant conditions. *Ethology.* 1979;40(3):225-249.
10. Czeisler CA, Allan JS, Strogatz SH, Rhonda JM, Sanchez R, Rios CD, Freitag WO, Richardson GS, Kronauer RE. Bright light resets the human circadian pacemaker independent of the timing of the sleep-wake cycle. *Science.* 1986;233(4764):667-671.
11. Duffy JF, Kronauer RE, Czeisler CA. Phase-shifting human circadian rhythms: Influence of sleep timing, social contact and light exposure. *J Physiol.* 1996;495:289-297.
12. Shneerson JM, Ohayon MM, Carskadon MA. Circadian rhythms. Available at: http://www.sleep.health.am/sleep/more/circadian-rhythms. Accessed September 22, 2011.
13. Regestein QR, Pavlova M. Treatment of delayed sleep phase syndrome [abstract]. *Gen Hosp Psychiatry.* 1995;17:335–345.
14. Thirsk R, Kuipers A, Mukai C, Williams D. The space-flight environment: the International Space Station and beyond. *CMAJ.* 2009;180:1216–1220.
15. Cassone VM, Warren WS, Brooks DS, Lu J. Melatonin, the pineal gland, and circadian rhythms. *J Biol Rhythms.* 1993;8(suppl): S73–S81.
16. Benloucif S, Guico MJ, Reid KJ, Wolfe LF, L'hermite-Balériaux M, Zee PC. Stability of melatonin and temperature as circadian phase markers and their relation to sleep times in humans. *J Biol Rhythms.* 2005;20:178–188.
17. Klerman EB, Gershengorn HB, Duffy JF, Kronauer RE. Comparisons of the variability of three markers of the human circadian pacemaker. *J Biol Rhythms.* 2002;17:181–193.
18. de Weerth C, Zijl R, Buitelaar J. Development of cortisol circadian rhythm in infancy. *Early Hum Dev.* 2003;73:39–52.
19. Semjonova, M. Healthy lighting, from a lighting designer's perspective. Available at: http://www.enlightermagazine.com/images/2009/01/healthyLighting.pdf. Accessed October 2, 2013.
20. Newman LA, Walker MT, Brown RL, Cronin TW, Robinson PR. Melanopsin forms a functional short-wavelength photopigment. *Biochemistry.* 2003;42:12734–12738.
21. Figueiro MG, Rea MS, Bullough JD. Does architectural lighting contribute to breast cancer? *J Carcinog.* 2006;5:20.
22. Martino TA, Oudit GY, Herzenberg AM, et al. Circadian rhythm disorganization produces profound cardiovascular and renal disease in hamsters. *Am J Physiol Regul Integr Comp Physiol.* 2008;294:R1675–R1683.
23. Strai K, Baan R, Grosse Y, et al. Carcinogenicity of shift-work, painting, and fire-fighting. *Lancet Oncol.* 2007;8:1065–1066.
24. Pilcher JJ, Michalowski KR, Carrigan RD. The prevalence of daytime napping and its relationship to nighttime sleep. *Behav Med.* 2001;27(2):71–76.
25. Rolston E, Sandlin JR, Sandlin M, Keathley R. Power-napping: effects on cognitive ability and stress levels among college students. Available at: http://aahperd.confex.com/aahperd/2007/finalprogram/paper_10353.htm. Accessed September 23, 2011.
26. Figueiro MG, Bierman A, Plitnick B, Rea MS. Preliminary evidence that both blue and red light can induce alertness at night. *BMC Neurosci.* 2009;10:105. doi: 10.1186/1471-2202-10-105.
27. Sloane PD, Figueiro MG, Cohen L. Light as therapy for sleep disorders and depression in older adults. *Clin Geriatr.* 2008;16(3):25–31.
28. Aschoff J. Circadian rhythms in man. *Science.* 1965;148:1427–1432.
29. Cromie WJ. Human biological clock set back an hour. *Harvard Gazette.* July 15, 1999. Available at: http://news.harvard.edu/gazette/1999/07.15/bioclock24.html. Accessed September 23, 2011.

30. Foster R, Kreitzman L. *The Rhythms of Life: The Biological Clocks That Control the Daily Lives of Every Living Thing*. New Haven, CT: Yale University Press; 2004.

31. Colin J, Timbal J, Boutelier C, Houdas Y, Siffre M. Rhythm of the rectal temperature during a 6-month free-running experiment. *J Appl Physiol*. 1968;25:170–176.

32. Michels J. ALPA Weighs in on pilot fatigue. *Aviation Week*. February 3, 2009. Available at: http://www.aviationweek.com. Accessed September 22, 2011.

33. Strauss S. Pilot fatigue. Available at: http://aeromedical.org/Articles/Pilot_Fatigue.html. Accessed September 22, 2011.

34. Chen S. Pilot fatigue is like "having too much to drink." *CNN*. Available at: http://www.cnn.com/2009/TRAVEL/05/15/pilot.fatigue.buffalo.crash/index.html. Accessed September 22, 2011.

9

Dreams

Julie M. Hereford, PT, DPT

Dreams have been the topic of philosophical and religious inquiry and scientific speculation throughout recorded history, but the study of dreams has experienced a recent resurgence in scientific inquiry, especially in an attempt to understand the neurobiological underpinnings of this phenomenon. Attempts to understand sleep and dreaming have been crucial to humankind's developing concept of mind and consciousness. As early as the 8th century BC, sleep was described by Hesiod as "the brother of death."[1]

Dream interpretation has been going on nearly since the dawn of perception. Archeologists have found 5000-year-old clay tablets from Mesopotamia that contain records of dreams. The Greeks and Romans believed that dreams were direct messages from the gods. In fact, the Greek god Morpheus is the god who sent warnings and prophecies to those who slept at shrines and temples, in a practice known as *dream incubation*. Morpheus is the Greek root of *morphine*, a potent narcotic that is known to cause hallucinatory-like dreams. Antiphon, an ancient Greek, wrote the first known book about dreaming in the 5th century BC. Hippocrates developed a dream theory in the 4th century BC, which stated that during the day, the soul receives images and during the night the soul produces images in dreams. Aristotle, in the 3rd century BC, connected dreams with physiological activities and believed that dreams could offer insight into illness and disease. During the 4th and 3rd centuries BC, the Chinese and Indian cultures were developing similar theories into the meaning of dreams independent of the Roman and Greek cultures. In the Americas, Native Americans saw dreams as messages from ancestors predicting the future. In fact, some Native American tribes engaged in a kind of dream incubation known as a *vision quest* in order to seek out knowledge and wisdom from the ancient ones.[2-6]

Religion also has played a role in dream interpretation, with all 3 Abrahamic religions recording dream sequences in the Old Testament, the New Testament, and the Koran, attributing dreams to messages from one God (Figure 9-1). It seems that many cultures throughout history have attached some meaning to dreams.[7-9]

Others saw sleep and dreaming as less a suspension of life and more of believing that it was a chance to engage in a freer form of mental activity. This is evidenced in Shakespeare's *Hamlet*: "To sleep, perchance, to dream"[10] (Figure 9-2), and the dream sequences in *Macbeth* that say that sleep "knits up the raveled sleave of care, ... balm of hurt minds. ..."[11] Shakespeare even offered a theory of the psychology of dreams in *Richard III* in which he rationalizes his behavior and ensuing dream, "... conscious is but a word that coward's use ... march on if not to heaven then hand in hand to hell."[12] These themes can easily be seen in the context of Freudian dream analysis.

Medieval times saw a change in the interpretation of the meaning of dreams, concluding that they were evil temptations from the devil. This led to the belief that the devil could enter the human mind during dream sleep and corrupt it with harmful thoughts. In fact, Martin Luther, the leader of the Protestant movement, was plagued by dreams that he believed to be the work of the Devil.[13] Dreams were also seen as directives. A number of Catholic saints around the same time period believed that dreams helped them determine the course of their lives.[14]

In 1900, the Austrian neurologist Sigmund Freud expanded the view that dreams are an altered but

Hereford JM. *Sleep and Rehabilitation:*
A Guide for Health Professionals (pp 77-84).
© 2014 Taylor & Francis Group.

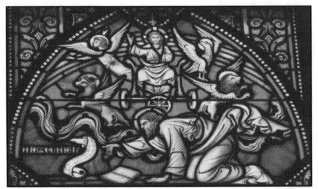

Figure 9-1. The prophet Ezekiel was visited by God in a dream. Dreams and dream interpretation are part of all major world religions. (From Fotolia.com)

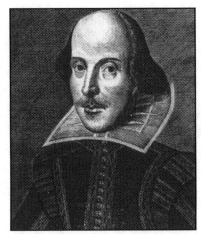

Figure 9-2. William Shakespeare analyzed the role of dreams in several of his works. (From Fotolia.com)

meaningful form of mental activity in *The Interpretation of Dreams.*[15] In this classical work, Freud categorized the mind into the id, the ego, and the superego. The id deals with basic instincts, primal impulses, and unchecked urges. The ego is concerned with conscious, rational thoughts and self-awareness. The superego acts as a censor to the id and a moral police for the ego. In the waking state, the superego suppresses the impulses and unchecked urges of the id, but during sleep, the superego is quiescent and the id can play. Freud believed that the primal desires of the id are the stuff that dreams are made of.[15]

Dreamscapes have been depicted in art and literature. For example, Rousseau's last painting was "The Dream"; Thomas Cole's series of paintings of "The Journey" depict a dreamscape across a lifetime. Goya etched "The Sleep of Reason Produces Monsters," Salvador Dali painted "Dream Caused by the Flight of a Bee Around a Pomegranate a Second Before Awakening," and Pablo Picasso painted *"Le Reve"* ("The Dream"). All of these works depicted various interpretations of dreamscapes. Dream worlds appear in literature, most notably probably Lewis Carroll's *Alice's Adventures in Wonderland* and *Through the Looking Glass* (Figure 9-3) or H. P. Lovecraft's *Dream Cycle* and Michael Ende's *The Never-Ending Story*. Movies regularly depict dream sequences in such films as *Spellbound* (1945), *The Manchurian Candidate* (1962, 2004), *Dreamscape* (1984), and *Inception* (2010). [16–23]

Dreams are generally made up of a succession of images and emotions and, to this date, the content and purpose of dreams is still not definitively understood. Although usually associated with rapid eye movement (REM) sleep, dreams occur during every stage of sleep. REM sleep dreams are usually more vivid and memorable.[24] Dreams can last for a few seconds or as long as 20 to 30 minutes. The dreams most likely to be remembered are those that occur immediately prior to awakening. The average sleeper has about 3 to 5 dreams per night, but some have as many as 7 dreams in one night's sleep. Dreams last longer later in the night's sleep, and the average time spent dreaming is about 2 hours per 8 hours of nighttime sleep. Most REM sleep dreams are mundane and ordinary; however, they can become surreal and truly bizarre. The events contained within the dream are generally outside the control of the sleeper, with the exception of lucid dreams in which the sleeper is self-aware.[25]

THE NEUROBIOLOGY OF DREAMING

Dreaming is most strongly associated with REM sleep (Figure 9-4). Dream narratives on awakening seem to match the period of coinciding REM sleep recorded preceding awakening. It is not clear where dreams originate in the brain or whether they originate in multiple areas. It is also not clear what the precise purpose for dreaming is. It is clear that there is a close correlation of REM sleep and the dream experience and that dreams occur nightly, even if they are not remembered by the sleeper. Dreams occur during high-frequency REM activity within each sleep period at predictable intervals throughout the life span.

REM sleep and REM dreams increase in length across a night's sleep. The last dream sequence in the night may consist of multiple dream episodes because of momentary awakenings that may begin to occur toward the end of the sleep cycle.

A number of theories regarding the source and function of dreaming have been put forth. These include the activation synthesis theory proposed by Hobson and McCarley in 1975.[26] This theory assumes that the same structures that induce REM sleep also generate sensory information. Research by Solms found that dreams are generated in the forebrain rather than the brain stem.[27] The continual activation theory—in which he proposed that dreaming is a result of brain activation and synthesis and that REM sleep and dreaming are controlled by 2 different brain mechanisms—was first presented by Zhang. Zhang further hypothesized that the function of sleep is to process and

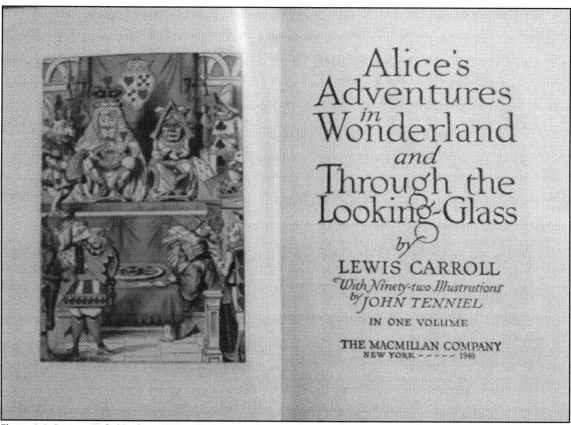

Figure 9-3. Dreams are fodder for paintings, literature, and movies. (Reprinted with permission from V. Mebruer.)

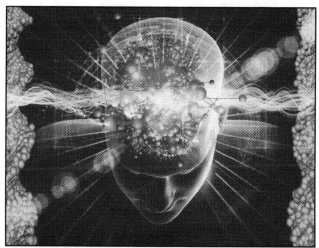

Figure 9-4. REM sleep may be likened to a computer defragmentation program in which informational errors are erased from memory. It is possible that these informational fragments are acted on by the frontal cortex, which generates the sometimes bizarre images and "stories" that are associated with dreaming. (From Fotolia.com)

consolidate short-term memory into long-term storage. Non-rapid eye movement (NREM) sleep processes conscious or declarative memory, and REM sleep processes unconscious or procedural memory. This processing is able to occur because of the disconnection from inputs from the sensory system. Zhang also proposed that this pulse-like

brain activation is the inducer of each individual dream and that the dream is maintained by the sleeper's own thinking until the next pulse of memory insertion. This is why a dream may be continuous or may oscillate suddenly between 2 different dreams.[28,29]

Tarnow[30] suggested that dreams are excitation of long-term memory and the strangeness of the dreamscape occurs because of the format of long-term memory storage. During waking, the higher executive function of the brain is able to place these memories in context and interpret them. However, the same process during sleeping, with the suppression of executive function, creates the out-of-context feel of the dreamscape.[30]

In 2001, research began to look at the illogical locations, characters, and story flow as a way in which the brain strengthens links and consolidation of semantic memories. Stickgold et al[31] and Payne et al[32] found that the flow of information between the hippocampus and neocortex is reduced during REM sleep, thus allowing for consolidation of distant but related memories. Increased levels of cortisol that normally occur in later sleep produce this decreased information flow.[31,32]

Crick and Mitchison's[33] reverse learning theory stated that dreams were cleanup operations, like a defragmentation function in a computer, in which off-line, informational errors that have been encoded and accumulated throughout the day are gathered and deleted as a component of the process of memory consolidation. This theory was further elaborated upon by Evans and Newman.[34] Hennevin and Hars[35] suggested that dreams are the result of spontaneous neural firing patterns that occur during the process of memory consolidation during REM sleep and therefore are a by-product of memory processing rather than a process unto itself.

Psychological theories of dreaming have been presented since Freud put forth his work *The Interpretation of Dreams*.[15] Alfred Adler, a contemporary of Freud, suggested that dreams were emotional practice for problem solving of real-life situations in which the residual feeling from the dream may either reinforce or reject a contemplated response. More recent theories suggest that dreams play a central role in improving the mind's ability to meet the needs of the individual while awake. This theory suggests that there is a mental phase and an emotional selection phase in which an idea for action is developed and played out in the dreamscape in order to test out its efficacy. In this way, adaptive ideas may be retained in memory while maladaptive actions are deleted, thus preparing the sleeper to act on the situation upon awakening, having practiced solutions to the problem.[36]

Evolutionary psychologists reject the theories of the usefulness of individual dreams and suggest rather that they are simply an epiphenomenon that does not serve any significant purpose.[37-39] They do, however, believe that dreams serve some adaptive function for survival, perhaps through rehearsal of threatening scenarios in order to better prepare for real-life threats, although the precise nature of this theory has not been well delineated.[36,40] Griffin[41,42] presented the expectation fulfillment theory, which suggests that dreaming metaphorically completes a pattern of emotional expectations in the autonomic nervous system, thereby lowering stress levels.

Lucid dreaming is another category of dreaming in which the sleeper has conscious perception of his or her dream state and may have some degree of control over actions within the dream. Dream control is reported to improve with practice and may be one way to manipulate dreams to "improve the outcome," especially in disturbing dreams. This is a tactic that is sometimes used in psychological counseling when the patient is troubled by recurrent disturbing dreams. This phenomenon of lucid dreaming has been validated by scientific methodology.[43,44]

There are multiple neurobiological and psychobiological theories of the function of dreams but, in reality, the precise nature and function of dreams remain an area of speculation.

Dream interpretation is another aspect of the study of dreams, but because neither the neurobiology nor the psychobiology is clear, it seems unlikely that the symbolism that some attach to various themes and images in dreams

has a great deal of validity. In general, however, it is apparent that as humans continue to strive for meaning they will continue to turn to dreams for answers and explanations.

Scientific inquiry into dreaming has been difficult because of the constraints presented in such study. Observational reports of individuals who sustained a traumatic brain injury have given some initial data. For instance, in 1951, Humphrey and Zangwill[45] reported on 2 cases of individuals who had sustained left parieto-occipital injuries with some hemianopia. Both of these individuals reported decreased visual capacity and disturbances in visual memory while awake. They also reported complete cessation of dreaming. Evidence from these cases was the first suggestion of a link between the visual system and the ability to dream and was the first time that dreaming was associated with the forebrain.[45] Other than these observational studies, it is difficult to obtain clear objective data regarding dreams. First, researchers must rely on verbal reports from subjects. These may contain pseudo-sensory, emotional, and motor elements. Dream narratives are also difficult to capture precisely because of forgetting and editing and censoring of dream content.[46] Data collection for dream research often occurs in a sleep lab, which is an unnatural sleep environment and is likely to affect the quality and quantity of sleep. Some have suggested that there are statistical concerns in dream research due to relatively small samples of data. Technical limitations of the electroencephalogram (EEG) cannot measure precise areas of the brain that are known or suspected of being important components of the neurological processes that make up dreaming. Neuroimaging has proven to be a more reliable tool in this area, however, and is offering some important new information in the study of dreams.

It is known that dreaming may occur in both REM and NREM sleep. Awakenings from REM sleep offer more frequent dream reports than awakenings from NREM sleep. REM sleep dream narratives tend to be longer, more perceptual and emotional, and less representative of waking life. NREM dream narratives on awakening tend to be more mundane, day-to-day imagery.[47] In REM sleep that is not lucid, the sleeper believes him- or herself to be awake. Usually these dreams are multimodal, containing any and all sensory modalities, and tend to be more visual than motor activities. Dream imagery can change quickly from the relatively common to the truly bizarre. There is less self-awareness and self-reflection in these dreams. They tend to be strewn across time and place in an incongruous fashion and have a certain organizational instability. REM dreams form a single narrative that explain and integrate all of the apparently unrelated elements of the dream.[48] On the contrary, NREM dream narratives can be thought-like depictions of current concerns.[45]

Dreams 81

NEUROANATOMY OF RAPID EYE MOVEMENT SLEEP DREAMING

REM sleep has been found to be generated by the pons in the brain stem, which releases acetylcholine and projects to the forebrain. Cholinergic neurons in the forebrain are thought to be responsible for the random imagery that is part of REM dreams. Cognitive areas in the forebrain attempt to exert sense or structure into the meaningless activation of REM dreams, but do not play a causal role in the production of REM dream sleep. REM sleep, and therefore REM dreaming, is switched off by norepinephrine and serotonin, which are also released in the brain stem. This has been shown in lesion studies in which the pons is intact but disconnected with higher brain centers and REM dream sleep is maintained.[49,50] This follows Hobson and McCarley's theory that dreams are activated in the brain stem and passively synthesized by the forebrain[26] (Figure 9-5).

This theory does not adequately account for dream reports that occur on awakening from NREM sleep. Mechanisms that control REM sleep and, theoretically, REM dreams, are not the same mechanisms that control the onset and maintenance of NREM sleep. This suggests that dreaming is controlled by a different area of the brain. Clinical research in which subjects with brain lesions suffered dream cessation showed that brain damage is not in the brain stem; rather, loss of dreaming only occurred when lesions were in higher brain centers, even while REM sleep was maintained. These findings led to a theory that REM sleep is controlled by cholinergic neurons, but dreaming may be controlled by dopaminergic neuronal activity in the limbic system and frontal cortex.

Mesolimbic and mesocortical dopaminergic pathways project between frontal and limbic structures. The pathway runs from the ventral tegmental area, ascends through the lateral hypothalamus, the nucleus basalis, stria terminalis, and nucleus accumbens of the basal forebrain, and terminates in the amygdala, anterior cingulate gyrus, and frontal cortex. Damage to this dopaminergic pathway can cause cessation of dreaming, as well as loss of motivating behavior.[48] Chemical stimulation of the pathway with L-dopa, for example, can increase the frequency and vividness of dreams without changing REM sleep.[49] Antipsychotic drugs that block this pathway also reduce excessive and vivid dreaming.

Another brain area implicated in the generation of dreams is the parieto-occipito-temporal junction. This area is responsible for the highest level of perceptual processing and converts perceptions into abstract thoughts and memories. It is also vital for mental imagery. Damage to this area can cause complete cessation of dreaming, but loss of lower perceptual areas results in muted perceptual imagery in dreams. These data seem to indicate a reverse

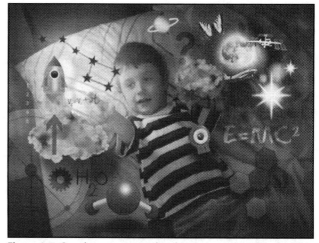

Figure 9-5. One theory suggests that dreams are activated in the brain stem and passively synthesized by the forebrain, which accounts for the random, disconnected, and sometimes bizarre nature of dream imagery. (From Fotolia.com)

order of perceptual processing during dreaming. Activation of the motivational mechanisms of the brain that help produce dreaming disallows action because of the atonia that is a hallmark of REM sleep. Since there cannot be physical acting out of the dream sequence because the motor system is inhibited, activation appears to move backward toward the perceptual area so that actions and motivated behaviors are imagined rather than acted out. Inactivation of the reflective areas in the limbic brain also leads the sleeper to mistake the dream for reality. Damage to this area of the brain may cause inability to distinguish dreams from reality during the waking state.

The neurobiology of dreaming appears to entail cholinergic activation from the brain stem during REM sleep that activates the motivational system of the mesolimbic and mesocortical dopaminergic pathways. Activation moves backward to the perceptual areas in the parieto-occipito-temporal junction to create the abstract imagery that usually occurs during dreaming. This activation is not restricted to REM sleep but can occur during all stages of NREM sleep as well. Even with the increasing understanding of the neuroanatomical underpinnings of dream sleep, understanding the functional content of dreams remains elusive.

In healthy adults, REM periods occur approximately every 90 to 110 minutes. About 85% to 90% of awakenings from REM sleep result in a dream report. REM sleep dream narratives appear to be as long as the REM sleep period and can last from a few minutes to as long as 30 minutes. Dreams that occur during REM sleep are predictable, frequent, and prolonged. However, dreaming is not limited to REM sleep. Frequent dreaming also occurs at sleep onset in the absence of REM sleep, which explains why an individual may report dreaming if awakened shortly after falling asleep or dream reports that occur during an afternoon nap that are not long enough to progress to REM sleep.

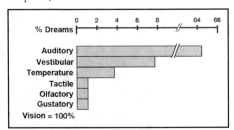

Figure 9-6. Graphic representation of the sensory content of dreams.

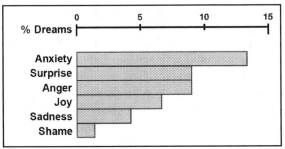

Figure 9-7. Graphic representation of the emotional content of dreams.

When subjects are in a quiet, darkened room with their eyes closed, approximately 25% of those aroused from this state of relaxed wakefulness will report dreamlike imagery, which are hallucinated, dramatic events even though EEG tracings reveal that they were not asleep. In fact, frequent and often prolonged dreaming can occur in all states of EEG-defined consciousness, including relaxed wakefulness at sleep onset, and during all stages of NREM sleep and REM sleep.

Dream content gathered from awakenings from on-the-spot dream retrieval in a sleep lab suggests, however, that most dreams come from REM sleep. The majority of these dreams are typically mundane, realistic experiences in which the dreamer has modest feelings appropriate to the dream situation and usually speaks with language that is similar to how he or she communicates during wakefulness. Dreams are not faithful reproductions of memories; rather, they are novel experiences with a thematic coherence like an invented story or narrative. However, in a single night, a sleeper may have several REM and NREM dream reports that are usually not thematically related like chapters in a book. The thematic coherence within each dream is so regular and persistent that it seems unlikely that dreams could be the product of a disorganized and randomly firing brain.

The typical dream is a REM sleep narrative that is relatively long, primarily a visual experience that is somewhat emotional, and not usually connected with the current life of the sleeper (Figures 9-6 and 9-7). Compared to the REM narrative, the typical NREM narrative is usually shorter, less perceptual, and a more thought-like mentation with less emotion and a connection to the current life of the sleeper.

Dreams that occur at sleep onset are remarkably similar to REM sleep dream reports. Compared to REM sleep dreams, these are shorter thematic sequences that may manifest sexual or aggressive content that is hedonic and bizarre.

NREM and REM narratives of dream length, vividness, emotionality, and distortion correlate positively with psychopathology scores on the Minnesota Multiphasic Personality Inventory.[51] It seems that emotional activation or tone during sleep parallels emotional activation or tone during wakefulness. Over the menstrual cycle in normal women, waking mood changes correlate positively with mood changes in REM sleep narratives. Depressed patients tend to have a depressive tone in their REM sleep narratives, and schizophrenic patients have disorganized, incoherent REM sleep reports similar to periods of hallucinations during wakefulness. These findings support a continuity hypothesis that dreams continue certain formal characteristics of waking mental life. Contrary to common belief, presleep stimuli and stimuli presented during sleep have only a minimal effect on dream content.

Dreaming is not usually present and reported regularly before 7 to 9 years of age. Across this age range, differences in dream reports are more strongly related to certain cognitive skill development than to psychosocial or emotional status. In other words, construction of dreams seems to be dependent on the presence of cognitive abilities to analyze, manipulate, and construct visuospatial images or ideas. Classical psychoanalytical theory postulates that emotional processes construct dreams, and that dreams are instigated by the relatively infrequent, unpredictable, forbidden unconscious that may exert its influence during sleep, when the rational brain is not in control (see Figures 9-6 and 9-7). In this theory, the dream is a hallucinated, disguised fulfillment of a wish. This theory further suggests that dream distortion is a virtually universal feature of adult dreams because it serves to distinguish the forbidden wish. Because children have not yet developed a conscience, their dreams are clear wish fulfillments without distortion.

The classical psychoanalytical theory presents some flaws in its argument in that the theory cannot easily explain the frequent and predictable nature of REM sleep dreams. Its reliance on dream distortions does not explain the usual mundane, undistorted quality of most adult dreams and the absence of undisguised wishes in children's dreams. Nor does the theory account for the abundant dreaming that occurs throughout all states of consciousness and the differences between REM sleep dreams and NREM sleep dreams.

Summary

A summary of the current scientific understanding of dreams reveals that there is an abundance of dreaming in all states of consciousness from wakefulness and sleep onset to all stages of NREM and REM sleep. There is an unexpected thematic coherence of dream content across dreams but not between episodes of dreams. There is an isolation of dreams from other mental and physical events just prior to sleep onset and during sleep. Cognitive skill rather than emotional needs drive dream construction.

Dreams are generated in the forebrain and can exist in the absence of REM sleep, contrary to long-held beliefs that REM sleep is the only time in which an individual dreams. The neurological pathways involved in the dream state appear to be dopaminergic and progress in a bottom-up manner in order to generate the perceptual content of the dream without acting out the motivation, behavioral part of the dream. This is due to a blocking of the motor system, which prevents sleepers from acting out their dreams.

In addition, although current research has been able to better delineate the neurobiological substrate of dreams, the function and content analysis of dreams continue to be somewhat of a mystery.

References

1. Gilliand M. Laudator Temporis Acti. Sleep and Death. Available at: http://laudatortemporisacti.blogspot.com/2004/06/sleep-and-death.html. Acessed July 2, 2013.
2. Lewis CS. *The Discarded Image*. Cambridge, UK: Cambridge University Press; 1964.
3. Callois R. Logical and philosophical problems of the dream. In: *The Dream and Human Societies*. Berkeley, CA: University of California Press; 1966;23-50.
4. Lincoln JS. *The Dream in Primitive Cultures*. London, UK: Cressett; 1935.
5. Gackenbach J, Sheikh A, eds. Languages of dreaming: anthropological approaches to the study of dreaming in other cultures. In: Gackenbach J, Sheikh A, eds. *Dream Images: A Call to Mental Arms*. Amityville, NY: Baywood; 1991:103-224.
6. Tedlock B. Quiche Maya dream interpretation. *Ethos*. 1981;9:313-350.
7. Bulkeley K. *Dreaming in the World's Religions: A Comparative History*. New York, NY: New York University Press; 2008.
8. O'Neil CW. *Dreams, Culture and the Individual*. San Francisco, CA: Chandler & Sharp; 1976.
9. Edgar IR, Henig D. Istikhara: the guidance and practice of Islamic dream incubation through ethnographic comparison. *Hist Anthropol*. 2010;21:251-262.
10. Shakespeare W. *Hamlet*. Act 3, scene 1, line 57.
11. Shakespeare W. *Macbeth*. Act 2, scene 2, line 37.
12. Shakespeare W. *Richard III*. Act 5, scene 2, line 327-330.
13. Thinkquest. Dream history. Available at: http://library.thinkquest.org/11189/nfhistory.htm. Accessed May 18, 2012.
14. Catholic Online. Lives of the saints. Available at: http://www.catholic.org/saints/stindex.php. Accessed May 18, 2012.
15. Freud S. *The Interpretation of Dreams*. New York, NY: Avon; 1900.
16. Carrol L. *Alice in Wonderland and Through the Looking Glass*. Classic Books International. 2009. New York, NY.
17. Lovecraft HP. *Dreams of Terror and Death: Dream Cycle of HP Lovecraft*. A Del Rey Book. New York, NY: Ballantine Books; 1995.
18. Ende M. *The Neverending Story*. Dutton Children's Books. New York, NY: Penguin Putnam Inc; 1984.
19. Hitchcock A. (Director). (1945). *Spellbound* [Film]. Los Angeles: United Artists.
20. Frankenheimer J. (Director). (1962). *The Manchurian Candidate* [Film]. Los Angeles: United Artists.
21. Demme J. (Director, Producer). (2004). *The Manchurian Candidate* [Film]. Los Angeles: Paramount Studios.
22. Ruben J. (Director). (1984). *Dreamscape*. [Film]. Los Angeles: 20th Century Fox.
23. Nolan C. (Director, Producer). (2010). *Inception*. [Film]. Los Angeles: Warner Bros. Pictures.
24. Kelly DD. Sleep and dreaming. In: Kandel E, Schwartz J, Jessell T, eds. *Principles of Neural Science*. 4th ed. New York, NY: McGraw-Hill Medical; 2000;936-947.
25. Domhoff GW. *The Scientific Study of Dreams: Neural Networks, Cognitive Development, and Content Analysis*. Washington, DC: American Psychological Association Press; 2003.
26. Hobson JA. McCarley R. The brain as a dream state generator: an activation-synthesis hypothesis of the dream process. *Am J Psychiat*. 1977;134(12):1335-1348.
27. Solms M. Dreaming and REM sleep are controlled by different brain mechanisms. *Behav Brain Sci*. 2000;23:793-1121.
28. Zhang J. Memory process and the function of sleep. *Journal of Theoretics*. 2004;6. Available at: http://citeseerx.ist.psu.edu/viewdoc/download?doi=10.1.1.65.4332&rep=rep1&type=pdf. Accessed October 2, 2013;2-3.
29. Zhang J. Continual-activation theory of dreaming. *Dynamical Psychology*. 2005. Available at: http://www.goertzel.org/dynapsyc/2005/ZhangDreams.htm. Accessed November 11, 2011;vol 6-6.
30. Tarnow E. How dreams and memory may be related. *Neuro-Psychoanalysis*. 2003;5. Available at: http://cogprints.org/2068/1/DreamsAndMemoryTarnow.pdf. Accessed November 11, 2011;3-16.
31. Stickgold R, Hobson JA, Fosse R, Fosse M. Sleep, learning, and dreams: off-line memory reprocessing. *Science*. 2001;294:1052-1057.
32. Payne JD, Nadel L. Sleep, dreams, and memory consolidation: the role of the stress hormone cortisol. *Learn Mem*. 2004;11:671-678.
33. Crick F, Mitchison G. The function of dream sleep. *Nature*. 1983;304:111-114.
34. Evans C, Newman E. Dreaming: an analogy from computers. *New Sci*. 1964;419:577-579.
35. Hennevin E, Hars B. Post-learning paradoxical sleep: a critical period when new memory is reactivated? In: Will BE, Schmidt P, Dalrymple-Afford JC, eds. *Brain Plasticity, Learning and Memory*. New York, NY: Plenum; 1985:193-203.
36. Coutts R. Dreams as modifiers and tests of mental schemas: an emotional selection hypothesis. *Psychol Rep*. 2008;102:561-574.
37. Revonsuo A. The reinterpretation of dreams: an evolutionary hypothesis of the function of dreaming. *Behav Brain Sci*. 2000;23:877-901.
38. Franklin M, Zyphur M. The role of dreams in the evolution of the human mind. *Evol Psychol*. 2005;3:59-78.
39. Blackmore S. *Consciousness: An Introduction*. New York, NY: Oxford University Press; 2004.
40. Blechner M. *The Dream Frontier*. Hillsdale, NJ: The Analytic Press; 2001.
41. Griffin J. The origin of dreams: how and why we evolved to dream. *Therapist*. 1997;4(3):24-28.

42. Griffin J, Tyrrell I. *Dreaming Reality: How Dreaming Keeps Us Sane or Can Drive Us Mad*. UK: Human Givens Publishing; 2004.

43. Watanabe T. Lucid dreaming: its experimental proof and psychological conditions. *J Int Soc Life Inf Sci*. 2003;21:159-162.

44. The Lucidity Institute. Lucid dreaming FAQ. Available at: http://www.psychwww.com/asc/ld/faq.html. Accessed November 11, 2011.

45. Humphrey ME, Zangwill OL. Cessation of dreaming after brain injury. *J Neurol Neurosurg Psychiatry*. 1951;14:322-325.

46. Schwartz S, Maquet P. Sleep imaging and the neuro-psychological assessment of dreams. *Trends Cogn Sci*. 2002;6:23-30.

47. Hobson JA, Pace-Schott EF, Stickgold R. Dreaming and the brain: toward a cognitive neuroscience of conscious states. *Behav Brain Sci*. 2000;23:793-842.

48. Hobson JA. *The Dreaming Brain: How the Brain Creates Both the Sense and the Nonsense of Dreams*. New York, NY: Basic Books; 1988.

49. Solms M. The interpretation of dreams and the neurosciences. Available at: http://www.psychoanalysis.org.uk/solms4.htm. Accessed November 12, 2011.

50. Solms M. Dreaming and REM sleep are controlled by different brain mechanisms. *Behav Brain Sci*. 2000;23:843-850.

51. Antrobus JS, Bertini M. *The Neuropsychology of Sleep and Dreaming*. Hillsdale, NJ: Lawrence Erlbaum Associates Inc; 1992:248.

The Function of Sleep

Julie M. Hereford, PT, DPT

The human mammal spends one third of life sleeping, and other members of the animal kingdom may spend substantially more or less. Sleep is such a persistent and regular activity, yet the reason why humans sleep remains unclear. It is difficult to find a clear answer when sleeping subjects themselves are so difficult to study, because they are unable to report on their state while in the process. A multitude of studies have been undertaken to find answers about the function of sleep. Observational studies that look at the effects of sleep deprivation on healthy subjects have shown that even short-term sleep deprivation can cause physiological changes associated with the development of disease. Short-term sleep deprivation causes increased stress, increased blood pressure, impaired control of blood sugar, and increased inflammation. Cross-sectional epidemiological studies of populations that report decreased habitual sleep duration or habitual increased sleep duration (greater than 9 hours per night) show an increased prevalence of hypertension, diabetes, and obesity than their regular-sleeping counterparts. Finally, long-term studies have been undertaken to track sleep habits that may be associated with the development of disease. Thus far, these observational and epidemiological studies universally indicate that sleep is a vital function, and chronic sleep loss is associated with the development of certain diseases such as hypertension, cardiovascular disease, and diabetes, but they do not clarify a precise reason for why humans sleep.

Sleep appears to be a function of the brain rather than a function of the body. Sleep may influence cognition in many ways including the removal of toxic by-products of wakefulness or the restoration of neural substances needed for mental processes. It has also been suggested that sleep promotes brain plasticity. Sleep is regulated in much the same way that feeding, thirst, and breathing are regulated. This suggests that sleep serves a similar critical role in health and well-being.

Although the reason for sleep is not completely clear, a good night's sleep makes one feel more alert, energetic, happy, and better able to function. Going without adequate sleep makes one feel worse. As with good nutrition, good sleep is a staple of optimal health. If one compares sleep with other life-sustaining processes such as feeding, one can see it has significant similarities. For instance, hunger is a protective mechanism that has evolved to ensure that the organism consumes the proper nutrients that it needs to grow, repair, and function properly. Both eating and sleeping are regulated by internal drives. Going without food produces the uncomfortable sensation of hunger and increases the drive to obtain food. Similarly, going without sleep causes overwhelming sleepiness and increases sleep drive until the need is fulfilled. Sleep is a biological imperative, and yet its precise function is not completely clear.

Studies designed to answer the question of the function of sleep have taken a number of tacks. Because of the inherent difficulty in studying sleep, some of the ideas regarding the function of sleep are conjecture. Some conclusions have been drawn by observing the consequences of sleep deprivation in both humans and animals. Although a number of theories have been developed, it is likely that no one theory will adequately explain the function of sleep but, rather, find that there are multiple functions. This chapter will explore a number of the most commonly held theories that answer the question of why we sleep.

Hereford JM. *Sleep and Rehabilitation: A Guide for Health Professionals* (pp 85-89). © 2014 Taylor & Francis Group.

INACTIVITY OR PRESERVATION THEORY

One of the earliest theories of the function of sleep suggests that sleep developed as an adaptive or evolutionary process. This ecological hypothesis of foraging and predator avoidance suggests that suppression of motor activity during the sleep period is an adaptation that serves a survival function by keeping the animal safe from attracting the attention of predators that are active when the animal might be particularly vulnerable to predation[1]. It seems unlikely that such a complex physiological process as sleep would have evolved merely to keep animals out of harm's way when waking; behavioral inactivity would serve the same purpose. The preservation theory does not explain why the brain disengages from the external environment during normal sleep. In fact, animals subject to predation are more vulnerable to predation while sleeping because of their decreased sensitivity to external stimuli during sleep, so prey animals sleep less than predators. It is always safer to remain conscious in order to be able to react to an emergency, even if lying still in the dark at night. Therefore, the inactivity/preservation theory does not seem to illustrate an advantage of being unconscious and asleep if safety is paramount. This theory does not address the animal's drive for sleep, causing it to alter behavior in order to obtain sleep. It also fails to explain why carnivores at the top of the food chain, such as lions, sleep more than animals lower in the chain. Clearly, they are not hiding from predators. Some aquatic mammals sleep while moving in an elaborate adaptation that is designed to allow them to sleep with one-half of their brains at a time. Continuous movement is necessary so that the animal can come up for air as necessary, even while sleeping. This adaptation keeps these animals alive but certainly does not hide them from predators, providing more evidence against the inactivity/preservation theory. Animals that are deprived of sleep will undergo a period of recovery sleep regardless of the increased vulnerability to predation. Though the inactivity/preservation theory may account for some aspects of the function of sleep, overall this theory does not seem sufficient to explain the complexities of sleep.

ENERGY CONSERVATION THEORY

One of the strongest factors in natural selection is competing for and gathering food and effectively utilizing energy resources. The energy conservation theory suggests that the primary function of sleep is to reduce the animal's energy demands and expenditures during part of the day or night, especially at times when it is least efficient to forage for food.

The energy conservation theory of sleep suggests that sleep serves to reduce the metabolic rate and body temperature in warm-blooded animals and birds during periods

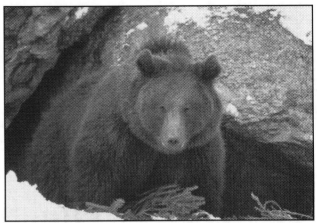

Figure 10-1. Hibernation—a long winter's nap? Then why do animals emerge so tired? (From Fotolia.com)

of rest to offset the high energetic costs of endothermy. Research has shown that energy metabolism is significantly reduced during sleep by as much as 10% in humans and even more in other species.[2] When humans, other mammals, and birds fall asleep, the metabolic rate decreases and heat is dissipated from the body through peripheral vasodilatation, which leads to a 1 to 2°C reduction in body temperature. This reduction in body temperature is controlled, at the onset of sleep, through the reduction in the thermosensitivity of neurons of the preoptic nucleus of the hypothalamus below the waking threshold. The preoptic nucleus acts like a thermostat in the brain. During sleep, both body temperature and caloric demand decrease compared to wakefulness. This supports the proposition that one of the primary functions of sleep is to help conserve energy resources. This theory is related to the inactivity theory. A drawback to this theory is that the reduction in basal metabolic rate produced during sleep is not enough to offset the energy expenditure while the animal is active during the day.

An argument can be made that energy conservation and restoration could just as well be accomplished by resting quietly without sleep, which could expose the unaware animal to dangerous situations of predation. Another example is found in the hibernating animal, which is clearly resting and has decreased energy requirements during the period of hibernation. The animal will wake from hibernation and go immediately into rebound sleep because of the lack of sleep during hibernation (Figure 10-1). Clearly, sleep serves an additional function other than energy conservation.

RESTORATIVE THEORY

This theory suggests that sleep serves to reverse and/or restore physiological processes that are progressively degraded during prior wakefulness (Figure 10-2). Sleep provides an opportunity for the body to repair and

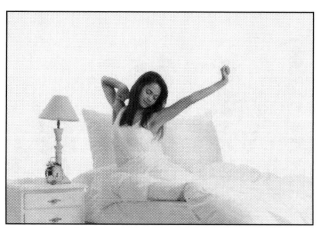

Figure 10-2. Is the purpose of sleep to repair and restore the body and mind? (From Fotolia.com)

rejuvenate itself. Animals deprived entirely of sleep lose all immune function and the ability to regulate body temperature; this would cause them to die within a matter of weeks. This theory is also supported by findings that many of the major restorative functions in the body such as muscle growth, tissue repair, protein synthesis, and human growth hormone release occur mostly, or in some cases only, during sleep.

Other rejuvenating aspects of sleep are specific to brain and cognitive function. While awake, neurons in the brain produce adenosine, a by-product of the cells' activities. The buildup of adenosine in the brain is thought to be one factor that leads to the perception of being tired. This feeling can be counteracted by the use of caffeine, which blocks the actions of adenosine in the brain and keeps it alert. The buildup of adenosine during wakefulness may promote the drive to sleep. As long as the individual is awake, adenosine accumulates and never declines. During sleep, the body has a chance to clear adenosine from the system and, as a result, the individual feels more alert on awakening.

There are several pieces of evidence that support the restorative theory. First, there are widespread detrimental psychological and behavioral effects that are experienced with the loss of sleep. Increased human growth hormone secretion occurs immediately following sleep onset, which remains synchronized with sleep even when normal sleep patterns are inverted. There is an increased amount and "intensity" of sleep during a period of sleep recovery after 24 hours of sleep deprivation in humans and most other mammals. On the contrary, the fact that there is a decrease rather than an increase in protein synthesis during sleep in humans does not seem to support this theory.

Restoration and repair of the body occur during sleep. Wound healing has been shown to be affected by sleep.[3] Animal studies have shown that sleep deprivation has a detrimental impact on white cell count.[4] Sleep also appears to enhance an endogenous antioxidant mechanism in the brain, which helps reduce the accumulation of free radicals in the brain.[1] Not only does sleep loss impair immune function, but challenges to the immune system in the form of viral illnesses alter sleep in order to improve immune function.[5] The metabolic phase during sleep is anabolic. Anabolic hormones such as human growth hormone are preferentially secreted during sleep. Duration of sleep appears to be inversely related to animal size and directly related to basal metabolic rate. For example, rats, which have a very high basal metabolic rate, sleep for up to 14 hours per 24-hour period, but elephants and giraffes, which have much lower basal metabolic rates, sleep far less. In fact, giraffes sleep the shortest amount of time per 24-hour period, averaging just 1.9 hours.[6,7]

MEMORY PROCESSING

There is an increasing body of literature that links sleep to memory processing and memory consolidation. Working memory—or that which keeps information actively available for further processing and is used to support higher level functions including decision making and reasoning—has been shown to be affected by sleep deprivation.[8] Memory is affected differently by certain stages of sleep. For example, in a study conducted by Born et al,[9] subjects were taught a novel task, and their skill was tested after being awakened at different stages of the sleep cycle. Testing occurred on awakening from the early cycle, which is associated with slow-wave sleep (SWS), and again during the late cycle, which is associated with rapid eye movement (REM) sleep. The early-night test group performed 16% better on declarative memory tasks than the control group that awakened naturally. The late-night test group scored 25% better on the procedural memory part of the memory test compared to the control. Conclusions of this study indicate that declarative memory, also known as *explicit memory*, benefits from SWS that occurs early in the night.[9] This appears to allow consolidation during sleep of memories learned during the daytime, which can then be consciously recalled. *Procedural memory* or *implicit memory* refers to that part of memory for how things are done and involves both cognition and motor skills. This type of memory seems to benefit from late-cycle REM sleep.

It is important to keep in mind that memory processing and both cognitive and motor memory are consolidated during sleep. Sleep disruption can interfere with both cognition and motor skill acquisition.

BRAIN PLASTICITY THEORY

Sleep is correlated to changes in the structure and organization of the brain. This phenomenon, known as *brain plasticity*, is not entirely understood, but its connection to sleep has several critical implications. Sleep appears to play

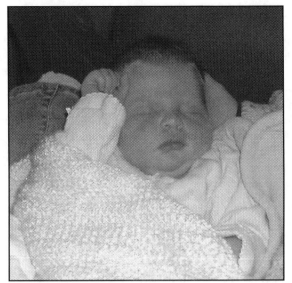

Figure 10-3. Sleep is critical to brain development. (Reprinted with permission from J. Hoskins.)

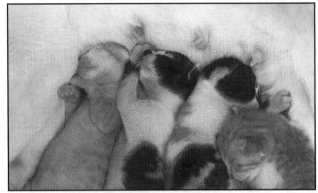

Figure 10-4. Mammals that are more immature at birth, such as the kittens shown, spend more time in REM sleep than those animals that are more mature at birth, such as a calf or foal. Since humans are more immature at birth, newborns spend more time in REM sleep. (From Fotolia.com)

a critical role in brain development in infants and young children (Figure 10-3). Infants spend about 14 to 16 hours per day sleeping and approximately 50% of that sleeping time is REM sleep. A link between sleep and brain plasticity has been found in adults as well. This is seen in the effect that sleep and sleep deprivation have on a person's ability to learn and perform a variety of tasks.

Numerous speculations exist to explain the evolution of REM sleep. It seems likely that REM sleep evolved from non-rapid eye movement (NREM) sleep. Studies have identified a key role that the hypothalamus plays in sleep and wakefulness. Damage to the posterior hypothalamus causes profound somnolence, and damage to the anterior portion induces insomnia. This indicates that the posterior hypothalamus is involved in the maintenance of wakefulness and the anterior hypothalamus is involved in the production of sleep. The hypothalamus is also involved in temperature regulation, and neurons that regulate both sleep and thermoregulation have been identified.[10] Because of this connection, one theory suggests that sleep evolved from a more primitive thermostat mechanism. This dual function offers evidence of the evolution of sleep from primitive mechanisms involved in temperature regulation.

REM sleep has also been implicated in brain growth, fine-tuning of the binocular oculomotor system, consolidation of memory, erasure of inappropriate memories, and harmless discharge of strong emotions during sleep that would otherwise intrude into waking behavior. The prodigious amounts of REM sleep that occur during fetal and infantile developments seem especially compelling arguments for the ontogenetic role of REM sleep. It has also been suggested that the maintenance of homeothermy of the brain is a function of REM sleep during early stages of life when thermoregulatory mechanisms are incompletely developed.

Other evidence of the importance of REM sleep or active sleep during the neonatal period comes from studies that show that the effects of sleep deprivation can result in behavioral problems, permanent sleep disruption, decrease in brain mass, and an abnormal degree of neuronal destruction.[11,12] The importance of REM sleep seems evident because it occupies the majority of neonatal and infant sleep (Figure 10-4). In fact, the more immature an animal is at birth, the greater the percentage of sleep spent in the REM stage. Because of the atonia characteristic of REM sleep, the increased amount of REM sleep may allow for brain development without interference from motor activity.

Roffwarg et al[13] speculated that the spontaneous, repetitive firing of neural circuits during REM sleep in fetal life facilitates neuronal circuitry development and maintenance. This theory led to the development of a model called the *dynamic stabilization of neural circuitry*. This model helps to explain the mechanisms that enhance and maintain synaptic capability that is involved in processing and consolidation of memory. It occurs during spontaneous oscillations in the brain during sleep. Dynamic stabilization is a necessary element involved in the development of neural circuitry, as well as its maturation, fine-tuning, and maintenance. It occurs almost exclusively in REM sleep in fetal life. In infancy and childhood, which are marked by intense episodes of new learning and development of the brain, there is an extensive amount of dynamic stabilization of neural circuitry that occurs primarily during sleep. In fact, evidence suggests that dynamic stabilization that occurs during sleep helps to maintain inherited (phylogenetic) and ontogenetic memories in children and adult humans. Ontogenetic memories are described as those that are acquired through experience.[14,15] Research by Margoliash[16] suggested the possibility of a signal gate that allows signal strengthening and refinement of newly learned information in an off-line scheme of memory consolidation that occurs during sleep.

During NREM sleep, muscle tone is reduced, but it is completely absent during REM sleep. Atonia during REM sleep is usually speculated to be an inhibitory mechanism that keeps the sleeper from acting out his or her dreams. However, it is more likely that it has evolved to inhibit motor function during motor circuit reinforcement as occurs in dynamic stabilization during REM sleep.[17]

SUMMARY

Though various theories have been published regarding the function of sleep, it is increasingly clear that sleep has multiple functions ranging from stress reduction to disease prevention rather than a single function such as energy conservation. It is further known to be necessary to the preservation and restoration of the organism. All mammals, birds, and most amphibians, fish, and reptiles sleep. Sleep appears to have evolved from a mechanism of rest, and REM sleep is believed to have evolved from NREM sleep. Such an elaborate and complex system is vital to the survival of creatures that sleep. This is evidenced by the illness and degeneration that can occur in situations of chronic sleep deprivation. In fact, experimental models have shown that when a rat is deprived of sleep, it will eventually lose its capacity to maintain body temperature and die.

Sleep has a mutual relationship with and connection to brain plasticity, which refers to alterations in neural pathways and synapses related to changes in an organism's behavior, environment, or biological processes. It plays a critical role in the brain development of infants and children as well as the ability of adults to learn and perform motor tasks.

In humans, sleep has been linked to proper hormonal and immune function and cardiovascular health. There is an increasing body of literature that links sleep to learning and memory consolidation. Sleep deprivation or the presence of a sleep disorder adversely impacts an individual's ability to properly learn and recall a task or motor skill. This function of sleep is very important for the rehabilitation clinician to understand because sleep loss may contribute to poor rehabilitation outcomes. Conversely, it may be possible to manipulate sleep to optimize the rehabilitation process.

REFERENCES

1. Live Science. New theory questions why we sleep. Available at: http://www.livescience.com/10579-theory-questions-sleep.html. Accessed July 12, 2011.
2. Zepelin H, Rechtschaffen A. Mammalian sleep, longevity, and energy metabolism. *Brain Behav Evol.* 1974;10:447-470.
3. Gumustekin K, Seven B, Karabulut N, et al. Effects of sleep deprivation, nicotine, and selenium on wound healing in rats. *Int J Neurosci.* 2004;114:1433-1442.
4. Zager A, Andersen ML, Ruiz FS, Antunes IB, Tufik S. Effects of acute and chronic sleep loss on immune modulation of rats. *Regul Integr Comp Physiol.* 2007;293:R504-R509.
5. Cirelli C, Tononi G. Is sleep essential? *PLoS Biol.* 2008;6(8):e216.
6. Capellini I, Barton RA, McNamara P, et al. Phylogenetic analysis of the ecology and evolution of mammalian sleep. *Evolution.* 2008;62:1764-1776.
7. Energetics and metabolism. Available at: http://www.cartage.org.lb/en/themes/sciences/zoology/animalphysiology/energeticsmetabolism/energeticsmetabolism.htm. Accessed July 11, 2011.
8. Turner TH, Drummond SPA, Salamat JS, Brown GG. Effects of 42 hr sleep deprivation on component processes of verbal working memory. *Neuropsychology.* 2007;21:787-795.
9. Born J, Rasch B, Gais S. Sleep to remember. *Neuroscientist.* 2006;12:410-424.
10. Parmeggiani PL. Thermoregulation and sleep. *Frontiers Biosci.* 2003;8:s557-s567.
11. Morrissey M, Duntley S, Anch A, Nonneman R. Active sleep and its role in the prevention of apoptosis in the developing brain. *Med Hypotheses.* 2004;62:876-879.
12. Jenni OG, Molinari L, Caflisch JA, Largo RH. Sleep duration from ages 1 to 10 years: variability and stability in comparison with growth. *Pediatrics.* 2007;120:e769-e776.
13. Roffwarg HP, Muzio JN, Dement WC. Ontogenetic development of the human sleep–dream cycle. *Science.* 1966;152:604-619.
14. Kavanau JL. Sleep and dynamic stabilization of neural circuitry: a review and synthesis. *Behav Brain Res.* 1994;63:111-126.
15. Mahowald MW, Schenck CH. Evolving concepts of human state dissociation. *Arch Ital Biol.* 2001;139:269-300.
16. Margoliash D. Sleep, learning and birdsong. *ILAR J.* 2010;51:378-386.
17. Kavanau JL. Memory, sleep and dynamic stabilization of neural circuitry: evolutionary perspectives. *Neurosci Biobehav Rev.* 1996;20(2):289-311.

Section II

Basic Science of Disordered Sleep

11

Manifestations of Disordered Sleep

Julie M. Hereford, PT, DPT

A sleep disorder is defined as any abnormal pattern that interferes with a normal sleep cycle. Sleep disorders may be mild, such as light snoring that does not interfere with breathing, or may be serious enough to interfere with normal physical function, mental acuity, or psychological well-being. The American Academy of Sleep Medicine has identified as least 84 separate sleep disorders.[1]

Sleep disruption may be caused by a wide variety of anatomical, neurological, and environmental factors including nocturnal teeth grinding (bruxism), change in light exposure, night terrors, or central or obstructive sleep apnea. Sleep disorders may occur that are characterized by difficulty in initiation or maintenance of sleep without a clear physiological cause; this is known as *primary insomnia*. Those related to circadian rhythm involve inability to stay awake, to fall asleep, or to awaken at a socially acceptable time but do not involve any problem with maintenance of sleep. Transient or situational circadian rhythm disorders include jet lag and shift work sleep syndrome. Disordered sleep may result in excessive daytime sleepiness, which may culminate in falling asleep spontaneously, but unwillingly, at inappropriate times or places.

Parasomnias are disruptive sleep-related events involving inappropriate actions during sleep and include sleepwalking, night terrors, periodic limb movements, restless leg/legs syndrome, hypnic jerk, or nocturnal myoclonus, and rapid eye movement (REM) behavior disorder.

Sleep-related breathing disorders include central and obstructive sleep apnea, in which there is insufficient respiratory effort to effectively ventilate the sleeper, and hypopnea syndrome, in which there is abnormally shallow breathing or slow respiratory rate during sleeping.

Sleep disorders can also be categorized by those that are intrinsic (ie, caused by factors from within the body), extrinsic (ie, causes that are attributed to environmental conditions or pathological conditions) and disturbances of circadian rhythm. Table 11-1 summarizes these conditions.

MANIFESTATIONS OF SLEEP DISORDERS

Sleep-related disorders are quite common in the general population and can present in a variety of ways. Individuals with disordered sleep may experience job or school performance problems. They may have a history of accidents at work or while driving. They may report depression or mood disorders or have developed problems with interpersonal relationships. Disordered sleep may contribute to the development of or exacerbation of medical, neurological, or psychiatric problems.

Individuals who have disordered sleep may describe symptoms of insomnia or difficulty initiating or maintaining sleep. They may report excessive daytime sleepiness or report frequent awakenings during a night's sleep. They may report abnormal movements or behaviors while asleep or on awakening during the night. Interviewing the individual's bed partner may also provide important information, because the one with disordered sleep may not be aware of the signs of disordered sleep such as snoring, momentary cessation of breathing, gasping, or abnormal limb movements during sleep. These symptoms may occur in isolation or might be combined. The individual suffering

Hereford JM. *Sleep and Rehabilitation: A Guide for Health Professionals* (pp 93-102). © 2014 Taylor & Francis Group.

Table 11-1.

Summary of Intrinsic and Extrinsic Sleep Disorders

Insomnia	May be a symptom of a mood disorder such as emotional stress, anxiety, or depression or may be caused by an underlying health condition such as asthma, diabetes, heart disease, pregnancy, or certain neurological conditions.
Narcolepsy	Chronic neurological condition caused by inability within the brain to control sleep and wakefulness.
Sleep-related breathing disorders	Includes central sleep apnea, obstructive sleep apnea, and mixed sleep apnea. Also includes snoring and upper airway resistance syndrome.
Restless leg/legs syndrome	Sleep disorder that involves an irresistible, uncomfortable urge or need to move the legs.
Periodic limb movement disorder	Repetitive movement of the arms and legs causing a disruption in sleep.
Hypersomnia	Recurrent hypersomnia including Kleine-Levin syndrome; posttraumatic hypersomnia; "healthy" hypersomnia.
Circadian rhythm sleep disorders	Delayed sleep phase syndrome; advanced sleep phase syndrome; non–24-hour sleep-wake syndrome.
Parasomnias	Sleep disorders that involve abnormal movements, behaviors, or perceptions; includes REM sleep behavior disorder, night terrors, sleepwalking, bruxism, bedwetting, sleep talking, and exploding head syndrome.
Medical or psychiatric conditions that may produce sleep disorders	Psychosis such as schizophrenia, mood disorders such as depression or anxiety, panic disorders, or alcoholism.

from disordered sleep may also report a variety of other symptoms that indicate disordered sleep.

Insomnia

Insomnia is one of the most frequently reported manifestations of disordered sleep. It is described as a complaint of difficulty initiating or maintaining sleep or of nonrefreshing sleep that leads to excessive daytime sleepiness and diminution of performance of daily tasks.[2] According to the National Sleep Foundation, 58% of adults in the United States experience symptoms of insomnia a few nights per week or more frequently.[3] Insomnia may accompany several sleep disorders as well as medical and psychiatric disorders. Insomnia is typically followed by some degree of impaired function during the daytime. It may be transient, acute, or chronic.

Transient insomnia is usually related to an event or situation, such as depression or severe stress, or by changes in the sleep environment that disrupt sleep for one or more nights. With transient insomnia, the sleeper will experience consequences similar to sleep deprivation, such as sleepiness or impaired psychomotor performance, but is able to return to a normal sleep pattern even after one night of sleeplessness.[4] Acute insomnia is described as the inability to sleep well consistently for a period less than 1 month. This difficulty initiating and/or maintaining sleep or poor-quality sleep occurs despite adequate opportunity and

circumstances for sleep. Acute insomnia will also interfere with daytime function. It is often related to stress or significant life-changing events but is not ongoing for longer than 1 month.[1] Chronic insomnia is that which has been going on for more than 1 month and may be a source of marked distress to the individual suffering from the disorder.[5] Chronic insomnia may be a primary disorder or may result from another medical, psychiatric, or environmental issue. Individuals with high levels of stress hormones or shifts in the levels of cytokines are more likely to suffer from chronic insomnia.[6]

This section will primarily deal with the problem of chronic insomnia, because transient and acute insomnia are, by definition, self-limiting. Chronic insomnia may manifest itself at any age but occurs with increasing frequency in older adults and tends to occur more frequently in adult women than in adult men. Insomnia is often subdivided into free-standing primary insomnia, which is insomnia not attributable to any other medical, psychiatric, or environmental cause; primary insomnia comorbid with other condition(s); or insomnia secondary to another condition.[7]

Insomnia may manifest as difficulty initiating sleep, which may also be a symptom of an anxiety disorder or of delayed sleep phase disorder. It may also manifest as frequent or prolonged awakenings in the middle of the night or as awakening very early in the morning and being unable to return to a sleep state, known as *terminal insomnia*.

Middle-of-the-night insomnia may be a symptom of a pain problem or an illness. Terminal insomnia is often a characteristic of clinical depression, in particular, a serotonin deficit (J. P. Rutledge, MD; personal communication, March 2011).

Poor-quality sleep may be a symptom of an underlying sleep disorder such as restless leg/legs syndrome, sleep apnea, or it may be a symptom of major depression. Major depression may lead to a functional alteration of the hypothalamic-pituitary-adrenal axis causing excessive release of cortisol, which interferes with normal sleep. Nocturnal polyuria may also disrupt sleep and is a frequent complaint of an individual who suffers from disordered sleep. It is more likely, however, that the individual's sleep architecture is such that he or she does not fully inhibit detrusor muscles in the bladder during sleep and therefore is more prone to this stimuli intruding upon his or her sleep as opposed to true awakening solely because of the sensation of a full bladder. In other words, the individual arouses to a state in which they become aware of bladder distention rather than bladder distention causing the awakening. An individual who reports poor sleep quality often fails to reach restorative sleep levels, called *delta sleep* or *slow-wave sleep* (SWS).

Sometimes, a self-report of insomnia is not truly insomnia but rather a sleep-state misperception. In this state, the individual actually sleeps for a normal duration and usually displays normal sleep architecture but severely overestimates the time it takes to fall asleep. They may also have the sense that they slept very little, although on polysomnographic (PSG) analysis, they are shown to have normal sleep patterns. Individuals with sleep-state misperception are generally in good health but may have excessive fear and concern associated with their misperception and fear of negative consequences of insomnia, rather than from actual sleep loss.[8,9]

Symptoms of insomnia can be caused by or can be comorbid with a significant number of disorders or behaviors. These may include the use of psychoactive drugs and stimulants including caffeine, nicotine, cocaine, amphetamines, methylphenidate (Ritalin), aripiprazole (Abilify), MDMA (ecstasy), and modafinil (Provigil), or excessive alcohol intake (Figure 11-1). Withdrawal from opioids and benzodiazepines may result in insomnia. Use of fluoroquinolones, a family of synthetic broad-spectrum antibiotics, has been associated with more severe and chronic types of insomnia.[10] Use or abuse of over-the-counter sleep aids can also cause rebound insomnia.

Other conditions that may lead to insomnia or poor sleep quality include restless leg/legs syndrome, which may cause sleep onset insomnia because of uncomfortable sensations in the legs or other body parts that cause the individual to feel like they have to move them constantly. Periodic limb movement occurs during sleep and the sleeper is usually unaware of this occurring, even though it may cause

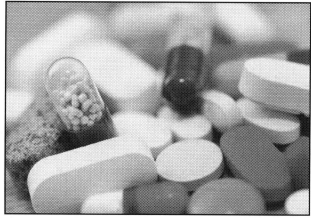

Figure 11-1. Certain medications can lead to or aggravate insomnia. (From Fotolia.com)

arousal from sleep. Often, the bed partner is aware of this symptom and may report it as, "kicking" in his or her sleep.

Pain is a common cause of disrupted or poor-quality sleep. It may manifest itself as initial insomnia, in which the individual has difficulty finding a comfortable position in which to fall asleep, or it may cause frequent awakenings as the sleeper changes positions or as pain increases because of a static position that irritates the injury or condition. The clinician should carefully question an individual who reports pain during sleep to determine the nature of the pain-disrupted sleep. For example, initial insomnia is often associated with an inflammatory condition that has been irritated all day and requires time and rest to settle to a point at which the individual can fall asleep. Sometimes, anti-inflammatory medications are needed or utilized to allow the individual to fall asleep more quickly.

The second type of pain-disrupted sleep is that which arouses or even awakens the individual from sleep during the night. It is important to discern the nature of this kind of painful condition. If the sleeper reports that he or she develops a sharp pain or ache that disrupts sleep but is able to change position, massage the area, or take some pain medication and then return to sleep fairly readily, this may be more indicative of a deranged joint or damaged muscle or ligament. Finally, in evaluating nocturnal pain, what is most important is the type of pain that awakens a sleeper and whether it is described as deep, moderate to severe, or unrelenting aching pain that does not respond to positional change or other attempts to relieve pain. This type of pain usually causes the sleeper to get up and seek some sort of pain relief, which may not be possible or may take a significant amount of time to relieve enough to allow return to sleep. This type of pain is a sign of serious disease and must be further evaluated to discover its source. Metastatic disease, especially bone metastasis, often presents in this fashion and must be addressed immediately.

Hormone shifts such as those that precede menstruation may cause transient insomnia, and those that occur during menopause may lead to chronic insomnia. Significant life events, especially those that induce fear, stress, or anxiety, can cause transient, acute, or chronic insomnia. Emotional turmoil, work stress, financial stress, dealing with an infant child or illness in a family member, and bereavement may also be sources of distress that may lead to periods of insomnia. Mental disorders including clinical depression, anxiety disorders, posttraumatic stress disorders, bipolar disorder, schizophrenia, or dementia may cause chronic insomnia.[11,12]

Disturbances in circadian rhythm such as those that occur in shift workers or travelers experiencing jet lag may cause insomnia and excessive sleepiness during the period in which the individual is supposed to be awake. This situation may present danger to the worker because of impairment in judgment and functional performance of work tasks due to excessive sleepiness. When suffered over a long period, this condition may also contribute significantly to related medical conditions including cardiovascular disease, diabetes, and metabolic syndrome.

Certain medical and neurological conditions may contribute to chronic insomnia such as brain lesions or traumatic brain injury. Hyperthyroidism and rheumatoid arthritis are also known to cause chronic insomnia. Parasomnias such as nightmares, sleepwalking, night terrors, and REM behavior disorder may cause poor sleep quality because of the disruptive effect on sleep. A rare genetic condition can cause a form of insomnia that is eventually fatal, known as *fatal familial insomnia.*[13]

Finally, one of the more common causes of chronic insomnia is induced by poor sleep hygiene. Poor sleep hygiene may be described as habits prior to going to bed for sleep that are not conducive to proper rest. These habits may include imbibing hard liquor, tobacco products, or late-night meals or snacks immediately prior to bedtime. A sedentary lifestyle or excessive daytime napping may also lead to poor quality of sleep or insomnia. Vigorous physical exercise less than 2 hours prior to bedtime may also interfere with sleep and increase sleep latency.

Other habits that encompass poor sleep hygiene may be inattention to time or deliberately staying up too late to accomplish a task. This is seen in students but is increasingly seen in individuals who engage in "screen time," playing video games or surfing the Internet immediately prior to bedtime (Figure 11-2). These habits can have a deleterious impact on the quality and quantity of sleep.

Studies have shown that people who experience sleep disruption have elevated nighttime cortisol and adrenocorticotropic hormone and will have an elevated metabolic rate during the night and during the day compared to normal sleepers. It is not known whether this is a cause or an effect of insomnia (Figure 11-3).[14]

Insomnia is usually diagnosed based on patient report and physical and behavioral findings. Care should be taken to determine whether the patient is suffering from

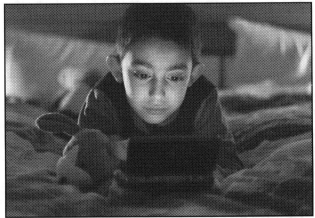

Figure 11-2. Screen time is impinging on sleep time, especially in children. (From Fotolia.com)

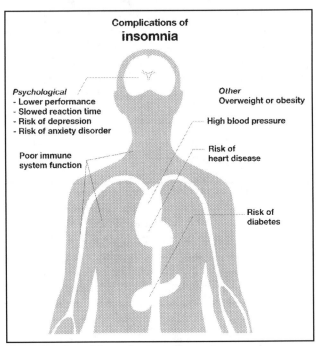

Figure 11-3. Potential complications of insomnia.

primary insomnia or whether there are comorbid factors that contribute to the symptoms. Certain circadian rhythm disorders may be misdiagnosed as primary insomnia. For example, delayed sleep phase syndrome is characterized by difficulty getting to sleep, but once sleep is established, the sleeper shows normal sleep architecture. Comorbidities of insomnia are most frequently other disease processes, side effects from medication, or psychological or psychiatric disorders.[15] Nearly half of all diagnosed cases of insomnia are related to psychiatric disorders such as depression. In depression in particular, the insomnia may predate the onset of other depressive symptoms and is seen as a risk factor in the development of subsequent depression.[13]

Effective treatment for insomnia requires an appropriate history and physical examination to rule out medical and psychological factors that may contribute to the symptoms.

If they are present, insomnia may be effectively combatted by treating the comorbidities. In primary insomnia, however, issues surrounding sleep hygiene should be evaluated and addressed first. This is superior to pharmacological approaches to treatment because of the side effects, dependence, and eventual tolerance to hypnotics and other sleep-promoting agents. Nonpharmacological strategies may include such things as biofeedback, stimulus control therapy, cognitive behavioral therapy, sleep restriction therapy, paradoxical intention therapy, and relaxation therapy (see Chapter 26).

Excessive Daytime Sleepiness

Excessive daytime sleepiness is characterized by unintended falling asleep or falling asleep in inappropriate settings. This persistent sleepiness and sometimes accompanying lack of normal energy during periods when one should be awake and engaged in activity is a symptom of a sleep disorder. Excessive daytime sleepiness can vary in degree and may manifest as a tendency to fall asleep while quietly reading a book. Excessive sleepiness may also intrude more significantly in daytime life, pushing the urge to sleep to an irresistible level and causing an individual to fall asleep while working or driving. These episodes may put the individual in substantial danger of an accident (Figure 11-4). They may also impair quality of life in that the drive for sleep becomes so overwhelming that it interferes with normal daily function. As the compulsion to sleep intensifies, task performance diminishes sharply and may even give an appearance similar to alcohol intoxication. In fact, drowsy driving is at least as dangerous and probably contributes to more motor vehicle accidents than intoxicated driving.[16]

Excessive daytime sleepiness is at its most clinically significant as narcolepsy, in which an individual will suffer sleep attacks that cause sudden onset of sleep that the individual is not able to control.

Diagnosis of excessive daytime sleepiness is usually identified by using one of a number of simple tools, such as the Epworth Sleepiness Scale[17] or the Stanford Sleepiness Scale[18] (see Chapter 28). These tools grade the level of interference that sleepiness has on the individual's normal daily function and, based upon the score, can suggest the need for further evaluation.

Excessive daytime sleepiness may also be evaluated clinically by use of the Multiple Sleep Latency Test[19], also called a *nap study*, which is performed in a sleep lab and is used to measure sleep latency, or the length of time it takes from the start of a daytime nap period to the first signs of sleep. This test is often performed following a full PSG evaluation and will measure sleep latency across multiple trials. The sleepier an individual is, the faster he or she will tend to fall asleep. Following a normal night's sleep, an individual

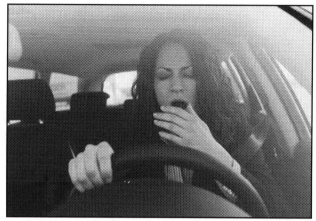

Figure 11-4. Sleep disorders can be extremely dangerous to the patient and others. (From Fotolia.com)

should have difficulty falling back to sleep after he or she has been awake for an hour or more.

Excessive daytime sleepiness can be a symptom of a number of sleep disorders or may be related to coexisting factors. The primary reason for excessive daytime sleepiness is insufficient quantity or quality of sleep the night before. This may be because of another sleep disorder such as sleep apnea or restless leg/legs syndrome or may be related to circadian factors such as jet lag or shift work. There may be psychiatric factors that contribute to excessive daytime sleepiness such as clinical depression or drug addiction. Medical factors may also be involved and may include tumor, head trauma, anemia, kidney failure, hypothyroidism, or central nervous system disorders.

Because of the emphasis on work ethic and the often negative connotations associated with daytime napping, excessive daytime sleepiness can be seen as willful behavior that is a sign of disinterest or laziness. In fact, it is usually a manifestation of an underlying disorder, not an indication of a behavioral problem. It is particularly important for educators to understand that if a student regularly falls asleep in the classroom, it is not a reflection on the student's interest or the teacher's ability; it is likely related to a treatable issue. Proper diagnosis and treatment will help mitigate sleep behavior and will likely improve performance.

In some instances, even after the underlying disorder is treated, excessive daytime sleepiness remains. In these situations, certain medications have been proven to be effective in treating the symptom, including modafinil (Provigil) or armodafinil (Nuvigil).

Sleep Apnea

Sleep apnea is one of the most common sleep disorders and is characterized by abnormal pauses in breathing during sleep. The cost of untreated sleep apnea can be great both in terms of financial responsibility and long-term health. The average untreated sleep apnea patient's annual health care costs are estimated to be $1336 more than the individual without sleep apnea. This results in an annual bill of $3.4 billion in the United States alone.[20]

Apneic episodes may last for a few seconds to several minutes and may occur many times during the course of 1 hour. An individual may also experience decreased respiratory effort, called *hypopnea*, during sleep. These apneic and hypopneic episodes can be documented during PSG or a sleep study and analyzed along with electroencephalogram (EEG), electromyogram (EMG), and electrooculogram (EOG) information in order to identify sleep apnea or other sleep disorders. Sleep apnea may be centrally mediated, in which there is a loss of respiratory drive and thus a cessation of breathing. That is, the central mechanisms that cause breathing are disrupted and do not drive respiratory effort and thus result in the cessation of breathing. Breathing is reestablished not because of the drop in oxygen saturation but rather because of the rise in CO_2 level. Obviously, this situation will result in sequelae of physiological activity (see Chapter 17).

Sleep apnea may also be obstructive, in which respiratory drive continues but there is a loss of respiratory effort. In this situation, there is a structural component in the upper airway that results in airway collapse that the respiratory drive is not able to overcome. This obstructs respiration, and the brain continues to send impulses to drive respiratory effort, but with insufficient force to overcome the collapse of the airway. Generally, this situation causes arousal from sleep, disrupting sleep architecture, but allowing additional respiratory effort to overcome the obstruction, and the sleeper goes back to normal sleep. This process tends to repeat itself over and over across a night's sleep, resulting in sleep disturbance. It is sometimes witnessed as snoring or as an irregular breathing pattern by a bed partner (Figure 11-5). Over time, this process will result in decline of sleep efficiency and efficacy. An individual with sleep apnea may become conditioned to excessive daytime sleepiness and fatigue and may not be able to identify this with disordered sleep. He or she may also have a number of other sequelae of disordered sleep that are being treated but have not been identified as associated with an underlying sleep disorder (see Chapter 12).

Apnea may also manifest itself as a mixed apnea, which is a combination of central and obstructive disorders. Approximately 0.4% of all sleep apnea is said to be only centrally mediated, 84% is obstructive, and 15% is mixed apnea.

Signs and symptoms of sleep apnea occur in both adults and children. Those with sleep apnea are likely to complain about excessive daytime sleepiness, functional performance impairment, and issues with alertness. It can lead to daytime fatigue, slowed reaction time, and vision problems. Individuals with sleep apnea may experience difficulties with executive functions, such as planning and initiating tasks. They may experience problems with attention to the

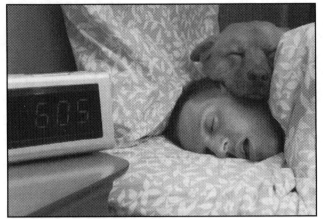

Figure 11-5. Untreated sleep apnea can have both physical and emotional consequences. (From Fotolia.com)

task, working effectively and efficiently, and appropriately processing incoming sensory data. Learning and memory may also be affected by sleep apnea. Because of excessive daytime sleepiness and the potential of microsleeps that disrupt the daytime cognitive state, behavioral effects may also be present. These may include moodiness, irritability, and a decrease in attentiveness and motivational drive. Ongoing problems with sleep apnea and its consequences may lead to the development of depression.

Diagnosis of sleep apnea is based on clinical evaluation and the results of a formal sleep study or PSG. PSG will analyze sleep across the night using EEG, EMG, and EOG data. This will give information regarding the apnea–hypopnea index and/or the respiratory disturbance index, which will help to qualify the existence of and severity of sleep apnea. It can also determine the type of sleep apnea; whether it is central, obstructive, or mixed. PSG is open to some interpretation, and currently most sleep labs use the guidelines revised by the American Academy of Sleep Medicine in 2007.[19] For instance, this sets the criteria for apnea in an adult as a minimum of 10-second intervals between breaths with either a neurological arousal measured by a 3-second or greater shift in EEG frequency, measured at C3, C4, O1, or O_2, or a blood oxygen saturations of 3% to 4% greater, or both arousal and O_2 desaturation. Multiple criteria may be utilized to make a clinical decision regarding the existence of and/or severity of a sleep disorder. These criteria are open to some interpretation and sometimes conflicting guidelines[21-23] (see Chapter 16).

Pulse oximetry may also be utilized in the patient's home overnight, and according to a study conducted by Sériès et al,[24] it proved to be a sensitive test and an easy alternative to a formal sleep study such that if readings were normal, sleep apnea is unlikely. Home pulse oximetry may also be useful in guiding prescription for automatically self-adjusting continuous positive airway pressure (CPAP) therapy.[25]

Once obstructive sleep apnea is identified, the most effective treatment is CPAP therapy. This device basically splints the airway open during sleep by means of a flow of pressurized air into the throat. Although CPAP is extremely effective and often substantially less expensive that other more invasive treatments for sleep apnea, compliance with treatment can be an issue.[26–28] For this reason, other less-effective treatments may need to be tried. These include behavioral therapy and also cautioning the patient to avoid alcohol, sleeping pills, and other sedatives that can relax upper airway dilatory musculature and contribute to airway collapse during the night.

Oral appliance therapy may be an effective alternative when CPAP is not successful. There are many different types of oral appliances, which are custom-made mouthpieces that usually advance the mandible and thus open the airway. This can be a successful treatment for mild-to-moderate sleep apnea but less so for severe cases. Care must be taken to protect the jaw joint and occlusion with this type of therapy. It is extremely important that the patient have this device fabricated by a dentist who understands occlusal position as it pertains to healthy functional maxillary–mandibular relationships; otherwise, the temporomandibular joint may be compromised. A compromised joint can lead to a significant pain problem and may in fact worsen symptoms of obstructive sleep apnea (see Chapter 22).

Because the consequences of chronic sleep apnea can be widespread and profound, it is important to find an effective treatment solution. The rehabilitation professional may be able to assist in this area by improving the mechanics of respiration during wakefulness, which has been shown to improve respiration during sleep (see Chapter 27). Rehabilitation providers may also be able to improve sleep by working with sensory integration issues in the child and the adult that contribute to disordered sleep (see Chapter 23).

Narcolepsy

Narcolepsy is a sleep disorder that is characterized by excessive daytime sleepiness and sleep attacks that occur at inappropriate times and in inappropriate places, such as during work (Figure 11-6). Individuals who suffer from narcolepsy often experience nighttime sleep disturbances and abnormal daytime sleep that is confused with insomnia. A hallmark of narcolepsy is the rapid onset of REM sleep within 5 minutes of falling asleep. Normally, REM sleep latency is 75 to 90 minutes into a single night's sleep.

Narcolepsy occurs in 0.04% to 0.07% of the population, with the typical onset of the disorder during adolescence and young adulthood.[29] The cause of narcolepsy is not yet completely understood, but there appears to be a strong genetic link. The genetically mediated dysfunction in cholinergic–dopaminergic interactions has been implicated in its pathophysiology. Variations in the human leukocyte antigen complex appear to increase risk of an autoimmune response to hypocretin or orexin neurons, which

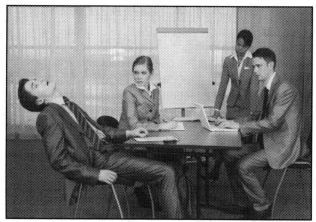

Figure 11-6. Narcolepsy can be extremely disruptive but can be treated. (From Fotolia.com)

are responsible for controlling appetite and sleep patterns. Narcoleptics usually have a decreased number of these protein-producing neurons.

Narcolepsy usually includes excessive daytime sleepiness with sleep attacks but may also include cataplexy, sleep paralysis, and vivid hypnagogic or hypnopompic hallucinations. The excessive daytime sleepiness leads to an irresistible urge to sleep known as a *sleep attack*. The narcoleptic may sleep for 20 to 40 minutes and awaken feeling refreshed but becomes irresistibly sleepy again in 2 to 3 hours. Cataplexy, sleep paralysis, and sleep hallucinations will be described in more detail. Other symptoms that accompany narcolepsy may be present at the onset of the disorder but diminish in frequency and intensity over time; however, narcolepsy is a chronic condition.

Treatment for narcolepsy is symptomatic. Stimulants such as modafinil (Provigil) are commonly used for treatment of excessive daytime sleepiness associated with narcolepsy. Stimulant use may allow the narcoleptic to engage in daytime activity, but sustained use of a stimulant may itself worsen the condition by interfering with SWS.

Treatment should also be directed toward lifestyle changes that reduce stress and encourage exercise. Obstructive sleep apnea must be treated in these patients. As much as possible, the narcoleptic should adjust his or her lifestyle to coincide with his or her natural sleep cycle. In addition to medication, the narcoleptic is well served to schedule brief naps of 15 to 20 minutes 2 to 3 times per day to help control excessive sleepiness and allow the individual to remain as alert as possible. These daytime naps, however, are not a replacement for nighttime sleep. It is important that the narcoleptic engage in very good sleep hygiene.

Sleep Paralysis

Sleep paralysis is defined as an inability to move associated with the onset of sleep (hypnagogic) or upon awakening (hypnopompic). It may occur in a healthy individual as isolated sleep paralysis or may be associated with narco-lepsy, cataplexy, or hypnagogic hallucinations. An episode of sleep paralysis may last for a few seconds up to a few minutes.[29] Because of the hallucinatory experience of sleep paralysis, the sleeper may interpret it as a particularly vivid dream, and these experiences have been proposed as expla-nations for such things as reports of alien abductions and ghost encounters.[30,31]

Survey studies have shown that sleep paralysis is reported to occur in up to 60% of people at least once in their lifetime.[32,33] However, it is more persistent in approxi-mately 6% of the general population. In those individuals, its occurrence is reported to increase with supine sleeping, increased stress, sudden environmental or lifestyle changes, or excessive consumption of alcohol coupled with sleep deprivation. In an individual with persistent symptoms, narcolepsy must be ruled out.

Other sensory experiences are often associated with sleep paralysis such as humming, hissing, and buzzing noises. This happens when REM atonia is initiated earlier than usual, before the individual is fully asleep, or when REM atonia persists after the individual has fully awoken. Other symptoms that accompany this disorder may include the feeling of being crushed or suffocated, electric tingling or vibrations, imagined speech, and imagined presence of visible entities. These experiences may also be accompanied by intense emotions such as fear or euphoria. It is relatively easy to see how these associated experiences, along with inability to move, could be mistaken for a paranormal experience.

Sleep Hallucinations

Sleep hallucinations have been interpreted as visions, premonitions, apparitions, and inspirations. This phenom-enon occurs in the transitional state between wakefulness and sleep (hypnagogia) or sleep and wakefulness (hypno-pompia). At this threshold of consciousness, an individual may experience lucid dreaming, hallucinations, out-of-body experiences, and sleep paralysis. It is a state in which the individual experiences being half-awake or half-asleep. This may occur in the normal course of a night's sleep and be a brief experience or it can be extended by a sleep dis-turbance. It can also be deliberately induced during certain meditation practices.

The transition between sleep and wakefulness is often accompanied by a wide variety of sensory experiences that may vary from minimally perceptible to vividly hallucina-tory.[34] These sensory experiences include visual phenom-ena that may be abstract flashes or more identifiable images but differ from visual imagery that accompanies dreams in that they are fleeting and rapidly changing and lack a narrative.[35]

Individuals who have engaged in a repetitive activ-ity prior to sleep, particularly a novel activity such as a computer game, may find that the imagery of that activity dominates as they drift to sleep, known as the *Tetris effect.* This experience can involve a variety of sensory aspects of an activity from the feel of snow in an individual who has been skiing all day, to a chess player who sees a chess match in the hallucinatory state experienced at the transition between wakefulness and sleep.

Sounds may also be present during this state and may vary in intensity and quality; visual sensations may range from faint sounds to loud crashing or banging as occurs in what is called *exploding head syndrome.* It is during this state that an individual may imagine that he or she hears the doorbell or some snippets of speech.

Sleep paralysis may also be a component of hypnagogia or hypnopompia. There may also be other random sensory experiences such as tactile, gustatory, olfactory, or thermal sensations. There have been reports of out-of-body experi-ences during sleep hallucinations. One of the most common experiences of this state is the experience of feeling like one is falling and the associated hypnic jerk that most people occasionally feel as they drift off to sleep.[36]

There are unique cognitive and affective phenomena associated with the transition between wakefulness and sleep, with a certain amount of "loosening of ego boundar-ies."[37] Cognition is suggestible, illogical, and characterized by fluid ideation compared to normal alert thought pro-cesses. In studies, subjects in this state are more receptive to suggestion and can more readily incorporate external stimuli into thought processes and subsequent dreams.[37] Thought processes during this state are relatively absent of repression or censorship. They may allow for insight into a problem, as was famously related in Kekulé's discovery of the structure of the benzene ring.[37] History is also replete with stories of writers, composers, and scientists who credit this state of sleep for their creativity; thus, the adage "let me sleep on it."[38]

The physiology of sleep hallucinations has been studied and has led to multiple findings. One study found that this state is associated with N1 sleep, but may also occur dur-ing the alpha wave state that occurs immediately prior to sleep onset. In fact, one study showed that sleep hallucina-tions began to occur just as alpha wave activity began to decrease.[39] Another study concluded that sleep hallucina-tions have distinct EEG and behavioral characteristics, and yet another suggested that the EEG findings during this state have characteristics of both REM sleep and the alpha wave state associated with quiet wakefulness.[40,41] Hori et al[42] further suggested that there are 9 EEG stages that define sleep, including alpha (stages 1 to 3), suppressed waves of less than 20 μV (stage 4), theta ripples (stage 5), proportions of sawtooth waves (stages 6 and 7), and pres-ence of spindles (stages 8 and 9). It appears that sleep hal-lucinations occur mainly in these sleep-onset stages 4 and 5.[43] These episodes differ from microsleep episodes that are related to sleep deprivation or from daydreaming that may intrude on alert wakefulness.

Nocturnal Dyspnea

Paroxysmal nocturnal dyspnea is an attack of severe shortness of breath and coughing that generally occurs at night. This usually awakens the sleeper and can be rather alarming to the individual. Often, simply changing positions, such as sitting on the side of the bed and dangling the legs, may relieve the symptoms. Sometimes, however, coughing and wheezing may persist even with a change in position.

This manifestation of disordered sleep is more common in individuals with interstitial lung disease and reduced pulmonary compliance. Paroxysmal nocturnal dyspnea may be caused by the depression of the respiratory center that occurs during sleep. The redistribution of blood volume from the lower extremities and splanchnic beds to the lungs results in a reduction of arterial oxygen tension. Though this generally does not affect normal individuals, in an individual who is compromised, the additional blood volume cannot be pumped out by the left ventricle, and the reduction in vital capacity and pulmonary compliance leads to shortness of breath. In an individual with congestive heart failure, the pulmonary circulation may already be overloaded because of the failing left ventricle and then is suddenly unable to match the output of the right ventricle, causing pulmonary congestion. This additional stress can lead to right-sided failure. Pulmonary congestion decreases when the individual sits on the side of the bed and dangles the legs, thus reducing the blood volume load and relieving the symptoms.

Treatment for this condition depends on the underlying cause, but options include nocturnal oxygen, diuretics, antihypertensive medication, and bronchodilators to decrease wheezing.

Nocturnal Pain

Chronic pain is the chief source of sleep disturbance in many medical disorders. Pain may arise from sleep-related headaches, cancer, and rheumatologic conditions including fibromyalgia. Individuals with fibromyalgia often complain of chronic fatigue, nonrestorative sleep, and generalized muscle discomfort. Nocturnal cardiac ischemia, left ventricular failure, sleep-related gastrointestinal reflux, peptic ulcer disease, or primary respiratory disorders such as chronic obstructive pulmonary disease may also produce nocturnal chest pain that disrupts sleep and increases anxiety. Increased anxiety makes return to sleep and maintenance of sleep difficult.

Nocturnal Physical Phenomena

Nocturnal physical phenomena include obstructive sleep apnea with forceful arousals in which the sleeper awakens suddenly with the sensation of choking or gasping for air. This is an extremely disturbing symptom and often evokes fear and increased anxiety on the part of the sleeper, further disrupting the sleep pattern. Physical phenomena that may also disrupt sleep include periodic limb movement disorder, confusional arousals, night terrors, rhythmic movement disorder, sleep starts, nocturnal leg cramps, nightmares, and bruxism, among other disorders.

SUMMARY

Sleep disorders are abnormal sleep patterns that interfere with normal sleep. They can be intrinsic, or arising from physiological factors; extrinsic, arise from environmental causes; or the result of disturbances of circadian rhythm. For example, insomnia can be the result of stress (an extrinsic cause) or diabetes (an internal cause), and shift work sleep disorder is a disturbance of circadian rhythm.

Sleep disorders are fairly common and can be manifested in various ways. One of the most common symptoms of sleep disorder is excessive daytime sleepiness. This sleepiness may occur from sleep fragmentation as a result of sleep apnea or may be caused by short sleep as may occur in insomnia. It may also be a result of environmental factors such as changes in schedule or in the amount of light a person is exposed to. The person may report difficulty staying awake during class or meetings or falling asleep at inappropriate times or places. Other manifestations include job or school performance problems or a history of accidents at work or while driving. It appears that regardless of the cause of sleep disturbance, the manifestations remain the same.

Insomnia is the most common sleep disorder and may be caused by medical, psychological, or environmental issues. It may present as either an inability to fall asleep or an inability to stay asleep. Insomnia can be either acute, lasting less than 1 month, or chronic, which would last for longer than 1 month. Pain is a common cause of insomnia. Other causes that a rehabilitation professional should be aware of are hormone shifts due to pregnancy or menstruation, significant life events, poor sleep hygiene, and mental disorders.

Sleep apnea is another common sleep disorder characterized by abnormal pauses in breathing during sleep. It is diagnosed based on the results of PSG. The most effective treatment is the use of a CPAP machine that keeps the airway open during sleep. The consequences of sleep apnea are profound and can have a significant impact on rehabilitation.

Narcolepsy, sleep paralysis, and other sleep disorders may interfere with neurocognitive function. They may lower immune response and aggravate other systemic health issues, including cardiovascular disease. Sleep disorders may cause insulin resistance, thus increasing the occurrence of diabetes and, further, may contribute to weight gain and obesity. They should be evaluated because of the significant impact they can have on physiological, neurocognitive, and psychological well-being.

REFERENCES

1. American Academy of Sleep Medicine. Clinical guidelines. Available at: http://www.aasmnet.org/practiceguidelines.aspx. Accessed August 13, 2011.
2. Roth T. Insomnia: definition, prevalence, etiology, and consequences. *J Clin Sleep Med.* 2007;3(5 suppl):S7–S10.
3. National Sleep Foundation. 2002 Sleep in America poll. Available at: http://www.sleepfoundation.org/sites/default/files/2002SleepInAmericaPoll.pdf. Accessed August 13, 2011.
4. Roth T, Roehrs T. Insomnia: epidemiology, characteristics, and consequences. *Clin Cornerstone.* 2004;5(3):5–15.
5. Morin CM. The nature of insomnia and the need to refine our diagnostic criteria. *Psychosom Med.* 2002;62:483–485.
6. Ramakrishnan K, Scheid DC. Treatment options for insomnia. *Am Fam Physician.* 2007;76:517–526.
7. Erman MK. Insomnia: comorbidities and consequences. *Prim Psychiatry.* 2007;14(6):31–35.
8. Case K, Hurwitz TD, Kim SW, Cramer-Bornemann M, Schenck CH. A case of extreme paradoxical insomnia responding selectively to electroconvulsive therapy. *J Clin Sleep Med.* 2008;4:62–63.
9. Trajanovic N, Radivojevic V, Kaushansky Y, Shapiro C. Positive sleep state misperception—a new concept of sleep misperception. *Sleep Med.* 2007;8(2):111–118.
10. Lawrence KR, Adra M, Keir C. Hypoglycemia-induced anoxic brain injury possibly associated with levofloxacin. *J Infect.* 2006;52(6):e177–e180.
11. Gelder M, Mayou R, Geddes J. *Psychiatry.* 3rd ed. New York, NY: Oxford; 2005.
12. Mendelson WB. New research on insomnia: sleep disorders may precede or exacerbate psychiatric conditions. *Psychiatr Times.* 2008;25(7):29–41.
13. Schenkein J, Montagna P. Self-management of fatal familial insomnia. Part 1: what is FFI? *MedGenMed.* 2006;8(3):65.
14. Mendelson WB. New research on insomnia: sleep disorders may precede or exacerbate psychiatric conditions. *Psychiatr Times.* 2008;25(7):29–41.
15. Wilson S, Nutt D, Alford C, et al. British Association for Psychopharmacology consensus statement on evidence-based treatment of insomnia, parasomnias and circadian rhythm disorders. *J Psychopharm.* 2010;24:1577–1601.
16. Blazejewski S, Girodet PO, Orriols L, Capelli A, Moore N. Factors associated with serious traffic crashes: A prospective study in southwest France. *Arch Intern Med.* 2012;172(13):1039-1041.
17. Johns MW. A new method for measuring daytime sleepiness: the Epworth Sleepiness Scale. *Sleep.* 1991;14:540–545.
18. Hoddes E, Zarcone V, Smythe H, Phillips R, Dement WC. Quantification of sleepiness: a new approach. *Psychophysiol.* 1973;10(4):431-436.
19. Iber C, Ancoli-Israel S, Chesson A, Quan SF. The AASM Manual for the Scoring of Sleep and Associated Events: Rules, Terminology
20. Kapur V, Blough DK, Sandblom RE, et al. The medical cost of undiagnosed sleep apnea. *Sleep.* 1999;22:749–755.
21. AASM Task Force. Sleep-related breathing disorders in adults—recommendations for syndrome definition and measurement techniques in clinical research. *Sleep.* 1999;22:667–689.
22. Ruehland WR, Rochford PD, O'Donoghue FJ, Pierce RJ, Singh P, Thornton AT. The new AASM criteria for scoring hypopneas: impact on the apnea hypopnea index. *Sleep.* 2009;32(2):150–157.

23. Penzel T, Schobel C, Sebert M, Diecker B, Fietze I. Revised recommendations for computer-based sleep recording and analysis. *Conf Proc IEEE Eng Med Biol Soc.* 2009;7099–7101.
24. Séries F, Marc I, Cormier Y, La Forge J. Utility of nocturnal home oximetry for case finding in patients with suspected sleep apnea hypopnea syndrome. *Ann Intern Med.* 1993;119:449–453.
25. Whitelaw WA, Brant RF, Flemons WW. Clinical usefulness of home oximetry compared with polysomnography for assessment of sleep apnea. *Am J Respir Crit Care Med.* 2005;171(2):188–193.
26. National Heart, Lung, and Blood Institute. How is sleep apnea treated? Available at: http://www.nhlbi.nih.gov/health/health-topics/topics/sleepapnea/treatment.html. Accessed May 13, 2012.
27. Hsu AA, Lo C. Continuous positive airway pressure therapy in sleep apnea. *Respirology.* 2003;8:447–454.
28. Barbé F, Durán-Cantolla J, Sánchez-de-la-Torre M, et al. Effect of continuous positive airway pressure on the incidence of hypertension and cardiovascular events in nonsleepy patients with obstructive sleep apnea: a randomized controlled trial. *JAMA.* 2012;307:2161–2168.
29. Murphy G, Egan J. Sleep paralysis and hallucinations: what clinicians need to know. *Irish Psychol.* 2010;36(5):95-98.
30. McNally RJ, Clancy SA. Sleep paralysis, sexual abuse, and space alien abduction. *Transcult Psychiatry.* 2005;42:113–122.
31. Blackmore SJ, Parker JJ. Comparing the content of sleep paralysis and dream reports. *Dreaming.* 2002;12:45–59.
32. Spanos NP, McNulty SA, DuBreuil SC, Pires M. The frequency and correlates of sleep paralysis in a university sample. *J Res Pers.* 1995;29:285–305.
33. Friedman S, Paradis C. Panic disorder in African-Americans: symptomatology and isolated sleep paralysis. *Cult Med Psychiatry.* 2002;26(2):179–198.
34. Mavromatis A. *Hypnagogia: The Unique State of Consciousness Between Wakefulness and Sleep.* London, UK: Routledge and Kegan Paul; 1987.
35. Vaitl D, Birbaumer N, Gruzeller J, et al. Psychobiology of altered states of consciousness. *Psychol Bull.* 2005;131:98–127.
36. Cheyne JA. Sleep paralysis and the structure of waking-nightmare hallucinations. *Dreaming.* 2003;13(3):163–179.
37. Rothenberg A. Creative cognitive processes in Kekulé's discovery of the structure of the benzene molecule. *Am J Psychol.* 1995;108:419–438.
38. Krippner S. Altered and transitional states. In: Runco MA, Pritzker SR, eds. *Encyclopedia of Creativity. Vol 1.* San Diego, CA: Academic Press; 1999:63–64.
39. Foulkes D, Schmidt M. Temporal sequence and unit composition in dream reports from different stages of sleep. *Sleep.* 1983;6:265–280.
40. Hori T, Hayashi M, Morikawa T. Topographical EEG changes and hypnagogic experience. In: Ogilvie RD, Harsh JR, eds. *Sleep Onset: Normal and Abnormal Processes.* Washington, DC: American Psychological Association Press; 1993:237–253.
41. Nielsen T, Germain A, Ouellet L. Atonia-signalled hypnagogic imagery: comparative EEG mapping of sleep onset transitions, REM sleep, and wakefulness. *Sleep Res.* 1995;24:133.
42. Hori T, Hayashi M, Morikawa T. Topographical EEG changes and hypnagogic experience. In: Ogilvie RD, Harsh JR, eds. *Sleep Onset: Normal and Abnormal Processes.* Washington, DC: American Psychological Association Press; 1993:237–253.
43. Germain A, Nielsen TA. EEG power associated with early sleep onset images differing in sensory content. *Sleep Res Online.* 2001;4(3):83-90.

12

Consequences of Sleep Deprivation

Julie M. Hereford, PT, DPT

Sleep deprivation may result from short sleep or fragmented sleep in which the individual does not get enough sleep to meet the requirements of physiological and neurocognitive function. Approximately 1 in 5 people in this country fail to get enough sleep on any given night. This state may be acute or chronic. It may also be purposeful, such as a college student cramming for an exam, or that same college student celebrating into the early hours after an exam. Voluntary behavior that leads to unintentional chronic sleep deprivation is a type of hypersomnia known as *behaviorally induced insufficient sleep syndrome* (Figure 12-1A and B). It involves a restricted sleep pattern that is persistent for at least 3 months. Sleep deprivation may also be an unintended consequence because of personal obligations that restrict sleep, such as a parent of a new baby or a chronically ill child. Some occupations or work schedules can lead to chronic sleep deprivation. A common example is the individual who works second or third shift and also has a family at home who are on a normal sleep cycle. Chronic sleep deprivation may occur as a consequence of an underlying medical or psychiatric disorder or may be the result of a comorbid sleep disorder such as obstructive sleep apnea.

Risk groups for chronic sleep deprivation include males and females of all ages, though adolescents are more likely to have self-inflicted sleep deprivation.

Chronic sleep deprivation can result in persistent fatigue, excessive daytime sleepiness, clumsiness, and weight gain. It can affect cognitive function and alter brain function and neuronal firing patterns.[1-4] Although there are those who boast of lack of sleep—in fact, it is not uncommon for a patient, especially one who has a painful condition, to report that he or she has not slept at all in days—complete sleep deprivation is not possible for humans to achieve for long periods of time. Only in a tragic condition known as *fatal familial insomnia* does this occur; otherwise, the drive for sleep is so powerful that brief bouts of microsleep cannot be avoided, even by one who is testing his or her limits. A *microsleep* is described as a very brief period, lasting from 1 second to as long as 30 seconds, in which the brain shuts down, falling into a sleep state. The individual falls asleep no matter what activity is being performed. These episodes are similar to blackouts; the individual experiencing them is unaware that they are occurring. Animal studies have shown that these microsleeps occur for as short as 80 ms but as frequently as 40 times a minute. Even though the animal appeared awake, neurons shut down and performance was negatively impacted.[5] In fact, long-term total sleep deprivation has caused death in lab animals.[6]

Sleep deprivation experimentation in animals has been shown to increase the homeostatic sleep drive with sleep rebound following the period of sleep deprivation. This sleep rebound included an increase in behavioral quiescence, increased slow-wave sleep (SWS), and increased rapid eye movement (REM) sleep. During experimentally induced total sleep deprivation, a change in metabolism was noted with a decrease in anabolic hormone, weight loss despite high amounts of food intake, and an increase in the metabolic neuroendocrine abnormalities, especially increased plasma norepinephrine levels. Animals were also noted to have impaired response to infectious agents, skin lesions including hyperkeratosis and ulcerations, increased heart rate, and a decrease in body temperature with a

Hereford JM. *Sleep and Rehabilitation:*
A Guide for Health Professionals (pp 103-112).
© 2014 Taylor & Francis Group.

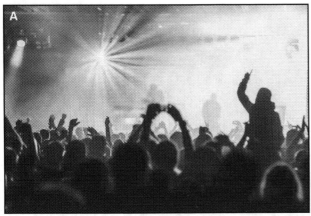
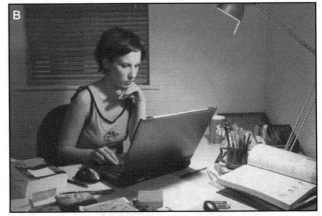

Figure 12-1. Behaviorally induced insufficient sleep syndrome is brought on voluntarily by poor sleep hygiene. (From Fotolia.com)

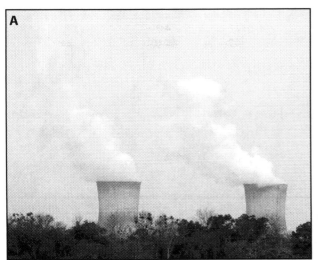
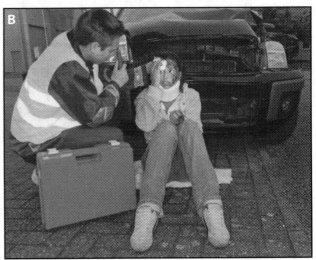

Figure 12-2. Sleep deprivation has contributed to fatal accidents, from (A) Three Mile Island to (B) car accidents. (From Fotolia.com)

failure of thermoregulation, eventually leading to death of the animals.

Consequences of sleep deprivation, sleep disorders, and shift work in humans pose a significant economic and health threat in the world. In fact, some of the most devastating human and environmental disasters have been linked to sleep deprivation and related performance failures (Figure 12-2A and B). Disasters known to be directly linked to human error due to sleep deprivation include the chemical plant disaster in Bhopal, India, in 1984; the nuclear reactor meltdowns at Three Mile Island in 1979 and Chernobyl in 1986; the grounding of the *Star Princess* cruise ship in 2012; and the *Exxon Valdez* oil tanker accident in 1989. Sleep deprivation of the engineers working on the NASA space shuttle *Challenger*, which exploded on lift-off in 1986, was a contributing factor in that accident. A number of airplane and freight train accidents have been investigated, and it was found that sleep deprivation of the pilots and conductors was a significant factor in the incidents. Each of these incidents resulted in loss of life and cost millions of dollars to clean up. Many of them have also had a long-term impact on the environment and the health of the local

community. According to the American Academy of Sleep Medicine's "Drowsy Driver Fact Sheet," 80,000 drivers fall asleep while driving each year, and sleep deprivation is a factor in 250,000 motor vehicle accidents each year on American roads. A survey showed that 9 out of 10 police officers stopped at least 1 driver whom they suspected of driving while intoxicated only to find out that they were sleepy drivers, which can be just as dangerous.[7]

Equally as important, but less visible, are the consequences of chronic sleep deprivation that impact the health of the population. Sleepiness has been shown to impact mortality, morbidity, academic performance, work productivity, quality of life, and family well-being. It has also been implicated in the rising cost of health care, because the consequences of chronic sleep deprivation increase health care utilization.[8]

Sleep deprivation is fairly rampant in today's society. It may be driven by home and family situations, social factors, or economic needs that result in persistent short sleep. It is often exacerbated by the ubiquitous nature of electronic devices including computers, television, cell phones, tablets, video games, and social media. Regardless of the cause, sleep deprivation has been linked to many mental, psychological, and medical disorders. Additionally, certain disorders can be the cause of sleep deprivation. In fact, disordered sleep may be brought on by a medical or anatomical disorder and may lead to complications of the underlying disorder or to other health threats.

This complex interplay makes it important for all health care providers to be able to at least recognize the signs and symptoms of a sleep disorder and to direct the patient to appropriate evaluation and treatment. The rehabilitation professional is often in a unique position to recognize this and must understand its impact. In fact, the rehabilitation provider may be dealing with the consequences of disordered sleep as a barrier to reaching rehabilitation goals. This may be evident in a slow-healing injury or a persistently recurring neuromusculoskeletal dysfunction.

Disordered sleep may interfere with a patient's ability to engage in the rehabilitation process. A patient who has poor motor control or who has great difficulty performing a corrective exercise technique may have an underlying sleep disorder that interferes with motor learning. A compliant patient who is unable to show carryover of an exercise program from one treatment session to the next may have disordered sleep that interferes with motor memory consolidation. A patient who has persistent pain despite the skilled application of appropriate therapeutic interventions may have an underlying sleep disorder that does not allow proper healing or maintains the inflammatory process beyond its useful phase.

These situations can be frustrating to the rehabilitation professional and to the patient alike. If the therapist is able to recognize the potential contribution of a sleep disorder to the health and welfare of the patient, the therapist may be able to improve patient outcomes and therefore decrease health care utilization. Because of the frequency and length of time that the rehabilitation professional has with the patient, the therapist is in a unique position to recognize signs and symptoms of disordered sleep and to direct the patient to obtain help. The appropriate provider can have a thorough sleep assessment done and provide subsequent treatment for patients presenting with disordered sleep.

GENERAL CONSEQUENCES OF DISORDERED SLEEP

Acute and chronic sleep deprivation may arise from different sources. Regardless of the cause, sleep deprivation may produce a variety of signs and symptoms affecting various different systems throughout the body.

Acutely sleep-deprived individuals obviously may present with sleepiness and fatigue. They may also report aching muscles, confusion, memory lapses, moodiness,

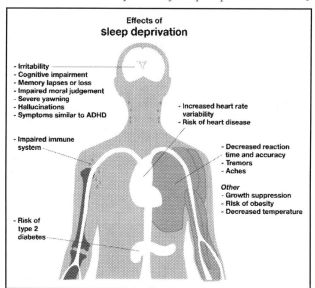

Figure 12-3. Effects of sleep deprivation.

headaches, and malaise. They may appear to have blood-shot eyes and periorbital puffiness (or "bags") under the eyes and may yawn frequently. They may be irritable and display low energy. Some may even have cold sensitivity or a slight hand tremor. Sleep-deprived children (and sometimes adults) may have temper tantrums.

When an individual is more chronically sleep deprived, he or she may have the symptoms described, but may have had them so long that the patient discounts the impact that these symptoms have on his or her day-to-day life. As sleep deprivation becomes more chronic, the individual can begin to develop more systemic consequences including increased blood pressure, increased stress hormones, increased risk of fibromyalgia, and diabetes (Figure 12-3). Increased incidence of obesity—particularly abdominal obesity and development of metabolic syndrome—have been linked to chronic sleep deprivation.

Sleepiness

Sleepiness is associated with an increase in homeostatic sleep drive and a propensity to fall asleep. Microsleep or brief lapses into sleep can occur during wakefulness due to heightened sleep pressure. When an individual who is sleep deprived undergoes polysomnography (PSG), the Multiple Sleep Latency Test, or the Maintenance of Wakefulness Test, he or she displays a decrease in sleep latency.[9] The greater the sleep deprivation, the shorter the sleep latency. Individuals who report that they have no trouble falling asleep or that they are asleep as soon as they hit the pillow may, in fact, be sleep deprived. Transitioning into sleep is an active process and should take 10 to 20 minutes to occur. A very rapid descent into a sleeping state is sometimes an indication of chronic sleep deprivation (see Chapter 16).

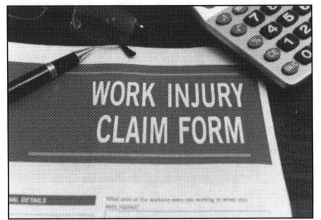

Figure 12-4. Sleep is often a factor in costly workplace injuries. (From Fotolia.com)

Excessive daytime sleepiness can be assessed with a number of easily administered clinical tools, such as the Epworth Sleepiness Scale[10] or the Stanford Sleepiness Scale[11] or any of the available fatigue scales[12,13] (see Chapter 28). The use of these instruments is an easy method for the rehabilitation professional to get a clearer picture of the amount of interference that sleepiness and fatigue are having in the life of a patient. It should be noted, however, that sleepiness and fatigue are different qualities and may represent different problems clinically. For example, an individual who has an underlying sleep disorder may have excessive daytime sleepiness, and an individual with fibromyalgia or another rheumatologic disorder may have fatigue but not sleepiness. This distinction may be an important factor in treatment planning.

General Health

Sleep deprivation is associated with an increase in morbidity and mortality. Increased mortality has been observed in individuals who regularly sleep less than 6.5 hours per 24-hour period or more than 9 to 10 hours per 24-hour period. The mechanisms responsible for the association between duration of sleep and elevated mortality are complex.

In addition to the effects of excessive daytime sleepiness, which increases the likelihood of an individual falling asleep in a quiet or monotonous situation, such as sitting in a meeting or attending a lecture, sleep deprivation can be a safety hazard leading to increased workplace injury and factoring into auto accidents (Figure 12-4).

Sleep deprivation, particularly restriction of non-rapid eye movement (NREM) sleep, has been shown to interfere with wound healing in animal models.[14,15] Sleep deprivation is known to increase the risk of certain medical conditions such as hypertension, cardiovascular disease, obesity, diabetes, and metabolic syndrome. It alters neurological function by interfering with cerebral glucose metabolism.

Symptoms of this may be ptosis, nystagmus, slurring of speech, hyperactive gag reflex, or tremors. Corneal reflexes become sluggish and deep tendon reflexes may become hyperactive. Pain sensitivity can increase significantly.

Endocrine function and metabolism are affected by sleep deprivation. Sleep deprivation can produce an increase in sympathetic activation and increased cortisol and ghrelin levels. It blunts the sleep-dependent secretion of human growth hormone and prolactin the following day because of the reduction in SWS. Sleep deprivation enhances the activity of the hypothalamic-pituitary-adrenal axis, which controls reaction to stress and regulates digestion, immune function, mood, sexual behavior, and energy level.[16] An increase in stress hormones may reduce new cell production in the adult brain, which limits cellular repair caused by free radical production while awake.

Levels of thyroxine and leptin may decrease. Low leptin levels, especially combined with increased ghrelin levels, stimulate appetite and suppress satiation, which may lead to weight gain and obesity.[17]

Immunity and inflammatory responses are affected by sleep deprivation. There is a decreased febrile response to endotoxins and antibody titers to influenza vaccine during states of sleep deprivation. It can alter levels of cytokines, interleukin-6 and tumor necrosis factor-alpha, leukocytes, and affects the function of natural killer cells. There is also a decrease in granulocytes and lymphocytes in response to antigens as a result of sleep deprivation.

Mood

Acute sleep deprivation is strongly associated with irritability, emotional lability, and lack of motivation. Chronic sleep deprivation also has a negative impact on mood and can give rise to nervousness and impulsivity. Chronic sleep deprivation has been correlated with depression, anxiety, and mental distress. Over time it can cause symptoms of depression. Studies of experimentally induced sleep deprivation have shown that subjects who slept 4.5 hours per night reported feeling more stressed and mentally exhausted and were more prone to sad or angry reactions to situations that normally would not bother them.[18] Another study of experimentally induced sleep deprivation showed that subjects who experienced short sleep showed decreased optimism and socialization as the length of sleep deprivation increased. All of these subjects returned to normal when they were allowed to return to a normal sleep cycle.[19,20]

Cognition and Performance

Sleep deprivation results in diminished attention, concentration, and alertness. It can cause a decrease in vigilance and an increase in reaction time, which will lead to an increased error rate in even simple tasks. It can interfere with cognition, learning, memory consolidation, psychomotor performance, and executive function. Focus and attention become impaired, and the individual becomes more distractible, also leading to increased confusion, poorer decision making, and poor performance.

Functional magnetic resonance imaging studies have shown that the prefrontal cortex in the sleep-deprived brain shows increased activity during the performance of a simple verbal task. The sleepier the brain is, the greater the activity in the prefrontal cortex when attempting a simple task. It was postulated that this activity is an attempt of the brain to compensate for the negative effects of sleep deprivation. The temporal lobe, which is involved in language processing, was active in control subjects in the same study.[21] The parietal lobe, however, which is associated with short-term memory, is more active in sleep-deprived subjects than in well-rested controls.[21]

Another study[22] conducted at Harvard and the University of California–Berkley used functional magnetic resonance imaging to investigate brains of individuals who were sleep deprived. This study found that the sleep-deprived brain becomes incapable of putting emotional content into proper perspective and is incapable of producing a controlled and appropriate response. This helps in understanding the often irrational responses and sometimes almost psychotic behavior in the seriously sleep deprived. According to Walker,[22] an investigator in the study, it appears that the sleep-deprived brain reverts to a more primitive level of function.

Another study shows the reduction in cerebral glucose metabolism in the prefrontal thalamic network by prolonged sleep deprivation causes a decrease in alertness and cognitive performance.[19] This study showed that increases in visual and motor areas show the brain's effort to remain awake and perform despite the increasing sleep pressure.

Work conducted at the University of California–Los Angeles suggested that NREM sleep allows neurotransmitters to turn off in order to regain sensitivity that allows improved function of monoamines.[23] This effect improves pathway function that is involved in mood and learning. This study also suggested that REM sleep deprivation does not allow the natural reduction of monoamines that may alleviate clinical depression because decreasing REM sleep mimics the action of selective serotonin re-uptake inhibitors. NREM sleep may allow repair of damage caused by free radicals. In addition, this study found the first evidence of brain damage as a result of prolonged sleep deprivation in rats.[19]

Attention and working memory are also affected by sleep deprivation and it is this parameter that may be most critical in choice reaction time tasks that have led to auto accidents and industrial disasters. These deficits cause life-and-death mistakes. Attention and reaction time can be measured in sleep-deprived subjects using the psychomotor vigilance task, which requires the subject to press a button

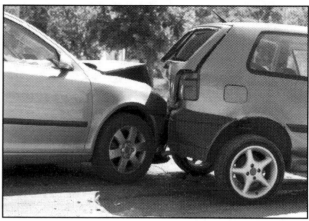

Figure 12-5. Sleep-deprived subjects often underestimate their level of impairment, causing them to make poor judgments. (From Fotolia.com)

in response to a light at pseudorandom intervals. Failure to press the button is recorded as an error attributable to microsleeps that occur in sleep-deprived individuals. When sleep-deprived subjects were questioned, they were often grossly unaware of their level of impairment (Figure 12-5).[24] This is true for the acutely sleep-deprived research subject and the chronically sleep-deprived citizen. In fact, the chronically sleep deprived generally judge themselves to be less impaired than the acutely sleep-deprived subject.

This is a finding similar to what is seen in individuals who are impaired due to alcohol or drugs. Studies that have compared subjects who drove after being awake for an average of 18 hours to those who tested at a 0.05% blood alcohol level found that the drowsy drivers performed worse than the tipsy drivers.[25,26] Overall, sleep deprivation can cause an individual to fall asleep even in the face of known life-and-death danger.

Academic performance has also been shown to be adversely affected by acute or chronic sleep deprivation. There is a growing body of data that shows a relationship between normal sleep and school performance.[27–30] A study of college students found that students get an average of 6.7 hours of sleep each night, which adversely affects academic performance. Sleep deprivation is shown to be worst in the first year of college, which is most likely due to the stress of adjusting to a new academic and social life.[31] Other studies have shown that adolescent and teenage students perform better when the school day begins later, compared to those who begin the school day earlier. Those who start the school day at a later time also tend to get more sleep overall. One in four high school students report falling asleep during the school day at least once a week.[33] This change in academic performance with a late school start is supported by what is known about the changes in circadian rhythms that occur in adolescence and the teenage years.[32,33] School schedules are often incompatible with normal adolescent sleep patterns that typically display a delayed sleep onset. This can lead to chronic sleep deprivation in school-age children, particularly adolescents, and has been linked to a decline in academic performance.[31]

Because of the powerful effects of sleep deprivation, it is used as a method of altering the defenses of an individual from whom an authority figure wishes to extract information. This is used regularly as a method of questioning suspects in criminal investigations. In one interrogation technique, a subject is kept awake for an extended period of time, sometimes over a period of several days. In this situation, the individual's ability to sort out information becomes more compromised as cognitive function declines. In more severe forms of interrogation, a subject may be kept awake for days and then allowed to fall asleep, only to be suddenly awakened and questioned again. This process may continue until the subject is so sleep deprived that he or she is prone to significant cognitive distortion. The intended purpose of this technique is to reduce defenses in order to extract information; however, because of the cognitive distortions and dysfunction, suggestive capacity, and outright hallucinatory thought processes that occur during severe sleep deprivation, the veracity of the information extracted is questionable. It has been described as torture by individuals who have undergone such interrogation techniques, saying that they would have been willing to say anything, even admitting to horrendous atrocities, in order to be allowed to sleep. They have reported that no other sensory experience, including hunger, thirst, or even pain, compares.[34-37] There has been significant debate regarding the ethics of these techniques and whether or not they are considered torture. Amnesty International has declared that "... sleep deprivation is cruel, inhumane and degrading. If used for prolonged periods of time, it is torture."[38]

Extrapolating from these data, one might consider how an individual with chronic sleep deprivation may have enough cognitive dysfunction to interfere with a rehabilitation program. If a neurological injury is superimposed upon a chronically sleep-deprived individual, his or her ability to fully engage in the rehabilitation process may be impaired. Therefore, it is important that the rehabilitation provider is able to recognize signs and symptoms of chronic sleep deprivation and able to understand appropriate intervention. This will likely improve patient outcomes.

Risk of Other Systemic Health Problems

Chronic sleep deprivation, as occurs in an individual with an underlying sleep disorder such as obstructive sleep apnea, can increase the risk of a number of other health problems.

There is an increasing body of literature linking insufficient sleep and sleep apnea to weight gain, particularly abdominal obesity. Individuals who chronically sleep less than 6 hours per night have a higher body mass index than those who sleep approximately 8 hours per night. Disordered sleep appears to be a potential risk factor for obesity in conjunction with the other commonly known factors of overeating and decreased activity level.

Hormones that control appetite, satiation, energy metabolism, and glucose metabolism are secreted during particular phases of sleep. Chronic sleep deprivation, as may occur with obstructive sleep apnea, also increases the production of cortisol, a stress hormone. Cortisol is associated with increased secretion of insulin, which regulates glucose metabolism and promotes fat storage. Higher levels of insulin are associated with weight gain. This cascade of metabolic events increases the risk of diabetes.

Insufficient sleep has been shown to be associated with decreased leptin levels and increased ghrelin levels.[39] Leptin acts on receptors in the hypothalamus to inhibit appetite by counteracting the effects of neuropeptide Y, a potent feeding stimulant secreted by cells in the gut and in the hypothalamus. It also counteracts the effects of anandamide, a feeding stimulant that binds to the same receptors as tetrahydrocannabinol (THC), the principal psychoactive constituent of marijuana, and promoting the synthesis of a-MSH (melanocyte stimulating hormone), an appetite suppressant. Leptin allows long-term appetite suppression, as opposed to the rapid inhibition caused by cholecystokinin.

Leptin plays an important role in regulating energy intake and energy expenditure in appetite and metabolism. It is one of the most important adipose-derived hormones. It produces satiation when present at higher levels.

Ghrelin is a hunger-stimulating peptide that is produced mainly by P/D1 cells lining the fundus of the stomach and epsilon cells of the pancreas. Ghrelin levels increase before meals and decrease after feeding.[40,41] Chronically elevated levels of ghrelin, in turn, increase food intake and may lead to higher fat mass through its action on the hypothalamus, where its neurons are both ghrelin and leptin sensitive.[42,43] Ghrelin activates the mesolimbic cholinergic–dopaminergic reward link that reinforces the reward link of food intake.[44-46] There is evidence that ghrelin modulates appetite peripherally, thus enhancing satiety by decreasing the sensitivity of gastric vagal afferents so that they are less responsive to gut distention and therefore lead to overeating.[47]

A state of chronic sleep deprivation has been found to decrease leptin and increase ghrelin. This change in leptin–ghrelin ratio results in food cravings even after satiety should have been reached based on caloric need. The chronically sleep deprived are more likely to crave foods with higher sugar content for their quick energy boost, because of the perception of decreased satiety created by the decreased leptin level. The chronic sleep deprivation may also leave the individual too tired to exercise in order to burn off the extra caloric intake.

Short sleep has been linked to alterations in the manner in which the body metabolizes glucose and thus may be linked to an increased incidence of type 2 diabetes. A number of studies have been conducted to explore the connection between sleep and diabetes.[48–51] In one such study, subjects restricted sleep by half for a short period of time and were found to have interferences in normal metabolism of glucose compared to normal sleep or long sleep periods.[52] Studies of individuals with obstructive sleep apnea have shown impaired glucose metabolism and insulin resistance, which is a precursor to type 2 diabetes. Epidemiological studies have shown that individuals who habitually sleep fewer than 5 hours per night have a significantly increased risk of developing type 2 diabetes.[53]

Chronic insufficient sleep has been linked to increased risk of hypertension and cardiovascular disease. Individuals who have just a single night of disrupted sleep and have pre-existing hypertension often show increased blood pressure the following day. Habitual short sleep of less than 6 hours per day and long sleep of greater than 9 hours per day have been linked with increased risk of cardiovascular disease, particularly in women. Individuals who suffer from obstructive sleep apnea also experience sudden surges of blood pressure associated with episodes of airway obstruction. Heart rate may also become substantially unstable and, over time, may increase the risk of cardiovascular disease.

In experimental investigations, rats that experienced prolonged, complete sleep deprivation increased food intake and significantly increased energy expenditure with a net effect of weight loss and ultimately death.[39] It is hypothesized from this and several other studies that moderate chronic sleep deprivation associated with habitual short sleep in humans is associated with increased appetite and food intake and some increased energy expenditure; however, the increased energy expenditure is not generally as great as the caloric intake.[54–56] In Western societies where high-calorie foods are freely available, the propensity to have chronic short sleep leads to weight gain.[1–3,57,58] One conclusion suggests that chronic moderate sleep deprivation may disrupt hormones that regulate glucose metabolism and appetite.[59] This, in turn, leads to increased caloric intake and weight gain. The problem with chronic sleep deprivation and obesity appears to occur with the highest frequency between young adulthood into middle age. Another contributor to this problem is obstructive sleep apnea, which further disrupts appetite and satiation hormones as well as those that govern glucose metabolism. It disturbs endocrine regulation of energy homeostasis. Obstructive sleep apnea occurs with increasing frequency across young adulthood and middle age.

A sleep study was conducted in 9 normal-weight healthy men studied over 3 nights, the first in which the men obtained 7 hours of sleep, the second in which they only obtained 4.5 hours total sleep time, and the third in which they had total sleep deprivation. Subjects reported markedly higher hunger symptoms after total sleep deprivation than after 7 or 4.5 hours of total sleep time. Ghrelin levels were higher after total sleep deprivation compared to 7-hour or 4.5-hour total sleep time, although morning serum leptin concentrations remained the same. These data suggest that sleep loss affects endocrine regulation of energy homeostasis. It is further suggested that this may be the mechanism that leads to weight gain and obesity.[60]

There is evidence that individuals who are habitually sleep deprived are more likely to develop impaired glucose tolerance and type 2 diabetes.[61] Another study found that glucose tolerance and thyrotropin levels are lower in those with chronic sleep deprivation compared to those in a fully rested condition.[62] Evening cortisol concentration was elevated and sympathetic nervous system activity was increased in individuals with short sleep.[63,64]

Immune Function

When an individual becomes sick with a virus such as the common cold or influenza, it is natural for him or her to sleep more. In fact, immune factors that are produced by the immune system to fight infection also cause fatigue. It is thought that the immune system developed sleepiness-inducing factors because inactivity and sleep assist in fighting the infection or sickness. Those who sleep more when they develop an infection are better able to fight that infection than those who do not sleep as much. Experimental studies show that animals that get deep sleep following microbial infection have a better chance of survival.[65,66]

Life Expectancy

Based on the aforementioned adverse health effects of chronic sleep deprivation, it is apparent that it is associated with decreased life expectancy. Epidemiological studies have shown that sleeping 5 hours or less per night increases the risk of mortality by up to 15%.[63,64,67] This chapter has shown that the effects of sleep deprivation are far-reaching and can be severe. It is also known that sleep deprivation can exacerbate existing medical and psychological/psychiatric disorders. Even with this knowledge, the medical community usually does not ask patients about their sleep habits. Patients are often unaware of the significant contribution that chronic sleep deprivation has on their physical and psychological functioning. It is very important that every health care provider understand the dramatic importance that sleep has in normal health and well-being. Chronic sleep deprivation impacts other medical and psychiatric functions. The general lack of awareness of the impact of sleep dysfunction has a significant and costly impact on public health.

STRATEGIES FOR COUNTERACTING THE EFFECTS OF SLEEP DEPRIVATION

When an individual is suffering from acute sleep deprivation, caffeine—which is an adenosine blocker—may be used over short periods to improve wakefulness. However, if caffeine is used regularly it becomes less effective. Other strategies that may help counteract sleep deprivation are a prophylactic nap before the period of sleep deprivation or the use of other stimulants. These strategies can be helpful to manage short-term acute sleep deprivation; however, chronic sleep deprivation is more complex, and its cause must be evaluated and treated. The cognitive dysfunction that occurs with short-term acute sleep deprivation generally recovers on return to normal sleep patterns. Chronic sleep deprivation, however, requires some time for the body to restore normal function and to recover from the deficits that can occur because of the deprivation. Recovery may not occur without good management of the causes of chronic sleep deprivation. Recovery sleep in the sleep-deprived person is generally more efficient than normal sleep with shorter sleep latency and increased amounts of SWS and REM sleep. There are a number of treatments that can be tried to restore sleep. Continuous positive airway pressure is a very effective treatment for obstructive sleep apnea; however, there are often problems with patient compliance. Treatment for other causes of sleep loss can be more complex and may be less effective. The only certain way to resolve sleep deprivation is to increase nighttime sleep time to an amount that satisfies the individual biological need; there is no substitute for getting a sufficient amount of sleep. One way to determine an individual's biological sleep need is to allow free sleep during a period when there is no need for a specific awakening time. The patient should go to sleep at a normal time and allow him- or herself to sleep until natural awakening for several days. Assuming that the individual is not chronically sleep deprived, the amount of sleep that one gets in this natural situation is the individual's biological sleep need. Going-to-bed time should be adjusted accordingly in order for the individual to get adequate sleep according to his or her individual needs.

Caffeine is probably the most commonly utilized substance to counteract sleep. It provides improved alertness by blocking adenosine receptors and is usually effective in doses of 75 to 100 mg after acute sleep restriction. Higher doses are needed with more protracted sleep loss, but frequent use can lead to tolerance and decreased efficacy. There are also negative side effects from withdrawal after habitual use.

Sleep prior to sleep deprivation, which may include getting extra sleep the night before a period of known sleep loss or taking a short nap prior to an anticipated late engagement, may be a successful strategy to alleviate the consequences of sleep deprivation. The downside of a longer nap is that it may produce a period of sleep inertia or grogginess that persists for some time upon awakening. Taking a nap and then ingesting caffeine may be additive and will provide improved alertness over a longer period.

Other stimulants are sometimes used in particular situations. Stimulants such as modafinil (Provigil) may be used to treat excessive daytime sleepiness that persists despite well-titrated continuous positive airway pressure use. In certain situations when recovery sleep is not possible, the use of other stimulant medications may be tried. These medications may be associated with some side effects and potential risks and have the potential to be abused. These may include amphetamines, methylphenidate, and methamphetamines. These should only be utilized in specific situations under close supervision by a physician.

SUMMARY

Sleep deprivation may result from short sleep or fragmented sleep in which the individual does not get enough sleep to meet the requirements of physiological and neurocognitive function. This sleep deprivation may be caused by voluntary behavior, whereby the sleeper shortens the sleep period because of family or social obligations; or involuntary behavior caused by disordered sleep. Neurocognitive consequences of sleep deprivation may include cognitive impairment and memory dysfunction, decreased reaction time, and reduced physical performance. It is also thought to be a contributing cause of attention–deficit/hyperactivity disorder (ADHD) in children.

Sleep deprivation can impede immune function and alter antibody response to vaccination. It is known to increase heart rate variability and contribute to the development of heart disease. It alters insulin metabolism, which may lead to insulin resistance, weight gain, and diabetes. Sleep deprivation increases pain sensitivity and interferes with tissue regeneration, which may become contributing factors in the development of chronic painful conditions such as fibromyalgia.

The consequences of sleep deprivation are widespread; however, effective treatment of the cause of sleep deprivation—such as addressing upper airway resistance issues—can reverse these consequences and restore more optimal health.

REFERENCES

1. Taheri S, Lin L, Austin D, Young T, Mignot E. Short sleep duration is associated with reduced leptin, elevated ghrelin, and increased body mass index. *PLoS Med.* 2004;1(3):e62.

2. Alhola P, Polo-Kantola P. Sleep deprivation: impact on cognitive performance. *Neuropsychiatr Dis Treat.* 2007;3:553–567.

3. Kushida CA. *Sleep Deprivation.* New York, NY: Informa Health Care; 2005.

4. Hasler G, Buysse DJ, Klaghofer R, et al. The association between short sleep duration and obesity in young adults: a 13-year prospective study. *Sleep.* 2004;27:661–666.

5. Vyazovskiy VV, Olcese U, Hanlon EC, Nir Y, Cirelli C, Tononi G. Local sleep in awake rats. *Nature.* 2011;472:443–447.

6. Rechtschaffen A, Bergmann B. Sleep deprivation in the rat by the disk-over-water method. *Behav Brain Res.* 1995;69:55–63.

7. American Academy of Sleep Medicine. AASM drowsy driver fact sheet. Available at: http://www.aasmnet.org/resources/factsheets/drowsydriving.pdf. Accessed February 23, 2012.

8. Colten HR, Altevogt BM, eds. Sleep disorders and sleep deprivation: an unmet public health problem. Available at: http://www.nap.edu/catalog/11617.html. Accessed June 15, 2012.

9. Iber C, Ancoli-Israel S, Chesson A, Quan SF. The AASM Manual for the Scoring of Sleep and Associated Events: Rules, Terminology and Technical Specifications. Westchester, IL: American Academy of Sleep Medicine; 2007.

10. Johns M. *Epworth Sleepiness Scale.* Available at: http://epworthsleepinessscale.com. Accessed February 23, 2012.

11. Stanford Sleepiness Scale. Available at: http://www.stanford.edu/~dement/sss.html. Accessed February 20, 2012.

12. Fatigue Severity Scale. Available at: http://www.saintalphonsus.org/documents/boise/sleep-Fatigue-Severity-Scale.pdf. Accessed October 2, 2013.

13. Friedber F, Jason LA. Selecting a fatigue rating scale. Available at: http://www.cfids.org/archives/2002rr/2002-rr4-article02.asp. Accessed June 15, 2012.

14. Mostaghimi L, Obermeyer WH, Ballamudi B, Martinez-Gonzalez D, Benca RM. Effects of sleep deprivation on wound healing. *J Sleep Res.* 2005;14:213–219.

15. Gümüştekín K, Seven B, Karabulut N, et al. Effects of sleep deprivation, nicotine, and selenium on wound healing in rats. *Int J Neurosci.* 2004;114:1433–1442.

16. Vgontzas AN, Mastorakos G, Bixler EO, Kales A, Gold PW, Chrousos GP. Sleep deprivation effects on the activity of the hypothalamic-pituitary-adrenal and growth axes: potential clinical implications. *Clin Endocrinol.* 1999;51:205–215.

17. Patel SR, Palmer LJ, Larkin EK, et al. Relationship between obstructive sleep apnea and diurnal leptin rhythms. *Sleep.* 2004;27(2):235–239.

18. Durmer JS, Dinges DF. Neurocognitive consequences of sleep deprivation. *Semin Neurol.* 2005;25:117–129.

19. Thomas M, Sing H, Belenky G, et al. Neural basis of alertness and cognitive performance inpairments during sleepiness. Effects of 24 h of sleep deprivation on waking human regional brain activity. *J Sleep Res.* 2000;9:335–354.

20. Post RM, Kotin J, Goodwin FK. Effects of sleep deprivation on mood and central amine metabolism in depressed patients. *Arch Gen Psychiatry.* 1976;33:627–632.

21. Brain activity is visibly altered following sleep deprivation. *Science Daily.* February 2000. Available at: http://www.sciencedaily.com/releases/2000/02/000209215957.htm. Accessed May 3, 2012.

22. Walker MP, Stickgold R. Sleep, memory, and plasticity. *Ann Rev Psychol.* 2006;57:139–166.

23. Ramanathan L, Gulyani S, Nienhuis R, Siegel JM. Sleep deprivation decreases superoxide dismutase activity in rat hippocampus and brainstem. *Neuroreport.* 2002;13:1387–1390.

24. Van Dongen HA, et al. The cumulative cost of additional wakefulness: dose–response effects on neurobehavioral functions and sleep physiology from chronic sleep restriction and total sleep deprivation. *Sleep.* 2002;26(2):117–126.

25. Williamson AM, Feyer AM. Moderate sleep deprivation produces impairments in cognitive and motor performance equivalent to legally prescribed levels of alcohol intoxication. *Occup Environ Med.* 2000;57:649–655.

26. Dawson D, Reid K. Fatigue, alcohol and performance impairment. *Nature.* 1997;388:235.

27. Mitchell H, Breedlove D, Askew E. Sleep deprivation and school performance. Available at: http://www.lagrange.edu/resources/pdf/citations/2009/24Nursing_Mitchell_Breedlove_Askew.pdf. Accessed April 22, 2012.

28. Wolfson AR, Carskadon MA. Understanding adolescents' sleep pattern and school performance: a critical appraisal. *Sleep Med Rev.* 2003;7:491–506.

29. Sadeh A, Gruber R, Raviv A. The effects of sleep restriction and extension on school-age children: what a difference an hour makes. *Child Dev.* 2003;74:444–455.

30. Sadeh A, Gruber R, Raviv A. Sleep, neurobehavioral functioning and behavior problems in school-age children. *Child Dev.* 2002;73:405–417.

31. Tsai LL, Li SP. Sleep patterns in college students; gender and grade differences. *J Psychosom Res.* 2004;56:231–237.

32. Giedd JN. Linking adolescent sleep, brain maturation, and behavior. *J Adolesc Health.* 2009;45:319–320.

33. American Academy of Sleep Medicine. Sleep deprivation fact sheet. Available at: http://www.aasmnet.org/Resources/FactSheets/SleepDeprivation.pdf. Accessed April 23, 2012.

34. BBC News. Binyam Mohamed torture appeal lost by UK government. Available at: http://news.bbc.co.uk/2/hi/uk_news/8507852.stm. Accessed April 2, 2012.

35. Begin M. *White Nights: The Story of a Prisoner in Russia.* San Francisco, CA: Harper & Row; 1979.

36. Mazzetti M, Shane S. Explaining and authorizing specific interrogation techniques. *The New York Times.* April 2009. Available at: http://www.nytimes.com/interactive/2009/04/17/us/politics/20090417-interrogation-techniques.html. Accessed April 12, 2012.

37. Australian Associated Press. Sleep deprivation is torture: amnesty. *The Sydney Morning Herald.* October 2006. Available at: http://www.smh.com.au/news/National/Sleep-deprivation-is-torture-Amnesty/2006/10/03/1159641317450.html. Accessed April 2, 2012.

38. Hassan T. Sleep deprivation remains red-hot question [transcript]. *PM.* 2006. http://www.abc.net.au/pm/content/2006/s1754821.htm. Accessed July 8, 2013.

39. Taheri S, Lin L, Austin D, Young T, Mignot E. Short sleep duration is associated with reduced leptin, elevated ghrelin and increased body mass index. *PLOS Medicine.* 2004;3(1):210–217.

40. Inui A, Asakawa A, Bowers CY, et al. Ghrelin, appetite, and gastric motility: the emerging role of the stomach as an endocrine organ. *FASEB J.* 2004;18:439–456.

41. Castañeda TR, Tong J, Datta R, Culler M, Tschöp MH. Ghrelin in the regulation of body weight and metabolism. *Front Neuroendocrinol.* 2010;31:44–60.

42. Lall S, Tung LY, Ohlsson C, Jansson JO, Dickson SL. Growth hormone (GH)-independent stimulation of adiposity by GH secretagogues. *Biochem Biophys Res Commun.* 2001;280:132–138.

43. Tschöp M, Smiley DL, Heiman ML. Ghrelin induces adiposity in rodents. *Nature.* 2000;407:908–913.

44. Hewson AK, Tung LY, Connell DW, Tookman L, Dickson SL. The rat arcuate nucleus integrates peripheral signals provided by leptin, insulin, and a ghrelin mimetic. *Diabetes.* 2002;51:3412–3419.

45. Jerlhag E, Egecioglu, E, Dickson SL, Andersson M, Svensson L, Engel JA. Ghrelin stimulates locomotor activity and accumbal dopamine-overflow via central cholinergic systems in mice: implications for its involvement in brain reward. *Addict Biol.* 2004;11:45–54.

46. Jerlhag E, Egecioglu E, Dickson SL, et al. Ghrelin administration into tegmental areas stimulates locomotor activity and increases extracellular concentration of dopamine in the nucleus accumbens. *Addict Biol.* 2007;12:6–16.

47. Page A, Slattery J, Milte C, et al. Ghrelin selectively reduces mechanosensitivity of upper gastrointestinal vagal afferents. *Am J Physiol Gastrointest Liver Physiol.* 2007;292:1376–1384.

48. Gottlieb DJ, Punjabi NM, Newman AB, Resnick HE, Redline S, Baldwin CM, Nieto FJ. Association of sleep time with diabetes mellitus and impaired glucose tolerance. *Arch Intern Med.* 2005;165(8):863-867.

49. Katano S, Nakamura Y, Nakamura A, Murakami Y, Tanaka T, Takebayashi T, Okayama A, Katsuyki M, Okamura T, Ueshima H. Association of short sleep duration with impaired glucose tolerance or diabetes mellitus. *J Diabetes Invest.* 2011;2(5):366-372.

50. Tauma C, Pannain S. Does lack of sleep cause diabetes? *Cleveland Clinic J Med.* 2011;78(8):549-558.

51. Iyer SR. Sleep and type 2 diabetes mellitus – clinical implications. *JAPI.* 2012;60:42-47.

52. Ip M, Mokhlesj B. Sleep and glucose intolerance/diabetes mellitus. *Sleep Med Clin.* 2007;2(1):19-29.

53. Knutson KL, VanCauter E. Associations between sleep loss and increased risk of obesity and diabetes. *Ann NY Acad Sci.* 2008;1129:287-304.

54. Horne J. Short sleep is a questionable factor for obesity and related disorders: statistical versus clinical significance. *Biol Psychol.* 2008;77(3):266-276.

55. Nedelteheva AV, Kilkus JM, Imperial J, Kasza K, Schoeller DA, Penev PD. Sleep curtailment is accompanied by increased intake of calories from snacks. *Am J Clin Natr.* 2009;89(1):126-133.

56. Spiegel K, Tasali E, Leproult R, Van Cauter E. Effects of poor sleep on glucose metabolism and obesity risk. *Natr Rev Endocrinol.* 2009;5:253-261.

57. Everson CA, Bergmann BM, Rechtschaffen A. Sleep deprivation in the rat: III. Total sleep deprivation. *Sleep.* 1989;12:13–21.

58. Bristol University. Does the lack of sleep make you fat? Available at: http://www.bris.ac.uk/news/2004/582. Accessed May 3, 2012.

59. Gangwisch JE, Malaspina D, Boden-Albala B, Heymsfield SB. Inadequate sleep as a risk factor for obesity: analyses of the NHANES I. *Sleep.* 2005;28:1289–1296.

60. Schmid SM, Hallischmid M, Jauch-Chara K, Born J, Schultes B. A single night of sleep deprivation increases ghrelin levels and feelings of hunger in normal-weight healthy men. *J Sleep Res.* 2008;17:331–334.

61. Gottlieb DJ, Punjabi NM, Newman AB et al. Association of sleep time with diabetes mellitus and impaired glucose tolerance. *Arch Intern Med.* 2005;165:863–867.

62. Spiegel K, Leproult R, L'Hermite-Baleriaux M, Copinschi G, Tenev PD, Van Cauter E. Leptin levels are dependent on sleep duration: relationships with sympathovagal balance, carbohydrate regulation, cortisol, and thyrotropin. *J Clin Endocrinol Metab.* 2004;89(11):5762-5768.

63. Hublin C, Partinen M, Koskenvuo M, Kaprio J. Sleep and mortality: a population-based 22-year follow-up study. *Sleep.* 2007;30:1245–1253.

64. Patel SR, Ayas NT, Malhotra MR, et al. A prospective study of sleep duration and mortality risk in women. *Sleep.* 2004;27:440-444.

65. Bryant PA, Trinder J, Curtis N. Sick and tired: does sleep have a vital role in the immune system? *Nat Rev Immunol.* 2004;4:457–467.

66. Moldofsky H, Lue FA, Davidson JR, Gorczyski R. Effects of sleep deprivation on human immune functions. *FASEB J.* 1989;3:1972–1977.

67. Sigurdson K, Ayas N. The public health and safety consequences of sleep disorders. *Can J Physiol Pharmacol.* 2007;85:179–183.

Parasomnias and Abnormal Sleep-Related Movements

Julie M. Hereford, PT, DPT

Parasomnias are conditions that are characterized by complex behaviors that occur during the sleep period without conscious awareness. An individual with a parasomnia as evidenced by polysomnography (PSG) usually does not complain of excessive daytime sleepiness or difficulty sleeping. Parasomnias are not characteristic of a specific state of sleep or wakefulness but rather are often found in a mixture of sleep states. These states are not mutually exclusive, and one state can intrude on another, resulting in a condition commonly known as a *parasomnia*. For example, disorders of arousal are a mixture of wakefulness and non-rapid eye movement (NREM) sleep; rapid eye movement (REM) behavior disorders are a mixture of wakefulness and REM sleep. A parasomnia can manifest itself as activation of the autonomic nervous system or of skeletal musculature during sleep. These episodes are usually intermittent. Parasomnias are generally divided into disorders of arousal from NREM, movement disorders associated with REM sleep, or other parasomnias according to the American Academy of Sleep Medicine.[1]

Disorders of arousal include confusional arousals, sleepwalking, and night terrors, also called *sleep terrors*. Parasomnias associated with REM sleep include REM sleep disorder, sleep paralysis, and nightmare disorder. Other parasomnias that do not fit in the previous categories include sleep-related dissociative disorder, sleep-related hallucinations, sleep enuresis, catathrenia or sleep groaning, exploding head syndrome, and sleep-related eating disorder.

Parasomnias are usually further categorized as primary or secondary. Primary parasomnias are disorders that arise from the sleep state, whereas secondary parasomnias are those that emerge during sleep but are not necessarily of the sleep state.

Unlike parasomnias, which are relatively complex, there are other relatively simple, stereotypical, and seemingly purposeful movements that occur during sleep. These sleep-related movement disorders usually cause sleep disturbance, but the sleeper may not even be aware that they are occurring. These include periodic limb movement disorder (PLMD), sleep-related bruxism, sleep-related leg cramps, sleep-related rhythmic movement disorder, and restless leg/legs syndrome.

This chapter will describe many of these parasomnias and other abnormal sleep-related movement disorders, especially those that are most likely to be encountered by the rehabilitation professional; however, this is not intended to be an exhaustive list and will not delve into in-depth neuropathophysiology, causative factors, or treatment regimens for these disorders. Rather, this is intended to be a basic overview of parasomnias and other abnormal sleep-related movement disorders (Table 13-1).

DISORDERS OF AROUSAL

Disorders of arousal are those parasomnias thought to be caused by dysfunction in the neurological processes involved in arousal in which motor activity is restored without a return to normal full consciousness. These disorders occur during NREM sleep, particularly in slow-wave (SWS) or N3 and N4 sleep, which normally occurs during the first part of a normal night's sleep and are significantly more common in childhood. These disorders rarely manifest

Hereford JM. *Sleep and Rehabilitation: A Guide for Health Professionals* (pp 113-120). © 2014 Taylor & Francis Group.

Table 13-1.

Predisposing Factors for Parasomnias

Nightmare Disorder	Night Terror Disorder	Sleepwalking Disorder	Rapid Eye Movement Sleep Behavior Disorder	Restless Leg Syndrome and Periodic Limb Movement Disorder
• Personality disorders (most frequently schizotypal) • Relationship difficulties • Other stressors • Levodopa, beta-adrenergic agents, and withdrawal of REM-suppressing medications	• Fever • Sleep deprivation • CNS-depressing medications	• Possible hereditary or familial trend • Thioridazine, fluphenazine, perphenazine, desipramine, chloral hydrate, lithium • Fever • Sleep deprivation and obstructive sleep apnea • Other disorders that disrupt slow-wave sleep • Internal stimuli (eg, distended bladder) • External stimuli (eg, noises)	• Dementia • Subarachnoid hemorrhage • Ischemic cerebrovascular disease • Olivopontocerebellar degeneration • Multiple sclerosis • Brain stem neoplasms	• Iron-deficiency anemia • Pregnancy, menstruation, and menopause • Chronic renal failure • Osteoarthritis of the hips and knees • Drugs: caffeine, TCAs, SSRIs, and dopamine receptor–blocking drugs • Neurologic disorders • Peripheral neuropathies (diabetic, idiopathic, or toxic) • Various causes of myelitis • Postpolio syndrome • Spinal cord pathology (eg, syringomyelia or radiation-induced myelopathy) • Lumbar or sacral radiculopathy

themselves during naps. The frequency of disorders of arousal lessen with increasing age as the amount of N3 and N4 sleep diminishes. There also appears to be a familial pattern to the occurrence of these types of disorders.[2]

Behaviors of disorders of arousal are more likely to occur during a febrile illness, following sleep deprivation or an irregular sleep schedule, emotional stress, alcohol consumption, menstruation, or pregnancy. Partial arousals can be provoked by obstructive sleep apnea, PLMD, or nocturnal seizures. In some cases, other sleep environmental factors such as distended bladder may play a role. Sometimes the behavior of disorders of arousal may be medication induced, especially with sedatives, hypnotics, major tranquilizers, stimulants, and antihistamines, often if used in combination with one another.

The etiology of disorders of arousal is not completely clear, but it appears that there is a combination of genetic factors and sleep environmental factors that contribute to the manifestation of the disorder. There is an increase in the prevalence of disorders of arousal in family members of an affected individual and a significant increase in these disorders in monozygotic twins.[3] It appears that rapid oscillation between components of wakefulness,

NREM sleep, and REM sleep can result in intrusion of elements of one state into another, which may be a component of these disorders. Evaluation of disorders of arousal may present a challenge because a single normal polysomnogram does not exclude the presence of a parasomnia. A parasomnia may be suspected because of complaints of excessive daytime sleepiness, unusual presentation, or significant sleep disturbance, especially if reported by a bed partner or of an individual who has a history of sleep disturbance in which injury to self or other has occurred. PSG should also be performed if underlying seizure activity is suspected. Additional electrode placement is necessary in order to detect abnormal signal activity associated with seizures.

Confusional Arousals

Confusional arousals are usually seen in children, occurring in 17%, although they occur in approximately 4% of adults.[2] Confusional arousals are characterized by excessive movement during sleep, occasionally rising to the level of thrashing about and/or inconsolable crying. The individual usually has diminished vigilance and response to external stimuli. Signs of fear or autonomic hyperactivity are generally minimal. Disorientation and confusion during the event and amnesia for the event on awakening are common. These arousals may be precipitated by sleep deprivation, shift work, forced awakenings from deep sleep, obstructive sleep apnea, or PLMD.

Sleepwalking

Sleepwalking, or somnambulism, is most prevalent in childhood, peaking at the age of 11 to 12 years, although it may also occur in nearly 4% of adults. Sleepwalking can be calm or agitated, and actions carried out during it may have varying levels of complexity and duration. Some sleepwalkers have been reported to have driven an automobile or walked away from home. Sleepwalking generally occurs during the first part of a night's sleep and typically occurs during NREM stage 3 and 4 sleep. Any factors that increase slow-wave sleep may increase the incidence of sleepwalking in affected individuals. SWS is most commonly exacerbated by sleep deprivation but may also be increased by obstructive sleep apnea, febrile illness, stress, and use of alcohol. Research has shown that sleepwalkers have activation of thalamocingulate pathways and persistent deactivation of other thalamocortical arousal systems.[4,5] There is no association between psychopathology and sleepwalking. Treatment using scheduled awakenings—that is, awakening the child just before the typical time of the sleepwalking episode—has been shown to be effective in treating this disorder and has a beneficial effect 3 to 6 months after the treatment period.[6]

Night Terrors

Night terrors are the most dramatic disorder of arousal and are distinguished from nightmares. Night terrors are frequently initiated by a loud, blood-curdling scream associated with extreme fear and panic. This is usually followed by significant activity including hitting, thrashing about, or running around, and this activity has been known to result in physical damage to the sleeper or those in the vicinity or may include property damage. The universal feature of a night terror is inconsolability. Although the individual appears to be awake, he or she cannot be drawn out of the confusional state and efforts to do so can prolong or intensify the episode. Amnesia for the event is typical. Night terror events appear to be provoked by stimuli such as snoring, irregular breathing, apneic or hypopneic events, leg movements, noise, or touch. Night terrors are typically seen in childhood but may persist into adulthood. Once thought to be an indication of significant psychopathology, it is now believed that there is no link between the existence of a disorder of arousal such as night terrors and psychological disorder. In fact, the sufferer of night terrors should be reassured that these events lack psychological significance and will tend to diminish over time. Night terrors should be distinguished from nightmares, which may be intense and may, on the other hand, have psychological significance. Night terrors generally emerge from NREM Stage 3 and 4 sleep and occur during the first part of the night. Treatment is usually not necessary, because these events will tend to diminish over time.

PARASOMNIAS ASSOCIATED WITH RAPID EYE MOVEMENT SLEEP

Rapid Eye Movement Sleep Behavior Disorder

REM sleep behavior disorder is a somewhat bizarre disorder in which the sleeper essentially acts out his or her dreams. Rather than the typical atonia of skeletal musculature that normally accompanies REM sleep, individuals with this disorder do not have this paralysis during REM sleep and therefore may act out components of their dreams. The supraspinal mechanisms responsible for REM atonia normally transmit descending inhibitory projections that result in postsynaptic inhibition of skeletal musculature. REM sleep behavior disorder is characterized by a disruption of the multisynaptic pathways in the brain stem responsible for normal suppression of muscle tone associated with REM sleep. Loss of REM atonia alone is insufficient to generate REM behavior disorder. It has been suggested that it is a problem in the pedunculopontine nucleus or other brain stem structures associated with basal ganglia pathology or may be caused by abnormal afferent signals in the basal ganglia leading to dysfunction in the midbrain. Impaired cortical activation during wakefulness and REM sleep has been reported with this disorder.[7] There is also disinhibition of motor pattern generators and behavioral release that results in the typical behavior of the disorder.

The behavior is often a violent acting-out of dreams that may be injurious to the sleeper or to the bed partner. This disorder may be acute or chronic. The acute disorder is almost always induced by medications or withdrawal of sedatives. Acute REM behavior disorder can also be triggered by withdrawal from alcohol, amphetamines, barbiturates, cocaine, and meprobamate (Equanil). The chronic disorder is more prevalent in males over the age of 50 years. It appears that individuals with this disorder do not act out normal sedate dreams, but act out more vivid, action-packed dreams that involve confrontation, aggression, and violence. The behavior acted out in the dream state is usually discordant with the individual's waking personality. REM behavior disorder has been associated with certain neurological disorders such as Parkinson's disease, multiple system atrophy, Shy-Drager syndrome, and Lewy body dementia.

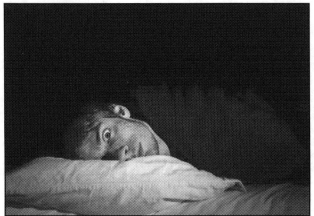

Figure 13-1. Sleep paralysis is usually associated with fear and profound anxiety. (From Fotolia.com)

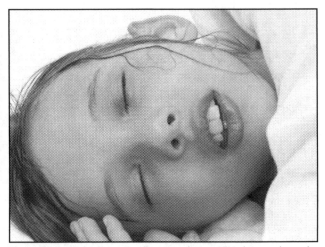

Figure 13-2. Nightmares usually occur during REM sleep and may be accompanied by increased heart rate, rapid respiration, and sweating. (From Fotolia.com)

PSG features of REM behavior disorder include excessive electromyogram (EMG) activity during REM sleep associated with abnormal movement. Limb EMG may also be increased during NREM sleep. REM sleep density is often increased and occasionally NREM stages 3 and 4 are also increased but, otherwise, sleep architecture is essentially normal.

The acute form of the disorder is generally self-limiting and will resolve once the offending medication is removed or withdrawal from sedatives is complete. Individuals with chronic REM behavior disorder, on the other hand, require treatment in order to protect themselves and/or others from harm. Approximately 90% of patients with the disorder respond positively to administration of clonazepam (Klonopin) prior to sleep.

Sleep Paralysis

Sleep paralysis is characterized by a transient inability to move the body, but respiration and eye movement are spared (Figure 13-1). The paralysis includes areflexia. The condition occurs either at sleep onset or upon awakening, but most episodes occur at sleep onset. It is usually associated with fear, profound anxiety, and hallucinations, but consciousness and memory are unaffected. Paralysis spontaneously resolves after seconds or minutes. Predisposing factors include sleep deprivation, irregular sleep patterns, stress, and sleeping in a supine position. PSG features include a REM-wake stage with increased alpha wave activity and persistence of muscle atonia into wakefulness. This is a benign condition by itself, and treatment includes reassurance and encouragement of a regular sleep cycle. The condition may, however, be associated with narcolepsy or cataplexy, and if symptoms associated with these disorders—such as excessive daytime sleepiness or sleep attacks during periods of intended wakefulness coexist—further evaluation is warranted.

Nightmares

Nightmares are described as sometimes frightening, usually unpleasant dreams that often involve threats to safety and security. These occur during REM sleep and commonly result in abrupt awakening from sleep and may involve some minor autonomic activation such as increased heart rate or respiration. They usually occur later in a night's sleep. Nightmares can erupt in NREM sleep, but these are usually associated with acute stress disorders or posttraumatic stress disorder (Figure 13-2). Recurrent nightmares can result in insomnia or sleep avoidance, excessive daytime sleepiness, and/or anxiety. PSG features of nightmare syndrome include abrupt awakening from REM sleep, REM sleep abnormalities such as decreased REM sleep latency, or increased REM sleep density and increased percentage of REM sleep.

Certain medications are known to induce nightmares in susceptible individuals. These include medications that affect neurotransmitters norepinephrine, serotonin, and dopamine such as antidepressants and antihypertensive agents, particularly beta-blockers or dopamine agonists. Withdrawal from REM-sleep suppressants such as tricyclic antidepressants, (TCAs) selective serotonin re-uptake inhibitors (SSRIs), benzodiazepines, and barbiturates can cause nightmares.

Nightmares should be distinguished from night terrors and from REM sleep behavior disorder. Nightmares tend to occur in the latter half of the night and are associated with REM sleep, whereas night terrors occur in the first half of the night and emerge from NREM stage 3 and 4 sleep. Individuals whose sleep has been disrupted by nightmares are awake and alert, but those disrupted by night terrors are generally confused and disoriented. Memory of a nightmare episode is usually complete, whereas night terrors

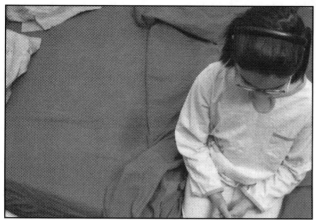

Figure 13-3. Nocturnal enuresis is more prevalent in children with ADHD. (From Fotolia.com)

usually leave the sleeper with often total amnesia to the event. Return to sleep from a nightmare may be delayed, whereas return to sleep from a night terror is usually rapid. Night terrors usually leave the sleeper with only vague imagery or a single pervasive thought such as being trapped or chased, whereas nightmares usually include a vivid, although sometimes bizarre, story line.

The occurrence of frequent and persistent nightmares may be termed a *nightmare disorder*. Treatment for nightmare disorder is varied and sometimes controversial, but reduction of anxiety through medication and/or psychotherapy may be considered. Medications that contribute to nightmares should be changed. Use of REM sleep suppressant agents such as SSRIs or TCAs may offer some relief.[8] In the case of posttraumatic stress disorder nightmares, psychotherapy to address the underlying issues should be undertaken.

OTHER PARASOMNIAS

Nocturnal Enuresis

Nocturnal enuresis is described as recurrent involuntary wetting of the bed during sleep after the age of 5 years (Figure 13-3). It can occur at any time of the night during any stage of sleep, but tends to occur in the first part of the night. A number of factors appear to contribute to this disorder, including failure to arouse in response to bladder distention, impaired ability to delay bladder contraction when the need to void develops, and increased urine production during sleep. Organic factors that may contribute to this condition should be ruled out by a physician. An organic cause should be suspected if urgency or abnormality in urinary flow is present or if involuntary voiding occurs during wakefulness, in addition to at night.

Generally, nocturnal enuresis can be subcategorized into two types with different etiologies. These include

functional bladder disorder, in which there is a failure of arousal to bladder distention stimuli due to very deep sleep, or maturational delay in nocturnal arginine vasopressin secretion. While there are pharmacologic treatments, it appears that the most effective treatment for primary nocturnal enuresis is a bed-wetting alarm.[9]

Nocturnal enuresis can be primary or secondary. Primary enuresis is described as bed wetting in a child older than 5 years or an adult who wets the bed at night at least twice a week for at least 3 months after having maintained dryness for at least 6 consecutive months. It is more common in boys than in girls and is more prevalent in children with attention-deficit/hyperactivity disorder (ADHD).[10,11] Secondary nocturnal enuresis can occur at any age and is associated with increased production of urine due to the use of diuretics, ingestion of caffeine, or impairment in the ability to concentrate urine. Urinary tract infection and urinary tract anomalies can lead to secondary nocturnal enuresis. Psychosocial stressors, depression, obstructive sleep apnea, congestive heart failure, dementia, seizures, and chronic constipation may also contribute to secondary nocturnal enuresis. Effective treatment of the underlying disorder may be effective in treating secondary nocturnal enuresis.

Parasomnias Related to Other Sleep Disorders

Parasomnias related to other sleep disorders may include abnormal movement behaviors that are particularly associated with obstructive sleep apnea. These disorders can sometimes be difficult to distinguish from disorders of arousal or REM sleep behavior disorder. Essentially, these disorders are movement behaviors that may be engaged in as an arousal from an apneic or hypopneic event. The function of such a disorder may be to restore normal respiration.

Some parasomnias are related to particular medications, rather than being a primary dysfunction in a neurological pathway. For example, β-adrenergic receptor–blocking agents have been associated with sleep hallucinations. A number of medications and substances have been known to trigger REM sleep behavior disorder, including bisoprolol (Zebeta), monoamine oxidase inhibitors, SSRIs, TCAs, and others, in susceptible individuals. Parasomnias are relatively common clinical complaints, and a formal PSG evaluation may be indicated for them, especially if accompanied by excessive daytime sleepiness or if the behavior is potentially harmful or excessively disruptive.

Restless Leg/Legs Syndrome

Restless leg/legs syndrome (RLS) is characterized by abnormal and unpleasant paresthesias or dysethesias in the lower extremities that become apparent or worsen at rest, especially during the evening at bedtime. Symptoms are often relieved, at least transiently, with movement.

Sensations often involve both legs but can be unilateral or may alternate between either lower extremity. Abnormal sensations are described as creeping, crawling, tingling, wormy, throbbing, pulling, burning, or increased tension deep in the legs, as opposed to a superficial feeling. Pain is not a common complaint but may sometimes be part of the description. Symptoms increase at rest with sitting or lying down and tend to increase at night, although they may also be associated with prolonged periods of immobility such as during an extended car trip or airline flight. There is usually an irresistible urge to move, and this may provide temporary relief of symptoms.[12]

RLS is reported in between 1% and 15% of the normal population and is more frequently reported during pregnancy and in individuals with comorbidities of uremia, anemia, and rheumatoid arthritis. The prevalence is lower in people of Asian descent than in those of northern and western European descent. It is more commonly reported in females than in males. It can occur at any age but increases in frequency of report with aging and is generally chronic in nature, although spontaneous remissions are known to occur.[13]

RLS is classified into primary, which is generally idiopathic, and secondary, which is associated with iron, folate, or cobalamin deficiency; uremia; pregnancy; or neurological disorder. Primary RLS can be further subclassified into early onset, which begins before the age of 40 to 45 and often gets progressively worse with age, and late onset, which generally begins rather suddenly and is often associated with a specific medical condition or administration of certain medications. Some medications can precipitate or worsen symptoms of restless leg/legs syndrome, including SSRIs, TCAs, sedating antihistamines, neuroleptic agents, lithium, dopamine antagonists, and calcium channel blockers.

The cause of RLS is not clear, but there appears to be a genetic link. One study indicated that approximately 92% of individuals diagnosed with primary RLS reported a positive family history for the disorder. This study also found that 13% of individuals diagnosed with secondary RLS reported a positive family history.[14] Most research seems to suggest that the mechanism of RLS is connected to dopamine production and iron metabolism. In individuals with RLS, dopamine and iron-related markers have been found in the cerebrospinal fluid (CSF) and low iron levels in the substantia nigra have also been noted.[15-17] Iron deficiency is most commonly associated with RLS. There is a link between RLS and PLMD, because both of these syndromes are related to the dopamine system. It has also been suggested that there is a link between RLS and PLMD and ADHD.[18]

The consequence of RLS is sleep disturbance. Depending on the severity of symptoms, the degree of sleep disturbance can be substantial. Symptoms may interfere with an individual's ability to get to sleep or may result in difficulty returning to sleep following awakenings. Sleep fragmentation can be significant and can lead to excessive daytime sleepiness. Symptoms of RLS are not a common reason to perform a PSG by itself, but if it is in the constellation of symptoms and a PSG is performed, sleep latency is usually prolonged and leg movements are often noted during wakefulness prior to sleep onset. Periodic limb movements during wakefulness greater than 15 per hour suggests RLS.

Periodic Limb Movement Disorder

PLMD is characterized by stereotypical intermittent repetitive movements, usually of the legs but occasionally of the arms during sleep. The stereotypic movement involves extension of the great toe, fanning of the lateral toes, partial dorsiflexion of the foot, and flexion of the knee and hip. In the upper extremity, it usually involves flexion at the elbow. This movement pattern may also occur while sitting or lying during restful wakefulness but is usually unnoticed by the individual.

Because PLMD does not awaken the sleeper, he or she is usually unaware that he or she has the condition unless it is noted by a bed partner or found during a PSG undertaken for other symptoms. Research suggests PLMD has approximately 5% prevalence in the general population. It is rarely diagnosed in children, but a link has been found between it and ADHD. It is suggested that the sleep disturbance associated with PLMD may contribute to the onset of symptoms of ADHD and further has been suggested that relief of these symptoms in children may ameliorate symptoms of ADHD.[19,20] The prevalence of PLMD increases with age, and it has been suggested that one third of adults over the age of 60 have the disorder.[21]

The etiology of PLMD appears to be related to the mechanism of disease in RLS and the genesis of RLS may trigger or aggravate symptoms of PLMD. Conditions that are associated with PLMD include low iron levels, peripheral neuropathy, renal failure, Parkinson's disease, and certain medications, including SSRIs, TCAs, monoamine oxidase inhibitors, and dopamine antagonists. Excess caffeine and alcohol or withdrawal from certain sedating medications can worsen symptoms.

Periodic limb movement symptoms can emerge after the application of continuous positive airway pressure for treatment of obstructive sleep apnea, although the mechanism for this is unknown. This is usually a transient finding and no treatment is necessary; however, if sleep disturbance or excessive daytime sleepiness continue despite optimal continuous positive airway pressure therapy, other treatment may be required.

PSG features of periodic limb movement include detection of limb movements on surface EMG over the tibialis anterior. Movements are considered as diagnostic of PLMD if they occur during sleep, have an amplitude of 25% greater than that of baseline, have duration of 0.5 to 5 seconds, and occur in a series of 4 or more contractions. Intervals between movements must be 5 to 90 seconds from the onset of one limb movement to the onset of the next. Muscle contraction can occur in one leg or in both and arousals usually occur within 3 seconds of the limb movement. Arousals can occur before, during, or after the muscle contraction. Limb movements that occur in conjunction with sleep-related breathing arousals are not scored as periodic limb movements, and stereotypical limb movements that occur during wakefulness are also considered separately. The periodic limb movement index (PLMI) is defined as the total number of periodic limb movements divided by the total sleep time in hours. A PLMI of greater than 5 in children and greater than 15 in adults is usually considered abnormal. It is often difficult to get a clear picture of this disorder on a single PSG because there can be considerable night-to-night variability. PLMD is a clinical syndrome that consists of sleep disturbance related to excessive limb movements, which is measured by the PLMI. Use of a dopaminergic agent is often considerably effective in improvement of clinical symptoms associated with PLMD.

Pathophysiology of Restless Leg/Legs Syndrome and Periodic Limb Movements of Sleep

It has been postulated that RLS and PLMD may be 2 different clinical manifestations of the same central nervous system dysfunction. The neurobiology of this is not completely clear, but it appears that areas involved include the cerebellum, thalamus, red nucleus, brain stem reticular area, pons, and diencephalon. It is possible that there is a dysregulation of the dopaminergic system with decreased receptor binding or dopaminergic hypofunction that generates these disorders. PLMD has a specific periodicity, which suggests that a central nervous system pacemaker function is involved. The movement disorder appears to originate in subcortical regions and is regulated by rhythmic fluctuations at the brain stem level.[22] When the central nervous system processes become disinhibited, the characteristic behaviors of RLS and PLMD emerge. PSG demonstrates periodic arousal stimuli leading to K-complexes followed by alpha wave activity, which is followed by limb movements. Impaired dopamine mechanisms create deficiency at dopamine-binding sites. Administration of dopamine or dopamine agonists is usually an effective treatment for RLS and PLMD and the efficacy of these drugs may be seen as diagnostic of the problem.[23]

There are a number of conditions that may have secondary RLS as a symptom. These conditions include end-stage renal disease and pregnancy, and it may be associated with gastric surgery. These conditions all have iron deficiency in common. In these conditions, there may be abnormal iron uptake or impaired iron transport across the blood–brain barrier. Iron, which is stored and transported in the form of ferritin, is transported into cells by transferrin through the transferrin receptor. When iron levels are low, ferritin is decreased, but transferrin levels are increased in an attempt to best utilize what is available. Ferritin and transferrin can be measured in CSF and serum, and in RLS; CSF ferritin levels are low and transferrin levels are high. This is important because iron plays a role in dopamine function. Iron is required for tyrosine hydroxylation, a rate-limiting step in dopamine synthesis. Decreased serum ferritin levels less than 50 mg/L decreases CSF concentrations of ferritin. This, in turn, leads to decreased iron concentration in the putamen and substantia nigra and the red nucleus and is associated with increasing severity of RLS, because these areas of the brain are not able to access sufficient iron for proper function. Impaired iron metabolism with ferritin deficiency is also associated with abnormalities in the endogenous opioid system. Interactions between the opioid system and the dopamine system in the basal ganglia, brain stem, and spinal cord all appear to be involved in the development of RLS and PLMD.[24]

RLS and PLMD can be successfully treated by resolving any underlying problems and secondary causes such as iron deficiency. Other metabolic imbalances should be evaluated and corrected. RLS that is associated with end-stage renal disease has been shown to resolve after kidney transplantation. RLS associated with pregnancy often resolves or is at least significantly diminished after delivery.

Correction of improper sleep habits that lead to chronic sleep deprivation and reduction of other contributing factors can help reduce symptoms. Avoiding exacerbating factors such as stress, strenuous activity close to bedtime, alcohol, caffeine, and certain medications may help reduce symptoms. Massage, stretching, moderate exercise, or application of heat may also help to reduce symptoms and should be considered, especially to reduce sleep-onset insomnia due to symptoms of RLS.

Medications that are commonly used for treatment of RLS or PLMD include dopaminergic agents such as dopamine precursors (carbidopa/levodopa) and dopamine agonists such as pramipexole (Mirapex) or ropinirole (Requip). These medications can produce sudden-onset severe sleepiness, which can limit their efficacy.

Benzodiazepines can be used to treat insomnia and arousals associated with symptoms of periodic limb movements of sleep, but do not change the frequency of the abnormal movements. These medications can improve sleep quality in those with RLS, but the side effects of these medications, including sedation, development of tolerance, risk of dependency, and increased fall risk in older adults, should be included in a risk–benefit analysis. Certainly iron supplementation may be considered in some patients, but must be monitored for efficacy and improvement. This treatment can be problematic because it may cause abdominal discomfort and significant constipation. Opioids may be considered in individuals with severe disease in which other treatments have not been helpful. Other medications that have been tried include anticonvulsant drugs, alpha-2 adrenergic agonists, and anti-inflammatory medications with varying degrees of success.

SUMMARY

It is important to recognize the symptoms of parasomnias, abnormal sleep-related movements, RLS, and PLMD. These conditions may cause sleep disruptions that may interfere with the rehabilitation process. Understanding these symptoms should help the clinician to direct a patient to appropriate evaluation and treatment. It is also important to understand some factors that may predispose an individual toward parasomnias and other sleep-related movement disorders in order to assist them in achieving optimal health.

REFERENCES

1. American Academy of Sleep Medicine. *The International Classification of Sleep Disorders: Diagnostic and Coding Manual.* 2nd ed. Westchester, IL: American Academy of Sleep Medicine; 2005.
2. Ohayon MM, Guilleminault C, Triest RG. Night terrors, sleepwalking and confusional arousals in the general population: their frequency and relationship to other sleep and mental disorders. *J Clin Psychiatry.* 1999;60:268-276.
3. Perlis ML, Lichstein KL, eds. *Treating Sleep Disorders: Principles and Practice of Behavioral Sleep Medicine.* Hoboken, NJ: John Wiley & Sons; 2003.
4. Crisp AH, Matthews BM, Oakey M, Crutchfield M. Sleepwalking, night terrors, and consciousness. *BMJ.* 1990;300:360-362.
5. Bassetti C, Vella S, Donati F, et al. SPECT during sleepwalking. *Lancet.* 2000;356:484-485.
6. Frank NC, Spirito A, Stark L, Owens-Stively J. The use of scheduled awakenings to eliminate childhood sleepwalking. *J Pediatr Psychol.* 1997;22:345-353.
7. Schenck CH, Mahowald MW. REM sleep behavior disorder: clinical, developmental, and neuroscience perspectives 16 years after its formal identification in sleep. *Sleep.* 2002;25(2):120-138.
8. Aurora RN, Zak RS, Auerbach SH, et al. Best practice guide for the treatment of nightmare disorder in adults. *J Clin Sleep Med.* 2010;6:389-401.
9. Thiedke CC. Nocturnal enuresis. *Am Fam Physician.* 2003;67:1499-1506.
10. Crimmins CR, Rathbun SR, Husmann DA. Management of urinary incontinence and nocturnal enuresis in attention deficit hyperactivity disorder. *J Urol.* 2003;170(4 pt 1):1346-1350.
11. Baeyens D, Roeyers H, Hoebeke P, et al. Attention deficit hyperactivity disorder in children with nocturnal enuresis. *J Urol.* 2004;171(6 pt 2):2576-2579.
12. Earley CJ. Restless legs syndrome. *N Engl J Med.* 2003;348:2103-2109.
13. National Institute of Neurological Disorders and Stroke. Restless legs syndrome fact sheet. Available at: http://www.ninds.nih.gov/disorders/restless_legs/detail_restless_legs.htm. Accessed June 22, 2012.
14. Lavigne GJ, Montplaisir JY. Restless legs syndrome and sleep bruxism: prevalence and association among Canadians. *Sleep.* 1994;17:739-743.
15. Clemens S, Rye D, Hochman S. Restless legs syndrome: revisiting the dopamine hypothesis from the spinal cord perspective. *Neurology.* 2006;67:125-130.
16. Earley C, B Barker P, Horska A, Allen R. MRI-determined regional brain iron concentrations in early- and late-onset restless legs syndrome. *Sleep Med.* 2006;7:458-461.
17. Allen RP, Connor JR, Hyland K, Earley CJ. Abnormally increased CSF 3-ortho-methyldopa (3-OMD) in untreated restless legs syndrome (RLS) patients indicates more severe disease and possibly abnormally increased dopamine synthesis. *Sleep Med.* 2009;10:123-128.
18. Cortese S, Konofal E, Lecendreux M, et al. Restless legs syndrome and attention deficit hyperactivity disorder: a review of the literature. *Sleep.* 2005;28:1007-1013.
19. Pincchiette DL, England SJ, Walters AS, et al. Periodic limb movement disorder and restless legs syndrome in children with attention deficit hyperactivity disorder. *J Child Neurol.* 1998;13:588-594.
20. Walters AS, Mandelbaum DE, Lewin DS, et al. Dopaminergic therapy in children with restless legs. Periodic limb movements in sleep and ADHD. Dopaminergic Therapy Study Group. *Pediatr Neurol.* 2000;22(3):182-186.
21. Ohayon MM, Roth T. Prevalence of restless legs syndrome and periodic limb movement disorder in the general population. *J Psychosom Res.* 2002;53:547-554.
22. Stiasny-Kolster K, Trenkwalder C, Fogel W. Restless legs syndrome—new insights into clinical characteristics, pathophysiology, and treatment options. *J Neurol.* 2004;251(suppl 6):39-43.
23. Eisensehr I, Ehrenberg BL, Noachtar S. Different sleep characteristics in restless legs syndrome and periodic limb movement disorder. *Sleep Med.* 2003;4(2):147-152.
24. Eisensehr I, Linke R, Tatsch K, et al. Increased muscle activity during rapid eye movement sleep correlates with decrease of striatal presynaptic dopamine transporters. IPT and IBZM SPECT imaging in subclinical and clinically manifest idiopathic REM sleep behavior disorder, Parkinson's disease. *Sleep.* 2003;26:507-512.

Daytime Sleepiness and Alertness

Julie M. Hereford, PT, DPT

Sleepiness is a basic physiological need state that can be likened to hunger or thirst and that does not become evident until it is most severe and persistent. Like hunger or thirst, deprivation induces the need; that is, sleep deprivation induces sleepiness and sleep fulfills the need and reverses the need state. Even when the sleep drive is severe, the subjective experience of sleepiness and its behavioral indicators such as nodding, yawning, and eye rubbing can be reduced in conditions of high motivation, excitement, or competing needs. How easily the need for sleep can be put off depends on how long it has been since the previous episode of sleep. However, at some point, as the period of time from the last sleep episode increases, sleep pressure also increases to a point at which sleep becomes impossible to avoid. Sleep is compelling and at times cannot be avoided, even though the consequences of sleep may put an individual at considerable risk. This is seen in drowsy driving and in industrial accidents in which an individual fell asleep, leading to disastrous results (Figure 14-1).

Periodic sleepiness is a normal part of life; however, when sleepiness becomes excessive and persistent, it is indicative of a serious and sometimes life-threatening condition. Severe sleepiness can manifest itself precipitously as sudden sleep attacks, episodes of microsleep, or automatic behavior during which there is no memory for the activity. Many have experienced this when driving a car and, suddenly being miles down the road, have no memory for the immediate past activity of driving. Microsleep can be suspected in this situation. Excessive sleepiness should be distinguished from fatigue and exhaustion, which carry similar characteristics but are different entities (Figure 14-2). Excessive sleepiness is defined as a condition in which an individual is unable to consistently achieve and sustain wakefulness and alertness in order to accomplish desired activities of daily living. In this condition, adults may fall asleep unintentionally and at inappropriate times and places. This condition may be experienced as hyperactivity when it occurs in children. According to WedMD, fatigue is a "state following a period of mental or bodily activity, characterized by a lessening capacity or motivation for work and reduced efficiency of accomplishment, usually accompanied by a feeling of weariness, irritability or loss of ambition."[1] It may also be described as a period after which the energy expenditure exceeds the restorative processes of the body or of a single region of the body or a single organ. This term should be distinguished from sleepiness in clinical practice.

In a normal sleep–wake cycle, maximal sleepiness occurs during the middle of the night. For example, if an individual is forced to awaken in the middle of the night, that individual will experience fatigue, weariness, difficulty concentrating, and memory lapses. Similar symptoms can be experienced during the day when physiological sleepiness becomes severe enough to intrude on waking activity. If an individual has had good quality and quantity of sleep and is well rested, he or she should be alert and should not experience sleepiness during the day even if he or she is in a soporific situation such as being in a warm room, on a long monotonous car ride, or in a boring lecture.

Changes in the electroencephalogram (EEG) may begin to occur in individuals with severe acute sleep deprivation or in those who are chronically sleep deprived. The EEG tracing may show increased alpha and theta activity which indicate the onset of sleep even though the individual

Hereford JM. *Sleep and Rehabilitation:*
A Guide for Health Professionals (pp 121-126).
© 2014 Taylor & Francis Group.

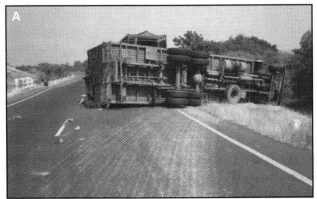 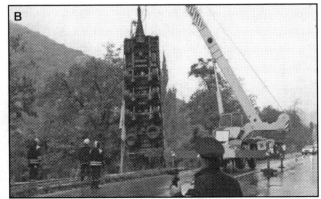

Figure 14-1. Daytime sleepiness is a particular danger in professions such as truck driving, sometimes leading to disastrous results. (From Fotolia.com)

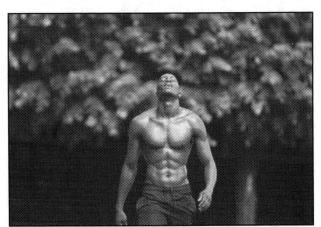

Figure 14-2. It is important to differentiate excessive sleepiness from fatigue. (From Fotolia.com)

appears behaviorally awake. These are known as episodes of microsleep. This is usually experienced as excessive daytime sleepiness. Sleepiness is often clinically measured using the Epworth Sleepiness Scale or the Stanford Sleepiness scale, while fatigue can be clinically measured using the Fatigue Severity Scale.[2-4]

DETERMINANTS OF SLEEPINESS

The degree of sleepiness is directly related to the quantity of the previous episode of sleep. The quantity of sleep is affected by the quality of sleep as well. If sleep is fragmented by sleep apnea or another sleep disorder, it will decrease the quantity of sleep. Total sleep deprivation and even modest sleep restriction reduces the average sleep latency in a systematic manner. The effects of sleep restriction accumulate over successive days.

Excessive daytime sleepiness can be screened for quickly in a clinical setting utilizing the Epworth Sleepiness Scale. This is an 8-item scale in which the individual rates likeliness to fall asleep during situations encountered in normal everyday life. A score of 0 to 9 is considered normal, but

a score above 10 suggests that the level of daytime sleepiness warrants further evaluation. A score of 11 to 15 has been correlated with increased incidence of moderate sleep apnea, and a score above 15 has been correlated with severe sleep apnea or narcolepsy.[2] Scoring of the Epworth Sleepiness Scale may vary slightly from clinic to clinic.

Sleepiness is considered mild when it occurs occasionally during times of rest or when little attention is required, such as when reading or watching television. Sleepiness is designated as moderate when it occurs daily and occurs during physical activities that require some degree of attention, such as attending a group participation meeting. Moderate sleepiness is usually associated with some impairment in social or work-related functions. Severe sleepiness is that which occurs daily and occurs during physical activities that require a moderate degree of attention and participation, such as during conversation, eating, or driving. This level of sleepiness is associated with a significant amount of impairment in social and/or work-related functions.

The consequences of excessive daytime sleepiness can be profound. It has been linked to automobile accidents, industrial disasters, and probably countless unreported household incidents. Excessive daytime sleepiness has been linked to decreased work productivity, poor academic performance, and increased absenteeism from both work and school. It has been known to contribute to mood disorders and increase irritability.

Excessive daytime sleepiness is usually caused by either inadequate duration of sleep or by sleep fragmentation due to frequent awakenings (Figure 14-3). Insufficient sleep duration may be voluntary and is, of course, the easiest condition to treat successfully. One needs only to provide for adequate opportunity for sleep, which for nearly all humans is 7 to 9 hours in a 24-hour period. Regardless of the sometimes firmly held belief that one can get by with less, the human requirement for sleep is a biological imperative and cannot be cheated without consequences. There are, however, rare genetic conditions in which an individual requires less than 7 hours of sleep or requires

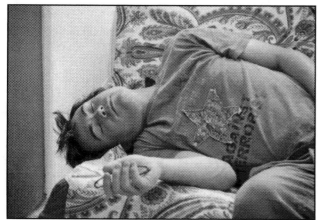

Figure 14-3. Excessive daytime sleepiness can result from any number of sources, including time zone or shift work changes, caring for a new baby or sick family member, or withdrawal from medications or stimulants. (From Fotolia.com)

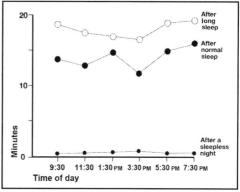

Figure 14-4. Repeated attempts to fall asleep during the day, after long sleep, normal sleep, and a sleepless night. The subjects lie down at 2-hour intervals between 9:30 AM and 7:30 PM. If they fall asleep, they are immediately awakened. The amount of time required to fall asleep is used as a measure of sleep propensity. After an extended sleep during the preceding night, the participants take a longer time to fall asleep; after a night without sleep, the time is greatly reduced.

more than 9 hours of sleep. Other than in those conditions, both chronic sleep deprivation and chronic oversleeping have been linked to illness, complications of illnesses, and premature death.

Sleep fragmentation may occur for a number of reasons, including pathology in the central nervous system pathways that disturb the sleep–wake cycle. Disruption in the sleep cycle may be caused by such conditions as obstructive sleep apnea, upper airway resistance syndrome, or periodic limb movement disorder. Environmental changes, such as change of time zone or change in lighting, shift work, or an irregular sleep–wake pattern as might occur if one is caring for a new baby or sick family member, may create abnormalities in the circadian system that impact the timing of the sleep–wake cycle. Certain medications, such as hypnotics and sedating medications, may cause sleep disruption that can lead to excessive daytime sleepiness. Withdrawal from stimulant agents or adverse reactions to certain medications may also contribute to excessive daytime sleepiness.

In addition to standard overnight polysomnography (PSG), an individual who has reported excessive daytime sleepiness may also be referred for a Multiple Sleep Latency Test (MSLT),[5] also known as a *nap study*. This test is usually performed on the morning following a standard overnight PSG. The assumption of this testing is that if an individual has normal quantity of sleep in the previous sleep episode and is well rested, he should not be able to easily fall back to sleep during the day. MSLT utilizes PSG to measure an individual's propensity to fall asleep when all competing motives are minimized. This test will therefore help to identify an individual's state of physiological sleepiness. In this test, at 2-hour intervals throughout the day, the subject is permitted to fall asleep while lying in a quiet, dark bedroom and the tendency to fall asleep is measured repeatedly using standard polysomnographic procedures (Figure 14-4). Extension of nighttime sleep time or increasing sleep

time with daytime napping increases the average sleep latency on the MSLT. Extension of sleep time through pharmaceutical means also produces an increase in sleep latency on the MSLT.

The quantity and continuity of sleep fragmentation affects daytime sleepiness. When sleep is disrupted by frequent, brief arousals of 3 to 15 seconds, characterized by EEG alpha activity or EEG desynchronization with low-voltage fast activity and sometimes accompanied by skeletal muscle tone increases, thus fragmenting sleep but not necessarily shortening the sleep episode, excessive daytime sleepiness can occur. This increases the amount of non-rapid eye movement (NREM) Stage 1 sleep and can increase the frequency of shifts between sleep stages.

Certain medications can have a profound effect on sleepiness and alertness. Central nervous system depressant medications tend to increase sleepiness. Benzodiazepines, barbiturates, and alcohol have been shown to decrease sleep latency and facilitate the action of gamma aminobutyric acid (GABA), which is a major inhibitory neurotransmitter in the central nervous system. H_1 antihistamines increase daytime sleepiness and the sedating effects related to their differential liposolubility and penetration into the central nervous system.

Certain antihypertensive agents, particularly the beta adrenoceptor blockers, also have differential liposolubility and penetration into the central nervous system. Presumably these effects are due to a blocking of the diffuse forebrain noradrenergic system, which maintains cortical activation.

Stimulant drugs reduce sleepiness and increase alertness. Amphetamine (Adderall), methylphenidate (Focalin), and pemoline (Cylert), which are given to treat the excessive sleepiness of narcolepsy and attention–deficit/hyperactivity disorder (ADHD), have been found to reduce sleepiness. These drugs facilitate catecholaminergic activity and thereby enhance and prolong wakefulness. Caffeine is a commonly used stimulant found widely in beverages and foods and has been shown to increase alertness as measured by the MSLT. Caffeine is an adenosine antagonist. Adenosine promotes the onset of sleep.

There are several conditions that may have their first manifestation as excessive daytime sleepiness.[6] These conditions include narcolepsy, cataplexy, hypersomnia, and insufficient sleep syndrome. Because of these, it is important to evaluate this complaint and to distinguish it from fatigue. There are also some conditions experienced by women during the normal course of the female cycle that can cause excessive daytime sleepiness.

INSUFFICIENT SLEEP SYNDROME

Insufficient sleep syndrome is defined as habitual, chronic, but voluntary loss of sleep time. This is usually done to try to maintain social, academic, or work activities. Some individuals, males more frequently than females, are unaware of sleep requirements or sleep habits. If an individual reports excessive daytime sleepiness, other causes of this symptom should be ruled out. PSG in individuals with chronic short sleep include decreased sleep latency, increased sleep efficiency, increased total sleep time, increased NREM Stage 3 and 4 sleep, and increased rapid eye movement (REM) sleep. The consequences of chronic insufficient sleep syndrome are predisposition toward accidents and neurocognitive impairment. It can also worsen symptoms of underlying sleep disorders.

NARCOLEPSY

Narcolepsy is a neurological disorder that is characterized by excessive daytime sleepiness and is hallmarked by the eruption of REM sleep atonia during wakefulness. Symptoms of narcolepsy generally begin during late adolescence or early adulthood, and the disorder tends to occur more frequently in men than in women.

Narcolepsy may also be accompanied by cataplexy, sleep paralysis, and sleep hallucinations. Individuals with narcolepsy may also display automatic, seemingly meaningless behavior during a sleep episode with no recall for the event. This is differentiated from sleepwalking or REM sleep behavior disorder in that the individual is otherwise physiologically awake. Sleep disturbance with frequent awakenings and poor-quality sleep are typical in narcoleptics.

PSG in individuals with narcolepsy usually include sleep fragmentation and repetitive awakenings. There is usually a shortened sleep latency of less than 10 minutes and a significantly shortened REM sleep latency, usually less than 20 minutes. REM sleep actually occurs at sleep onset in approximately 50% of individuals with narcolepsy and should always be suspected if this occurs. NREM stage 1 sleep is increased, but total sleep time and percentage of REM sleep are often normal.

The MSLT, discussed previously, is usually performed immediately following overnight PSG. This test rules out other sleep disorders and ensures adequate duration of the previous night's sleep in order to get an accurate evaluation of sleep pressure. Characteristic findings in MSLT seen in narcolepsy include a shortened mean sleep latency of less than 8 minutes with at least 2 sleep-onset REM periods. Normal sleepers usually have a mean sleep latency of 10 to 11 minutes and do not have REM sleep periods during sleep episodes in the MSLT.

Differential diagnosis of narcolepsy includes insufficient sleep syndrome, chronic sleep deprivation, hypersomnia, and substance abuse. Treatment for narcolepsy generally is pharmacologic and includes use of stimulant agents for excessive daytime sleepiness and administration of selective serotonin re-uptake inhibitors and/or tricyclic antidepressants (TCAs) for prevention of cataplexy and other symptoms associated with the disorder. Behavior modification and support are also important to manage the symptoms of this disease.

HYPERSOMNIA

Hypersomnia is a rare disorder that consists of excessive sleepiness, extended sleep time in a 24-hour sleep–wake cycle, and a persistent feeling of non-refreshing sleep, even in the immediate period after awakening. Hypersomnia may be primary idiopathic hypersomnia or recurrent hypersomnia. Symptoms of these 2 types of hypersomnia are the same but the frequency of occurrence is different.

Individuals with hypersomnia have recurring episodes of excessive daytime sleepiness. They tend to nap frequently throughout the day, often at unintended times and inappropriate places such as during work or while driving. Unfortunately, these nap periods do not afford relief from symptoms of excessive sleepiness. This disorder usually causes impaired social, academic, and/or occupational function.

Diagnosis of hypersomnia is made on the basis of history and exclusion of other causes of excessive daytime sleepiness. PSG usually reveals normal sleep architecture, but these individuals may have decreased sleep latency and increased total sleep time. Sleep latency is usually significantly reduced to as little as 3 minutes on the MSLT, but individuals with hypersomnia do not have REM sleep at sleep-onset episodes.

Treatment for this disorder includes administration of stimulant agents, although the response to them is generally less predictable. Behavioral modification is very important in management of symptoms of this disorder.

Menstrual-Related Hypersomnia

Recurrent and transient sleepiness is a frequent symptom during the premenstrual period and sometimes causes significant impairment in social, academic, or work functions. Excessive daytime sleepiness usually normalizes following menses. The cause of this symptom is not completely clear. PSG performed during this point in the menstrual cycle demonstrated decreased NREM stage 3 and 4 sleep.

Posttraumatic Hypersomnia

Posttraumatic hypersomnia is a sleep disturbance that occurs following traumatic brain injury. Studies conducted by Guilleminault et al[7,8] indicated that more than 98% of patients complained of some degree of posttraumatic hypersomnolence, which led to impairment in daytime functioning. Epworth Sleepiness Scale scores were elevated, and sleep latency on the MSLT was 5 minutes or less.[8] Several studies have shown that sleep disruptions are more likely to occur in individuals who suffer mild head trauma—that is, concussion—than in those who suffer more significant head injuries.[9,10] A study by Guilleminault et al[7] suggested that adolescents who suffer mild traumatic brain injuries such as concussions are at significantly greater risk of developing chronic sleep disorders. Other data have shown that sleep architecture changes from pre-injury patterns. This may involve difficulty initiating and maintaining sleep and excessive daytime sleepiness.[11–13] This suggests that concussions such as those suffered during collision injuries in sports are probably not as benign as had previously been thought. Disordered sleep may negatively affect response to rehabilitation processes including tissue regeneration and motor learning. The clinician should be aware of this and monitor such a patient for signs and symptoms of posttraumatic hypersomnolence.

This change in sleep pattern and the onset of hypersomnolence is especially important to note in individuals who suffer from mild concussions such as those that may result from whiplash, an auto accident, or a collision during athletics. These patients are often seen in the rehabilitation setting. Even though they have not necessarily been diagnosed with a concussion, a patient who suffers a blow to the head or who is in an auto accident often has complaints consistent with a mild traumatic brain injury. These patients may complain of pain at night that causes disruption of sleep. Sleep-disordered breathing is also a common finding in patients who have sustained a whiplash injury. Studies have shown that a high prevalence of sleep-related breathing disorders are a consequence of mild traumatic brain injuries.[14–16] Research shows that this behavior is often a new finding after the accident. Individuals who had preexisting excessive daytime sleepiness often showed severe impairment in performance of activities of daily living posttraumatically.[7,17–19] It is apparent that changes in sleep patterns and development of disordered sleep may persist well after the onset of the injury.[20,21]

Treatment of disordered sleep following a concussion or other traumatic brain injury requires good patient education and behavioral modification. These individuals should take precautions to avoid insufficient sleep. Excessive daytime sleepiness that persists may need further evaluation with a polysomnography and MSLT. These individuals may require medication and/or a continuous positive airway pressure device to manage the symptoms of disordered sleep. It is important to attain adequate sleep following a concussion or other traumatic brain injury in order to achieve optimal recovery from the injury.

SUMMARY

Excessive daytime sleepiness may be a symptom of an underlying sleep disorder and therefore should be thoroughly evaluated. The rehabilitation professional can distinguish between the symptoms of sleepiness and fatigue using the Epworth Sleepiness Scale and/or the Fatigue Severity Scale. Both of these instruments are brief, easily administered, and quickly scored. They help to identify individuals who may require further evaluation for disordered sleep. They can also help the clinician to direct treatment and thus help the patient improve overall sleep health.

Further evaluation of excessive daytime sleepiness should include a thorough history with inquiries into nighttime and daytime sleep habits. This evaluation involves estimation of sleep latency, duration of nighttime sleep, and frequency of awakenings among other things. Daytime alertness should be evaluated by discussing the overall level of alertness, inquiry into episodes of sleepiness including timing of sleepiness episodes and activity engaged in when they occur. Changes in cognition and performance and any incidence of accident should be discussed. Frequency and duration of napping and the use of stimulants including caffeine and other medications need to be evaluated in order to determine the extent of the problem.

It is important to understand the most frequent causes of excessive daytime sleepiness: disordered sleep, obstructive sleep apnea, narcolepsy, cataplexy, and hypersomnia. It is also important for the clinician to discuss normal sleep behavior and habits with the patient to help identify incidences of insufficient sleep syndrome. In this instance, the patient should be counseled on the importance of good sleep habits to overall health and the importance of sleep during the rehabilitation process.

REFERENCES

1. Fatigue. *WebMD Medical Dictionary*. Available at: http://dictionary.webmd.com/terms/fatigue. Accessed May 2, 2012.

2. Johns MW. A new method for measuring daytime sleepiness: the Epworth Sleepiness Scale. *Sleep*. 1991;14:540–545.

3. Stanford Sleepiness Scale: Hoddes E, Zarcone V, Smythe H, Phillips R, Dement WC. Quantification of sleepiness: a new approach. *Psychophysiology*. 1973;10:431-436.

4. Fatigue Severity Scale: Fatigue Severity Scale. Available at: http://www.sarme.org/pdf/sleep-Fatigue-Severity-Scale.pdf. Accessed April 19, 2011.

5. Iber C, Ancoli-Israel S, Chesson A, Quan SF. *The AASM Manual for the Scoring of Sleep and Associated Events: Rules, Terminology and Technical Specifications*. Westchester, IL: American Academy of Sleep Medicine; 2007.

6. Moline ML, Broch L, Zak R, Gross V. Sleep in women across the life cycle from adulthood through menopause. *Sleep Med Rev*. 2003;7(2):155-177.

7. Guilleminault C, Faull KF, Miles L, van den Hoed J. Posttraumatic excessive daytime sleepiness: a review of 20 patients. *Neurology*. 1983;33:1584–1589.

8. Guilleminault C, Yuen KM, Gulivich MG, et al. Hypersomnia after head–neck trauma. A medicolegal dilemma. *Neurology*. 2000;54:653.

9. Orff HJ, Avalon L, Drummond SP. Traumatic brain injury and sleep disturbance: a review of current research. *J Head Trauma Rehabil*. 2009;24(3):155–165.

10. Castriotta RJ, Murthy JN. Sleep disorders in patients with traumatic brain injury: a review. *CNS Drugs*. 2011;25(3):175–185.

11. Kaufam Y, Tzischinsky O, Epstein R, Etxioni A, Lavie P, Pillar G. Long-term sleep disturbance in adolescents after minor head injury. *Pediatr Neurol*. 2001;24(2):129–134.

12. Ayalon L, Caplan B, Drummond SP, Orff HJ. Traumatic brain injury and sleep disturbance: a review of current research. *J Head Trauma Rehabil*. 2009;24(3):155–165.

13. Mahmood O, Rapport LJ, Hanks RA, Fichtenberg NL. Neuropsychological performance and sleep disturbance following traumatic brain injury. *J Head Trauma Rehabil*. 2004;19:378–390.

14. Castriotta RJ, Wilde MC, Lai JM, Atanasov S, Masel BE, Kuna ST. Prevalence and consequences of sleep disorders in traumatic brain injury. *J Clin Sleep Med*. 2007;3:349–356.

15. Clinchot DM. Defining sleep disturbance after brain injury. *Am J Phys Med Rehabil*. 1998;77:291–295.

16. Bassiri AG, Guilleminault C. Clinical features and evaluation of obstructive sleep apnea–hypopnea syndrome. In: Kryger MH, Roth T, Dement WC, eds. *Principles and Practice of Sleep Medicine*. Philadelphia, PA: Saunders; 2005;1043-1052.

17. Watson NF, Dikmen S, Machamer J, et al. Hypersomnia following traumatic brain injury. *J Clin Sleep Med*. 2007;3:363–368.

18. Vaumann CR, Werth E, Stocker R, Ludwig S, Bassetti CL. Sleep-wake disturbances 6 months after traumatic brain injury: a prospective study. *Brain*. 2007;130:1873–1883.

19. Castriotta RJ, Lai JM. Sleep disorders associated with traumatic brain injury. *Arch Phys Med Rehabil*. 2001;82:1403–1406.

20. Chaput G, Lavigne G, Paquet J, et al. Time course prevalence of sleep disturbances and mood alterations after mild traumatic brain injury: a preliminary report. *Sleep*. 2007;30(suppl):A302.

21. Rao V, Rollings P. Sleep disturbances following traumatic brain injury. *Curr Treat Options Neurol*. 2002;4(1):77–87.

Sleep and Other Medical and Psychiatric Disorders

Julie M. Hereford, PT, DPT

RESPIRATORY DISORDERS AND SLEEP

Asthma

Asthma is characterized by episodes of shortness of breath and wheezing, reversible bronchoconstriction, and airway hyperactivity that occur in response to a variety of specific and nonspecific stimuli. Asthmatic patients sometimes experience sleep disturbance such as complaints of early morning awakenings or excessive sleepiness (Figure 15-1). Research demonstrates that 3 out of 4 asthmatics report nighttime awakenings that occur at least once per week with asthma-related symptoms.[1] Sleep in patients with nocturnal asthma is characterized by poor sleep quality with frequent arousals. These individuals report awakening due to coughing, shortness of breath, wheezing, and chest discomfort. Complaints of insomnia and excessive daytime sleepiness are also regularly reported. They may have nocturnal bronchoconstriction and sleep-related hypoxemia.[2]

Respiratory airflow varies according to circadian rhythm, with the greatest airflow occurring in the late afternoon and the lowest occurring in the morning. Expiratory flow rate also varies with sleep, and function residual capacity, minute ventilation, and tidal volume decrease during sleep. These functions may be further compromised in the individual who suffers from asthma. Circadian rhythms play a role in increased airway responsiveness, increased airway secretions, and changes in vagal tone, body temperature, cortisol production, epinephrine, and inflammatory mediator production. This may lead to a cellular inflammatory response with an increase in total leukocyte count, neutrophils, and eosinophils in individuals with nocturnal asthma.

Polysomnographic features of nocturnal asthma demonstrate decreased sleep efficiency and total sleep time and an increase in wake time after sleep onset (WASO) and frequency of awakenings. Non-rapid eye movement sleep (NREM) stage 3 and 4 may be reduced, and hypoxemia may be evident.

Treatment of nocturnal asthma may include the use of inhaled corticosteroids and long-acting bronchodilators. Anticholinergic agents may also be an effective therapy. Corticosteroid administration can diminish the circadian variability in airway tone. Nocturnal symptoms reverse rapidly with administration of bronchodilators, but unfortunately the use of short-acting beta-agonists may actually increase nighttime awakenings.

Chronic Obstructive Pulmonary Disease

Chronic obstructive pulmonary disease (COPD) is characterized by an increased inflammatory response in the airway as a response to smoking, noxious gases or fumes, heavy amounts of secondhand smoke, pollution, and frequent use of cooking fire without proper ventilation that causes injury to the bronchioles and alveoli. COPD is usually progressive and is not fully reversible. Types of COPD include chronic bronchitis in which there is airway narrowing and excessive mucus production, along with emphysema in which the alveoli are destroyed and the lungs lose capacity for efficient air exchange. Chronic cough and

Hereford JM. *Sleep and Rehabilitation: A Guide for Health Professionals* (pp 127-153). © 2014 Taylor & Francis Group.

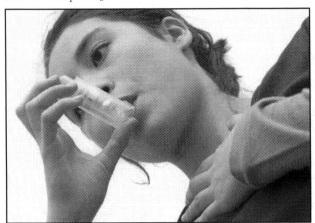

Figure 15-1. Three out of four asthma patients report nighttime awakenings. (From Fotolia.com)

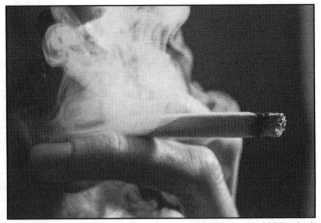

Figure 15-2. Sleep disorders are common in patients with COPD, which is commonly caused by smoking. (From Fotolia.com)

shortness of breath are the most common complaints in individuals with COPD. As the disease advances, hypoxemia and hypercapnea can occur during both wakefulness and sleep (Figure 15-2).[3]

Nocturnal cough and shortness of breath are usually associated with COPD and lead to insomnia, sleep disruption, frequent awakenings, nonrestorative sleep, and excessive daytime sleepiness. Additionally, medications such as methylxanthines and beta-adrenergic agonists are known to cause sleep disturbances.[4]

Cystic Fibrosis

Cystic fibrosis is an autosomal recessive congenital multisystemic disease that is characterized by abnormal sodium and chloride transport across the epithelium in exocrine tissues. This causes increased concentration of salt in sweat and thick viscous secretions in the lungs, pancreas, intestine, liver, and reproductive tract. Patients with cystic fibrosis may develop bronchiectasis and bronchiolectasis, exocrine pancreatic insufficiency, intestinal dysfunction, abnormal sweat gland function, and urogenital dysfunction.[5]

Patients who suffer from cystic fibrosis frequently report poor sleep quality and are noted to have increased sleep fragmentation. They often have coughing spells at night and frequently show oxygen desaturation. Patients with cystic fibrosis may have low forced expiratory volume (FEV_1) on spirometry, which is the amount of air that can be forcibly exhaled from the lungs in the first second of exhalation. They also often have low oxygen saturation during wakefulness, and this is likely to worsen during sleep. Sleep disturbances with this population can worsen during exacerbations of the disease, although they usually have normal sleep latency and normal sleep efficiency.

Restrictive Pulmonary Disease

Restrictive pulmonary disease is characterized by decreased lung volume and diffusion capacity caused by pathology involving the lung parenchyma or alteration in the chest wall, pleura, or neuromuscular apparatus of respiration.

Restrictive pulmonary diseases consist of those interstitial lung diseases that are most commonly thought of when considering this pathology. Patients with interstitial lung diseases often demonstrate transient or sustained oxygen desaturation during rapid eye movement (REM) sleep. This is characterized by an increase in the frequency of arousals and a decrease in the quality of sleep. There is an increase in NREM stage 1 sleep and a decrease in total REM sleep time.

There may also be musculoskeletal reasons why the thoracic cage is unable to achieve normal expansion and thus may result in restriction in the ability of the lungs to provide sufficient oxygen exchange with the normal respiratory apparatus (see Chapter 27). It is suggested that this is an often overlooked, yet critical area of concern and one in which the rehabilitation professional may be able to provide appropriate therapeutic intervention to maximize mechanical restrictions that limit chest expansion. Faulty mechanics of respiration may be caused by poor postural habits, accessory respiratory breathing patterns, kyphosis and scoliosis, ankylosing spondylitis, pregnancy, obesity, obstructive sleep apnea (OSA), chest wall injury, or chest wall deformity.

Additionally, many systemic disorders that affect connective tissue result in decreased segmental mobility in the thoracic cage. While a single level of restriction is unlikely to cause significant limitation of lung expansion, multiple levels of restriction and increasing severity of restriction often cause some reduction in respiratory expansion capacity. This restriction may also lead to increased muscular tone in the accessory respiratory musculature, which, in turn, alters the mechanics of respiration and adversely affects normal respiratory expansion. When muscle tone is decreased during sleep, these restrictions may contribute to the sleep-related breathing disorders, as respiratory drive is only able to overcome so much restriction in the mechanics of the system.

Patients with restrictive pulmonary disorders exhibit rapid, shallow respiratory patterns. Chronic hyperventilation occurs in an effort to overcome the effects of decreased respiratory capacity, whether it is because of reduced lung capacity and compliance or restrictions in the thoracic cage. Shortness of breath with exertion in patients with restrictive pulmonary disease often progresses to shortness of breath at rest. This can lead to fatigue of respiratory musculature and result in inadequate alveolar ventilation and carbon dioxide retention. This eventually leads to hypoxemia, which is a hallmark of respiratory disorders.

A variety of sleep-related breathing syndromes can develop in patients with kyphoscoliosis, which may include OSAs and hypopnea. These may become significant enough to cause episodes of severe central sleep apnea. Patients with restrictions in the mechanics of respiration may complain of disturbed sleep, frequent awakenings, unrefreshing sleep, and excessive daytime sleepiness.

Obesity may be a significant contributing factor to OSA because of increased fat deposits in the retropharyngeal region. OSA is found in more than 50% of severely obese individuals, and nocturnal hypoventilation occurs in more than 29% of severely obese individuals. Sleep latency is usually normal, but sleep efficiency is decreased. REM sleep latency is usually normal, but the total amount of REM sleep is often reduced in the obese sleeper.

During pregnancy, polysomnography (PSG) usually demonstrates a decrease in sleep efficiency and an increase in the frequency of awakenings. NREM stage 1 sleep is often increased and REM sleep is decreased, resulting in complaints of deterioration in the quality of sleep. During pregnancy, there may be a new onset of snoring, but significant OSA is uncommon unless it was present prior to pregnancy.

Overall, with restrictive pulmonary diseases, there is sleep disturbance and nonrestorative sleep reported. There often are frequent awakenings and sleep-related breathing disorders in addition to nocturnal oxygen desaturation. These occurrences at night generally lead to excessive daytime sleepiness.

NEUROMUSCULAR DISORDERS AND SLEEP

Ventilator compromise may be a complication of neuromuscular disorders, and these problems can be further complicated during sleep. Several neuromuscular disorders are commonly associated with sleep-related breathing disorders. These include muscular dystrophy, myotonic dystrophy, amyotrophic lateral sclerosis, poliomyelitis, and myasthenia gravis. Sleep-related breathing disorders, including alveolar hypoventilation, can precede abnormalities during wakefulness by months or years. Symptoms of sleep disorders often manifest themselves prior to overt symptoms of neuromuscular disorders. Symptoms can include insomnia, sleep disturbance, excessive daytime sleepiness, fatigue, morning headaches, nocturnal dyspnea, and new onset of snoring. It is unknown if sleep disturbance plays a role in the development of neuromuscular disorder. On the contrary, individuals with neuromuscular disorders often have decreased respiratory function, which is more pronounced during sleep. Sleep-related oxygen desaturation is greater in individuals with maximal inspiratory pressure less than 60 cm H_2O and forced vital capacity less than 50% of predicted.

Specific neuromuscular disorders have some characteristic findings on PSG. These changes in sleep patterns may be contributing factors in expression of the disorder or may be a contributing factor in the rapidity of progression of these disorders. Because of this, it is important for rehabilitation professionals to understand the relationship between sleep disorders and neuromuscular disorders. The rehabilitation professional should be able to recognize signs and symptoms of disordered sleep and be prepared to direct the patient toward appropriate resources and sleep specialists in order to identify and effectively treat sleep disorders. This will help the overall course of the disease process and positively impact rehabilitation outcomes.

Duchenne Muscular Dystrophy

Duchenne muscular dystrophy (DMD) is a neuromuscular disorder characterized by muscle wasting that begins in the lower extremities and pelvis and progresses to shoulder and neck musculature. As this degenerative disease progresses, there is loss of musculature in the arms and, finally, loss of respiratory musculature. Signs and symptoms may be present at birth, but usually are evident prior to the fifth birthday. The disease is progressive and fatal, with an average life expectancy of 25 years. DMD is a recessive x-linked mutation affecting 1 in 3600 boys. While both sexes can carry the mutation, females very rarely exhibit signs of the disease.[6] It is caused by a mutation in the dystrophin gene, which is involved in generation of the protein dystrophin. Dystrophin connects the cytoskeleton of each muscle fiber to the underlying basal lamina. When it is absent, excess calcium can penetrate the sarcolemma. The change in this signaling pathway allows water to enter into the mitochondria and causes them to burst. Mitochondrial dysfunction amplifies stress-induced cytosolic calcium signals and reactive-oxygen species production. This leads to a complex and not clearly understood cascade of events that leads to damage to the sarcolemma and eventually muscle cell death. Necrotic muscle fibers are replaced with adipose and connective tissue.

Individuals with DMD can present with both central sleep apnea and obstructive sleep apnea. PSG may reveal an increase in the frequency of arousals and a reduction in the total amount of REM sleep. These changes in sleep pattern during the natural course of DMD, if left untreated, may result in a more rapidly progressive disease.

Myotonic Dystrophy

Myotonic dystrophy is a chronic, slowly progressive, inherited, multisystemic disease characterized by muscle wasting and atonia, endocrine dysfunction, cardiac conduction defects, and cataract formation, but the presentation can be substantially variable. It occurs as a severe congenital form (DM1) and a milder form (DM2) that can occur at any age but usually begins in childhood. It is an autosomal dominant disease. DM1 patients often present with myotonia, distal weakness, and cognitive problems. They may have weakness in the face and jaw musculature, ptosis, and weakness of the musculature of the neck, hands, and lower legs. DM2 is generally milder and may also involve the smooth musculature especially in the gastrointestinal (GI) tract. DM2 patients usually present with muscle pain, stiffness, fatigue, and proximal muscle weakness.[7] Both forms of myotonic dystrophy are characterized by excessive daytime sleepiness, dysphagia, and respiratory insufficiency. Cognitive dysfunction may be manifested by problems with executive function including concentration and word-finding problems. Both forms are also associated with insulin resistance.

Physical therapy intervention calls for strengthening and aerobic training, which will promote cardiorespiratory function and prevent further disuse atrophy.[8-10] Patients with myotonic dystrophy may also require bracing and specific neuromuscular re-education to allow normal gait and other functional activities.

Individuals afflicted with myotonic dystrophy frequently have disrupted sleep including apneic and hypopnic events and hypoventilation-induced oxygen desaturation during REM sleep.

Amyotrophic Lateral Sclerosis

Amyotrophic lateral sclerosis (ALS) is characterized by a rapidly progressive muscle weakness, atrophy, and fasciculation and muscle spasticity. Eventually, individuals with ALS develop dysarthria, dysphagia, and respiratory disability. Muscle weakness and atrophy are caused by upper and lower motorneuron degeneration. As the disease progresses, the patient will lose the ability to control all voluntary movement, although bladder and bowel control and ocular movement are usually spared. Cognitive function is also usually preserved, as is the sensory system and autonomic function, leaving the patient virtually trapped in a progressively, and eventually completely, dysfunctional body in which they are still able to sense, feel, and understand what is happening. A very small percentage of ALS patients may also develop frontotemporal dementia.[11]

As the diaphragm and intercostal musculature weaken, FEV_1 and maximum inspiratory pressure, which is a measure of the respiratory muscles obtained by having the patient inhale as strongly as possible with the mouth against a mouthpiece (the maximum value is near the residual volume), decrease. Bilevel positive pressure ventilation or BiPAP can be utilized to support respiration and to reduce the energy expenditure of the increased respiratory effort. This is, however, only a temporary treatment, as eventually there is enough respiratory compromise rendering it ineffective, and the patient must be placed on long-term mechanical ventilation.

Physical therapy and occupational therapy for individuals with ALS include interventions and supportive techniques that are aimed at delaying loss of strength, maintaining endurance, limiting pain, preventing complications, and promoting functional independence. A treatment program should also consider appropriate adaptive equipment and assistive technology to enhance the patient's independence and safety throughout the course of the disease.[12]

ALS is the most common neuromuscular disease affecting all ethnicities. One to two out of 100,000 individuals are affected annually, with the most common age of onset between 40 and 60 years of age; men are affected slightly more frequently than women.[13]

OSA and hypopnea are predominantly seen during REM sleep of patients who suffer from ALS. The overall apnea hypopnea index (AHI) can be elevated, but may only be mildly so. As diaphragmatic dysfunction begins to develop, however, apneic and hypopnic events can cause marked nocturnal oxygen desaturation and can significantly complicate the disease and impact survival. REM sleep is also reduced and correlates with increasing diaphragmatic dysfunction.

The rehabilitation professional should be aware of the signs and symptoms of disordered sleep, especially those that may have pre-dated the diagnosis of ALS, and ensure that the patient receives appropriate screening. PSG is strongly recommended in any patient diagnosed with ALS especially during the early stages so that neuromuscular function can be preserved for as long as possible. Preexisting sleep-related breathing disorders increase energy expenditure and may allow a more rapid progression of the disease.

Poliomyelitis

Poliomyelitis or infantile paralysis is an acute infectious disease spread primarily via the fecal-oral route from person to person. Approximately 90% of polio infections pass with little or no obvious disease; however, in approximately 10% of the cases, the virus enters the central nervous system and approximately 5 per 1,000 cases develop preferential infection and destruction of the alpha motorneurons in the anterior column of the spinal cord or brain stem. This results in muscular weakness and acute flaccid paralysis. Polio has existed as an endemic pathogen for thousands of years until the 1880s when major epidemics swept Europe and then the United States. This led to development of a vaccination and near eradication of the disease, until the last 10 years when waning vaccination efforts have led to a resurgence of the disease, especially in third world counties.[14,15]

While the occurrence of acute flaccid paralysis from a new polio infection is unlikely in the United States, a rehabilitation professional is far more likely to encounter cases of postpolio syndrome. Studies have reported that 25% to 50% of individuals who have survived childhood paralytic polio will develop additional symptoms many decades after recovering from the acute infection. Postpolio syndrome is characterized by new muscle weakness and marked fatigue. This disorder is thought to be caused by failure of the oversized motor units created during recovery from childhood polio.[16-20] It appears that the risk of postpolio syndrome increases in relationship to the length of time passed since the acute polio infection. It also increases in the presence of permanent residual impairment after recovery from the acute illness due to both overuse and disuse of neurons.[16] It should be noted that individuals displaying symptoms of postpolio syndrome do not shed new polio virus and therefore cannot spread the virus any longer.[13]

As a lower motorneuron disease, poliomyelitis can involve respiratory motor nuclei and cause respiratory dysfunction because of weakness of the diaphragm and intercostal musculature that persists after recovery of the acute infection. This can set up an abnormal respiratory pattern with increased use of accessory respiratory musculature and disuse atrophy in the diaphragm. This respiratory pattern can become more entrenched and may worsen with the onset of postpolio syndrome.

Sleep-related breathing disorders may be more pronounced in this population and may include nocturnal hypoventilation, OSA, and hypopnea. Excessive daytime sleepiness is a common feature of postpolio syndrome. PSG findings may include decreased sleep efficiency and increased frequency of arousals. NREM sleep stage 1 may be increased, and total REM sleep time may be decreased. These sleep disorders may lead to increased progression of weakness. Disordered sleep and excessive daytime sleepiness may lead to impaired motor function and contribute to balance disorders, which, in turn, increase the risk of falls. It is important that the rehabilitation professional recognize signs and symptoms of disordered sleep and the consequences in this particular patient population.

Myasthenia Gravis

Myasthenia gravis is an autoimmune disease that affects the neuromuscular system leading to fluctuating muscle weakness and muscle fatigue. The disease is caused by antibodies that cause postsynaptic inhibition of the acetylcholine receptors at the neuromuscular junction. It is treated with acetylcholinesterase inhibitors or immunosuppressant medication. Thymectomy may also be considered in some cases.

Muscular involvement is variable, and the disease is classified accordingly. It may cause weakness in muscles that control eye muscles. It may present as a ptosis or paresis in muscles of facial expression or may present as difficulty chewing, talking, or swallowing. Respiratory muscles may be affected, and in some cases, there is weakness in the muscles of the neck and upper and lower extremities.[21] When respiratory musculature is involved, the patient may require assisted ventilation in order to sustain life. This may occur in patients who have a preexisting dysfunction in the mechanics of respiration. Exacerbations of the disease may be triggered by fever, infection, or emotional stress.[22]

Because of the fluctuating nature of the weakness and muscle fatigue symptoms associated with myasthenia gravis, patients with this disease should be educated regarding appropriate pacing, especially during exercise. Patients with myasthenia gravis also have a propensity to have weakness in muscular control of respiration, particularly inspiratory musculature. They should undergo specific rehabilitation to promote normal respiration and to strengthen the diaphragm and inhibit accessory respiratory musculature. Improving chest wall mobility and respiratory pattern and increasing respiratory endurance is also an important component of management of this disease.[23]

There is a higher incidence of OSA and hypopnea in patients with myasthenia gravis. They may also experience significant oxygen desaturation, particularly in REM sleep. The rehabilitation professional should be aware of the potential respiratory complications inherent in this disease and work to restore proper mechanics of respiration.

Diaphragm Paralysis

Diaphragm paralysis is a rare clinical problem that may occur in isolation or as part of a systemic disease, especially those that involve the phrenic nerve. Unilateral diaphragmatic paralysis is far more common than bilateral diaphragmatic paralysis. The former is most commonly caused by invasion of the phrenic nerve by malignant disease, particularly bronchogenic carcinoma. Bilateral diaphragmatic paralysis is most commonly caused by spinal cord injury, multiple sclerosis (MS), anterior horn disease, and muscular dystrophy.

In the incident of unilateral diaphragmatic paralysis, the hemidiaphragm elevates and compresses the hemithorax.

This consequently creates a restrictive lung disorder. A hemidiaphragm reduces vital capacity by approximately 20% in sitting and by nearly 40% in supine positions. Ventilation and perfusion of the lower lobe of the lung on the affected side is also reduced. This mismatch can increase the alveolar-arterial oxygen difference and produce a mild hypoxemia. Generally healthy adults may tolerate these changes fairly well, but patients who are obese or have underlying pulmonary disease are more likely to be symptomatic.[24]

It is clear from the description of this disorder that any further compromise to respiratory function will complicate the effects of this disorder. Unilateral diaphragmatic paralysis may lead to significant nocturnal hypoxemia due to positional restrictions. In the absence of underlying pulmonary disease, it does not usually cause chronic respiratory failure or cor pulmonale. Bilateral diaphragmatic paralysis, however, can contribute to sleep apnea. PSG in individuals with paralysis of the diaphragm can demonstrate an increase in NREM stage 3 and 4 sleep and a decrease in total sleep time. This, in turn, causes excessive daytime sleepiness and poor sleep efficiency, which will lead to the sequelae of disordered sleep discussed earlier in this section.

OTHER CENTRAL NERVOUS SYSTEM CONDITIONS

Dementia

Dementia is described as a loss of brain function that affects memory, judgment, perception, behavior, thinking, and sometimes language. Most types of dementia are degenerative. Alzheimer's disease is the most common form of dementia, but it accompanies a number of other diseases including Huntington's disease, MS, and Parkinson's disease. Dementia can be caused by changes in the vasculature in the brain or may be caused by a series of small strokes.

Sleep fragmentation and repetitive arousals and awakenings are common findings in sleep studies of individuals with dementia. This disordered sleep pattern is primarily due to the underlying dementia, but symptoms may also be worsened by sleep-related breathing disorders, periodic limb movement, or secondary depression. Individuals with dementia may also experience a phenomenon known as "sundowning" in which the individual displays symptoms of increased confusion, agitation, and wandering as the day passes into night. Individuals with dementia also often have an issue with a reversal of the normal sleep-wake cycle in which they experience nighttime insomnia and excessive daytime sleepiness. PSG often shows decreased sleep efficiency, decreased REM sleep, and decreased REM density.

Sleep disorders in patients with dementia can be challenging, especially in an institutional setting such as a long-term care facility. If factors that may be contributing to disordered sleep, such as depression, pain problems, or other disorders that disrupt sleep, receive adequate treatment, the sleep disorder may become significantly more manageable. If not, both the sleep disorder and the underlying problem may become worse. Careful management of proper sleep hygiene is also important and should include keeping a regular sleep schedule and reducing or eliminating daytime napping. Short-term hypnotics such as zolpidem, zaleplon, or eszopiclone may also provide short-term relief of insomnia.

Cerebrovascular Disease

Cerebrovascular disease is caused by disease in the blood vessels of the brain. The most likely contributor to cerebrovascular disease is hypertension, which damages the endothelium of the blood vessels, exposing underlying collagen and allowing platelets to aggregate in an effort to repair the damage. Sustained hypertension permanently changes the architecture of the vasculature, causing it to narrow and become stiffer, deformed, and more vulnerable to fluctuations in blood pressure. The changes in blood pressure during sleep can lead to marked decrease in blood flow in already narrowed vasculature, causing ischemic stroke early in the morning. Sudden rises in blood pressure due to excitation during the day can result in hemorrhagic stroke.

Patients who have suffered a stroke may develop sleep onset insomnia and frequent awakenings. If the stroke is hemorrhagic, it may cause excessive daytime sleepiness. OSA increases the risk of cerebrovascular disease and stroke. Stroke may also increase the risk of developing OSA.

Central Nervous System Infections

Central nervous system infections include encephalitis and meningitis. Fungal infections may include brain abscesses; protozoal infections include toxoplasmosis or malaria. Bacterial infections of the brain may occur as a result of tuberculosis, syphilis, bacterial meningitis, or late-stage Lyme disease. Viral infections of the brain may be those carried by mosquitoes or resulting from herpes simplex, rabies, measles, polio, or AIDS.

Central nervous system infections tend to increase excessive daytime sleepiness. In fact, this may be the initial presenting symptom.

Central Nervous System Neoplasms

Central nervous system neoplasms include solid tumors in the brain or spinal cord and malignancies in lymphatic tissue, blood vessels, cranial nerves, skull, pituitary gland, or pineal gland (Figure 15-3). Brain tumors may involve malignancy of the neurons or glial cells. They may be

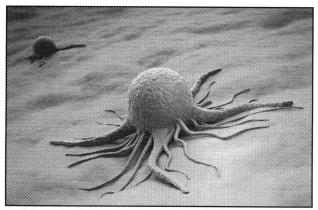

Figure 15-3. A cancer cell. Cancer is often associated with daytime sleepiness. (From Fotolia.com)

primary tumors or metastatic tumors in which the primary malignancy is elsewhere in the body. Primary brain tumors are most commonly located in the posterior cranial fossa in children and in the anterior two-thirds of the cerebral hemispheres in adults. The most common primary brain tumors are gliomas, which constitute more than 50% of all malignant tumors. Twenty percent of all primary brain tumors are meningiomas, 15% are pituitary tumors, and 8% are nerve sheath. Tumors of the central nervous system may manifest as either excessive sleepiness, hypersomnia, or insomnia. Hypersomnolence may be caused by increased intracranial pressure especially if the tumor involves midline structures such as the hypothalamus or brain stem. Nocturnal seizures or abnormal sleep-related movements may also be noted.

Encephalopathy

Encephalopathy is a global term used to generally describe a disorder or disease of the brain that is not one of the more clearly described disorders. Encephalopathy is not a single disease, but rather usually describes a syndrome of dysfunction that may be caused by a variety of different illnesses. The hallmark of encephalopathy is altered mental state, which may be a loss of cognitive function, personality changes, irritability, lethargy, and altered state of consciousness. There may be other neurological signs involved, including nystagmus, myoclonus, tremor, seizures, and respiratory abnormalities such as Cheyne Stokes respiration. Encephalopathy may manifest as excessive daytime sleepiness.

Multiple Sclerosis

MS is characterized by damage and ultimate demyelination and scarring of the myelin sheaths around axons of the brain and spinal cord. As myelin is lost, axons can no longer effectively conduct electrical impulses, leading to a variety of neurological symptoms. This disorder is most commonly diagnosed in young adult females. Its

prevalence is between 2 and 150 per 100,000.[25] The etiology is unknown, but theories include infection or genetic links and environmental risk factors.[26,27] MS may manifest as a slowly progressive disorder or may present as a relapsing-remitting disorder. The course of the disease is difficult to predict, and there is no known cure. Treatment is aimed at restoring function after an exacerbation, preventing relapse, and preventing disability.

MS may produce insomnia, which leads to excessive daytime sleepiness. Insomnia associated with MS may be initial insomnia, which is likely caused by side effects of certain medications used to treat symptoms of MS. Middle insomnia may be caused by high levels of daytime fatigue, which is a paradoxical but common occurrence. Middle insomnia may also be caused by nocturia or bladder dysfunction or may be because of muscle spasms and pain that are associated with MS. Terminal insomnia in individuals with MS is not well understood, but may be related to mood disorders or lack of normal sunlight exposure because of the level of disability causing a circadian rhythm dysfunction. It is important to sort out the nature of the insomnia in this patient population and help develop strategies to deal with the causes. Fatigue can be a significant factor affecting the quality of life in a patient with MS; therefore, adequate sleep and rest are very important in any disease management plan.

Myelopathy

Myelopathy is disease or injury involving the spinal cord, that may be caused by inflammation, known as myelitis; vascular disease, known as vascular myelopathy; or by trauma. It is defined clinically by the presence of bilateral upper motor neuron signs including paresis and hyperreflexia, bilateral sensory deficits, and bowel and bladder problems. Spinal cord disease can result in insomnia related to chronic pain and/or muscle spasms. Sleep-related breathing disorders can be exacerbated by paresis of respiratory musculature. Both of these situations can cause excessive daytime sleepiness.

Traumatic Brain Injury

Traumatic brain injury (TBI) occurs when an external force injures the brain. It may occur because of a direct impact to the head or may be caused by acceleration alone. TBI can take the form of a closed head injury or a penetrating head injury. The injury may occur in specific area of the brain or may cause widespread damage. Damage may be caused by the initial injury, changes in cerebral blood flow, or increases in intracranial pressure leading to secondary damage. TBI can cause a range of physical, cognitive, and emotional problems depending on the severity and location of the injury. It can cause a range of impairments in movement and motor control including spasticity, ataxia, and tremor. TBI can also cause impairments in cognitive function, ranging from memory loss to loss of attention and concentration, impaired judgment, insight and thought processes, decreases in processing speed, and loss of executive function such as abstract reasoning and problem solving. It may also cause communication difficulties from various forms of aphasia, depending on location and severity of injury, to loss of understanding of more subtle forms of communication such as body language. Ten to fifteen percent of individuals who have suffered a TBI also develop hypopituitarism as a result of the injury and may go on to develop diabetes insipidus or other hormonal or electrolyte imbalances because of a shearing injury to the stem of the pituitary as it sits in the sella turcica.[28]

TBI is associated with significant sleep disturbances including excessive daytime sleepiness and a new onset of sleep apnea. This should be a consideration for the rehabilitation provider in developing and implementing a treatment program. If the patient has a significant sleep disorder, it may impact his or her ability to fully engage in and progress through a rehabilitation program. It may be difficult to determine if symptoms are a direct result of the TBI or if they are exacerbated by either preexisting or new onset of disordered sleep. For example, attention and concentration may be impaired by sleep deprivation or may be a primary symptom of the TBI. Difficulty learning new motor tasks may also be complicated by disordered sleep. Therefore, it is important to understand the impact of disordered sleep in this patient population as it relates to memory and motor learning (see Chapter 21).

Postconcussion Syndrome

Another significant, but often overlooked, consequence of TBI is postconcussion syndrome, which is described as a set of symptoms that last beyond the immediate recovery period after the initial injury. These symptoms may include physical, cognitive, and behavioral problems such as headaches, dizziness, and loss of concentration, word-finding problems, and depression.[29-33] Repetitive TBI or concussion may also have a cumulative effect. A growing concern in TBI is second-impact syndrome, in which a young person with a still-developing brain sustains a second concussion before fully recovering from the first. After the second injury in this situation, the brain can swell catastrophically after even a relatively mild blow, resulting in significant debilitation or even death.[30] Repetitive concussions or mild TBI, like those experienced by 1 in 5 career boxers, can cause cognitive and behavioral impairments and may even result in dementia pugilistic and parkinsonism.[34]

TBI, particularly mild injury such as concussion, is known to cause excessive daytime sleepiness. It has also been linked to new onset of sleep-related breathing disorders.[35-38] TBI may also cause insomnia, which further contributes to excessive daytime sleepiness and may complicate the sequelae of the TBI. Sleep apnea and/or circadian rhythm sleep disorders, especially delayed phase sleep disorder, can develop.[34] PSG findings demonstrate increased sleep fragmentation marked by increased awakenings and decreased total sleep time.

NEURODEGENERATIVE DISORDERS AND SLEEP

Neurodegenerative disorders tend to have characteristic disturbances of sleep. These individuals usually demonstrate markedly disrupted sleep with muscular contractions and gross body movements that occur during sleep and may cause arousals or awakenings. They may have insomnia, which, in conjunction with the frequent awakenings, can cause excessive daytime sleepiness. These individuals may suffer from REM sleep behavior disorder. Polysomnographic features include reduced sleep efficiency, increased frequency of awakenings, decreased NREM stage 3 and 4 sleep, and decreased REM sleep.

Because of the postural deficits that may occur in neurodegenerative disorders, preexisting OSA may be significantly worse. Consideration should be given to the impact of disordered sleep on rehabilitation. Correction of sleep disorders may improve patient outcomes and improve compliance with the treatment program.

Huntington's Disease

Huntington's disease is a neurodegenerative disease that affects muscle coordination, causes abnormal involuntary writhing movements known as chorea, and usually causes a decline in cognitive function. It is a genetically mediated disorder that has a typical onset in middle-aged adults. The genetic mutation causes a mutant form of protein that gradually damages brain cells. It is most commonly found in people of Western European descent and is an autosomal dominant mutation of either copy of the Huntington gene. Symptoms of Huntington's disease can begin at any age, but people usually experience onset at 35 to 44 years of age. Symptoms vary, but usually the onset involves a subtle decline of mood or cognition. Gradually coordination and gait ataxia develop. As the disease progresses, movement becomes more uncoordinated and jerky until coordinated movement is extremely difficult. Cognitive abilities worsen, and behavioral and psychiatric functions decline into dementia. Life expectancy is usually approximately 20 years from onset due to complications such as pneumonia, heart disease, or sequelae from falls. There is currently no cure for Huntington's disease, and drug treatment is aimed at treating symptoms or slowing the progression of the disease.

The hallmark of sleep dysfunction in individuals with Huntington's disease is sleep fragmentation and insomnia.

Progressive Supranuclear Palsy

Progressive supranuclear palsy is a degenerative disease that results in gradual deterioration of specific regions of the brain. Approximately 6 in 100,000 are afflicted with the disease, and there is no gender or ethnic bias to its victims. Neuronal and glial cells are affected by forming neurofibrillary tangles in clumps of tau protein, which may bear some resemblance to those seen in the cerebral cortex in an Alzheimer's brain.[39,40] Areas usually affected in progressive supranuclear palsy include the basal ganglia, particularly the subthalamic nucleus, substantia nigra and globus pallidus, the brain stem, the frontal lobes of the cerebral cortex, dentate nucleus of the cerebellum, and the spinal cord, particularly bowel and bladder control areas.

Patients with progressive supranuclear palsy should receive rehabilitation for balance and gait disturbances.[41] Patients with this disease have a tendency to fall, especially backward, so assistive devices must be selected accordingly, with a weighted walker preferred over a cane. Rehabilitation will help improve independence as long as possible. Because of the progressive nature of the disease, however, patients with progressive supranuclear palsy will eventually be unable to walk and will become wheelchair bound.

The hallmark of sleep dysfunction in individuals with progressive supranuclear palsy is insomnia and significant sleep disruption.

Torsion Dystonia

Torsion dystonia is characterized by painful muscle contractions that result in uncontrollable postural distortions. The disease usually occurs in children at 11 to 12 years of age. It may affect a local area but will progress to involve the entire body and lead to a completely debilitated state usually within 5 years of onset of symproms. It is a genetic disorder with a mutation of the DYT1 gene that causes a deletion of the glutamic acid in the Torsin A protein. This defect causes a disruption in motor control.

The hallmark of disordered sleep in individuals with torsion dystonia is sleep deterioration and dystonia symptoms, which increase during sleep. Any pre-existing airway problem is likely to be significantly worse because of the postural constrictions caused by the torsional dystonia. This should be a consideration in treatment planning and referral to a functional dentist who understands the relationship between mandibular positioning and cervical function.

Parkinson's Disease

Parkinson's disease is a degenerative disorder of the central nervous system that results from destruction of dopaminergic cells in the substantia nigra of the basal ganglia. During the early course of the disease, there is a tremor at rest, muscular rigidity, difficulty in initiation of movement, and slowness of movement. There is also a characteristic gait pattern in which the individual may seem to have difficulty initiating walking, but then seems to lean forward and move rapidly but rigidly. As the disease progresses, cognitive and behavioral difficulties arise. Cognitive dysfunction often progresses into Parkinsonian dementia in the advanced stages of the disease. Other common symptoms of Parkinson's disease include sensory problems, emotional problems, and sleep disturbance. Parkinson's disease is more common in older adults, but can occur in younger individuals usually related to TBI or repetitive concussion. There are also cases reported related to street-drug use and exposure to certain pesticides. There is also a reduced risk of development of the disease reported among tobacco smokers.

Treatment for Parkinson's disease in its early stages includes managing motor symptoms through the use of levodopa and dopamine agonists. As the disease progresses and more and more dopaminergic neurons are lost, these medications become less effective. Deep brain stimulation has been shown to be effective in reducing motor symptoms in some individuals. New treatments are on the horizon and include gene therapy, stem cell transplants, and neuroprotective agents. Medication is also used to treat the non-motor symptoms that usually accompany Parkinson's disease such as sleep disturbances and emotional problems.

The hallmark of disordered sleep in individuals who suffer from Parkinson's disease is excessive sleepiness due to sleep fragmentation. These individuals also often suffer from insomnia and reversal of the sleep-wake cycle. Sleep disturbances in Parkinson's disease may be caused by muscle spasms, painful leg cramps, or tremors. These individuals also have decreased spontaneous body movements and difficulty moving in bed, especially turning because of muscular rigidity that can result in arousals from sleep. Patients with Parkinson's disease often also have circadian rhythm disorders. Concurrent Parkinsonian dementia, mood disorder, or pre-existing sleep problems can exacerbate symptoms of disordered sleep. Pharmaceutical agents used to treat Parkinson's disease may also cause sleep problems, most notably excessive daytime sleepiness. Disordered sleep in this patient population can have an adverse effect on the rehabilitative process, and the clinician should be aware of these potential complications.

SLEEP-RELATED HEADACHES

Headaches are usually related to sleep in some fashion. Headaches are associated with insomnia, either as a causative factor (ie, lack of sleep from insomnia triggers a headache) or resultant (ie, headache pain disrupts the ability to fall asleep and therefore causes disruption of sleep). Some headaches are characterized by their onset during particular stages of sleep. For example, migraines often occur during NREM stage 3 and 4 sleep or during REM sleep. Cluster headaches and chronic paroxysmal hemicrania that occur during sleep are associated with REM sleep.

Morning headaches are a very frequent symptom in patients with OSA prior to the administration of continuous positive airway pressure (CPAP) or another effective method of ameliorating the airway obstruction. Patients who report frequent morning headaches should be screened more carefully for indications of a sleep disorder. It is not uncommon for these individuals to position their head and neck such that they are able to maintain an airway during sleep but are hyperextending the head on the neck. This posture, especially if it is sustained over a night's sleep, can be the source of mechanical pain resulting in a headache.

Polysomnographic features of headache syndromes include increased frequency of arousals and decreased total sleep time.

Migraine Headaches

Migraine headaches are characterized by moderate to severe headaches that are usually unilateral. The individual may also report nausea, vomiting, and sensitivity to light and sound. Usually the headache requires the person to lie down in a dark room. Treatment can include use of analgesics for headache and antiemetic for nausea and learning to avoid triggers. The cause of migraine is unknown but is frequently thought to be neurovascular in nature. It has been theorized that hyperexcitability of the cerebral cortex and abnormal control of pain neurons in the trigeminal nucleus of the brain stem is a primary source of migraine headaches, although this is still under debate.[42]

Migraine headaches can be triggered by changes in sleep patterns. It is important that an individual who suffers from frequent migraine episodes understands the relationship between changes in sleep pattern, especially insufficient sleep, and the onset of a migraine. Migraine headaches may also be associated with NREM stage 3 and 4 sleep or REM sleep.

Cluster Headache

Cluster headache occurs in approximately 0.1% of the population and is found most frequently in men. It is characterized by a periodic sudden attack of very severe pain often reported as a stabbing, shocking, or crushing pain on one side of the head. An attack may last for seconds or minutes at a time, but an episode may last up to 3 hours. The attack is rapid, usually without the characteristic warning signs that occur with a migraine. It is called a cluster headache because episodes occur in clusters and then may remit spontaneously.[43]

Cluster headaches tend to occur during sleep, particularly during REM sleep. OSA is a known trigger for this form of headache.

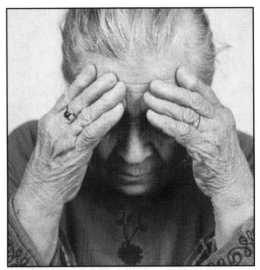

Figure 15-4. Hypnic headaches occur mostly in older adults and usually at the same time every night. (From Fotolia.com)

Chronic Paroxysmal Hemicrania

Chronic paroxysmal hemicrania is a debilitating headache that usually occurs in an area around the eye that consists of multiple severe short headache attacks usually on only one side of the head. This type of headache occurs more frequently in females than in males. It is can be very successfully treated by nonsteroidal anti-inflammatory drugs (NSAIDs), particularly indomethacin. This headache is most commonly associated with REM sleep.

Hypnic Headaches

Hypnic headaches are a type of headache that primarily affects older adults (Figure 15-4). They consist of a moderate, throbbing, bilateral or unilateral headache that wakes the individual from sleep once or multiple times a night. They can last for 15 minutes to several hours and usually occur at the same time every night. On PSG, it appears that these headaches are almost exclusively associated with REM sleep, particularly those that occur earlier in the night. They rarely occur in NREM stage 3 and 4 sleep. There are not usually any other symptoms associated with this type of headache. Treatment may include lithium carbonate, verapamil, indomethacin, or methylsergilide. It has also been shown that 1 to 2 cups of coffee or 100 to 200 mg of caffeine before bed may prevent hypnic headaches.[44] Sleep apnea may be a component of this type of headache. Other causes of headache should be ruled out before the diagnosis is made.

Exploding Head Syndrome

Exploding head syndrome is also known as *hypnagogic hallucination,* in which an individual has the sense of a sudden loud noise coming from within his or her own head that is likened to an explosion, gunshot, or screaming. This experience usually happens at sleep onset or within 1 to 2 hours of falling asleep. It is not usually associated with a dream. There is also a sense of fear or anxiety that accompanies the attack, as well as an elevated heart rate. Sleep paralysis may also accompany episodes of this syndrome.[45] This episode may be related to rapid withdrawal from certain selective serotonin reuptake inhibitor (SSRI) medications. The mechanism is not understood, but it has been suggested that it may be from the middle ear or may be a minor temporal lobe seizure.[46]

Exploding head syndrome usually occurs either during the transition from wakefulness to sleep or the transition from sleep to wakefulness. Occurrence is almost always the former rather than the latter.

SLEEP-RELATED EPILEPSY

Generally, nocturnal seizure activity has 2 peaks. The first occurs approximately 2 hours after sleep onset and the second occurs around 4 to 5 PM. Sleep-related seizures tend to occur more frequently during NREM stage 1 and 2 sleep than during REM sleep. Partial seizures (ie, frontal and temporal lobe events) occur more during NREM sleep, and generalized seizures tend to occur during awakenings from sleep. Sleep deprivation, irregular sleep patterns, or concurrent sleep disorders such as OSA can trigger a seizure.

Changes in sleep, architecture associated with seizure disorders that can be seen on PSG may include increased sleep latency, increased WASO, increased NREM stage 1 and 2 sleep, decreased NREM stage 3 and 4 sleep, and decreased REM sleep. Normal PSG does not necessarily rule out a seizure disorder. If seizure activity is suspected, additional encephalographic (EEG) electrodes are needed to capture frontal and temporal lobe activity (Figure 15-5).

Nocturnal Frontal Lobe Epilepsy

Nocturnal frontal lobe epilepsy is an autosomal dominant disorder that involves violent seizure activity during sleep. This form of seizure often involves complex movement patterns and vocalizations. It can be misdiagnosed as nightmares. Attacks usually first occur during childhood. It is thought that this type of seizure is caused by a malfunction in the thalamocortical pathway because this pathway is critical in sleep and this type of seizure originates in the frontal cortex. Both the thalamus and cortex receive cholinergic inputs and acetylcholine receptor subunits compose the 3 known causative genes for nocturnal frontal lobe epilepsy. K-complexes are almost invariably present at the start of this type of seizure. These receptor subunits are expressed presynaptically by neurons that release the inhibitory transmitter gamma-aminobutyric acid (GABA).

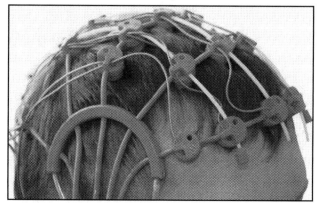

Figure 15-5. Electroencephalogram is used to identify epilepsy and special care is taken in electrode placement during sleep studies in which epilepsy is suspected. (From Fotolia.com)

Therefore, the mutation could lead to reduced GABA release, causing hyperexcitability.

The bed partner of an individual with nocturnal frontal lobe seizures may notice involuntary movements that appear no different than those typical during normal sleep. The individual with the seizure disorder may awaken in the morning with headache, having wet the bed, or having a bitten tongue or other injury. Other symptoms include unusual mental behaviors consistent with a postictal period.

MENTAL RETARDATION AND DEVELOPMENTAL DISORDERS

Disordered sleep is a common finding in individuals with mental retardation and developmental disorders.

Mental Retardation

Mental retardation is generally considered a developmental disability acquired from a problem with growth and development. This term includes congenital medical conditions that are characterized by significantly impaired cognitive functioning and deficits in 2 or more adaptive behaviors. Historically, it has been defined as an IQ score under 70.[47] Syndromic mental retardation is characterized by intellectual deficits associated with other medical and behavioral abnormalities. Intellectual disability may appear at any age and may be too mild to qualify as mental retardation; may be too specific, as in a specific learning disability; or may be acquired later in life through a TBI or a neurodegenerative disease.

Insomnia, particularly sleep-onset insomnia, and early morning awakenings and frequent nighttime awakenings are common features in mental retardation. Polysomnographic features include increased frequency of arousals and awakenings.

Developmental Disorders

Developmental disorders are conditions that appear during childhood development and delay normal development of one or more functions, such as language skill. These disorders encompass those that result in impairment in normal development of motor of cognitive skills before the age of 22. They are disorders that persist and have no cure. Developmental disorders may include psychological and physical disorders such as autism and dyslexia. Developmental disorders can be specific or pervasive.

There is a wide variety of thought about the causes of developmental disabilities that range from organic causes to environmental exposure, stress, genetics, or whether it is combination of any of these factors.[48]

Asperger Syndrome

Asperger syndrome is a disorder on the autism spectrum that is characterized by significant difficulties in social interaction and may also involve restricted and/or repetitive patterns of behavior or interest. It is different from other autism spectrum disorders in that language and cognitive development are preserved, although atypical use of language and physical clumsiness frequently accompany this condition. The cause of Asperger syndrome is unknown, but research suggests a genetic basis. Treatment is aimed at assisting in management of dysfunctional behaviors and improving deficits in communication skills, obsessive behaviors, and physical clumsiness.[49]

Disordered sleep in individuals with Asperger syndrome includes insomnia, usually characterized by decreased sleep time during the first part of the night. These individuals often also have REM sleep disruption.

Autism

Autism, like Asperger syndrome, is characterized by an impairment of social interaction and communication and restrictive and repetitive behavior, but is more pervasive. Autism affects how information is processed in the brain by altering how nerve cells and synapses connect and organize.[50] It has a strong genetic basis, but the mechanism is not well understood. Like with Asperger syndrome, there is controversy regarding the causes of autism, including suspicions that it is caused by heavy metal poisoning, pesticides, or childhood vaccines.[51,52] A discussion regarding the causative factors of these disorders is outside the scope of this book, but it remains an area of considerable controversy. The prevalence of autism spectrum disorders in the United States in 2008, according to the Centers for Disease Control and Prevention, was 11 per 1000.[53] The number of people diagnosed with autism has increased dramatically since the 1980s at least in part because of improved diagnostics, but whether there is actually an increase in prevalence is open to question.[54]

While many neurological disorders can be traced to a single pathway or brain region, autism spectrum disorders do not have a single clear mechanism, but rather autism appears to affect areas of the brain during development, disrupting resulting neural pathways.[55] Some studies suggest that the mechanism of autism results from changes in brain development in fetal life that begins a cascade of neural pathology leading to the disorder.[56] It has been found that the brains of some autistic infants tend to grow more rapidly compared to normally developing infants, but then that growth becomes relatively slower during childhood. The overgrowth appears to be greatest in brain regions associated with higher cognitive specialization.[57,58] Suggested mechanisms for this pathological development include excess neuronal growth causing local over-connectivity in key brain regions,[59] disturbances in neuronal migration in early gestation,[60] unbalance in excitatory-inhibitory networks, and abnormal formation of synapses and dendritic spines.[61] It is possible that these abnormalities in development are related to abnormalities in the early development of sleep during fetal life and infancy.

Individuals with autism may complain of poor sleep quality and nonrestorative sleep. They may also have somewhat fragmented sleep.

CARDIAC DISORDERS RELATED TO DISORDERED SLEEP

Hypertension

Sleep-related breathing disorder is a risk factor for hypertension independent of other known confounding factors. In the Sleep Heart Health Study,[62] mean systolic and diastolic blood pressures and the prevalence of hypertension increase significantly with increasing measures of sleep-related breathing disorder (eg, AHI and percent sleep time with oxygen saturation below 90%). The odds of developing hypertension were observed to increase by about 1% for each additional apneic event per hour of sleep and to increase by 13% for each 10% decrease in nocturnal oxygen saturation. In the Wisconsin Sleep Cohort Study,[63] in over 4 years of follow-up, subjects with an AHI of at least 15 events per hour had an odds ratio of 2.89 for the presence of hypertension compared with those with an AHI of 0 events per hour.

Typically, there is a drop in blood pressure during sleep that is usually observed in hypertensive patients without OSA. Some patients with OSA do not demonstrate this sleep-related drop in blood pressure. The risk of cardiovascular disease may be greater in this group compared to the former. It was found that 48% of this group had no change in systolic and 22% had no change in diastolic blood pressure at night. The respiratory index (RDI) was the only significant variable related to the lack of blood pressure drop during sleep.

A reduction in blood pressure was observed during administration of therapeutic CPAP, but not subtherapeutic CPAP in patients with coexisting OSA. The benefit was larger in patients with more severe OSA and in those taking drug treatments for high blood pressure. Reversal of OSA by CPAP was also noted to reduce nocturnal blood pressure in patients with refractory hypertension. However, some investigators have reported no significant beneficial effect of CPAP on blood pressure in patients with OSA and hypertension.

Sleep-Related Coronary Artery Ischemia

Sleep-related coronary artery ischemia shares many features in common with its daytime counterpart (Figure 15-6); that is, left-sided or retrosternal chest pressure, pain radiation to the jaw or left upper extremity, dyspnea, diaphoresis, nausea, and palpitations. This can potentially lead to similar complications including myocardial infarction, congestive heart failure (CHF), cardiac arrhythmias, and sudden cardiac death. Chest pain can awaken the patient from sleep. There may also be frequent arousals and awakenings.

Pathogenic mechanisms responsible for cardiac ischemia developing during sleep include marked sleep-related hypotension and sympathetic surges with increase in blood pressure and heart rate during arousals or awakenings from sleep. Hypertension may be particularly prominent during NREM stages 3 and 4 sleep. REM sleep can be associated with instability of heart rate and blood pressure. The risk of sleep-related cardiac events is increased in patients with OSA due, in part, to the hypoxemia that develops during apneic episodes and the post arousal increase in blood pressure and heart rate.

Electrocardiographic monitoring during PSG may reveal features consistent with myocardial ischemia such as depression or elevation of the ST segment, T-wave changes, or atrial or ventricular arrhythmias.

Cardiovascular Disease and Obstructive Sleep Apnea

Cardiovascular disease and OSA have been increasingly linked. A significant body of research has been dedicated to understanding this connection. The literature is clear that the risk of cardiovascular disease increases in middle-aged patients with untreated OSA.[64-66] This risk appears to be independent of age, body mass index, blood pressure, and smoking history. The risk of cardiovascular disease including myocardial infarction, angina, heart failure, and stroke is increased even in sleepers with mild OSA, but this risk is reduced very effectively with optimal CPAP application

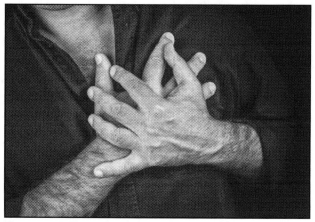

Figure 15-6. Sleep-related coronary artery ischemia is similar to the daytime counterpart and can cause frequent awakenings. (From Fotolia.com)

or an appropriate dental device that is shown to normalize AHI. Care must be taken to prove that OSA therapy is effective to adequately ameliorate cardiovascular risk from intervention. The only positive method currently available to prove this is a full laboratory PSG, despite the increasing popularity of the home sleep study devices.

Studies have been conducted to determine the mechanism responsible for the increased risk of cardiovascular disease in patients with untreated OSA, and multiple theories explaining this mechanism have been proposed.[66] Studies suggest that the change is related to changes in sympathetic tone in patients with OSA. It is known that there is a slight increase in sympathetic activity during sleep. Heart rate, blood pressure, and cardiac output are all reduced during normal sleep. However, in sleepers with OSA, the increase in sympathetic activity that is already elevated during wakefulness does not balance out with changes in parasympathetic tone but, in fact, increases further in sleep-related disordered sleep. Well-titrated CPAP therapy nearly completely attenuates this increased sympathetic activation and therefore normalizes heart rate, blood pressure, and cardiac output.[67-70]

Another theory suggests that proinflammatory cytokines including tumor necrosis factor-alpha (TNF-α), interleukin-6 and interleukin-8, and adhesion molecules including intercellular adhesion molecule-1 and vascular cell adhesion molecule-1 are increased in sleepers with OSA. Elevation of plasma level of C-reactive protein, a marker for inflammation, and of cardiovascular risk is related to the severity of OSA.[71]

One theory suggests that the elevated cardiovascular risk in sleepers with OSA may be related to an increase in coaguability because of elevated fibrinogen levels, increased platelet activity, and reduced fibrolytic in this population. CPAP therapy seems to decrease platelet activity and other clotting factors. Endothelial dysfunction has also been described in this population and seems to be revered with effective CPAP therapy.[72]

Oxidative stress is associated with OSA. Biomarkers of oxidative stress are higher in sleepers with OSA and these biomarkers are positively correlated with respiratory disturbance index. Oxidative stress is reversed with effective CPAP therapy.

Finally, a theory of the relationship between increased risk of cardiovascular disease and OSA is related to the increased incidence of insulin resistance found in individuals who have OSA. The AHI and decreased oxygen saturation in this population are also related to insulin resistance, which is a known risk factor for atherosclerosis.[73]

Congestive Heart Failure

CHF is the inability of the heart to effectively pump blood to meet the demands of the body. It causes shortness of breath, edema in dependent limbs, and intolerance to exercise. It can be diagnosed by echocardiogram and laboratory testing. Treatment usually consists of lifestyle changes including smoking cessation, light exercise designed to increase tolerance, decreased sodium intake and other dietary changes, and medications as needed. CHF may have a variety of causes including myocardial infarction or other forms of ischemic heart disease, hypertension, valvular disease, and cardiomyopathy.[74]

Patients with CHF may develop OSA or central sleep apnea. Both obstructive and central sleep apnea are prevalent in patients with left ventricular dysfunction without apparent heart failure. Left ventricular systolic dysfunction is an independent risk factor for sleep apnea in patients with CHF. Untreated severe sleep-related breathing disorders may further impair left ventricular function.

CHF causes sleep disruption and can cause Cheyne-Stokes respiration predominately in NREM stage 1 and 2 sleep. The cause of the development of central sleep apnea in CHF patients is not understood. Possible mechanisms for its development include pulmonary congestion or alteration in end-tidal carbon dioxide pressure. Another mechanism that has been suggested is a decrease in circulation time with a delay in response to changes in blood gas concentrations has been proposed as a pathogenetic mechanism of central OSA.

Cheyne–Stokes Respiration

Cheyne-Stokes respiration is an abnormal breathing pattern characterized by progressively deeper and sometimes more rapid breathing followed by gradual decreasing depth and rate of breathing and finally a temporary cessation of breathing or apneic event. This is a crescendo-diminuendo cycle of oscillatory breathing pattern and is also associated with changing serum partial pressures of oxygen and carbon dioxide.[75] Cheyne-Stokes respiration and periodic breathing are distinct from one another in that during the trough of ventilation, if there is an apneic event, it is Cheyne-Stokes respiration. If there is only hypopnea, it is identified as periodic breathing. It may be caused by damage to the respiratory centers or by physiological dysfunction such as CHF, but may also be seen in newborns with immature respiratory systems or those adjusting to high altitude breathing.[76]

Sleep disruption may occur with this respiratory pattern due to arousals associated with hypercapnea or hypoxemia. Cheyne-Stokes respiration is usually associated with NREM stages 1 and 2 sleep. Mortality in patients with CHF is higher in those who develop Cheyne-Stokes respiration during sleep than in those who do not. The prognosis is even more dismal in patients with both CHF and Cheyne-Stokes respiration and with an increased AHI.

Treatment for central sleep apnea and Cheyne-Stokes respiration in patients in CHF should include well-titrated CPAP therapy. This appears to improve cardiac function, especially left ventricular ejection fraction. Oxygen therapy may be used in conjunction with CPAP in this patient population, but oxygen alone does not appear to significantly improve the quality of sleep, nor does it improve cardiac function. Patients with CHF and OSA are at increased risk of progressing to cardiac dysfunction. CPAP therapy improves left ventricular systolic function and appears to improve quality of life.

Cardiac Arrhythmias

Cardiac arrhythmias describe a large and heterogeneous group of conditions that are characterized by an abnormal electrical activity in the heart. It may cause the heart to beat too fast, too slow, or skip beats. Some arrhythmias are life threatening and can cause cardiac arrest. Others cause symptoms such as palpitations, which are usually benign and annoying. Still others may not be noticed but may predispose an individual to potentially life-threatening conditions such as stroke or embolism.

Ventricular arrhythmias appear to increase during arousals from sleep due to the surge of sympathetic tone that is associated with these arousals. On the contrary, premature ventricular beats appear to decrease during sleep because of the higher prevalence of parasympathetic tone. In sleepers with OSA, the heart rate typically decreases at the onset of an apneic episode and increases after the termination of the event. OSA is also associated with ventricular tachycardia or fibrillation, complex ventricular ectopy, supraventricular tachycardia, sinus pauses, and second or third degree heart blocks. The severity of arrhythmias appears to be correlated with increased severity of OSA.

GASTROINTESTINAL DISEASES ASSOCIATED WITH SLEEP DISORDERS

Peptic Ulcer Disease

Peptic ulcer disease is the most frequently occurring GI ulceration. It is usually acidic and extremely painful. It is characterized by mucosal erosions equal to or greater than 0.5 cm. Seventy to ninety percent of peptic ulcers have a spiral-shaped bacterium known as *Helicobacter pylori* that thrive in the acidic environment of the stomach. These ulcerations are worsened by certain NSAIDs that contain cox-1 inhibitors such as aspirin and ibuprofen. Four times as many peptic ulcers occur in the duodenum than the stomach. Approximately 4% of peptic ulcers are caused by malignant tumors.[77,78]

Gastric acid secretion increases during sleep in sleepers with peptic ulcer disease. This population may display frequent arousal and awakenings because of abdominal pain, which usually occurs during the first 4 hours of sleep. The pain is usually described as dull, steady, or intermittent. It is localized to the epigastric region.

Gastroesophageal Reflux Disease

Gastroesophageal reflux disease (GERD) is caused by backflow of gastric acid and other gastric contents into the esophagus due to incompetent barriers at the gastroesophageal junction. This leads to irritation and damage to the esophageal mucosa which produces heartburn, pain, or discomfort in the retrosternal area and a sour or bitter taste.

In a survey conducted in the United States, 79% of individuals reported having heartburn symptoms every night; 75% of all respondents reported that sleep was adversely affected by heartburn and 63% reported heartburn did not allow them to sleep well.[79] The prevalence of GERD increases with age, and its course is generally chronic.

The primary mechanism for GERD is transient relaxation of the lower esophageal sphincter. In addition, pressure of the upper esophageal sphincter, which acts as an additional barrier to nocturnal regurgitation, diminishes during sleep. The presence of a hiatal hernia, poor esophageal clearance, delayed gastric emptying, and impaired mucosal defense factors also play into the symptoms of GERD. Although symptoms primarily occur during wakefulness, they also occur during sleep and may cause arousal during any stage of sleep.

Nocturnal GERD symptoms are associated with a more prolonged contact time with gastric acid, and esophageal acid clearance times are also increased during sleep, leading to increased symptoms. Production of saliva, which normally helps to neutralize acid reflux, ceases during sleep. Sleepers with nocturnal GERD symptoms often experience awakenings with substernal burning or discomfort, indigestion, and a bitter taste. Shortness of breath, coughing, and choking may also be reported. These symptoms may lead to complaints of insomnia or sleep fragmentation because of frequent arousals.

Complications of repeated nocturnal GERD symptoms include esophageal mucosal damage, asthma exacerbation, and sleep disruption. Reflux into the pharynx, larynx, and tracheobronchial tree can cause chronic cough, morning hoarseness, bronchoconstriction, pharyngitis, laryngitis, bronchitis, or pneumonia. Recurrent pulmonary aspiration as a result of GERD can cause aspiration pneumonia and pulmonary fibrosis. Esophageal complications include esophagitis, esophageal strictures, and Barrett esophagitis, a precancerous condition.

GERD may be related to "sleep-related laryngospasm," a condition characterized by sudden awakening with the sensation of suffocation and apnea lasting 5 to 45 seconds, followed by stridor. Breathing usually normalizes in a few minutes but can be quite alarming to the sleeper suddenly awakened with this sensation.

Nocturnal GERD appears to be common in sleepers with OSA. In one study, 50% of episodes of GERD occurring in sleepers with OSA were related to apneas or hypopneas.[80] In some studies, erosive reflux disease appears to be more frequent in patients with severe OSA, although this finding remains open to some controversy.

Polysomnographic findings in sleepers with GERD include repeated arousals followed by swallowing observed by increased electromyogram (EMG) activity in the chin electrode. Aside from an increased arousal index, a decrease in duration spent in deeper stages of sleep has been described.

Therapy may involve elevating the head of the bed, administration of histamine-2 antagonists or proton pump inhibitors, or anti-reflux surgery. CPAP therapy appears to decrease the frequency of nocturnal GERD symptoms not only in sleepers with OSA, but also in those without sleep-related breathing disorders. This anti-reflux activity may be due to elevation of intraesophageal pressure, as well as constriction of the lower esophageal sphincter. Higher CPAP pressures produce greater improvement in GERD.

Functional Bowel Disorders

Functional bowel disorders are characterized by chronic GI tract symptoms without significant anatomical, metabolic, or infectious abnormalities. These disorders include functional dyspepsia and irritable bowel syndrome. Patients with functional bowel disorders can have abnormalities of autonomic functioning, and measurements of autonomic functioning during sleep can differentiate these patients from normal controls.

Sleep disturbances including recurrent nighttime awakenings, poor sleep quality, nonrestorative sleep, and increased daytime fatigue are common in patients with functional bowel disorders. In one study of patients with sleep disturbances, there was a prevalence of 33% for irritable syndrome and 21% for functional dyspepsia.[81] Nighttime awakenings can be caused by abdominal aches. A significant proportion of patients report nighttime GI symptoms, but objective sleep abnormalities may be uncommon. In one study, no abnormalities in polysomnographic parameters such as sleep efficiency, sleep latency, number of arousals, and percentage of NREM stage 3 and 4 sleep were identified in patients with irritable bowel syndrome.[82]

RENAL DISORDERS AND DISORDERED SLEEP

Chronic Renal Disease

Chronic renal disease is characterized by a loss of kidney function that progresses over a period of months or years (Figure 15-7). Symptoms of declining kidney function may include a general feeling of not being well and a reduction in appetite. The disease is often found during routine screening of individuals who have known risk of kidney problems such as individuals with hypertension or diabetes. Chronic kidney disease may also lead to cardiovascular disease, anemia, or pericarditis.[83] In an individual suffering from chronic renal disease, creatinine levels are elevated indicating decreased glomerular filtration rate, which decreases the capacity of the kidneys to excrete waste products. Chronic renal disease guidelines classify the disease into 5 stages from stage 1, indicating mild disease, to stage 5 disease, also known as end-stage renal disease or chronic renal failure.[84] Treatment for chronic renal disease is aimed at managing any underlying contributing disease and, in more advanced stages, treating the effects of the disease. End-stage renal disease requires renal replacement therapy, which may include dialysis or, ideally, kidney transplant.[84]

Sleep disturbance is a very common occurrence in individuals on maintenance hemodialysis for end-stage renal disease. These individuals often complain of excessive daytime sleepiness, insomnia, and prolonged awakenings. The normal sleep-wake cycle is often reversed, and there is a high prevalence of primary sleep disorders such as OSA, restless leg/legs syndrome, and periodic limb movement disorder. Common polysomnographic features found in individuals who suffer from end-stage renal disease include increased sleep latency, decreased sleep efficiency, increased frequency of awakenings, and decreased total sleep time. NREM stages 1 and 2 sleep are generally increased, while slow-wave sleep (SWS) and REM sleep are decreased.

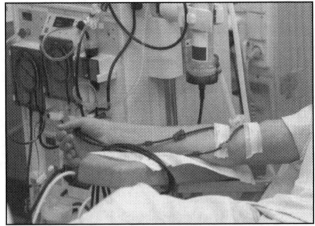

Figure 15-7. Patients with renal disease frequently suffer sleep disorders, including insomnia and restless leg/legs syndrome. (From Fotolia. com)

ENDOCRINE AND METABOLIC DISORDERS AND SLEEP

Hypothyroidism

Hypothyroidism is characterized by a low thyroid function. It may be caused by a number of factors including iodine deficiency, stress, loss of thyroid gland, and iodine-131 treatment.[85]

Hypothyroidism is generally classified as primary, secondary, or tertiary. Primary hypothyroidism is caused by thyroid gland malfunction. It is caused by an autoimmune disease known as Hashimoto's thyroiditis and is treated with radioiodine therapy. Secondary hypothyroidism originates in the pituitary when it does not produce enough thyroid-stimulating hormone (TSH). TSH stimulates the thyroid to produce thyroxine and triiodothyronine. Secondary hypothyroidism is usually caused by damage to the pituitary gland by tumor, radiation, or surgery, although sometimes the cause is not clear.[39] Secondary hypothyroidism accounts for approximately 5% to 10% of the cases.

Tertiary hypothyroidism originates in the hypothalamus when it fails to produce enough thyrotropin-releasing hormone. Thyrotropin-releasing hormone promotes pituitary production of TSH, which is why it is sometimes known as *hypothalamic-pituitary-adrenal axis* (HPA-axis) hypothyroidism. It accounts for less than 5% of the cases.[86]

Hypothyroidism is usually associated with sleep disorders including excessive daytime sleepiness and OSA. Central sleep apnea may also be present. Polysomnographic features include decreased SWS; however, this finding is usually reversed by adequate thyroid hormone replacement.

Acromegaly

Acromegaly is a disorder of the anterior pituitary gland in which it produces excessive growth hormone after epiphyseal end-plate closure. This disorder is most commonly caused by a pituitary adenoma and affects middle-aged adults. It can cause disfigurement and may lead to premature death if untreated. Because the disease is very slowly progressive, its symptoms may not lead to a clear diagnosis for years.

Sleep disorders occurring in individuals with acromegaly include both obstructive and central sleep apnea. Polysomnographic features include decreased SWS and REM sleep.

Cushing Syndrome

Cushing's syndrome is caused by high levels of cortisol. This can be caused by taking glucocorticoids or can be caused by disease processes that result in increased cortisol, adrenocorticotropic hormone (ACTH), or corticotropin-releasing hormone (CRH).[87] Cushing's syndrome is caused by dysfunction in the pituitary gland, such as a pituitary adenoma, which produces excess ACTH, thus causing the adrenal glands to produce an increased level of cortisol.[88]

Hallmarks of disordered sleep in Cushing's syndrome include insomnia and increased incidence of OSA. Polysomnographic features include increased sleep fragmentation, decreased SWS and REM sleep, and increased REM sleep density.

Metabolic Syndrome

Metabolic syndrome is a collection of symptoms and disorders that occur together and result in an increased risk of cardiovascular disease and diabetes. The prevalence of this syndrome has been on the increase, and it is estimated that up to 25% of the United States population has developed the disorder and the incidence increases with age.[89] The American Heart Association's criteria for metabolic syndrome includes waist circumference measured at more than 40 inches in men and more than 35 inches in women; elevated triglycerides of at least 150 mg/dL; reduced high density lipid (HDL), or protective cholesterol, in males less than 40 mg/dL and in females less than 50 mg/dL; hypertension at least 130/85 or the use of medication for hypertension; and elevated fasting glucose at least 100 mg/dL or use of medication for hyperglycemia.[90] Another finding in metabolic syndrome that appears to predict coronary vascular disease is elevated C-reactive protein level. This has also been used as a predictor for nonalcoholic fatty liver disease.[91] Increased stress levels also appear to play a role in development of the syndrome.

The mechanisms of this complex syndrome are not completely clear. It appears that there are genetic factors and endocrine factors that contribute.[92-95] In fact, women with

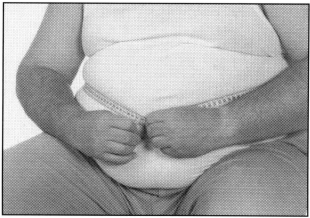

Figure 15-8. Obesity is frequently associated with sleep apnea. (From Fotolia.com)

polycystic ovary syndrome (POS) appear to be especially prone to developing the multitude of factors that make up metabolic syndrome.[96,97] Aging and a sedentary lifestyle are also linked to development of the syndrome, especially in the presence of other contributing factors.[98] Individuals with metabolic syndrome also appear to have increased systemic inflammatory markers including C-reactive protein and have increase fibrinogen, interleukin-6, and TNF-α.[99,100]

The increase in adipocytes with the development of excessive visceral fat causes increased plasma levels of TNF-α, which has been shown to cause increased production of inflammatory cytokines and trigger cell signaling by interaction with TNF-α receptor that may lead to insulin resistance.[101] In an animal study, rats were fed a diet of 33% sucrose. Initially, the animals developed elevated triglycerides, which caused increased visceral fat and eventually resulted in insulin resistance.[102] The increase in adipose tissue increases immune cells, which play a role in inflammation. Chronic inflammation contributes to hypertension, arthrosclerosis, and diabetes.[103]

One risk factor for the development of metabolic syndrome is stress. Prolonged stress can alter the hormonal balance of the hypothalamic-pituitary-adrenal axis (HPA-axis). This causes elevated cortisol levels, which raise glucose and insulin levels, which causes insulin-mediated effects on adipose tissue, promoting visceral adiposity, insulin resistance, dyslipidemia, and hypertension. This can, in turn, affect low turnover osteoporosis.[104,105] HPA-axis dysfunction may contribute to abdominal obesity and related cardiovascular disease, type II diabetes, and stroke.[106,107]

Central obesity is another risk factor in the development of metabolic syndrome (Figure 15-8). Increasing adiposity and particularly increased waist circumference are related to the development of the syndrome; however, individuals of normal weight and body mass index may also have insulin resistance and develop metabolic syndrome.[108] Decreased physical activity is also a predictor of cardiovascular disease and related mortality. Metabolic syndrome affects 44% of the United States population over 50 years old, and women are more affected than men.[58]

Individuals with metabolic syndrome tend to have higher incidence of cardiovascular disease than patients with type II diabetes or impaired glucose tolerance without metabolic syndrome. Hypoadiponectinemia has also been shown to increase insulin resistance and is a risk factor for developing metabolic syndrome.[58,109,110]

Approximately 50% of individuals with coronary artery disease also have metabolic syndrome; this occurs particularly in women. Lipodystrophy is also associated with metabolic syndrome. Lipodystrophy can be genetic or acquired, as occurs with human immunodeficiency virus (HIV)-related highly active antiretroviral therapy. This can cause a significant increase in severe insulin resistance and many of the components of metabolic syndrome.[51,60]

Metabolic syndrome is also seen with increased frequency in individuals who suffer from schizophrenia, schizoaffective disorder, or bipolar syndrome and is exacerbated by the sedentary lifestyle, poor dietary habits, and antipsychotic medication use seen in these syndromes.[111,112]

Rheumatologic disease also has been found to be related to the development of metabolic syndrome. This has particularly been found in systemic lupus erythematosus, psoriasis and psoriatic arthritis, and rheumatory arthritis.[113,114]

Other endocrine disorders that are associated with metabolic syndrome include hyperuricemia, nonalcoholic fatty liver disease, POS, and acanthosis nigricans.

Disordered sleep may be a contributor to the development of or a consequence of metabolic syndrome. Particularly, hypertension related to heart rate variability and changes in endothelial function and changes in leptin and ghrelin production, which lead to insulin resistance, central obesity, and diabetes, have been directly linked to disordered sleep. Successful treatment of disordered sleep may result in reversal of some of the symptoms of metabolic syndrome.

INFECTIOUS DISEASES AND DISORDERED SLEEP

Sleep can be disrupted in individuals with infectious disease processes and includes features such as excessive daytime sleepiness, decreased sleep efficiency, and increased arousals from sleep. REM sleep is also significantly reduced during the course of an acute infection; however, there is usually significant REM sleep recovery in the period immediately following the infectious period.[115] It is important for the rehabilitation professional to consider these factors when dealing with a patient with an acute infection or who is in the recovery period of acute infection. Chronic infections also have related sleep disorders. Several specific infectious diseases bear closer examination as they are likely to be seen in the rehabilitation setting.

Human Immunodeficiency Virus

HIV infection is a disease that interferes with immune system function, rendering its victims more likely to get infections, especially when it progresses to acquired immunodeficiency syndrome (AIDS). Individuals with AIDS are prone to opportunistic infections and tumors that do not usually affect those with healthy immune systems. HIV is transmitted primarily by sexual intercourse, including oral and anal sex; contaminated blood transfusions; sharing of hypodermic needles; and from mother to child during pregnancy, delivery, or breast feeding. It is not transmitted by other bodily fluids such as saliva or tears.[116] There is no known cure for HIV, but the development of antiretroviral medications can slow the course of the disease and lead to a near-normal life expectancy. However, antiretroviral drugs are very expensive and have significant side effects of their own.

HIV/AIDS is considered a pandemic, which is a disease outbreak that is present over a large area of the world and is actively spreading. As of 2010, approximately 34 million people are infected with the virus worldwide. Since the disease was first identified in 1981, it has caused over 30 million deaths worldwide. Genetic research has indicated that it originated in west central Africa as a mutation from a simian immunodeficiency virus. The United States Centers for Disease Control and Prevention reported the first case of AIDS in 1981 and its cause, HIV, was identified in the early 1980s.[117,118]

HIV infection is associated with insomnia, excessive daytime sleepiness, and recurrent arousals. Antiretroviral therapy used in the treatment of HIV infection and AIDS can also lead to disrupted sleep. In particular, efavirenz (Sustiva) is associated with insomnia, increased awakenings, vivid dreams, increased sleep latency, and decreased SWS. Zidovudine or azidothymidine (AZT) is also associated with insomnia. Polysomnographic features of HIV infection include decreased sleep latency and sleep efficiency, increased frequency of awakenings and arousals, and increased WASO. NREM stage 2 sleep is often decreased. In terminal stages of HIV/AIDS, SWS is often increased.

Lyme Disease

Lyme disease is an infectious disease caused by at least 3 species of *Borrelia* bacteria.[119] It was first identified in 1975 in Lyme, Connecticut, giving the disease its name. Early symptoms of this tick-borne disease include fever, headache, fatigue, depression, and a characteristic circular rash called *erythema migrans*.[120] Early identification and treatment for the infection with antibiotics usually leads to its cure. However, if treatment is delayed or inadequate, it can lead to more serious symptoms involving disorders in the joints, heart, and central nervous system. These treatments can be disabling and difficult to treat.[121]

Sleep disruptions associated with Lyme disease include insomnia, excessive daytime sleepiness, frequent awakenings, and restless leg/legs syndrome. Polysomnographic features include increased sleep latency, decreased sleep efficiency, and increased frequency of arousals and alpha wave intrusions into NREM sleep.

FIBROMYALGIA AND PAIN SYNDROMES AND SLEEP DISORDERS

Acute Pain

Acute pain is described temporally as that which lasts less than 30 days. In terms of tissue irritability, acute pain is known as that which occurs before one encounters restriction in a joint or muscle.

Acute pain is associated with insomnia because of pain and frequent sleep disruptions (Figure 15-9). Polysomnographic features include decreased SWS and decreased REM sleep.

Chronic Pain

Chronic pain syndrome is described temporally as that which lasts for more than 30 days. In terms of tissue irritability, it is that pain that comes on after one encounters restriction in a joint or muscle.

Individuals who report chronic pain also usually report poor and nonrestorative sleep quality. They may also have significant periods of sleep-onset insomnia, middle insomnia, and early awakenings because of chronic pain. Polysomnographic features include increased sleep latency, increased WASO, and decreased SWS, and alpha wave intrusions into NREM sleep.

Fibromyalgia

Fibromyalgia is characterized by widespread chronic pain and allodynia, or painful pressure points. Individuals with fibromyalgia generally also complain of debilitating fatigue, sleep disturbance, and joint stiffness. Some complain of other symptoms including bowel and bladder problems, variable numbness and tingling, and cognitive dysfunction.[122,123] There are a number of psychiatric conditions that seem to be associated with fibromyalgia including depression, anxiety, and stress-related disorders such as posttraumatic stress disorder (PSTD).[124,125]

Fibromyalgia affects 2% to 4% of the population, with only 1 of 10 individual's diagnoses being male. As its name indicates, it involves both muscle and connective tissue pain.[126] Fibromyalgia is sometimes considered a central sensitization syndrome caused by neurobiological abnormalities that act to produce physiological pain

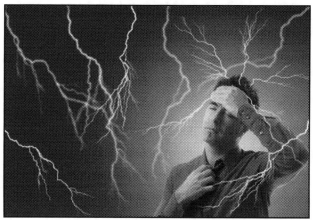

Figure 15-9. Lack of good quality sleep is frequently an aggravating problem for the pain patient. (From Fotolia.com)

and cognitive impairments, as well as neuropsychological symptomology.[127] Despite this, some health care providers do not consider fibromyalgia a disease because of the lack of abnormal findings on physical examination and laboratory findings and other objective diagnostic tests.[128,129]

Sleep disruptions are thought to be a major factor in the development of fibromyalgia, as well as a complicating factor during the course of the disorder. A hallmark of fibromyalgia is nonrestorative sleep. These individuals often report fatigue but do not tend to report excessive daytime sleepiness. Insomnia and early morning awakenings are common. Primary sleep disorders are often found on polysomnographic testing including OSA, restless leg/legs syndrome, and periodic limb movement disorder. Polysomnographic features include increased sleep latency with decreased sleep efficiency and decreased total sleep time. There are frequent arousals from sleep and increased WASO. NREM stage 1 sleep is may be increased, while SWS is significantly diminished. REM sleep is usually decreased. During NREM stage 2 sleep, the normally occurring sleep spindles are often markedly diminished or absent. There may be alpha wave intrusions into NREM sleep. Spectral EEG analysis demonstrates decreased delta frequency power and decreased alpha frequency bands.

SLEEP AND NEUROLOGICAL DISORDERS

Psychiatric and Behavioral Disorders and Sleep

A significant body of knowledge is accumulating on the role of sleep and sleep disruption in the cause and severity of symptoms in a variety of psychiatric disorders. It is well established that poor sleep can contribute to dysfunction of a number of systems. It is also clear that for some psychiatric disorders in which sleep is disrupted, adequate treatment of the sleep disorder may improve the prognosis.

Schizophrenia

Schizophrenia is a thought disorder characterized by disorganized speech and thinking, significant problems in social and/or occupational function, and poor emotional responsiveness. Those with the disorder often experience auditory hallucinations and/or paranoia, which contribute to chronic problems with behavior and emotion. In the US, the prevalence is approximately 0.3% to 0.7% and typically has onset of symptoms in young adulthood.[130] Schizophrenics are also likely to have comorbid conditions including depression and anxiety disorders with nearly 50% having substance abuse problems. The cause of schizophrenia is uncertain, but genetics, early environment, and psychological and social processes appear to be important contributory factors. Treatment usually consists of antipsychotic medication, which suppresses dopamine and sometimes serotonin.[131] Societal problems associated with schizophrenia include homelessness, unemployment, and poverty.

Sleep dysfunction is a very common feature in individuals diagnosed with schizophrenia. Symptoms of the disorder are often worsened with increased sleep disturbances, and excessive sleep disruption tends to aggravate schizophrenic psychosis. The normal sleep-wake cycle can become reversed with increased sleep during the daytime and insomnia at night. Sleep can become polyphasic, or an alternating pattern of sleeplessness and hypersomnolence may develop. Rebound sleepiness with increased sleep efficiency as schizophrenic symptoms abate may also occur. Weight gain associated with long-term neuroleptic therapy may lead to OSA and result in destabilization of symptoms. Polysomnographic features of schizophrenia include increased sleep latency and decreased sleep efficiency. There tends to be increased WASO and decreased total sleep time. SWS and REM sleep are decreased, and there is usually decreased REM sleep latency.

Mood and Behavior Disorders

Major Depressive Disorder

Major depressive disorder is characterized by a pervasive depressed mood the components of which include low self-esteem, loss of interest in usually pleasurable activities, poor attention and concentration, and often disrupted sleep pattern characterized by either insomnia or hypersomnia (Figure 15-10). It should be distinguished from nonclinical depression, which consists of a low mood; however, the individual does not suffer from the other disabling symptoms of major depression. The age of onset for a

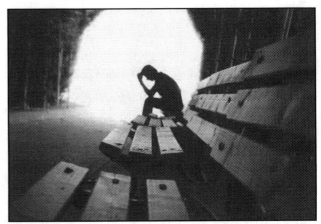

Figure 15-10. Depression can be associated with either insomnia or hypersomnia. (From Fotolia.com)

major depressive episode is usually between the ages of 20 to 30 years, and a second episode often occurs between 30 and 40 years of age.[132] The cause of major depression has been the subject of study across the centuries and has included psychological, psychosocial, hereditary, and neurobiological factors. Treatment approaches usually call for medications including monoamines such as serotonin, norepinephrine, and dopamine, while psychological treatments utilize techniques that include strengthening interpersonal communication and self-esteem.

The vast majority of individuals with major depression report disrupted sleep. Insomnia is the most common complaint; however, some individuals with major depression report hypersomnolence. Insomnia associated with major depression usually includes sleep-onset disruption, frequent or prolonged awakenings, or early morning awakenings. Polysomnographic features of major depression include increased sleep latency with decreased sleep efficiency and decreased total sleep time. There is increased WASO. NREM stage 1 sleep is increased, while SWS is decreased or absent. REM sleep latency can be significantly shortened, and REM density is increased. The duration of REM sleep is increased early in the sleep cycle with a delay of SWS until the second sleep cycle. Sleep disturbances may precede the onset of major depressive symptoms and may persist after remission of the episode has been accomplished. It is thought that this may put the patient at increased risk for recurrence of depression.

Dysthymic Disorder

Dysthymic disorder is characterized by chronic depression that is less severe but longer lasting than major depression. It is defined as depression that persists for at least 2 years but is less acute. Often, individuals with dysthymic disorder are thought to just have low self-esteem and low motivation as a general part of their character and thus the disorder may go unrecognized and untreated for years. Such individuals with mild dysthymia generally withdraw from stressful situations and avoid various opportunities and generally find little pleasure in normal activities.

The cause of dysthymic disorder is not completely understood. Because it may be linked to other disorders, it is uncertain if dysthymia is the cause or an effect of another disorder. Genetics likely play a role in the disorder, perhaps predisposing an individual to the symptoms. Other factors may also play a role, including stress and lack of social interaction or social isolation.[133]

Certain sleep disruptions are associated with dysthymic disorder. Patients with dysthymic disorder usually have increased sleep latency and increased wakefulness during sleep. Early morning awakening is also a characteristic symptom of dysthymic disorder. Patients with dysthymic disorder often display a decreased amount of SWS in the first half of the night. REM sleep latency, or the length of time from sleep onset to the first bout of REM sleep, is often decreased in patients with dysthymic disorder. The first episode of REM sleep is usually of a longer duration and REM density is increased, as is the overall increase in the percentage of REM sleep.

Seasonal Affective Disorder

Seasonal affective disorder (SAD), also known as the winter blues, is a mood disorder characterized by a repetitive depressive episode at a particular time of the year (Figure 15-11). Individuals with this disorder often begin to experience a depression in mood as the daylight hours decrease.[134] Symptoms may begin as early as late summer or early fall for those who are severely affected. Others experience severe depression in the middle of the winter when daylight hours are extremely short. Still others may experience symptoms with the change of any season. Those who experience the onset of symptoms in the summer often also experience an increase in anxiety symptoms.[135] Symptoms include a serious change in mood as the season changes with excessive sleep, decreased energy, and little interest in activities that usually engage them. When symptoms come on in the summer, they can be severe, but generally resolve. The prevalence of SAD varies by region in the United States, with a reported 1.4% in Florida and 9.7% in New Hampshire.[136] The precise mechanism for this disorder is unclear, although it is thought to involve the mechanisms of circadian rhythm. Treatment for classic winter SAD involves light therapy, in which the individual will sit in front of a special full-spectrum light for 45 to 60 minutes 1 to 2 times a day. This therapy has been shown to improve melatonin metabolism that is thought to be a depleted and is a causative factor in this disorder. Other treatments may include administration of antidepressants, specifically timed supplementation with melatonin,[137] cognitive behavioral therapy, and ionized air administration.[138]

There are no distinct polysomnographic changes apparent in this disorder, although some clinicians and patients describe an increase in total sleep time and decreased REM latency.

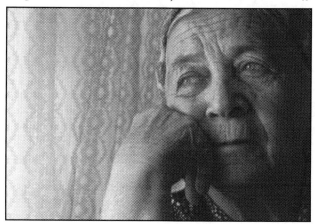

Figure 15-11. Seasonal affective disorder can have symptoms similar to those of depression. (From Fotolia.com)

Bipolar Disorder

Bipolar disorder is also known as manic-depressive disorder. It is a mood disorder characterized by episodes of abnormally elevated mood, energy level, and thought processes, also known as *mania*, often followed by episodes of moderate to severe depression. During manic episodes, the individual may have psychotic symptoms including delusions and hallucinations. Depressive episodes can present with an increased risk of suicide. These cycles are usually separated by periods of normal mood and behavior. The prevalence of bipolar disorder is approximately 1%.[139]

Symptoms usually begin in late adolescence or young adulthood, and diagnosis is based on self-report. Genetics appear to play a significant role in development of the disorder. Environmental factors may also contribute to expression of the disorder. Treatment is geared toward the use of mood-stabilizing medication and other psychotropic medications to manage symptoms of the disorder. Because of the severity of the episode, the individual with bipolar disorder may sometimes be at serious risk of injury to self or others. In this case, involuntary commitment may be required. This may be because of a severe manic episode that involves dangerous behavior or a severe depressive episode with suicidal ideation.

During the manic phase of this disorder, there is a decreased requirement for sleep and often a significant decrease in total sleep time. Polysomnographic features include increased awakenings, decreased SWS, decreased REM sleep latency, and increased REM density. Sleep disruption during the depressive phase of bipolar disorder is similar to other depressive episodes.

Anxiety Disorders

Anxiety disorders encompass acute anxiety reaction, generalized anxiety disorder, panic disorder, and PTSD. Anxiety disorders may be acute episodes that are psychological reactions that result from a traumatic or frightening event or may be a more chronic condition known as *generalized anxiety disorder.* An acute stress reaction is thought to be a discharge of sympathetic nervous system activity as a reaction to a threat or traumatic event. It is the first stage of a general adaptation that regulates stress responses. When exposed to a traumatic or stressful situation, the sensory cortex relays information through the thalamus to the brain stem. This increases norepinephrine activity in the locus coeruleus, causing the individual to become very alert and vigilant to the environment. Epinephrine and a lesser amount of norepinephrine are released from the medulla and adrenal glands. These hormones trigger increased heart rate and respiration and stress-related changes in vasculature. This physiological response is the acute stress reaction. Insomnia is the most commonly reported sleep disruption in anxiety disorders.

Generalized Anxiety Disorder

Generalized anxiety disorder is an anxiety disorder characterized by excessive and often irrational worry, disproportionate to the situation at hand. The worry is often about normal everyday things that are not usually a source of concern. This generalized anxiety often interferes with regular activities of daily living, and the individual may worry about impending disaster related to health, money, family issues, friends, work, and other relationships. Individuals with generalized anxiety disorder often also have a wide range of physical symptoms including agitation, restlessness, insomnia, headaches, and sweating. The American Psychiatric Association's *Diagnostic and Statistical Manual of Mental Disorders* (DSM-IV) lists the core criteria for the diagnosis of generalized anxiety disorder as excessive anxiety and worry on most days for at least the past 6 months in which the individual has difficulty controlling worry. In order to meet the criteria for generalized anxiety disorder, an individual must also have at least 3 physical symptoms including restlessness, fatigue, difficulty with concentration, irritability, muscle tension, and significant sleep disturbances including difficulty falling asleep or staying asleep and a history of nonrestorative sleep.

Between 50% and 70% of people with generalized anxiety disorder report trouble sleeping and often report difficulty falling asleep because they cannot stop thinking about things at bedtime. There is ample scientific evidence from PSG testing to indicate that anxiety disorders result in problems of falling asleep and problems staying asleep. There is also evidence that adequate treatment of the sleep problems in these patients results in improvement of the anxiety symptoms and general functioning.

The prevalence of generalized anxiety disorder is approximately 2%, and it is the most common cause of disability in the workplace in the United States.[140]

Insomnia and nonrestorative sleep are regular complaints in generalized anxiety disorder. Polysomnographic features of the disorder include increased sleep latency, decreased sleep efficiency, and decreased total sleep time. There are often increased WASO and a reduction in SWS.

Panic Disorder

Panic disorder is another type of anxiety disorder that is characterized by recurrent panic attacks that can occur in any environment or time of day. Panic attacks are recurrent and last for several minutes or longer. During a panic attack, the individual experiences overwhelming fear in the absence of danger. They also may feel like they are having a heart attack with symptoms that include a pounding or racing heart, sweating, hyperventilation, weakness, dizziness, numbness or tingling in the hands, or stomach pain.[141] A panic attack cannot be predicted, and therefore the individual suffering with the disorder may also have stress and anxiety because they do not know when the next attack will come. Panic disorder may be disabling because of the unpredictable nature of the disorder, but it usually can be successfully treated with anti-anxiety medication and psychotherapy. Panic attacks may be unexpected, situationally bound, or situationally predisposed.

Seventy percent of individuals with panic disorder often report being awoken from sleep by a panic attack in which they have a sensation of choking and gasping for breath. Other sleep complaints include insomnia, restlessness, and fragmented sleep. Treatment including a combination of medication and cognitive behavioral therapy has been proven to be highly effective.

Insomnia is a frequent complaint in panic disorder with both sleep-onset and middle and terminal insomnia. Panic attacks can strike during sleep, often in the transition from NREM stage 2 sleep to SWS, although occasionally panic attacks may occur during REM sleep. Awakenings from panic attacks during sleep are accompanied by significant sympathetic activation including tachycardia, chest pain, and shortness of breath. Return to sleep following a panic attack can be significantly delayed.

Posttraumatic Stress Disorder

PTSD is a severe anxiety disorder that develops as a response to exposure to a significant psychological trauma (Figure 15-12). It may be the result of a single event such as an accident or threat of death or exposure to repetitive traumas such as physical or sexual abuse. Regardless of the source of the trauma or the apparent objective severity of the trauma, an event that overwhelms an individual's ability to cope can create PTSD. PTSD is more enduring than an acute stress response. Its symptoms include re-experiencing the original trauma through flashbacks or nightmares. The individual with PTSD will usually avoid anything associated with the trauma. They may have increased arousal and hypervigilance as well as disrupted sleep. They also often experience significant impairment in social functioning and in their workplace environments.

PTSD may develop following a traumatic event that exceeds the body's capacity to cope by causing an excessive

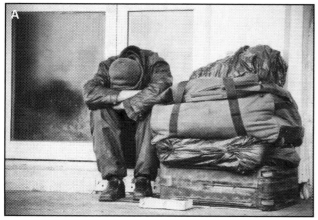
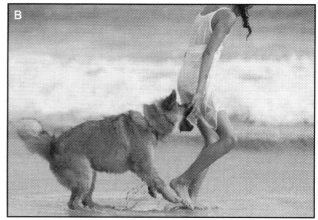

Figure 15-12. (A) PTSD can come from prolonged exposure to danger, such as abuse or war, (B) or can result from a single traumatic event such as a car accident or dog bite. (From Fotolia.com)

adrenaline response, that alters neurological firing patterns and these patterns may persist well after the cessation of the precipitation event. An individual diagnosed with PTSD usually has more of a response to a dexamethasone suppression test and may have decreased cortisol levels.[142] Catecholamine and corticotropin-releasing factor has been shown to be elevated, suggesting changes in the HPA-axis.[143] Some research further suggests that the PTSD response sets up a maladaptive learning pathway to fearful situations through hypersensitivity, hyperactivity, and hyper-responsiveness of the HPA-axis.[144] However, controversy exists regarding the relationship between cortisol production and the development of PTSD.[145] Other research suggests that cortisol, which is normally involved in restoration of homeostasis after stress, may be lower in some individuals, predisposing them to developing PTSD.[146]

PTSD appears to be a malfunction that occurs in the prefrontal cortex, the amygdala, and the hippocampus. The amygdala is particularly involved in the creation of fearful memories. It has been proposed that, when a susceptible individual is exposed to a traumatic event, there is a hyper-arousal of the amygdala that the prefrontal cortex and hippocampus are unable to suppress even after the traumatic event passes. The result is hyper-responsive and hyperactive symptoms that are associated with PTSD.[147]

Sleep disturbance is a significant factor in PTSD. Hyperarousal associated with PTSD contributes to sleep disruption and chronic insomnia. There are no consistent polysomnographic features associated with PTSD, but generally sleep is fragmented with frequent arousals and awakenings, delayed return to sleep, decreased SWS, and decreased REM sleep. Increased body movement has also been described. Re-experiencing of the original traumatic event can occur through frequent distressing dreams, nightmares, and night terrors. PTSD dreams can occur in both NREM and REM sleep. Full awakening and hyperalertness with recall of the preceding dream are typical in PTSD.

Attention-Deficit/Hyperactivity Disorder

Attention-deficit/hyperactivity disorder (ADHD) is characterized by problems with the coexistence of attentional problems and hyperactivity with each behavior occurring infrequently alone and symptoms starting before 7 years of age.[148] Impulsivity is another common feature of the disorder. It is diagnosed more frequently in boys than in girls. Treatment usually involves a combination of medication, behavioral modification, and counseling. The pathophysiology of ADHD is complex and not completely clear. Research has shown that children with ADHD have a reduction in brain volume, particularly in the left prefrontal cortex, suggesting it is a frontal lobe dysfunction. There also appears to be a delay in the development of the frontal cortex and the temporal lobe, which are associated with attention and a faster development of the motor cortex.[149] There also appears to be decreased neural activity as evidenced by decreased circulation and increased dopamine in the striatum, an area associated with planning ahead.[150]

Research has shown that sleep deprivation is linked to ADHD in children. A study by Cortese et al[151] found that children with ADHD had higher rates of daytime sleepiness than their normal peers. Golan et al[152] suggested that 50% of children with ADHD have symptoms of sleep-related breathing disorder compared to 22% of children without ADHD. Other research reports increased incidence of restless leg/legs syndrome and periodic limb movement disorder in children with ADHD.[153] It appears that poor quality sleep or not enough sleep is a contributing factor in the development of symptoms of ADHD. Improving sleep in children is vitally important because successful treatment of sleep problems in children, for example, improving airway resistance by excising hypertrophic tonsillar tissue, improves symptoms of ADHD. A study by Shur-Fen Gau[154] found that treating sleep problems may be enough to eliminate symptoms of ADHD in some children.

SUMMARY

Disordered sleep is known to be a contributing factory in decline in neurocognitive and psychological function. It has also been found to be a complicating factor in a number of medical illnesses. This chapter outlined the relationship between sleep and a number of particular medical, neurological, and psychiatric disorders.

REFERENCES

1. Brohadana AB, Hannhart B, Teculescu DB. Nocturnal worsening of asthma and sleep-disordered breathing. *J Asthma.* 2002;39(2):85–100.
2. Goodman CC, Boissonnault WG, Fuller KS. The respiratory system. In: Goodman CC, Boissonnault WG, Fuller KS, eds. *Pathology: Implications for the Physical Therapist.* 2nd ed. Philadelphia, PA: Saunders; 2002:574–581.
3. Goodman CC, Boissonnault WG, Fuller KS. The respiratory system. In: Goodman CC, Boissonnault WG, Fuller KS, eds. *Pathology: Implications for the Physical Therapist.* 2nd ed. Philadelphia, PA: Saunders; 2002:569–574.
4. McNicholas WT. Impact of sleep in COPD. *Chest.* 2000;117(2 suppl): 48S–53S.
5. Goodman CC, Boissonnault WG, Fuller KS. The respiratory system. In: Goodman CC, Boissonnault WG, Fuller KS, eds. *Pathology: Implications for the Physical Therapist.* 2nd ed. Philadelphia, PA: Saunders; 2002:591–598.
6. Kaneshiro NK, Seckler B, Jasmin L. Duchenne muscular dystrophy. Available at: http://www.nlm.nih.gov/medlineplus/ency/article/000705.htm. Accessed June 25, 2012.
7. Turner C, Hilton-Jones D. The myotonic dystrophies: diagnosis and management. *J Neurol Neurosurg Psychiatry.* 2010;81:358–367.
8. Cup EH, Pieterse AJ, ten Broek-Pastoor J, et al. Exercise therapy and other types of physical therapy for patients with neuromuscular diseases: a systematic review. *Arch Phys Med Rehabil.* 2007;88:1452–1464.
9. Orngreen MC, Olsen DB, Vissing J. Aerobic training in patients with myotonic dystrophy type 1. *Ann Neurol.* 2005;57:754–757.
10. Pandya S, Eichinger K. Role of physical therapy in the assessment and management of individuals with myotonic dystrophy. Available at: http://www.myotonic.org/sites/default/files/pages/files/Physical%20Therapy%20FINAL.pdf. Accessed May 5, 2012.
11. Sabatelli M, Madia F, Conte A, et al. Natural history of young-adult amyotrophic lateral sclerosis. *Neurology.* 2008;16:876–881.
12. Lewis M, Rushanan S. The role of physical therapy and occupational therapy in the treatment of amyotrophic lateral sclerosis. *NeuroRehabilitation.* 2007;22:451–461.
13. Brain and Nervous System Health Center. Amyotrophic lateral sclerosis. Available at: http://www.webmd.com/brain/tc/amyotrophic-lateral-sclerosis-als-topic-overview. Accessed June 28, 2012.
14. Atkinson W, Hamborsky J, McIntyre L, Wolfe S, eds. Poliomyelitis. In: Centers for Disease Control and Prevention. *Epidemiology and Prevention of Vaccine-Preventable Diseases (The Pink Book).* 11th ed. Washington, DC: Public Health Foundation; 2009:231–244.
15. Frauenthal HWA, Manning JVV. *Manual of Infantile Paralysis, With Modern Methods of Treatment.* Philadelphia, PA: FA Davis; 1914.
16. National Institute of Neurological Disorders and Stroke. Post-polio syndrome fact sheet. Available at: http://www.ninds.nih.gov/disorders/post_polio/detail_post_polio.htm. Accessed August 2, 2011.
17. Trojan D, Cashman N. Post-poliomyelitis syndrome. *Muscle Nerve.* 2005;31:6–19.
18. Ramlow J, Alexander M, LaPorte R, Kaufmann C, Kuller L. Epidemiology of the post-polio syndrome. *Am J Epidemiol.* 1992;136:769–786.
19. Lin K, Lim Y. Post-poliomyelitis syndrome: case report and review of the literature. *Ann Acad Med Singapore.* 2005;34:447–449.
20. Centers for Disease Control and Prevention. Update on vaccine-derived polioviruses. *MMWR.* 2006;55:1093–1097.
21. McGrogan A, Sneddon S, de Vries CS. The incidence of myasthenia gravis: a systematic literature review. *Neuroepidemiology.* 2010;34(3):171–183.
22. Conti-Fine BM, Milani M, Kaminski HJ. Myasthenia gravis: past, present, and future. *J Clin Invest.* 2006;116:2843–2854.
23. Cup EH, Pieterse AJ, ten Broek-Pastoor JM, et al. Exercise therapy and other types of physical therapy for patients with neuromuscular diseases: a systematic review. *Arch Phys Med Rehabil.* 2007;88:1452–1464.
24. Gibson GJ. Diaphragmatic paresis: pathophysiology, clinical features, and investigation. *Thorax.* 1989;44:960–970.
25. Rosati G. The prevalence of multiple sclerosis in the world: an update. *Neurol Sci.* 2001;22(2):117–139.
26. Compston A, Coles A. Multiple sclerosis. *Lancet.* 2002;359:1221–1231.
27. Ascherio A, Munger KL. Environmental risk factors for multiple sclerosis: Part I. The role of infection. *Ann Neurol.* 2007;61:288–299.
28. Aimaretti G, Ghigo E. Should every patient with traumatic brain injury be referred to an endocrinologist? *Nat Clin Pract Endocrinol Metab.* 2007;3:318–319.
29. Hall RC, Hall RC, Chapman MJ. Definition, diagnosis, and forensic implications of postconcussional syndrome. *Psychosomatics.* 2005;46(3):195–202.
30. Kushner D. Mild traumatic brain injury: toward understanding manifestations and treatment. *Arch Intern Med.* 1998;158:1617–1624.
31. Stone VE, Baron-Cohen S, Knight RT. Frontal lobe contributions to theory of mind. *J Cogn Neurosci.* 1998;10:640–656.
32. Kwasnica C, Brown AW, Elovic EP, Kothari S, Flanagan SR. Congenital and acquired brain injury: 3. Spectrum of the acquired brain injury population. *Arch Phys Med Rehabil.* 2008;89(3 suppl 1):S15–S20.
33. Brown AW, Elovic EP, Kothari S, Flanagan SR, Kwasnica C. Congenital and acquired brain injury: 1. Epidemiology, pathophysiology, prognostication, innovative treatments, and prevention. *Arch Phys Med Rehabil.* 2008;89(3 suppl 1):S3–S8.
34. Jordan BD. Chronic traumatic brain injury associated with boxing. *Semin Neurol.* 2000;20(2):179–185.
35. Pillar G, Averbooch E, Katz N, Peled N, Kaufman Y, Shahar E. Prevalence and risk of sleep disturbances in adolescents after minor head injury. *Pediatr Neurol.* 2003;29(2):131–135.
36. Kaufam Y, Tzischinsky O, Epstein R, Etxioni A, Lavie P, Pillar G. Long-term sleep disturbance in adolescents after minor head injury. *Pediatr Neurol.* 2001;24(2):129–134.
37. Ayalon L, Caplan B, Drummond SP, Orff HJ. Traumatic brain injury and sleep disturbance: a review of current research. *J Head Trauma Rehabil.* 2009;24(3):155–165.
38. Mahmood O, Rapport LJ, Hanks RA, Fichtenberg NL. Neuropsychological performance and sleep disturbance following traumatic brain injury. *J Head Trauma Rehabil.* 2004;19:378–390.

39. Amano N, Iwabuchi K, Yokoi S, et al. The reappraisal study of the ultrastructure of Alzheimer's neurofibrillary tangles in three cases of progressive supranuclear palsy [in Japanese]. *No to Shinkei.* 1989;41:35–44.

40. Keith-Rokosh J, Ang LC. Progressive supranuclear palsy: a review of co-existing neurodegeneration. *Can J Neurol Sci.* 2008;35:602–608.

41. Zampieri Cris, Di Fabio R. Progressive supranuclear palsy: disease profile and rehabilitation strategies. *Phys Ther.* 2006;86:870–880.

42. Dodick DW, Gargus JJ. Why migraines strike. *Sci Am.* 2008;299(2):56–63.

43. Beck E, Sieber WJ, Trejo R. Management of cluster headache. *Am Fam Physician.* 2005;71:717–724.

44. Evers S, Goadsby PJ. Hypnic headache: clinical features, pathophysiology, and treatment. *Neurology.* 2003;60:905–909.

45. Pearce JM. Clinical features of the exploding head syndrome. *J Neurol Neurosurg Psychiatry.* 1989;52:907–910.

46. Sachs C, Svanborg E. The exploding head syndrome: polysomnographic recordings and therapeutic suggestions. *Sleep.* 1991;14:263–266.

47. Daily DK, Ardinger HH, Holmes GE. Identification and evaluation of mental retardation. *Am Fam Physician.* 2000;61:1059–1070.

48. Karmiloff A. Development itself is key to understanding developmental disorders. *Trends Cog Sci.* 1998;2:389–398. Available at: http://ac.els-cdn.com/S1364661398012303/1-s2.0-S1364661398012303-main.pdf?_tid=b7632094-2a0d-11e3-b915-00000aabof01&acdnat=1380572595_ca50d98b9ceoa-51f5acf9f801e50918b. Accessed October 2, 2013.

49. National Institute of Neurological Disorders and Stroke. Asperger syndrome fact sheet. Available at: http://www.ninds.nih.gov/disorders/asperger/detail_asperger.htm. Accessed May 3, 2012.

50. Levy SE, Mandell DS, Schultz RT. Autism. *Lancet.* 2009;374:1627–1638.

51. Rutter M. Incidence of autism spectrum disorders: changes over time and their meaning. *Acta Paediatr.* 2005;94:2–15.

52. Gerber JS, Offit PA. Vaccines and autism: a tale of shifting hypotheses. *Clin Infect Dis.* 2009;48:456–461.

53. Centers for Disease Control and Prevention. Prevalence of autism spectrum disorders—autism and developmental disabilities monitoring network, 14 sites, United States, 2008. *MMWR Surveill Summ.* 2012;61(3):1–19.

54. Newschaffer CJ, Croen LA, Daniels J, et al. The epidemiology of autism spectrum disorders. *Annu Rev Public Health.* 2007;28:235–258.

55. Amaral DG, Schumann CM, Nordahl CW. Neuroanatomy of autism. *Trends Neurosci.* 2008;31(3):137–145.

56. Arndt TL, Stodgell CJ, Rodier PM. The teratology of autism. *Int J Dev Neurosci.* 2005;23(2–3):189–199.

57. Casanova MF. The neuropathology of autism. *Brain Pathol.* 2007;17:422–433.

58. Geschwind DH. Advances in autism. *Annu Rev Med.* 2009;60:367–380.

59. Courchesne E, Pierce K, Schumann CM, et al. Mapping early brain development in autism. *Neuron.* 2007;56:399–413.

60. Persico AM, Bourgeron T. Searching for ways out of the autism maze: genetic, epigenetic and environmental clues. *Trends Neurosci.* 2006;29:349–358.

61. Südhof TC. Neuroligins and neurexins link synaptic function to cognitive disease. *Nature.* 2008;455:903–911.

62. Shahar E, Whitney CW, Redline S, et al. Sleep-disordered breathing and cardiovascular disease—cross-sectional results of the Sleep Heart Health Study. *Am J Respir Crit Care Med.* 2001;163:19–25.

63. Peppard PE, Young T, Palta M, Skatrud J. Prospective study of the association between sleep-disordered breathing and hypertension. *N Engl J Med.* 2000;342:1378–1384.

64. Peker Y, Hedner J, Norum J, Kraiczi H, Clarlson J. Increased incidence of cardiovascular disease in middle-aged men with obstructive sleep apnea. A 7-year follow up. *Am J Respir Crit Care Med.* 2002;166(2):159–165.

65. Peker Y, Kraiczj H, Hedner J, Loth S, Johansson A, Bende M. An independent association between obstructive sleep apnea and coronary artery disease. *Euro Respir J.* 1999;14:179–184.

66. Shahar E, Whitney CW, Redline S, Lee ET, et al. Sleep-disordered breathing and cardiovascular disease. Cross-sectional results of the Sleep Heart Health Study. *Am J Respir Crit Care Med.* 2001;163:19–25.

67. Becker HF, Jerrentrup A, Ploch T, et al. Effect of nasal continuous positive airway pressure treatment on blood pressure in patients with obstructive sleep apnea. *Circulation.* 2003;107:68–73.

68. Mansfield DR, Gollogly NC, Kaye DM, et al. Controlled trial of continuous positive airway pressure in obstructive sleep apnea and heart failure. *Am J Respir Crit Care Med.* 2004;169:361–366.

69. Narkiewicz K, Kato M, Pillips BG, et al. Nocturnal continuous positive airway pressure decreases daytime sympathetic traffic in obstructive sleep apnea. *Circulation.* 1999;100:2332–2335.

70. Somers VK, Dyken ME, Clary MP, et al. Sympathetic neural mechanisms in obstructive sleep apnea. *J Clin Invest.* 1995;96(4):1897–1904.

71. Shamsuzzaman AS, Winnicki M, Lanfranchi P, et al. Elevated C-reactive protein in patients with obstructive sleep apnea. *Circulation.* 2002;105:2462–2464.

72. Ip MS, Tse HF, Lam B, et al. Endothelial function in obstructive sleep apnea and response to treatment. *Am J Respir Crit Care Med.* 2004;169:348–353.

73. Ip MS, Lam B, Ng MM, et al. Obstructive sleep apnea is independently associated with insulin resistance. *Am J Respir Crit Care Med.* 2002;165:670–676.

74. McMurray JJ, Pfeffer MA. Heart failure. *Lancet.* 2005;365(9474):1877–1889.

75. Kumar P, Clark M. *Clinical Medicine.* 6th ed. St Louis, MO: Elsevier-Saunders; 2005.

76. Francis DP, Willson K, Davies LC, Coats AJ, Piepoli M. Quantitative general theory for periodic breathing in heart failure and its clinical implications. *Circulation.* 2000;102:2214–2221.

77. Cullen DJ, Hawkey GM, Greenwood DC, et al. Peptic ulcer bleeding in older adults: relative roles of *Helicobacter pylori* and nonsteroidal anti-inflammatory drugs. *Gut.* 1997;41:459–462.

78. Goodman CC. The gastrointestinal system. In: Goodman CC, Boissonnault WG, Fuller KS, eds. *Pathology: Implications for the Physical Therapist.* 2nd ed. Philadelphia, PA: Saunders; 2003:628–666.

79. Dubois RW, Orr WC, Lange SM. GERD-related sleep impairment among individuals with nighttime versus daytime GERD. *Gastroenterology.* 2005;128(suppl 2):A288.

80. Orr WC, Goodrich S, Fremstrom P, Hasselgren G. Occurence of nighttime gastroesophageal reflux in disturbed and normal sleepers. *Clin Gastroent Hepatol.* 2008;6(10):1099–1104.

81. Fass R, Fullerton S, Tung S, Maer EA. Sleep disturbances in clinic patinets wit functional bowel disorders. *Am J Gastroenteol.* 2000;95:1195–1200.

82. Elsenbruch S, Harnish MJ, Orr WC. Subjective and objective sleep quality in irritable bowel syndrome. *Am J Gastroenterol.* 999;94:2447-2452.

83. National Kidney Foundation. K/DOQI clinical practice guidelines for chronic kidney disease. Available at: http://www.kidney.org/professionals/KDOQI/guidelines_ckd/toc.htm. Accessed June 25, 2012.

84. Levey AS, Coresh J, Balk E, et al. National Kidney Foundation Practice Guidelines for Chronic Kidney Disease: Evaluation, Classification and Stratification. *Ann Int Med.* 2003;139(2):137-147.

85. American Thyroid Association. Hypothyroidism. Available at: http://www.thyroid.org/what-is-hypothyroidism. Accessed June 2, 2012.

86. Agabegi ED, Agabegi SS. *Step-Up to Medicine*. Hagerstown, MD: Lippincott Williams & Wilkins; 2008.

87. Kumar V, Abbas A, Fausto N. *Robbins and Cotran Pathologic Basis of Disease*. 7th ed. New York, NY: Elsevier-Saunders; 2005.

88. Nieman LK, Ilias I. Evaluation and treatment of Cushing's syndrome. *Am J Med*. 2005;118:1340–1346.

89. Ford ES, Giles WH, Dietz WH. Prevalence of metabolic syndrome among US adults: findings from the third National Health and Nutrition Examination Survey. *JAMA*. 2002;287:356–359.

90. Grundy SM, Cleeman JI, Daniels SR, et al. Diagnosis and management of the metabolic syndrome: an American Heart Association/National Heart, Lung, and Blood Institute scientific statement. *Circulation*. 2005;112:2735–2752.

91. Kogiso T, Moriyoshi Y, Shimizu S, Nagahara H, Shiratori K. High-sensitivity C-reactive protein as a serum predictor of nonalcoholic fatty liver disease based on the Akaike information criterion scoring system in the general Japanese population. *J Gastroenterol*. 2009;44:313–321.

92. Pollex RL, Hegele RA. Genetic determinants of the metabolic syndrome. *Nat Clin Pract Cardiovasc Med*. 2006;3:482–489.

93. Poulsen P, Vaag A, Kyvik K, Beck-Nielsen H. Genetic versus environmental aetiology of the metabolic syndrome among male and female twins. *Diabetologia*. 2001;44:537–543.

94. Groop L. Genetics of the metabolic syndrome. *Br J Nutr*. 2000;83(suppl 1):S39–S48.

95. Bouchard G. Genetics and the metabolic syndrome. *Int J Obes Relat Metab Disord*. 1995;19(suppl 1):52–59.

96. Glueck CJ, Papanna R, Wang P, Goldenberg N, Sieve-Smith L. Incidence and treatment of metabolic syndrome in newly referred women with confirmed polycystic ovarian syndrome. *Metabolism*. 2003;52:908–915.

97. Essah PA, Nestler JE. The metabolic syndrome in polycystic ovary syndrome. *J Endocrin Invest*. 2006;29:270–280.

98. Katzmaryk PT, Leon AS, Wilmore JH, et al. Targeting the metabolic syndrome with exercise: evidence from the HERITAGE family study. *Med Sci Sports Exerc*. 2003;35:1703–1709.

99. Morinigo R, Casamitjana R, Delgado S et al. Insulin resistance, inflammation and the metabolic syndrome following Rouz-en-Y gastric bypass surgery in severely obese subjects. *Diabetes Care*. 2007;30:1906–1908.

100. Haffner SM. The metabolic syndrome: inflammation, diabetes mellitus and cardiovascular disease. *Am J Cardiol*. 2006;97(2A):3A–11A.

101. Hotamisligil GS, Arner P, Caro JF, et al. Increased adipose tissue expression of tumor necrosis factor-α in human obesity and insulin resistance. *J Clin Invest*. 1995;95:2409–2415.

102. Fukuchi S, Hamaguchi K, Seike M, Himeno K, Sakata T, Yoshimatsu H. Role of fatty acid composition in the development of metabolic disorders in sucrose-induced obese rats. *Exp Biol Med*. 2004;229:486–493.

103. Brunner EJ, Hemingway H, Walker BR, et al. Adrenocortical, autonomic, and inflammatory causes of the metabolic syndrome: nested case-control study. *Circulation*. 2002;106:2634–2636.

104. Gohill BC, Rosenblum LA, Coplan JD, Kral JG. Hypothalamic-pituitary-adrenal axis function and the metabolic syndrome X of obesity. *CNS Spectr*. 2001;6(7):581–589.

105. Tsigos C, Chrousos GP. Hypothalamic-pituitary-adrenal axis, neuroendocrine factors and stress. *J Psychosom Res*. 2002;53:865–871.

106. Rosmond R, Björntorp P. The hypothalamic-pituitary-adrenal axis activity as a predictor of cardiovascular disease, type 2 diabetes and stroke. *J Intern Med*. 2000;247:188–197.

107. Brunner EJ, Hemingway H, Walker BR, et al. Adrenocortical, autonomic, and inflammatory causes of the metabolic syndrome: nested case-control study. *Circulation*. 2002;106:2634–2636.

108. Ford ES, Giles WH, Dietz WH. Prevalence of the metabolic syndrome among US adults: findings from the Third National Health and Nutrition Examination Survey. *JAMA*. 2002;287:356–359.

109. Lara-Castro C, Fu Y, Chung BH, Garvey WT. Adiponectin and the metabolic syndrome: mechanisms mediating risk for metabolic and cardiovascular disease. *Curr Opin Lipidol*. 2007;18:263–270.

110. Renaldi O, Pramono B, Sinorita H, Purnomo LB, Asdie RH, Asdie AH. Hypoadiponectinemia: a risk factor for metabolic syndrome. *Acta Med Indones*. 2009;41:20–24.

111. John AP, Koloth R, Dragovic M, Lim SC. Prevalence of metabolic syndrome among Australians with severe mental illness. *Med J Aust*. 2009;190(4):176–179.

112. Narasimhan M, Raynor JD. Evidence-based perspective on metabolic syndrome and use of antipsychotics. *Drug Benefit Trends*. 2010;22(3):77–88.

113. Chung CP, Avalos I, Oeser A, et al. High prevalence of the metabolic syndrome in patients with systemic lupus erythematosus: association with disease characteristics and cardiovascular risk factors. *Ann Rheum Dis*. 2007;66:208–214.

114. Cohen AD, Sherf M, Vidavsky L, Vardy DA, Shapiro J, Meyerovitch J. Association between psoriasis and the metabolic syndrome: a cross-sectional study. *Dermatology*. 2008;216(2):152–155.

115. Toth LA, Opp MR. Sleep and Infection. In: Lee-Chiong TL. Sateia MJ. Carskadon MA. eds. *Sleep Medicine*. Philadelphia, PA: Hanley & Belfus, Inc; 2002:77-84.

116. Centers for Disease Control and Prevention. HIV and its transmission. Available at: http://web.archive.org/web/20050204141148/http://www.cdc.gov/HIV/pubs/facts/transmission.htm. Accessed June 1, 2012.

117. Sharp PM, Hahn BH. Origins of HIV and the AIDS pandemic. *Cold Spring Harbor Perspect Med*. 2011;1(1):1-22.

118. Gallo RC. A reflection on HIV/AIDS research after 25 years. *Retrovirology*. 2006;3(72):1-7.

119. Cairns V, Godwin J. Post-Lyme borreliosis syndrome: a meta-analysis of reported symptoms. *Int J Epidemiol*. 2005;34:1340–1345.

120. Smith RP, Schoen RT, Rahn DW, et al. Clinical characteristics and treatment outcome of early Lyme disease in patients with microbiologically confirmed erythema migrans. *Ann Intern Med*. 2002;136:421-428.

121. Fahrer H, Sauvain MJ, Zhioua E, Van Hoecke C, Gern LE. Longterm survey (7 years) in a population at risk for Lyme borreliosis: what happens to the seropositive individuals? *Eur J Epidemiol*. 1998;14(2):117–123.

122. Wolfe F, Smythe HA, Yunus MB, et al. The American College of Rheumatology 1990 criteria for the classification of fibromyalgia. *Arthritis Rheum*. 1990;33(2):160–172.

123. Wolfe F. Fibromyalgia: the clinical syndrome. *Rheum Dis Clin North Am*. 1989;15:1–18.

124. Buskila D, Cohen H. Comorbidity of fibromyalgia and psychiatric disorders. *Curr Pain Headache Rep*. 2007;11:333–338.

125. Schweinhardt P, Sauro KM, Bushnell MC. Fibromyalgia: a disorder of the brain? *Neuroscientist*. 2008;14:415–421.

126. Bartels EM, et al. Fibromyalgia, diagnosis and prevalence. Are gender differences explainable? *Ugeskr Laeger*. 2009;171:3588–3592.

127. Häuser W, Thieme K, Turk C. Guidelines on the management of fibromyalgia syndrome—a systematic review. *Eur J Pain*. 2009;14:5–10.

128. Wolfe F. Fibromyalgia wars. *J Rheumatol*. 2009;36:671–678.

129. Goldenberg DL. Fibromyalgia: why such controversy? *Ann Rheum Dis*. 1995;54:3–5.

130. van Os J, Kapur S. Schizophrenia. *Lancet*. 2009;374:635–645.

131. Buckley PF, Miller BJ, Lehrer DS, Castle DJ. Psychiatric comorbidities and schizophrenia. *Schizophr Bull*. 2009;35:383–402.

132. National Institute of Mental Health. Depression. Available at: http://www.nimh.nih.gov/health/publications/depression/complete-index.shtml/index.shtml. Accessed April 17, 2012.

133. Sansone RA, Sansone LA. Dysthymic disorder: forlorn and overlooked? *Psychiatry*. 2009;6(5):46–50.

134. Lurie SJ, et al. Seasonal affective disorder. *Am Fam Physician*. 2006;74:1521–1524.

135. Mayo Clinic. Seasonal affective disorder. Available at: http://www.mayoclinic.com/health/seasonal-affective-disorder/DS00195/DSECTION=symptoms. Accessed April 18, 2012.

136. Friedman RA. Brought on by darkness, disorder needs light. *New York Times*. December 18, 2007. Available at: http://www.nytimes.com/2007/12/18/health/18mind.html?_r=2&em&ex=1198213200&en=a955503f665508cf&ei=5087%0A. Accessed April 18, 2012.

137. National Institute of Mental Health. Properly timed light, melatonin lift winter depression by syncing rhythms. Available at: http://www.nimh.nih.gov/science-news/2006/properly-timed-light-melatonin-lift-winter-depression-by-syncing-rhythms.shtml. Accessed April 18, 2012.

138. Terman M, Terman JS. Controlled trial of naturalistic dawn simulation and negative air ionization for seasonal affective disorder. *Am J Psychiatry*. 2006;163:2126–2133.

139. National Institute of Mental Health. Bipolar disorder. Available at: http://www.nimh.nih.gov/health/publications/bipolar-disorder/complete-index.shtml. Accessed April 18, 2012.

140. Ballenger JC, Davidson JR, Lecrubier Y, et al. Consensus statement on generalized anxiety disorder from the International Consensus Group on Depression and Anxiety. *J Clin Psychiatry*. 2001;62(suppl 11):53–58.

141. National Institute of Mental Health. Panic disorder: when fear overwhelms. Available at: http://www.nimh.nih.gov/health/publications/panic-disorder-when-fear-overwhelms/panic-disorder-when-fear-overwhelms.shtml. Accessed May 4, 2012.

142. Yehuda R, Halligan SL, Grossman R, Golier JA, Wong C. The cortisol and glucocorticoid receptor response to low dose dexamethasone administration in aging combat veterans and holocaust survivors with and without posttraumatic stress disorder. *Biol Psychiatry*. 2002;52:393–403.

143. Yehuda R. Biology of posttraumatic stress disorder. *J Clin Psychiatry*. 2001;62(suppl 17):41–46.

144. Yehuda R. Clinical relevance of biologic findings in PTSD. *Psychiatr Q*. 2002;73(2):123–133.

145. Lindley SE, Carlson EB, Benoit M. Basal and dexamethasone suppressed salivary cortisol concentrations in a community sample of patients with posttraumatic stress disorder. *Biol Psychiatry*. 2004;55:940–945.

146. Aardal-Eriksson E, Eriksson TE, Thorell LH. Salivary cortisol, posttraumatic stress symptoms, and general health in the acute phase and during 9-month follow-up. *Biol Psychiatry*. 2001;50:986–993.

147. Jatko A, Rothenhofer S, Schmitt A, et al. Hippocampal volume in chronic posttraumatic stress disorder (PTSD): MRI study using two different evaluation methods. *J Affect Dis*. 2006;94:121–126.

148. Biederman J. Attention-deficit/hyperactivity disorder: a life-span perspective. *J Clin Psychiatry*. 1998;59(suppl 7):4–16.

149. Bush G, Valera EM, Seidman LJ. Functional neuroimaging of attention-deficit/hyperactivity disorder: a review and suggested future directions. *Biol Psychiatry*. 2005;57:1273–1284.

150. Lou HC, Andresen J, Steinberg B, McLaughlin T, Friberg L. The striatum in a putative cerebral network activated by verbal awareness in normals and in ADHD children. *Eur J Neurol*. 1998;5:67–74.

151. Cortese S, Konofal E, Yateman N et al. Sleep and alertness in children with attention-deficit/hyperactivity disorder: a systematic review of the literature. *Sleep*. 2006;29:504–511.

152. Golan N, Shahar E, Ravid S, Pillar G. Sleep disorders and daytime sleepiness in children with attention-deficit/hyperactive disorder. *Sleep*. 2004;27:261–266.

153. Sadeh A, Pergamin L, Bar-Haim Y. Sleep in children with attention-deficit hyperactivity disorder: a meta-analysis of polysomnographic studies. *Sleep Med Rev*. 2006;10:381–398.

154. Sur-Fen Gau S. Prevalence of sleep problems and their association with inattention/hyperactivity among children aged 6–15 in Taiwan. *J Sleep Res*. 2006;15:403–414.

Section III

Evaluation and Treatment of Disordered Sleep

16

Evaluation of Sleep and Sleep Disorders

Julie M. Hereford, PT, DPT

REVIEW OF MANIFESTATIONS OF DISORDERED SLEEP AND SLEEP DEPRIVATION

It is clear that sleep disorders have an impact not only on general functioning but also on long-term health and well-being. Sleep disorders may manifest themselves as insomnia, which is the inability to fall asleep or remain asleep. Individuals with insomnia may feel that sleep is short and inadequate. They may report that they are a "light sleeper" and that their sleep is easily disrupted. They usually report generally nonrestorative sleep.

Another characteristic manifestation of disordered sleep is excessive daytime sleepiness. Individuals with excessive daytime sleepiness report difficulty being able to consistently achieve and sustain wakefulness and alertness to accomplish the tasks of daily living. These individuals may also fall asleep unintentionally or at inappropriate times when they should be awake. This can be life-threatening when an individual with excessive daytime sleepiness falls asleep while driving or operating heavy machinery.

Sleep apnea may be the cause of disordered sleep. Sleep apnea is defined as the absence of air flow for 10 or more seconds. When air flow is diminished, but not absent, the event is known as *hypopnea*. Sleep apnea may be obstructive, in which the upper airway collapses during sleep but respiratory effort continues but is unable to overcome the restriction caused. Central sleep apnea (CSA) is a cessation of breathing and a loss of respiratory effort. Both obstructive sleep apnea (OSA) and CSA can result in either insomnia or excessive daytime sleepiness.

Pain can be exacerbated in an individual with disordered sleep. Disordered sleep may also lead to increased symptoms in other medical disorders. Sleep disorders may complicate headache syndromes. Cancer pain and pain from fibromyalgia and other rheumatologic conditions are often aggravated by disordered sleep. Individuals with disordered sleep often complain of chronic fatigue, nonrestorative sleep, and generalized muscle discomfort. Individuals with underlying heart disease, gastroesophageal reflux disease, or chronic obstructive pulmonary disease may report increased nocturnal chest pain. In short, disordered sleep has been considered as a causative or contributing factor or has been implicated in exacerbating the primary disease.

Acute and chronic sleep deprivation has widespread systemic consequences (see Chapter 12). Animal studies have shown that sleep deprivation increases the homeostatic sleep drive, with sleep rebound characterized by an increase in behavioral quiescence, slow-wave sleep, and paradoxical sleep. Animal studies also show changes in metabolism, with a decrease in anabolic hormones, weight loss despite high amounts of food intake, and an increase in metabolic rate.[1] A human study showed that with partial-night sleep deprivation or sleep deprivation from disordered sleep there is a decrease in slow-wave sleep. This may cause an increase in plasma norepinephrine levels, which, in turn, may increase cardiovascular disease.[2] Sleep deprivation may also impair response to infectious agents and, in animal studies, has been shown to cause increased skin lesions, including hyperkeratosis and skin ulcerations.[3]

Hereford JM. *Sleep and Rehabilitation:
A Guide for Health Professionals* (pp 157-168).
© 2014 Taylor & Francis Group.

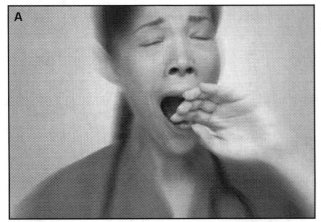
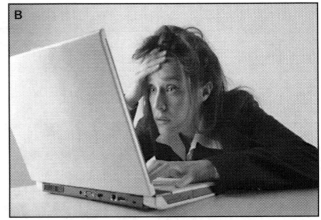

Figures 16-1. Sleep deprivation has physiological and psychological consequences. (From Fotolia.com)

Other studies have shown that acute and chronic sleep deprivation may cause increased heart rate and blood pressure.[4-6] Sleep deprivation may interfere with normal body temperature regulation, with a decrease in normal temperature and a failure of thermoregulation.[7,8] Animal studies have shown that prolonged total sleep deprivation will cause the aforementioned problems but will ultimately result in death.[9]

REVIEW OF THE CONSEQUENCES OF SLEEP DEPRIVATION

Sleepiness is the most obvious consequence of sleep deprivation (Figure 16-1). It is associated with an increase in homeostatic sleep drive and a propensity to fall asleep. Microsleeps or brief lapses into sleep can occur during wakefulness as a result of partial or total sleep deprivation or sleep loss from disordered sleep. These microsleeps are due to the heightened sleep pressure that overwhelm the individual and make it impossible to remain awake.

An individual who suffers from excessive daytime sleepiness as a consequence of disordered sleep will show decreased sleep latency on polysomnography (PSG). Sleep latency is defined as the length of time it takes from the time an individual goes to bed with the intention of sleeping to the point at which they fall asleep as evidenced by a change in electroencephalogram (EEG) pattern to a sleep pattern. These individuals also show decreased sleep latency in the Multiple Sleep Latency Test (MSLT) or nap study and on the Maintenance of Wakefulness Test.[10] It was also shown that the greater the degree of sleep deprivation an individual has, the shorter the sleep latency he or she will produce.

Consequences of sleep deprivation can also be seen on PSG. PSG demonstrates an increase in slow-wave activity and non-rapid eye movement (NREM) stages 3 and 4 sleep and a decrease in NREM stages 1 and 2 sleep following

periods of sleep deprivation. Rapid eye movement (REM) sleep may increase during the second recovery night after NREM stages 3 and 4 sleep has normalized. Wake time after sleep onset is reduced, alpha activity is decreased, and delta and theta activity is increased in recovery sleep following periods of sleep deprivation. It has been shown that following selective sleep deprivation as occurs in experimental models, rebound of specific sleep stages that are reduced during a study will occur with increased density during recovery sleep.[11] This indicates the specific need for each stage of sleep. EEG obtained during wakefulness following a period of sleep deprivation may show an increase in the slower theta and delta wave forms. Greater frequency of slow eye movements during wakefulness has been noted. Clearly, the changes in PSG and EEG patterns during wakefulness in the period following acute sleep deprivation offer evidence of the importance of each stage of sleep and highlight the changes that occur as a consequence of sleep deprivation.

Hyperactivity may paradoxically develop in children following periods of acute sleep deprivation. Chronic sleep deprivation from short sleep or from disordered sleep has been linked to attention-deficit/hyperactivity disorder.

Sleep deprivation can cause problems with general health. It is associated with an increase in morbidity and mortality. Excess mortality has been observed in individuals who sleep fewer than 6.5 hours or who sleep more than 9 or 10 hours per 24-hour period. The mechanism responsible for the association between sleep duration and increased mortality is not completely clear.

Sleep deprivation is also known to have a negative impact on mood and has been found to be a particular problem in adolescents; it can cause irritability, nervousness, and impulsiveness. Short sleep—that is, not getting as much sleep as is required for optimal neurocognitive function—is associated with diminished attention, alertness, and vigilance. This situation has been linked to increased incidence of motor vehicle accidents and industrial accidents. Sleep deprivation may interfere with memory and concentration, thinking, and learning. It may lead to confusion and is known to lead to increased error rate of both omission and commission.

Total sleep deprivation and partial sleep loss, as well as chronic disordered sleep, have been linked with a number of specific neurological disorders. It is associated with a decrease in cerebral glucose metabolism. Ptosis, nystagmus, slurring of speech, a hyperactive gag reflex, and tremors may develop as total sleep deprivation continues. Corneal reflexes become sluggish, and deep tendon reflexes may become hyperactive. Pain sensitivity is known to increase in relationship to sleep deprivation, but increased pain may also cause sleep disruption.

Chronic sleep deprivation, particularly as is seen in OSA, has been seen to cause an increase in cardiovascular morbidity. It has been linked to an increase in blood pressure and left-sided heart failure. Increased sympathetic activation that is a component of sleep deprivation may lead to increased heart rate.

Sleep deprivation can produce increased cortisol and ghrelin levels, which both may cause an increase in appetite. The hormone leptin, which is responsible for the sense of satiation, usually decreases in individuals with disordered sleep. These sleep-related changes in leptin and ghrelin are a proposed mechanism for weight gain and particularly abdominal obesity, which can be characteristic of an individual who suffers from chronic sleep deprivation. In extreme sleep deprivation, particularly total sleep deprivation produced in experimental models, the metabolic rate may increase and hypothermia may occur, even to the point of death.

Sleep deprivation decreases secretion of human growth hormone and prolactin. It has been reported to decrease the febrile response to endotoxins and change antibody titers following influenza vaccination. It has been shown to alter cytokine levels and interleukin-6 levels and cause changes in tumor necrosis factor-α and leukocytes. Further, it can affect the activity of natural killer cells. Lastly, there is a decrease in granulocytes and lymphocytes in response to antigens as a result of acute and chronic sleep deprivation.

There is increasing evidence that disordered sleep may also interfere with the rehabilitation process.[12-17] It may increase pain sensitivity, alter pain threshold, interfere with connective tissue healing, disrupt motor memory consolidation, and affect motor learning. In a patient with a chronic musculoskeletal injury, for example, disordered sleep may increase pain sensitivity, which may restrict tolerance to stretching. It may interfere with connective tissue healing, which will slow recovery. Disruption of particular sleep stages may change motor memory consolidation, making integration of practiced novel movement patterns in a therapeutic exercise program difficult to perform with precision. Faulty movement patterns that result may further irritate inflamed tissue. Disordered sleep and chronic sleep deprivation could interfere with motor

learning, making instruction in corrective movement patterns less effective, which would therefore lengthen the rehabilitation process.

HOW TO EVALUATE SLEEP

Because of its potential impact on the rehabilitation process, it is important that clinicians be able to recognize the signs and symptoms of disordered sleep and be able to use some tools to help identify individuals with a significant sleep problem. The rehabilitation professional should also know how to assist a patient in seeking further sleep evaluation and should understand appropriate treatments for disordered sleep.

In order to better understand the extent of the sleep disorder in an individual patient, it is important to thoroughly evaluate the problem. Identification of disordered sleep should begin with the initial visit. The rehabilitation professional should question the patient regarding sleep pattern in order to identify the quantity and quality of sleep. With a patient who is seeking rehabilitation for a painful condition, it is important for the rehabilitation provider to gather information regarding the relationship between sleep and pain. This data collection should include questions regarding normal times that the individual goes to bed and awakens in the morning. Total sleep time (TST) should be reported. The patient should report whether pain makes it difficult for him or her to fall asleep or whether he or she awakens with pain. If the patient is awakened because of pain, he or she should be questioned regarding the severity and nature of that pain because it may be a sign of serious illness. The patient should be questioned about what he or she must do to return to sleep and the length of time required for return to sleep. For example, the patient who awakens with pain and changes positions and is able to return to sleep immediately is in a different situation than the patient who has pain that makes it difficult for him or her to find a comfortable position, but once asleep he or she is able to stay asleep until normal morning awakening. The former is evidence of a joint derangement or dysfunction; the latter is more likely a sign of an inflammatory process. How pain interferes with sleep is an important part of the subjective evaluation and should play a role in treatment planning.

The rehabilitation professional should regularly inquire about the quality and quantity of sleep and be prepared to administer one of the instruments described in the following paragraphs to identify disordered sleep.

Sleep Questionnaires

Epworth Sleepiness Scale

The Epworth Sleepiness Scale[18] is a brief, easily administered instrument that was developed at Epworth Hospital in

Melbourne, Australia, in 1991 to help identify individuals who may have excessive daytime sleepiness. The instrument asks the subject to rate the probability of falling asleep in 8 different situations that are common in everyday life using a 0 to 3 scale.[18] The total numeric score is compiled. A score in the 0 to 9 range is considered a normal level of daytime sleepiness; however, a score above 9 is considered to indicate excessive daytime sleepiness, and further evaluation is recommended. A score of 11 to 15 has been correlated with an increased possibility of mild-to-moderate sleep apnea, and a score above 16 may indicate severe apnea, narcolepsy, or idiopathic hypersomnia. The instrument correlates with PSG findings, and certain questions appear to be predictors of specific sleep disorders. The instrument cannot be used as an accurate diagnostic tool but is likely to indicate the existence of a sleep disorder that requires further evaluation. This instrument may be used after a treatment regime such as continuous positive airway pressure (CPAP) has been introduced in order to document improvement of symptoms.

Stanford Sleepiness Scale

The Stanford Sleepiness Scale[19] is another instrument that is easily administered in a rehabilitation setting.[20] It is a very brief 7-point subjective measure of an individual's perception of sleepiness. This instrument may be used to track an individual's level of alertness over time. By measuring the level of alertness throughout the day, an individual may better recognize when he or she is likely to be more effective at cognitive and behavioral tasks. Most people have peaks of alertness and sleepiness or fatigue, and this can help to identify those. Peak alertness is likely to occur at about 9 AM and again at 9 PM, with the lowest level of alertness likely to occur at around 2 or 3 PM. An individual who is well rested should usually score 1 or 2 on this scale during much of the day. If an individual scores 3 when he or she should be feeling alert, it may be an indicator of acute or chronic sleep deprivation.

Fatigue Severity Scale

The Fatigue Severity Scale[21] is another tool that may be easily administered in the rehabilitation setting. It is a 9-item questionnaire in which the subject rates the level of agreement on a 7-point scale with questions regarding the manner in which fatigue interferes with normal function. Because sleepiness and fatigue are distinctly different qualities, it can be important to distinguish between the two. Fatigue may have a negative impact on quality of life and performance of normal tasks. Sleepiness may impair function until the sleep drive is satisfied, but then vitality is restored, at least temporarily. For example, patients who suffer from fibromyalgia often complain of fatigue and report that they have difficulty functioning on a regular basis because of it but are less likely to complain of sleepiness. This tool helps to distinguish between sleepiness and fatigue and may help direct a treatment program.

Polysomnography

PSG, which is also known as a sleep study, is a multiparameter evaluation of sleep used to diagnose the presence and severity of disordered sleep. The American Academy of Sleep Medicine (AASM) has defined at least 84 sleep disorders that may be identified with PSG. Often, a sleep study may be read as normal because, according to the AASM, the patient does not meet the strict criteria of OSA.[10] However, a PSG provides a wealth of information that can be utilized to assess a patient's function and may help to identify reasons the patient may have difficulties fully benefiting from a rehabilitation program. For example, if a patient does not show that he or she is getting any stage 3 or 4 sleep, identified together in a sleep study as N3, he or she may be slow to recover from a musculoskeletal injury. If the patient is not getting normal stage 2 sleep, he or she may not be able to encode and consolidate motor memory, which may impact the ability to successfully perform a neuromuscular re-education program. It is therefore important that the rehabilitation professional be able to evaluate a sleep study for some of these parameters and make adjustments to a treatment plan accordingly.

This section will describe the process of PSG and define the terms most commonly found in a sleep study report. A PSG may be ordered if a sleep disorder is suspected as identified by patient complaint of nonrestorative sleep, snoring, elevated score on the Epworth Sleepiness Scale, or witnessed snoring or apneic event, usually by a bed partner or parent in the case of a child. PSG may be used to diagnose or rule out a specific sleep disorder, usually OSA. It is also used to identify parasomnias and abnormal movement disorders during sleep that may be indicators of other systemic disease. PSG measures biophysiological changes that occur during the course of sleep. A comprehensive PSG is performed in a sleep laboratory; however, a home sleep study can be performed, although it is not as comprehensive and usually does not include EEG tracings. The PSG is usually performed at night when most people sleep, although some sleep labs will evaluate shift workers and individuals with circadian rhythm disorders such as delayed phase sleep disorder at other times of the day. The PSG monitors brain function with a selective EEG and other physiological parameters such as muscle activity; cardiac function, including heart rate and rhythm; eye movement with an electrooculogram (EOG); and respiratory function including air flow and respiratory effort by measuring thoracic and abdominal excursion during sleep. Oxygen saturation is measured by pulse oximetry.

In a standard PSG evaluation, the patient may be seen for evaluation by a physician who has attained certification in sleep medicine. A sleep specialist is often trained as a pulmonologist, neurologist, or psychiatrist prior to seeking additional training and certification in sleep medicine, although any physician, regardless of specialty, may become a board-certified sleep specialist. The initial evaluation will usually involve a complete history, particularly as it pertains to the quality and quantity of sleep. Past medical history, including comorbid conditions, is assessed. Indications of conditions that may be related to disordered sleep are noted. These may include, but are not limited to, cardiovascular disease, diabetes, weight gain or obesity, and depression. An Epworth Sleepiness Scale or similar instrument is usually administered and scored. The patient will receive a physical examination, with special attention given to the structure and function of the upper airway. Neck circumference is usually measured because there is a correlation between increased neck circumference and upper airway resistance. Body mass index is calculated to determine the impact that excess weight may have on the sleep pattern.

If, based upon the history and physical examination, it is determined that there is a reasonable suspicion of a sleep disorder, a PSG will be ordered. Depending upon the signs and symptoms, it may also be suggested that the patient undergo an MSLT.

The patient is asked to arrive at the sleep laboratory several hours prior to normal sleep time in order to accommodate to the sleep lab environment. A sleep lab is generally designed to have the look and feel of a comfortable hotel room. It is equipped with a video recording system and telemetry, in order for data to be collected during the course of the night. An hour or so prior to normal sleep time, a sleep technician will attach multiple sensors and monitors to the patient's head, face, throat, chest and abdomen, and legs so that multiple channels of data can be collected during sleep. Once the monitors have been attached, a biocalibration is performed to assure the integrity of the electrodes and amplifiers, including filters and sensitivity settings. This is done by having the patient follow a series of instructions such as lying still, eyes open, and looking straight ahead for 30 seconds to calibrate the EEG for attenuation of alpha activity, and then eyes closed for the presence of alpha activity and EOG for slow-rolling eye movements. The patient is instructed to clench to check electromyography (EMG) and to breathe in and breathe out then hold his or her breath for 10 seconds to calibrate air flow and respiratory effort monitors.

Patients are often very concerned about the ability to sleep while wired to so many monitors. Though there may be a "first-night effect" that limits the accuracy of the data collected, a single-night PSG is usually adequate to evaluate the quality of sleep and identify disordered sleep, particularly OSA. There can be variability in the quality of sleep from night to night in some patients, and there can be inter-scorer reliability variables, but usually the data collected are useful in determining disordered sleep. It is not uncommon for a patient to report that he or she "didn't sleep at all" during a sleep study; however, polysomnographic evidence demonstrates a relatively normal sleep episode.

During the sleep study, a technician monitors the patient while the instruments continuously record biophysiological data. During testing, a patient may be asked to turn onto his or her back; for instance, if data were not collected from that position during the study. Testing is usually completed by 7 AM, and the patient is discharged to home. The data collected are then analyzed by a sleep technician and the sleep specialist physician, and a report is generated.

If, during the course of the sleep study, the patient demonstrates excessive apneic events that meet particular criteria, the study may be interrupted and a CPAP device may be applied with a face mask. With this device in place, the patient is allowed to return to sleep, and air is forced through the device to the patient in an attempt to overcome the collapsibility of the upper airway. Air pressure is titrated according to the PSG data recording until the best pressure is identified to reduce apneic and hypopnic events to within acceptable parameters. This is known as a *split-night study*.

Upon completion of an overnight PSG evaluation, some patients may also undergo an MSLT. This test is generally performed if the patient reports excessive daytime sleepiness.

In some instances, because of expense or comfort or to ameliorate the first-night effect or because of the evaluator's preference, a patient may be prescribed a home sleep study. In this case, the patient is given equipment and instructed on application for testing while sleeping in his or her normal sleep environment. Home sleep study tools measure air flow using a thermistor and oxygen saturation using a pulse oximeter. Some of these devices also include EMG sensors to monitor muscular function. These devices are limited in the amount of information that they are able to provide; however, they can be used over several successive nights for a significantly reduced cost. Information retrieved from this type of monitoring may provide data gathered in a more natural environment and over a period of time and so may identify apneic or desaturation events that may not occur in a single night sleep lab setting. The at-home sleep study is thought to have particular value in confirming the efficacy of dental repositioning devices that are used to ameliorate less severe cases of OSA.

Polysomnographic Parameters

These are the most commonly found terms used on a typical sleep study report. This list is certainly not exhaustive but should give readers a good understanding of the terms and phrases found so they can understand the manner in which the information in a sleep study is presented. Understanding these terms will help clinicians to be able to discuss the findings of a sleep study from the content of the data presented rather than just from the impressions drawn

Table 16-1.

Polysomnographic Measures of Sleep Macroarchitecture

Polysomnographic Measure	Description
Sleep integrity and continuity	
Sleep latency	Time from lights-out to first occurrence of sleep stage 1, 2, 3, 4, or REM
TST	Number of minutes of sleep from lights out to lights on
Sleep efficiency	TST as a percentage of total recording time
Number of awakenings	Number of times the patient awoke within the total recording time
Global sleep-stage structure	
Wake after sleep onset	Total time spent awake during the night after having initially fallen asleep
Stage 1 sleep percentage	Percentage of TST scored as stage 1 sleep
Stage 2 sleep percentage	Percentage of TST scored as stage 2 sleep
Slow-wave sleep percentage	Percentage of TST scored as stage 3 or 4 sleep
REM sleep percentage	Percentage of TST scored sleep stage REM
REM sleep latency	Time from sleep onset to the appearance of REM sleep

by the report writer. It is often the case that the conclusions drawn from a sleep study reflect the existence and severity of OSA or upper airway resistance syndrome. Often, more subtle data contained in the sleep study reveal information that may be significant to the rehabilitation professional. Understanding the terms and meanings may influence decision making and treatment planning with a rehabilitation client.

Polysomnography Procedure Definitions

The following are terms that are found in the PSG report that describe the mechanics of the actual testing procedures and parameters. This list will help an individual new to reviewing a PSG report to understand the procedure (Table 16-1).

- **Bedtime** is the term used to describe the time when a person gets into bed and attempts to fall asleep. For the purposes of sleep medicine, bedtime does not include the time that a person lies on the bed while reading or watching television. It is specifically designated for the time dedicated to attempting to fall sleep.

- **Drowsiness** is defined as the period of wakefulness that commonly precedes sleep onset and is characterized by diffuse alpha EEG activity with the eyes closed.

- **Final wake-up** is defined as the time in which an individual awakens for the final time after a period of sleep.

- **Lights out** is defined as the time when sleep recording begins. Lights out does not coincide with when the subject actually goes to sleep. The period of time between lights out and the point at which the EEG shows changes that the individual has fallen asleep will include a period of drowsy wakefulness in which the EEG shows alpha and theta wave activity. This period is known as *sleep latency*.

- **Lights on** is defined as the point at which recording is ended. This usually also coincides with the final wake-up.

- **Time in bed** is defined as the duration of monitoring that takes place between lights out and lights on.

- **Total recording time** is defined as the time from sleep onset to final awakening. This will include the TST plus the wake time after sleep onset plus movement time.

- **Total sleep episode** is defined as the time available for sleep during a sleep study. It is the TST plus the wake time after sleep onset. This is also known as the *total sleep period* or *sleep period time*.

- **Total sleep time (TST)** is defined as the sum of all sleep stages including NREM stages 1–4 and REM sleep. It is reported in minutes and includes the total sleep episode minus wake time after sleep onset.

- **Wake time after sleep onset** is defined as the time spent awake during a particular sleep episode; that is, from sleep onset to the final awakening. This time may include awakenings but not arousals. Awakenings after sleep onset occur for a variety of reasons, including underlying sleep disorder, pain, or intrusions in the sleep environment.

Telemetry Used During Polysomnography

Electroencephalography

Electroencephalography is utilized during PSG to record particular brain wave activity in order to determine neurological events during sleep (see Figure 2-4). It is used to define particular stages of sleep and transitions from one stage to another. Disruptions in expected EEG patterns and sleep architecture are one of the measurement tools used to determine the existence of sleep disorders. The PSG EEG will generally use 6 exploring electrodes, applied to the frontal, central, and occipital regions and 2 reference electrodes placed over the mastoid processes. If a seizure disorder is suspected, other electrodes will be added to document activity from specific areas of the brain. Electrodes are applied according to the International 10-20 system of EEG electrode placement.[22] This means that electrodes are placed at 10% or 20% of the distance between specific landmarks.

Electrooculography

Electrooculography is defined as a technique for measuring the resting potential of the retina. It is also used to measure eye movements. Usually, pairs of electrodes are placed approximately 1 cm above the outer canthus of the right eye and 1 cm below the outer canthus of the left eye. The electrodes measure the electropotential difference between the relatively positively charged cornea and the relatively negatively charged retina. EOG is primarily used to help identify the onset of REM sleep, but there are characteristic eye movements associated with several different stages of sleep. Patterns of eye movements may be slow rolling movements or rapid movements.

Slow rolling movements consist of slow undulating waveforms that occur during drowsy wakefulness with eyes closed in which the EEG shows alpha or theta waves or during NREM stage 1 sleep or during brief arousals from sleep. These movement patterns disappear completely during NREM stage 2 sleep. Individuals who are taking particular antidepressant medications including selective serotonin re-uptake inhibitors (SSRIs) and tricyclic antidepressants (TCAs) may have eye movements during NREM sleep.

Rapid eye movements appear as sharp deflections that occur during wakefulness with eyes open or during REM sleep. REM density—that is, the increased occurrences of bursts of REM sleep—is decreased, with fewer episodes of REM sleep occurring earlier in the night and becoming progressively denser as sleep progresses.

Electromyography

EMG is a technique used to evaluate the electrical activity produced by skeletal musculature. It detects the electrical potential generated by muscle cells. This technique is used to analyze abnormalities in muscle activation, recruitment pattern, or biomechanical movement. EMG is used during PSG in order to monitor certain motor activity during sleep. Typically, electrodes are placed on the chin, with one above the jaw line and one below, and an electrode over the tibialis anterior muscle of each leg. The electrodes on the chin help determine the onset of REM sleep because during this stage of sleep there is a characteristic postsynaptic inhibition of skeletal musculature, which can be monitored by these electrodes. They also record the level of muscular relaxation that should accompany sleep. Electrodes on the tibialis anterior monitor leg movement and are used to record for excessive amounts of leg movements during sleep, which may indicate periodic limb movement disorder.

Electrocardiography

Electrocardiography (EKG) tracings used during PSG utilize 2 or 3 electrodes, rather than the 10 that are used in a typical EKG. Electrode placement is usually under the clavicle on the right and the left and another 6 inches above the waist on either side of the body. These electrodes measure P-wave, QRS-complex, and T-wave activity. Electrical activity in the heart during sleep, particularly during REM sleep, may become variable and somewhat unstable. Analysis of these data may indicate underlying cardiac disease or a dysfunction of cardiac rhythm.

Measurement of Air Flow

Air flow measurement consists of measurement of respiratory rate, rhythm, and effort utilizing several different instruments. Nasal and mouth air flow can be measured using pressure transducers and/or a thermocouple that is fitted into or near the nostrils. Respiratory effort is monitored in concert with nasal and oral air flow by the use of a belt that expands and contracts with thoracic and/or abdominal movement. These instruments provide indirect evidence of changes in air flow based upon changes in thermal and chemical characteristics of inspired and expired air. Use of pressure transducers and thermocouples is important because they are sensitive instruments that can accurately measure changes in air flow that may occur during an apneic or hypopneic event. Expired carbon dioxide sensors may be utilized to assist in evaluating for sleep apnea. If an individual shows an increase in the concentration of CO_2 in expired air, it may be an indication of hypoventilation.

Measurement of Respiratory Effort

Measurement of respiratory effort during PSG is usually accomplished by measuring surface EMG of the diaphragm or the use of thoracic and abdominal strain gauges and respiratory inductance plethysmography (Figure 16-2). Surface tracings from electrodes placed on the chest may infer diaphragmatic effort. Strain gauges attached to 2 belts placed around the thorax positioned below the axilla and

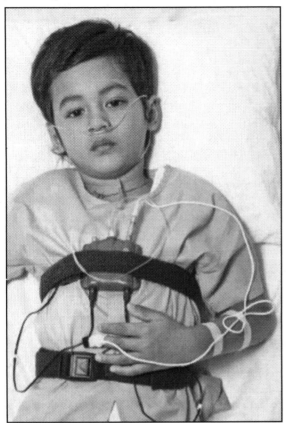

Figures 16-2. Typical arrangement of thoracic and abdominal belt used for polysomnography. (From Fotolia.com)

around the abdomen at the level of the umbilicus measure excursion. Each of these strain gauges can detect movement associated with respiration. If calibrated beforehand, quantitative measurements of volume changes of the thoracic and abdominal strain gauges can be obtained and can be used to estimate tidal volume and respiratory patterns during sleep. Technical difficulties may be encountered in this effort by changing positions of the strain gauges that may occur with changes of body position during sleep and movements during sleep. This may affect the strict accuracy of such quantitative measurements; however, useful information may be derived by monitoring thoracic and abdominal movement to detect apneic events. These instruments also cannot distinguish between obstructive and central apneic events.

Measurement of Oxygenation

Measurement of oxygenation can be accomplished by pulse oximetry. A pulse oximeter may be attached to either a fingertip or the earlobe and used to measure blood oxygen saturation levels during sleep. Oxygen desaturation is an indicator of disordered sleep but must be analyzed in conjunction with other parameters during the PSG.

Measurement of Snoring

Measurement of snoring is accomplished by attaching a small microphone to the anterior neck. Snoring is usually simply rated as mild, moderate, or loud snoring in a sleep study report. Snoring indicates some disruption in air flow and, evaluated with other findings during a PSG, may be an indicator of OSA or upper airway resistance syndrome.

Polysomnography Findings Definitions

These are terms found in a polysomnographic evaluation report used to describe particularly abnormal events that occur during the course of a sleep study.

Apnea Index

The *apnea index* is defined as the number of apneic events that occur per hour of sleep; that is, a period of respiratory cessation that lasts for at least 10 seconds per hour of sleep. These events are also associated with decreased oxygen saturation. This is a measure of the severity of sleep apnea.

Apnea–Hypopnea Index

The *apnea–hypopnea index* (AHI) is defined as the number of apnea plus hypopnea events that occur per hour of sleep. A hypopneic event is described as a period of shallow respiration or an abnormally low respiratory rate. It differs from apnea because some air flow remains. With moderate-to-severe hypopnea, sleep is disturbed, though the individual may report getting a full night's sleep but not feel rested. Hypopnea may cause oxygen desaturation, sleep fragmentation, and disruption of normal sleep architecture.

Combining apnea and hypopnea scores indicate the severity of sleep apnea. The score indicates the number of sleep disruptions and the degree of oxygen desaturation. AHI values are categorized as mild apnea if they are 1 to 15 events per hour. An AHI of 15 to 30 events per hour is considered a moderate disorder. An AHI greater than 30 events per hour is considered a severe sleep apnea.

Arousal

Arousal is a term used in PSG to define a sudden brief change in EEG that may last from 3 to 14 seconds. The change is from sleep to wakefulness or from a deeper stage of sleep such as NREM 3-4 to a lighter stage such as NREM 1–2. This change may be accompanied by an increase in EMG activity, body movements, or heart rate.

Arousals usually erupt during NREM sleep by an abrupt change in EEG frequency for at least 3 seconds. Arousals include alpha, theta, or beta activity but no spindles or delta waves. This disruption is followed by at least 10 seconds of continuous sleep. NREM sleep arousals are not necessarily accompanied by changes in chin EMG, but arousals from REM sleep are usually accompanied by an increase in amplitude measured on the chin EMG. Isolated increases in chin EMG amplitude without changes in EEG do not constitute an arousal. Movement arousal is defined as a body movement associated with an EEG arousal and may include an increase in alpha wave activity and a decrease in wave amplitude or paroxysmal high-voltage waveforms and an increase in EMG activity. The arousal index is calculated as the number or arousals per hour of sleep.

Awakening

The term *awakening* is distinguished from arousal in a sleep study. It is defined as an occurrence of an awake state from any state of sleep as indicated on EEG. The awakening usually produces alpha or beta EEG waves and an increase in chin EMG tone.

Epoch

An *epoch* is a standard period, usually 30 seconds in duration, of a recording during a sleep study that is assigned a specific sleep stage designation. For particular purposes, a longer or shorter time period can be selected.

Hypopnea

Hypopnea is defined as a reduction of air flow or amplitude of thoracoabdominal movement by at least 30% from the baseline, which lasts for at least 10 seconds. The Medicare guidelines also require the definition to be accompanied by an oxyhemoglobin desaturation of at least 4%.[23] Alternatively, the American AASM defines hypopnea as a reduction of air flow by at least 50% from the baseline lasting at least 10 seconds'.[10]

Movement Time

Movement time is defined as an epoch in which sleep stage scoring is not possible because more than 50% of the epoch is obstructed by movement artifact, if this time period occurs between 2 epochs of sleep. It is usually a period lasting more than 15 seconds in which the EEG and EOG tracings are obscured. An epoch is scored as "stage-wake" if it meets the criteria for movement time but is between 2 epochs of wakefulness.

Periodic Limb Movement Index

The *periodic limb movement index* is defined as the number of periodic limb movements that occur per hour of sleep. A periodic limb movement, also known as *periodic leg movement* or *nocturnal myoclonus*, is characterized by episodes of repetitive and stereotypic limb movements that occur during sleep. These movements are usually associated with arousal or awakening, even though the sleeper is usually unaware of the event or the sleep disruption. An individual may report nonrestorative sleep. Often, a bed partner may report that the individual kicks or flails in his or her sleep. There is often night-to-night variability in periodic limb movements, and a single-night PSG may not capture these events.

Rapid Eye Movement Sleep Latency

REM sleep latency is defined as the length of time in minutes from the onset of sleep to the first epoch of REM sleep as measured by EEG and EOG. In a normal healthy adult, this period may occur between 90 to 110 minutes after sleep onset. If an adult shows evidence of entry into REM sleep immediately after sleep onset, narcolepsy should be suspected. Significantly shortened sleep latency may be indicative of depression. Infants may enter directly into REM from wakefulness.

Respiratory Effort–Related Arousal

Respiratory effort–related arousal is defined as an arousal from sleep that is accompanied by a decrease in air flow and an increased inspiratory effort that lasts for at least 10 seconds but does not technically meet the criteria of either apnea or hypopnea and is not associated with a significant oxygen desaturation. A respiratory effort–related arousal is identified by a transient flattening of the nasal pressure signal or an increasingly negative deflection of esophageal pressure, followed by a sudden change in pressure accompanied by an arousal as indicated on EEG. It is a measure of an abrupt transition from a deeper stage of sleep to a shallower one.

Respiratory Disturbance Index

Respiratory disturbance index is a formula used in analysis of a polysomnogram to determine the degree to which changes in respiratory pattern disrupt sleep. It is defined as the number of apneic plus the number of hypopneic plus the number of respiratory effort–related arousals per hour of sleep. A respiratory disturbance index of greater than 5 is usually considered abnormal. This may also be known as the *respiratory arousal index*. An elevated respiratory disturbance index may be associated with excessive daytime sleepiness and has been shown to be more highly correlated with sleepiness than an increased frequency of oxygen desaturation during sleep.[24]

Sleep Efficiency

Sleep efficiency is defined as a ratio of the TST to the total time in bed (TIB). The formula utilized in PSG is usually (TST × 100)/TIB. For practical purposes, sleep efficiency is a term used to describe the effectiveness of sleep during a particular sleep episode expressed as percentage. It is an objective measurement that may be used to gauge the time spent asleep versus the time spent in bed as recorded during a polysomnogram. If the sleep efficiency is decreased, this may indicate the presence of a sleep disorder. Usually, sleep efficiency greater than 85% is considered normal and sleep efficiency less than 85% may indicate insomnia. A sleep efficiency score of greater than 95% is not considered normal and may be an indicator or narcolepsy or idiopathic hypersomnia. This measure is not necessarily an indicator of an individual's own assessment of the quality of his or her sleep.

Sleep Latency

Sleep latency, for the purposes of a polysomnogram, is defined as the time in minutes from lights out to sleep onset as indicated by EEG of the first epoch of any stage of sleep. Because sleep is an active process, as described earlier in this text, time is required to accomplish the events that are necessary to transition the brain from a period of alert wakefulness into a period of sleep. Normal sleep latency is between 15 and 30 minutes. Longer sleep latency—that is, greater than 30 minutes—is characteristic of sleep-initiation insomnia. Longer sleep latency may be seen in PSG because of the so-called first-night effect or sleeping in a new environment. Very rapid time to sleep onset or short sleep latency is indicative of excessive sleep pressure, which is seen in individuals with marked sleep debt. Practically speaking, when an individual indicates that he falls asleep as soon as his head hits the pillow, it may indicate sleep debt, rather than being a "good sleeper."

Sleep Apnea Definitions

Apnea

Apnea is defined as the absence of air flow at the nose and mouth for at least 10 seconds. For polysomnographic purposes, apnea is classified as obstructive, central, or mixed.

Obstructive Sleep Apnea

OSA is the absence of air flow that occurs despite respiratory effort. This usually occurs because of a structural problem in the upper airway that may cause narrowing, in conjunction with the decreased muscle tone associated particularly with certain stages of sleep, causing airway collapse during sleep that normal respiratory effort cannot overcome. The causes of OSA are loosening of tissue in the upper airway that occurs as a function of aging, increased soft tissue around the airway as may occur with weight gain or obesity, brain injury that changes the tone of musculature, and normal decrease in motor tone in the upper airway. Decreased muscle tone may be caused by drugs or alcohol or may be caused by neurological disorders. It has also been suggested that long-term snoring may cause vibrational injury to the motor nerves in the pharynx that help to maintain the patency of the upper airway.

In some individuals, there may be a craniofacial syndrome that causes unusual facial features that involve the nose, mouth, and jaw or there may be changes to the resting tone in the upper airway that places such an individual at increased risk for OSA.

Central Sleep Apnea

CSA is described as a condition in which there is an absence of air flow with an accompanying absence of respiratory effort. The apneic event typically lasts for 10 to 30 seconds and is often associated with decreased oxygen saturation. CSA occurs because the normal feedback mechanism that controls respiration is dysfunctional. Normally, carbon dioxide levels in the blood and the neurological feedback mechanism that monitors it does not react quickly enough to maintain a normal respiratory rate. Following the episode of apnea, the individual may experience increased rate of breathing, which is a compensatory mechanism that helps to blow off excess CO_2 and increase oxygen saturation. The neurological control for respiration fails to signal the brain to inhale. If the apneic event lasts long enough, the concentration of CO_2 increases, creating a condition known as *hypercapnia*, which usually is effective in restoration of respiratory rate.

Mixed Sleep Apnea

Mixed sleep apnea is defined as a period of apnea that consists of an initial central component of apnea that terminates with an obstructive apneic event. Sometimes when OSA has been severe and longstanding, CSA may develop.

Complex Sleep Apnea

Complex sleep apnea occurs when an individual with OSA who utilizes CPAP has persistent CSA despite its use.

FACTORS AFFECTING SLEEP ARCHITECTURE

Many factors can change sleep architecture by changing the relative percentages of sleep stages throughout a night's sleep. The most common factor affecting sleep architecture is age. Other factors that may cause a characteristic change in sleep architecture include medication, comorbid medical condition, neurological disease, or psychiatric disorder.

Aging is associated with an increase in NREM stages 1 and 2 sleep and a decrease in NREM stages 3 and 4 sleep. There is also diminished amplitude of delta waves during slow-wave sleep. There is generally no significant change in REM sleep after young adulthood.

Sleep architecture during recovery sleep following acute or chronic sleep deprivation usually reflects an increase in NREM stages 3 and 4 sleep and an increase in REM sleep. Antidepressants generally decrease REM sleep and increase REM sleep latency. Conversely, discontinuation of antidepressants can cause an increase in REM sleep and a decrease in REM sleep latency.

There are several factors that can affect REM sleep latency. These include an advance in bedtime or a first-night effect, such as may occur during polysomnographic testing. Increased alcohol consumption can increase REM sleep latency. Certain medications can also increase REM sleep latency, including clonidine, antidepressant medications such as monoamine oxidase inhibitors (MAOIs), SSRIs, TCAs, trazodone, and venlafaxine, and stimulant agents such as amphetamine.

Decrease in REM sleep latency can be caused by a delay in bedtime, depression, and certain medications such as bupropion (Wellbutrin); OSA, which causes sleep deprivation; schizophrenia; and sudden withdrawal from REM-suppressing agents, including the medications listed. Narcolepsy is also associated with a dramatic shortening of REM sleep latency and sometimes individuals with this disorder have sleep-onset REM periods.

Several antidepressant agents have been shown not to change REM sleep latency, including mirtazapine (Remeron) and nefazodone (Serzone).

Changes in the total amount of REM sleep can occur with certain medications. Medications that increase the percentage of REM sleep include bupropion, nefazodone, and reserpine. REM sleep percentages may be decreased by alcohol use, amphetamines, benzodiazepines, clonidine, lithium, MAOIs, methylphenidate (Ritalin), SSRIs, and TCAs. In fact, MAOIs are the most potent inhibitors of REM sleep. Mirtazapine and trazodone do not change REM sleep.

POLYSOMNOGRAPHIC FEATURES OF SLEEP DISORDERS

The most common reason for referral for a sleep study is suspicion of a sleep-related breathing disorder such as OSA. It is important to be able to identify the features in a PSG report that characterize some of the most common sleep disorders. The following are some sleep disorders and PSG features associated with them.

Obstructive sleep apnea
- Decreased sleep latency
- Decreased sleep efficiency
- Increased NREM stage 1 sleep
- Decreased NREM stages 3 and 4 sleep
- Decreased REM sleep
- Increased frequency of awakenings and microarousals

Narcolepsy
- Decreased sleep latency
- Decreased sleep efficiency
- Increased NREM stage 2 sleep
- Increased REM sleep
- Decreased REM sleep latency (<20 minutes)
- Increased frequency of awakenings and microarousals
- Increased wake time after sleep onset
- MSLT shows
  - Decreased sleep latency
  - Decreased REM sleep latency (sleep-onset REM periods)

Periodic limb movements of sleep
- Increased NREM stage 1 sleep
- Decreased NREM stages 3 and 4 sleep
- Increased frequency of awakenings and microarousals

Primary insomnia
- Increased sleep latency
- Decreased TST
- Decreased NREM stages 3 and 4 sleep
- Decreased REM sleep latency
- Increased REM sleep
- Increased wake time after sleep onset

For examples of full sleep studies, see Appendix A.

REFERENCES

1. Rechtschaffen A, Gilliland MA, Bregmann BM, Winter JB. Physiological correlates of prolonged sleep deprivation in rats. *Science.* 1983;221(4606):182-184
2. Irwin M, Thompson J, Miller C, et al. Effects of sleep and sleep deprivation on catecholamine and interleukin-2 levels in humans: clinical implications. *J Clin Endocrinol Metab.* 1999;84:1979-1985.
3. Kushida CA, Everson CA, Suthipinittharm P, et al. Sleep deprivation in the rat: VI. Skin changes. *Sleep.* 1989;12:42-46.
4. Ogawa Y, Kanbayashi T, Saito Y, et al. Total sleep deprivation elevates blood pressure through arterial baroreflex resetting: a study with microneurographic technique. *Sleep.* 2003;26:986-989.
5. Ewing DW, Neilson JMM, Shapiro CM, Stewart JA, Reid W. Twenty four hour heart rate variability: effects of posture, sleep, and time of day in healthy controls and comparison with bedside tests of autonomic function in diabetic patients. *Br Heart J.* 1991;65:239-244.
6. Bonnft MH, Arand DL. Heart rate variability in insomniacs and matched normal sleepers. *Psychosom Med.* 1998;60:610-615.
7. Sawka MN, Gonzalez RR, Pandolf KB. Effects of sleep deprivation on thermoregulation during exercise. *Am J Physiol.* 1984;246 (1 of 2):R72-R77.
8. Everson CA. Functional consequences of sustained sleep deprivation in the rat. *Behav Brain Res.* 1995;69:43-54.
9. Everson CA, Bergmann BM, Rechtschaffen A. Sleep deprivation in the rat: III. Total sleep deprivation. *Sleep.* 1989;12:13-21.
10. Iber C, Ancoli-Israel S, Chesson A, Quan SF. *The AASM Manual for the Scoring of Sleep and Associated Events: Rules, Terminology and Technical Specifications.* Westchester, IL: American Academy of Sleep Medicine; 2007.

11. Morden B, Nitchell G, Dement W. Selective REM sleep deprivation and compensation phenomena in the rat. *Brain Res.* 1967;339-349.

12. Lautenbachen S, Kundermann B, Krieg JC. Sleep deprivation and pain perception. *Sleep Med Rev.* 2006;10(5):357-369.

13. Smith R. Recovery and tissue repair. *Br Med Bull.* 1985;41(3):295-301.

14. Landis CA, Whitney JD. Effects of 72 hours sleep deprivation on wound healing in the rat. *Res Nursing Health.* 1997;20(3):259-267.

15. Stickgold R. Sleep-dependent memory consolidation. *Nature.* 2005;427:1272-1278.

16. Curcio G, Ferrara M, de Gennaro L. Sleep loss, learning capacity and academic performance. *Sleep Med Rev.* 2006;10(5):323-337.

17. Williamson AM, Feyer AM. Moderate sleep deprivation produces impairments in cognitive and motor performance equivalent to legally prescribed levels of alcohol intoxication. *Occup Environ Med.* 2000;57:649-655.

18. Johns MW. A new method for measuring daytime sleepiness: the Epworth Sleepiness Scale. *Sleep.* 1991;14:540–545.

19. Stanford Sleepiness Scale: Hoddes E, Zarcone V, Smythe H, Phillips R, Dement WC. Quantification of sleepiness: a new approach. *Psychophysiology.* 1973:10:431-436.

20. Dement WC. Stanford Sleepiness Scale. Available at: http://www.stanford.edu/~dement/sss.html. Accessed June 29, 2013.

21. Fatigue Severity Scale: Fatigue Severity Scale. Available at: http://www.sarme.org/pdf/sleep-Fatigue-Severity-Scale.pdf. Accessed April 19, 2011.

22. Immrama Institute. International 10-20 system of electrode placement. Available at: http://www.immrama.org/eeg/electrode.html. Accessed July 12, 2012.

23. Sleep apnea & Continuous Positive Airway Pressure (CPAP) therapy. Available at: http://www.medicare.gov/coverage/sleep-apnea-and-epap-therapy.html. Accessed September 28, 2013.

24. Verster JC, Pandi-Perumal SR, Steiner DL, eds. *Sleep and Quality of Life in Clinical Medicine.* Totowa, NJ: Humana Press; 2008.

Sleep-Related Breathing Disorders

Julie M. Hereford, PT, DPT

Several conditions can cause disorders of respiration during sleep. These include obstructive sleep apnea (OSA), central sleep apnea, and hypoventilation syndromes. Apnea is defined as the absence of nasal or oral air flow that lasts for at least 10 seconds. OSA syndrome is a sleep-related breathing disorder in which inadequate ventilation occurs despite continued efforts to breathe due to complete or near-complete obstruction of the upper airway. Central sleep apnea is characterized by an absence of air flow that lasts for at least 10 seconds, which results from absent or diminished respiratory effort. Sleep apnea may also be considered to be mixed. This is defined by an apneic pattern that begins with a centrally mediated episode that is followed by an obstructive event that is consistent with OSA.

Hypopnea is defined as a reduction of air flow such that ventilation is inadequate to perform necessary gas exchange. By definition, hypopnea is caused by an increased concentration of carbon dioxide or by hypercapnea and respiratory acidosis. Hypercapnea is a state in which partial pressure of arterial carbon dioxide ($PaCO_2$) is less than 45 mm Hg. The American Academy of Sleep Medicine defines hypopnea as a reduction in air flow or a decrease in the amplitude of thoracoabdominal movement by at least 30% from baseline, a decrease in air flow that lasts at least 10 seconds, and oxyhemoglobin desaturation of 4%.[1]

Another hypoventilation syndrome is known as *Cheyne-Stokes respiration*. This is defined as crescendo–decrescendo variability in respiratory rate and tidal volume. It is an abnormal breathing pattern characterized by progressively deeper and sometimes more rapid respiration, followed by a gradual decrease in breathing. The pattern ends with a temporary cessation of respiration or apneic event and then this cycle repeats itself. The cycle usually lasts for 30 seconds to 2 minutes.[2]

Sleep apnea may also have periods of arousals that are related to respiratory events characterized by a reduction of air flow that do not meet the criteria of either apnea or hypopnea and are not associated with significant oxygen desaturation. These types of arousals are characterized by increased respiratory effort or flattening of the nasal pressure waveform that leads to arousal from sleep. These so-called respiratory effort–related arousals (RERAs) can cause significant sleep fragmentation but do not meet the criteria of sleep apnea described. RERAs are often accompanied by a snort. Unfortunately, insurance carriers have a rigid definition of sleep apnea criteria that must be met before they will pay for adequate treatment of this type of sleep-related breathing disorder. Nonetheless, a significant RERA index may cause sleep fragmentation, which may result in excessive daytime sleepiness and/or other sequelae of disordered sleep.

Sleep-related breathing disorders tend to affect sleep quality and sleep architecture and may be characterized by excessive daytime sleepiness, fatigue, or diminished neurocognition and signs and symptoms of organ system dysfunction. Apneas and hypopnea have the same underlying mechanisms and are considered together in determining the severity of sleep-related breathing disorders.

Hereford JM. *Sleep and Rehabilitation:*
A Guide for Health Professionals (pp 169-180).

SLEEP-RELATED BREATHING DISORDER TERMS

- **Apnea index (AI)**: Total number of apneas per hour of sleep.

- **Apnea–hypopnea index (AHI)**: Total number of apneas and hypopneas per hour of sleep. This is the primary metric utilized in a polysomnographic report.

- **Respiratory disturbance index**: Total number of apneas, hypopneas, and RERAs per hour of sleep.

- **Oxygen desaturation**: The measure of oxygen desaturation is used to quantify the severity of disease. This measure usually consists of the minimum level of desaturation and the number of times that oxygen desaturation falls by more than 4% per hour of sleep. This measure may also indicate the fraction of time spent at each 10% level of desaturation and the mean oxygen saturation. These measures quantify the cumulative exposure to hypoxemia and may be inversely associated with the risk for cardiovascular disease and insulin resistance.

- **Arousal index**: Total number of arousals per hour of sleep.

OBSTRUCTIVE SLEEP APNEA

OSA is a chronic disorder of sleep that usually requires lifelong management. The cardinal features of OSA are a clinically significant number of apneas, hypopneas, and RERAs; daytime symptoms attributable to sleep disturbance, including excessive daytime sleepiness, fatigue, and diminished neurocognition; and reported or observed restless sleep, snoring, or resuscitative snorts during sleep (Table 17-1).

It is important to identify individuals with OSA. It has been shown that repeated arousals and hypoxemia during sleep occurring over months or years is a significant contributor to the development of systemic health issues. It has been associated with increased risk of mortality in patients with cardiovascular disease, especially in patients with untreated OSA with an AHI greater than 30 events per hour.

Epidemiologic data suggest that an estimated 26% of the adult population is at high risk for developing OSA. The prevalence in the general population is 20%, but only 9% of the population has an AHI greater than 5 events per hour with a report of at least one symptom of OSA. This indicates that most individuals who have OSA are probably asymptomatic for some time or may ignore or not recognize

Table 17-1.

Common Clinical Features Associated With Obstructive Sleep Apnea[a]

- Daytime sleepiness or fatigue

- Awakenings with a sensation of gasping or choking

- Witnessed apneas, gasping, or choking

- Impaired cognition (memory and concentration)

- Nonrestorative or unrefreshing sleep or naps

- Snoring

- Excessive body movements during sleep

- Restless sleep with frequent movements

- Insomnia

- Behavioral disorders
  - Decline in performance at work or school
  - Attention deficit (in children)
  - Hyperactivity (in children)
  - Changes in mood (eg, depression) or personality

- Dry mouth or sore throat upon awakening

- Morning headaches

- Gastroesophageal reflux disease

- Impotence or diminished libido

- Mouth breathing (in children)

- Hearing impairment

- Bed-wetting

- Shortness of breath at night (especially with pulmonary comorbidities)

[a]Common clinical features associated with OSA. During the initial interview with a patient, if he or she has a complaint of excessive daytime sleepiness, further questioning regarding other symptoms often associated with OSA may indicate the need for referral to a sleep specialist.

symptoms of snoring, excessive daytime sleepiness, or other sequelae of OSA as cause for concern.[3-5] OSA is most prevalent in males between the ages of 18 and 45 years old, although it may be diagnosed at any age in both males and females. OSA appears to occur with increasing frequency in individuals of African descent compared to Caucasians or Asians independent of body weight. This suggests that the greater risk may be related to differences in craniofacial structure.[5-8]

Risk Factors for Development of Obstructive Sleep Apnea

Certain individuals are at increased risk for developing OSA. Increased weight is the most widely documented risk factor for the development of OSA. The risk increases relative to the increase in body mass index. There is also a positive correlation between increased neck circumference, greater than 17 inches in males and greater than 16 inches in females and increased waist-to-hip ratios and increased risk for OSA. Weight loss has been shown to be an effective therapy in resolution of OSA, although OSA may also contribute to weight gain and interfere with weight loss attempts due to associated symptomology.

Abnormalities in the upper airway soft tissues, especially thickening in the retrolingual and retropalatal regions, increase the risk of OSA. This includes increased fat deposits in the soft tissues. Tonsillar or adenoid hypertrophy can be a significant factor in narrowing the airway. This is of particular concern in children because of the consequences of chronic sleep apnea in the developing brain. There is evidence that this can lead to changes in neurocognitive function, including poor academic performance and even the development of attention–deficit/hyperactivity disorder. Other abnormalities in the upper airway that are associated with OSA include choanal atresia, which is a congenital narrowing or blockage of the nasal airway by tissue, nasal obstruction, laryngomalacia, and tracheal stenosis.

Abnormalities in craniofacial structure including abnormal maxillary development, shortened mandible, or a widened craniofacial base may result in a narrowed airway and increase the risk of OSA. Correction of craniofacial abnormalities, including oral appliance therapy, has been shown to be an effective therapy in resolution of OSA.

Current smokers, but not past smokers, are almost 3 times more likely to develop OSA compared to individuals who have never smoked. However, smoking cessation has not been shown to resolve OSA. It is unknown whether this is contributory or coincident.

The nasal passages are the most frequent areas to be narrowed in individuals with OSA. Nasal congestion nearly doubles the prevalence of OSA, regardless of the cause of the congestion. More frequent apneic events in individuals with increased nasal congestion are likely due to airway resistance from decreased nasal patency. In children, this can be a source of mouth breathing, which can cause changes in the growth and development of the midface. In turn, this can lead to further narrowing of the upper airway. However, management of nasal congestion or septal deviation has not been shown to be effective in resolving OSA.

There are certain genetic syndromes that are associated with OSA (Table 17-2). Conditions that cause maxillary hypoplasia, or an underdeveloped midface, include

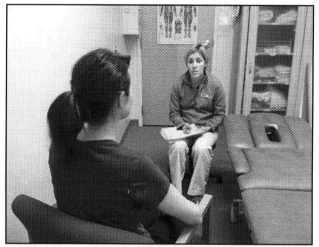

Figure 17-1. Questions about sleep should be included in all patient interviews. (Reprinted with permission from N. Hammond.)

Down's syndrome or trisomy 21 and cleft palate repair, among others. Mandibular hypoplasia can be part of a genetic syndrome or can exist alone and causes crowding of the upper airway, predisposing the affected individual to OSA. Several genetic syndromes produce macroglossia or enlargement of the tongue. This can be observed by noting the scalloping of the edges of the tongue that is too large to fit neatly inside the mandible. The scalloping is caused by sustained contact with the teeth of the lower jaw. An abnormally large tongue will narrow the upper airway, which is a predisposition for OSA. The genetic conditions that cause some to the anatomic features noted may also have neural consequences that lead to abnormal tone in the musculature of the upper airway or problems with timing of respiratory events that become more critical during sleep.

Clinical Presentation of Obstructive Sleep Apnea

When gathering a clinical history, it is important to ask a patient about sleep. The patient should be asked whether he or she snores or whether he or she has been witnessed to snore. Any patient who reports snoring should be asked whether he or she also experiences excessive daytime sleepiness. Reporting both of these symptoms should raise the suspicion of a sleep-related breathing disorder that requires further evaluation. Excessive daytime sleepiness is a common feature of OSA; however, if it is mild or chronic, an individual may underestimate its significance.

Sometimes, individuals will report fatigue rather than sleepiness, and it is important to distinguish between these 2 clinical complaints. Fatigue is generally more of a constitutional symptom, described as weariness or lack of physical or mental energy. Sleepiness, on the other hand, is a propensity to fall asleep in passive or monotonous situations. If an individual has mild disease, he or she may be

Table 17-2.

Physical Features Often Seen in Individuals Predisposed to Obstructive Sleep Apnea[a]

- Large neck circumference
- Obesity (BMI > 25)
- Nose
  - Chronic nasal congestion
  - Nasal septal deviation
  - Nasal turbinate hypertrophy
- Oral cavity
  - Enlarged tongue (macroglossia)—indicated by lateral scalloping
  - Low-lying soft palate
  - High, narrow, hard palate
  - Enlarged tonsils and adenoids, prominent tonsillar pillars (especially among children)
  - Large uvula
  - Dental malocclusion
  - Crowded posterior pharyngeal space
  - Narrow oropharynx (maxilla and mandible)
- Craniofacial features
  - Retrognathia—posterior positioning of the mandible
  - Micrognathia—undersized mandible
  - Brachyocephaly—shorter A/P dimension of the cranial base
- Lower extremity edema
- Chest wall or diaphragm disorders
  - Diaphragmatic paresis or paralysis
  - Chronic loss of zone of apposition of the diaphragm
  - Kyphoscoliosis
  - Severe obesity that restricts the excursion of the diaphragm

[a]Physical features often seen in individuals who are predisposed to obstructive sleep apnea (OSA). Correction of craniofacial structure and alignment has been shown to be effective in reversing OSA. Weight loss has also been shown to resolve the symptoms of OSA. Clinical experience has shown that correction of the dysfunction that may be associated with the mechanics of respiration particularly chest wall mobility and loss of the zone of apposition of the diaphragm are often effective in reducing the symptoms of OSA. This has been seen to be more effective if temporomandibular and dental contributions are effectively managed simultaneously.

unaware that falling asleep in situations other than in bed is not considered normal. Upon questioning, the patient may often report falling asleep while reading, watching television, or attending a lecture or religious service. Sometimes, the patient may even report marked drowsiness or falling asleep while driving. It is important to question the patient about the propensity to fall asleep away from the workplace because excessive daytime sleepiness can be masked by activity (Figure 17-1). The Epworth Sleepiness Scale is an effective tool for screening for evidence of excessive sleepiness that may require further clinical evaluation.[9]

In order to distinguish between sleepiness and fatigue, the clinician may also administer the Fatigue Severity Scale to gain more objective insight into the source of the patient's complaint.[10] Some conditions may cause fatigue but do not typically cause sleepiness. These include conditions such as chronic insomnia, depression, multiple sclerosis, fibromyalgia, and a number of other medical conditions.

Individuals who report excessive daytime sleepiness and present with an elevated score on the Epworth Sleepiness Scale should undergo further diagnostic evaluation for sleep apnea, which will likely include a polysomnogram.

Table 17-3.

Comorbidities Linked to Obstructive Sleep Apnea[a]

- Cardiac arrhythmias
- Systemic hypertension
- Congestive heart failure
- Ischemic heart disease
- Nocturnal seizures
- Pulmonary hypertension or cor pulmonale (severe disease)
- Insulin resistance
- Type 2 diabetes mellitus
- Polycystic ovarian syndrome
- Parasomnias
  - Confusional arousals
  - Sleepwalking, talking, or eating
  - Periodic limb movement disorder

[a]If a patient has one or more of these disorders and also complains of excessive daytime sleepiness or snoring, further evaluation should be undertaken to determine whether a sleep-related breathing disorder exists.

Other symptoms that are positively correlated with OSA include reports of awakening with a sensation of choking or gasping for air, nonrestorative sleep, and snoring or awakening with a dry mouth (from mouth breathing) or a mild sore throat, which may occur if snoring is so persistent that the vibration irritates the soft palate and pharynx. If there are witnessed episodes of cessation of breathing or periods of silence followed by loud snoring, OSA should be suspected. Frequently individuals with OSA may report moodiness, lack of concentration, or poor memory. Comorbidities of hypertension, cardiovascular disease, cerebrovascular disease, renal disease, type 2 diabetes, or gastroesophageal reflux disease may also point to the possibility of OSA (Table 17-3).

Morning headaches are also associated with OSA. Although it is suggested in some literature that this may be linked to rapid eye movement (REM) sleep, it is probably much more likely that morning headache or headache upon wakening is cervicogenic in nature. In an individual with OSA, increased upper cervical extension can help to mechanically increase the patency of the airway, much as this positioning is utilized to open the airway in an individual in respiratory arrest for rescue breathing. This marked cervical extension puts increased mechanical stresses on the upper cervical segments and may even compress the dorsal root ganglion of C_1. Positioning the upper cervical spine in extension can cause local facet irritation and changes in muscle tone that can generate morning headache. In addition, positioning to increase upper airway patency can contribute to upper cervical dysfunction. Upper cervical dysfunction is known to be a significant factor in temporomandibular dysfunction. These musculoskeletal problems can be a manifestation of OSA or can contribute to it. When screening a patient, especially one referred for evaluation of an upper quadrant problem, careful consideration should be given to the quality of the patient's sleep.

Differential Diagnosis

Excessive daytime sleepiness is often a result of OSA and may be the symptom that sends a patient for further evaluation. Although OSA is one of the most common causes of excessive daytime sleepiness, there can be other causes. For example, periodic limb movements of sleep, which are recurrent jerking movements of the legs and sometimes the arms, are associated with arousal from sleep and sleep fragmentation that can cause excessive daytime sleepiness. These movements sometimes do not manifest themselves until after OSA is successfully treated, although the mechanism for this is unknown. Shift work can lead to excessive daytime sleepiness, because the worker often tries to fit into a normal daytime schedule on days off from work, which increases the irregularity of the sleep schedule. This can lead to chronic sleep deprivation, which may manifest itself as excessive daytime sleepiness.

Upper airway resistance syndrome is considered a subtype of OSA. It is characterized by increased resistance in the upper airway, which decreases air flow and leads to arousals during sleep. This is seen on polysomnography (PSG) as increased frequency of RERAs. Individuals with upper airway resistance syndrome have few discrete apnea/hypopnea episodes and do not generally experience oxyhemoglobin desaturation.

Chronic obstructive or restrictive pulmonary diseases can cause excessive daytime sleepiness. Although the prevalence of OSA is higher in these individuals, these diseases may not have OSA as a component. These diseases may cause sleep-related oxyhemoglobin desaturation and sudden awakenings and dyspnea that limit OSA. Coughing that is consistent with chronic obstructive pulmonary disease (COPD) causes awakening and can result in significant sleep fragmentation. Poorly controlled asthma tends to be more symptomatic at night in which bronchospasm and coughing cause sleep fragmentation and paroxysmal dyspnea.

Individuals with neuromuscular diseases may have to use accessory respiratory musculature to breathe, and the normal postsynaptic inhibition of voluntary musculature that occurs during REM sleep may cause profound oxyhemoglobin desaturations, resulting in awakenings.

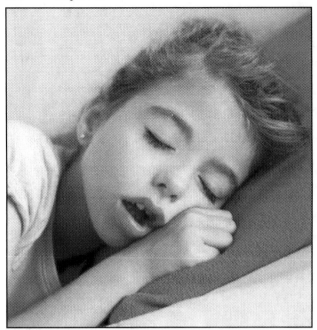

Figure 17-2. Snoring is often indicative of sleep apnea. (From Fotolia.com)

Finally, gastroesophageal reflux disease can mimic symptoms of OSA. If gastric secretions reflux into the esophagus and airway, they can induce coughing and a choking sensation and dyspnea that is similar to awakenings that may occur as part of the mechanism to restart respiration following cessation of breathing. These 2 conditions appear to be related, although the exact mechanism is not entirely understood. Both gastroesophageal reflux disease and OSA usually improve with successfully titrated continuous positive airway pressure (CPAP) therapy.

Obstructive Sleep Apnea— Spectrum of the Disorder

A healthy sleeper may experience occasional periods of respiratory disruption, especially at sleep onset or during REM sleep. These episodes are generally short, lasting fewer than 10 seconds, and are random and not repetitive. This is considered normal sleep and is not associated with any known sequelae. Snoring is a common and often benign occurrence of sleep; however, snorers are 7 times more likely to develop OSA than non-snorers, especially if the snoring becomes chronic (Figure 17-2).[11] If an individual's only symptom is snoring without complaints of excessive daytime sleepiness, he or she probably would not benefit from a complete workup including PSG. Snoring commonly increases with age as the soft tissues in the upper airway lose some of their elasticity.

Individuals with OSA, especially those who have an AHI of greater than 15 events per hour, are at an increased risk for developing hypertension. This increased risk occurs even if they are relatively asymptomatic; that is, they do not have complaints of excessive daytime sleepiness or have other sleep-related comorbidities.[12]

It is important to determine the extent and severity of OSA in order to manage symptoms and prevent the consequences of the disorder. OSA is categorized as mild, moderate, or severe.

Mild OSA is defined as that in which the PSG shows an AHI of 5 to 15 respiratory events per hour of sleep.[13] Individuals with this degree of sleep-related breathing disorder typically have passive daytime sleepiness, in which they may feel sleepy or have an increased propensity to fall asleep when they are sedentary and understimulated. This may occur while reading, watching television, or attending a lecture. Students with mild OSA may have a tendency to fall asleep during class; however, this propensity may also be related to chronic sleep deprivation. It is not possible to distinguish the cause of excessive daytime sleepiness that is caused by OSA versus that which is caused by sleep deprivation. In individuals with mild OSA, daytime sleepiness usually does not impair normal function and the patient may not recognize the problem until the symptoms improve. Sleep architecture is usually preserved and other systemic consequences of the disorder usually do not present with this level of disease. Improvement of mild OSA may occur by weight loss, abstinence from alcohol, reducing intake of sedating medications, or treatment of OSA through administration of a passive airway pressure device or an oral device during sleep.

Moderate OSA is classified as that which presents with an AHI of 15 to 30 respiratory events per hour of sleep.[13] Individuals with moderate OSA often report excessive daytime sleep apnea and the Epworth Sleepiness Scale is often predictive of the disorder. These individuals may also report taking steps to avoid falling asleep at inappropriate times, including taking naps or avoiding soporific situations. They may also avoid driving during certain periods of the day because they may be aware of their propensity to fall asleep or know the risks of drowsy driving. They may have relatively normal activities of daily living but perform at a reduced level because of the impact of excessive daytime sleepiness. They may be more prone to accidents, including motor vehicle accidents.[14] Individuals with mild OSA may have systemic hypertension. Sleep fragmentation is evident on PSG, and sleep architecture is often moderately disrupted. Individuals who suffer from moderate OSA respond well to application of CPAP and usually report significant improvement in daytime sleepiness and quality of life. They usually have improvement in systemic hypertension. Treatment with CPAP alone may improve systemic hypertension in a small but statistically significant way.[15–17] Even a small decrease in systemic blood pressure of 2 mm Hg is enough to significantly reduce the risk of cardiovascular disease.[18] Studies show that treatment with antihypertensive medication alone in patients who also have OSA is not as effective as treatment with CPAP and antihypertensive medication.[19,20]

Severe OSA is defined as that level of sleep disturbance as seen in PSG with an AHI of 30 or more respiratory events per hour of sleep and a oxyhemoglobin desaturation below 90% for more than 20% of the total sleep time.[13] Individuals with severe OSA usually have disabling excessive daytime sleepiness that interferes with normal activities of daily living. They are at significantly increased risk of accident and injury and have a marked propensity to fall asleep even during an activity, in a nontraditional sleep posture. They may have significant consequences of OSA, including cardiovascular disease, cardiopulmonary failure, nocturnal angina, or cor pulmonale, which is failure of the right side of the heart brought on by long-term high blood pressure in the pulmonary arteries and right ventricle of the heart. They may also have signs of polycythemia or erythrocytosis, which is a disease state in which the proportion of blood volume that is occupied by red blood cells increases as measured by the hematocrit level.

Individuals who have evidence of severe OSA during PSG usually undergo what is called a *split-night study*, in which treatment for OSA is instituted during the initial sleep study and titrated to a level of pressure in which the greatest reduction of respiratory events can be achieved. There is urgency to initiating treatment in these individuals because of the significant risk severe OSA poses to overall health and well-being. Effective positive airway pressure therapy provides significant benefit to these individuals and will improve daytime sleepiness, quality of life, hypertension, and possibly other hypoxemia-related abnormalities such as cor pulmonale and polycythemia.[21]

Pathophysiology of Obstructive Sleep Apnea

The upper airway maintains its patency by bony and cartilaginous structures surrounding the nasopharynx and the oropharynx in addition to 12 pairs of muscles that make up the muscular tube that extends from the hard palate to the larynx (see Figure 5-13).

It has been postulated that OSA is an anatomic disease because in individuals with OSA the upper airway is narrower and the cross-sectional area is reduced. The airway is often highly compliant in individuals with OSA. These individuals are more likely to have differences in the structure of the soft tissue surrounding the upper airway.[22]

The upper airway is designed to perform functional tasks including speech, swallowing, and respiration. A complex interaction between the anatomical structures and their neural controls has evolved in order to allow these functions. It has been suggested that because of the evolution of the airway and larynx, specifically that which allows for human speech, humans are at an increased risk of development of OSA.[23,24] This is because of the shortening of the craniofacial bones and the migration of the larynx to

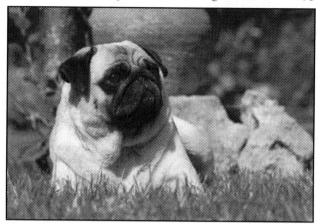

Figure 17-3. Humans and certain flat-faced dogs are the only animals who experience OSA. (From Fotolia.com)

a position inferior to the tongue, as opposed to behind it, as occurs in all other species.

The airway is a muscular tube that extends from the hard palate to the larynx and is without rigid bony support, which allows it to change shape and momentarily collapse. This arrangement allows for the complex mechanics required for control of the larynx and the tongue in order to form speech. It is also this arrangement that allows for the tongue to drop into a position that reduces the size of the upper airway when the human assumes a horizontal position, particularly when supine. This fact, coupled with the inherent increased collapsibility of the airway, especially during certain stages of sleep, particularly at sleep onset and during REM sleep, creates the possibility of OSA.[25,26]

Individuals at increased risk for OSA have been shown to have a narrower upper airway, making it more prone to collapsibility than a normal airway. There appears to be characteristic changes in the structure of the surrounding soft tissues in individuals with OSA.[23] This may be due to accumulation of fat in the soft tissues, mucosal swelling, or muscle hypertrophy. The most common sites of upper airway obstruction are the retropalatal and retrolingual airspaces. A study conducted by Isono observed an increased closing pressure in the airway in individuals with OSA under conditions of general anesthesia and muscle paralysis.[27] This further supports the theory that individuals with OSA have differences in anatomy that increases the susceptibility of the upper airway to collapse.[26]

During an apneic or hypopneic event, the forces that maintain upper airway patency, such as the activation of the dilator muscles, which include the genioglossus, tensor palatini, geniohyoid, and sternohyoid, are insufficient to counteract the factors that promote upper airway closure during sleep. These factors include negative intraluminal pressure, forces of gravity, and decreased neural drive. Diminished tone in the muscles that maintain upper airway patency is part of the generalized muscle hypotonia that occurs during sleep.

While awake, individuals with OSA compensate for the anatomical compromise that makes up their upper airway with increased activity of the upper airway dilator musculature including the genioglossus muscle to maintain airway patency.[28] At sleep onset, this tone is decreased, further reducing the patency of the airway in both healthy individuals and those with OSA. The normal loss of motor tone that occurs during sleep is further complicated in individuals with OSA. There is usually some degree of respiratory instability at the transition from wakefulness to sleep. In individuals with OSA, apneic and hypopneic events occur during this transition which can lead to cortical arousal. Cycling from sleep onset to apneic/hypopneic events to cortical arousal can result in increased difficulty achieving deeper stages of sleep. In order to achieve non-rapid eye movement (NREM) stage 3 and 4 sleep, the individual with OSA must have increased muscular activity to stabilize breathing.[29,30]

The genioglossus muscle is controlled by the central respiratory drive, as well as mechanoreceptors within the muscle that respond to negative pharyngeal pressure.[31] The reflexive response, once thought to be diminished during NREM sleep in healthy individuals, has more recently been shown to be maintained in NREM sleep, especially when gravitational collapse of the airway is maximal, such as occurs in the supine position. The genioglossus reflex appears to become impaired, suppressed rather than inhibited, in individuals with OSA.[32,33] Research into the neurophysiology of the upper airway dilator musculature, particularly the genioglossus musculature, has led to the suggestion that one might be able to develop training exercises to improve the function and patency of the upper airway in individuals with OSA.[10,34,35]

It has been established that, in normal healthy sleepers, the upper airway narrows during sleep. Normal airway patency is maintained by a balance of inward and outward forces, which favors airway patency during wakefulness. During normal sleep, there is some upper airway narrowing caused by decreased neural drive to the muscles normally involved in respiration and a reduction in the compensatory reflexes of the upper airway. Supine sleep position can add increased gravitational forces.

Brain stem nuclei coordinate the ventilatory actions of the upper airway musculature, the musculature of the thorax, and the diaphragm. During sleep, there is a normal reduction in drive to the dilator muscles of the upper airway and the diaphragm and accessory respiratory musculature. When this occurs, there is decreased tone in the dilator musculature in the upper airway, resulting in narrowing. This narrowing is made worse during inspiration because the mechanics of inspiration of the inspiratory musculature and the accessory musculature generates a negative intraluminal pressure.[36–38]

Decreased activity in the brain stem motor neurons during sleep, especially as part of the atonia that characterizes REM sleep, is thought to be due to decreased activity of the neurotransmitter serotonin. Serotonin is known to be excitatory to the motor neurons that subserve the muscles of the upper airway, and serotonin antagonists decrease this activity and therefore increase the susceptibility of the upper airway to collapse.[39,40]

The decreased neural drive to the respiratory musculature appears to affect tonic musculature; that is, musculature of expiration, as opposed to phasic musculature, or musculature of inspiration that responds more rapidly to stimulation. Decreased neural drive to tonic musculature appears to be accompanied by increased esophageal pressure and decreased air flow, which is thought to increase resistance during inspiration.[37,41]

Upper airway dilator musculature activity is generally increased during wakefulness, especially in individuals with OSA to compensate for forces that narrow the airway. Sleep normally reduces activity in the genioglossus, which is a primary dilator of the airway. In OSA, activity of the genioglossus may be decreased or absent. If the genioglossus dilating response to a collapsing airway is decreased, delayed, or absent, the result can be narrowing or collapse of the upper airway during sleep. This will result in an apneic or hypopneic event.[42–44]

Maintenance of the upper airway depends not only on normal neural activity but on appropriate timing of muscle firing during inspiration. For example, the upper airway musculature must maintain enough tone to preserve airway patency against the suction forces created by the diaphragm and chest wall musculature involved in respiration. Further, the upper airway dilator musculature must fire before the diaphragm, chest wall, and accessory respiratory musculature contract in order to maintain upper airway patency. If the diaphragm, chest wall, and accessory musculature fire prior to genioglossus activation, the suction force may be enough to overcome the dilatory efforts of the musculature of the upper airway and result in partial or complete collapse of the upper airway.[45,46] This is one of the mechanisms of upper airway obstruction during sleep. The consequent apnea/hypopnea respiratory event often leads to arousal from sleep in order to reestablish the patency of the airway. Disruption of sleep may further reduce upper airway muscle activation and result in a recurring cycle of airway collapse, followed by reestablishment of the airway, but the increased resistance can lead to another collapse and the subsequent apneic/hypopneic event and arousal. When this pattern occurs repetitively, it may cause sleep fragmentation and eventually excessive daytime sleepiness. Over time, OSA can worsen.

Studies have suggested other mechanisms that may influence the neural control of respiration during sleep and in individuals with OSA. For example, hormonal levels and increased inflammatory processes may play a role in respiratory depression, decreased upper airway patency, and contractibility of the upper airway dilator musculature.[47,48]

The position of the body can also have an influence on the caliber of the upper airway, the degree of upper airway resistance, and the propensity to collapse. The soft tissues that surround the upper airway can move into the upper airway because of the effects of gravity in the supine position. This position also favors narrowing of the retropalatal and retrolingual spaces, which are often found to be already narrowed in individuals with OSA.

Once an obstructive apneic or hypopneic event begins, with the collapse of the upper airway, a sequence of events begins that leads to arousal in order to reestablish the airway and allow sleep to continue. O_2 saturation may drop during the hypopneic–apneic phase. Respiratory efforts against an occluded upper airway result in decrease intrathoracic pressure. This, in turn, gives rise to reduction in blood pressure and cardiac output. Systemic and pulmonary artery blood pressure then rises as apnea progresses, reaching their peak in the immediate post apneic period. Relative bradycardia may develop during airway obstruction followed by tachycardia during termination of apnea. After a variable period of time, the apneic episode is terminated by an arousal that manifests as gross body movement, loud grunting, gasping, or choking. This brief arousal reestablishes airway patency. O_2 saturation generally returns to its baseline level with resumption of normal respiration and sleep then resumes and the cycle repeats itself. Respiratory events occur more frequently during REM sleep than during NREM sleep. Events occurring during REM sleep tend to be longer in duration and are associated with greater falls in O_2 saturation.

Several factors determine the severity of the oxyhemoglobin desaturation that occurs in OSA. If oxygen saturation is decreased while awake and in the supine position, the degree of desaturation while asleep is likely to be more severe. If the baseline oxygen saturation at sleep onset is decreased, desaturation that occurs during a sleep-related breathing event will be worse. Increased duration of apnea/hypopnea episodes or the percentage of sleep time with apneic/hypopneic events, as well as a decreased time between apneic events, is likely to increase the severity of the oxyhemoglobin desaturation because there is less time for recovery after reestablishment of normal respiration before the next event begins. Oxyhemoglobin desaturation also tends to be more severe during REM sleep than during NREM and tends to be more severe with OSA than during central sleep apnea. Finally, decreased functional residual capacity and expiratory reserve volume and/or the presence of comorbid lung disease or neuromuscular disease usually lead to more severe oxyhemoglobin desaturation.

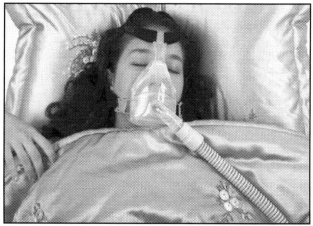

Figure 17-4. Sleep apnea is frequently treated with positive airway pressure, most commonly CPAP. (From Fotolia.com)

TREATMENT OF SLEEP-RELATED BREATHING DISORDERS

Management of sleep-related breathing disorders is almost always a lifelong undertaking. Though it is possible to resolve OSA with correction of craniofacial structural and functional disorders, by weight loss and maintenance of optimal body mass index, and by avoiding sedative medications and alcohol, these measures are not always successfully attained or maintained.

It is first important to establish the severity of the disorder when it exists. Mild and moderate disease have more flexibility in treatment options than does severe disease. When severe sleep apnea is found, application of positive airway pressure is the most effective treatment and should be initiated immediately in order to reduce the risk of developing or exacerbating systemic consequences of sleep-related breathing disorder (Figure 17-4).

Once the severity of the disease has been established, it is important that the patient receive education regarding the risk factors and consequences of OSA. The patient should also be warned about the potential consequences of driving or operating dangerous equipment while sleepy. The patient should be warned to avoid activities that require special attention or vigilance if he or she is experiencing excessive sleepiness. The patient should understand that excessive daytime sleepiness is not normal and can usually be quite effectively treated. He or she should also understand the potential consequences of allowing sleep-related breathing disorders to remain untreated.

In clinical practice, it is not uncommon for a patient who has been diagnosed with a moderate or severe form of sleep-related breathing disorder to refuse effective treatment because it is inconvenient or costly. It is important to impress upon him or her the dangers inherent in allowing the disorder to remain untreated. This is also true for individuals who suffer from excessive daytime sleepiness because of voluntary, avoidable sleep deprivation. Patients should come to understand that sleep debt, regardless of its cause, sleep apnea, or sleep deprivation from other causes can have substantial, long-term, and even deadly consequences. Although the cost of management of the disorder can be significant (a CPAP device may cost several thousand dollars, and supplies may cost several hundred dollars each year), the cost and inconvenience of treating the consequences of sleep-related breathing disorders are much higher. It cannot be stressed enough how important it is that a patient is completely informed of the cost–benefit of effective management of the disorder. In addition to reducing or even eliminating risk to long-term health, improved sleep quality and quantity also substantially improve quality of life.

Behavior Modification

Behavior modification is an important aspect of management of all patients who have sleep-related breathing disorders. General measures include weight reduction and maintenance and avoidance of alcohol, muscle relaxants, and sedative agents. Smoking cessation is always a good health decision, but the literature does not show that stopping smoking effectively changes sleep-related breathing disorders, although it may improve neurotransmitter function. Precipitating factors that may contribute to sleep-related breathing disorders, such as hypothyroidism, should be addressed.

Positional Therapy

Positional therapy may be utilized successfully, especially if polysomnographic evaluation indicated increased apnea in a particular position, nearly always in supine. There are a number of specialty pillows and other techniques that can promote lateral sleeping, including pillow placement to interfere with turning supine during sleep. Another technique that is often effective is to sew a golf ball or tennis ball into a pocket on the back of sleepwear. The proprioceptive stimulus of rolling onto the ball can shape sleep behavior over time such that the sleeper can train themselves to become a lateral sleeper. Prone sleeping should be avoided because of the excessive cervical rotation that is required. It is possible that this may aggravate underlying cervical dysfunction.

Treatment that is specific to OSA generally includes application of some sort of positive airway pressure device, oral appliance therapy, or surgical correction of upper airway abnormalities.

Positive Airway Pressure Devices

Positive airway pressure devices act to splint the upper airway open by forcing air into it in order to counteract the forces that are acting on it to cause its collapse. Positive airway pressure therapy is generally the most effective treatment of OSA and upper airway resistance syndrome. However, there can be a significant patient compliance factor that compromises the efficacy of this treatment. Different delivery systems have been developed to meet the needs of individuals with a variety of different clinical needs in order to improve patient compliance. These include CPAP, bi-level positive airway pressure (BPAP), autotitrating positive airway pressure (APAP), and adaptive servo-ventilation.

CPAP is probably the most commonly utilized device for individuals managing OSA. It is the simplest of the available devices. As its name implies, it provides a constant air pressure throughout the respiratory cycle. A pressure relief setting that lowers the air pressure at the onset of exhalation is sometimes added to improve comfort and tolerance to the device. Optimal pressure is determined during PSG as the lowest pressure at which abnormal respiratory events cease during sleep. Once normal respiration is established, sleep architecture may return to a more normal pattern and the consequences of OSA may resolve, particularly snoring, excessive daytime sleepiness, and systemic hypertension.

BPAP delivers a preset inspiratory pressure and an expiratory pressure based upon titration established during PSG. This device is often used to improve patient comfort and tolerance and, therefore, compliance. The superiority of BPAP over CPAP has not been established.

APAP provides airway pressure that increases or decreases according to the changes in resistance measured in patient air flow. This may occur during a vibratory snore or other factors that alter the respiratory pattern during sleep. Although APAP has not been shown to improve the efficacy of positive airway pressure devices compared to CPAP, it is usually preferred by patients. Improved comfort may improve tolerance and compliance with positive airway pressure therapy.

Adaptive servo-ventilation provides a varying amount airway pressure during inspiration but has an underlying low level of CPAP. This device is often the therapy of choice for patients who have central and OSA. It is also utilized in patients who require medication for other conditions that suppresses respiration, such as opiates, because it appears to compensate for central sleep apnea episodes.

Oral Appliance Therapy

Oral appliance therapy is being used with increasing frequency for several reasons. First, there appears to be increasing evidence of its efficacy and, secondly, patient compliance can be much better with oral appliance therapy because of ease of use and portability. Oral appliance therapy can be an effective alternative to positive airway pressure therapy, especially in mild-to-moderate sleep-related breathing disorders. It is a less optimal choice in moderate-to-severe disease. There are 2 main types of oral appliance, although there is a dizzying array of brands and manufactures. Basically, one type acts to advance the mandible, and the other retains the tongue or holds it in a more anterior position. Both of these techniques are aimed at reducing the narrowing of the upper airway. They also act to hold the soft tissues of the oropharynx away from the posterior pharyngeal wall and therefore improve upper airway patency. Oral devices have been shown to decrease the frequency of respiratory events, arousals, and oxyhemoglobin desaturation. These devices are generally well tolerated by patients and many prefer them to positive airway pressure therapy because of ease of use, portability, and use during travel because they do not require a power source. It is sometimes suggested that oral appliance therapy is also less expensive; however, the initial cost of positive airway pressure therapy and oral appliance therapy is about the same. Ongoing costs may vary, as the appliance must be replaced, and positive airway pressure devices require replacement of the mask, usually at least annually.

Surgical Treatment

Surgical treatment of abnormalities of the upper airway is most effective in a situation in which an individual has a severe obstructing lesion. The most commonly performed surgery that has a positive impact on the size and shape of the airway is tonsillectomy and adenoidectomy. This is a very effective treatment in children who have OSA due to hypertrophy obstructing the pharyngeal airway. There does not appear to be consensus regarding the efficacy of surgical treatment of the upper airway in the absence of an obstructive lesion. Uvulopalatopharyngoplasty, which involves resection of the uvula, redundant retrolingual soft tissue, and palatine tonsillar tissue, is the most commonly performed procedure, but it does not appear to provide a cure for OSA. There are myriad other surgical procedures that have been performed in an attempt to improve signs and symptoms of OSA, but thus far, results are inconsistent and fail to demonstrate benefit.

SUMMARY

Sleep-related breathing disorders are among the most frequently diagnosed sleep problems. The upper airway is subject to collapse because of the effects of gravity and the decreased tone during NREM sleep and atonia during REM sleep. An individual may already have a compromised airway due to hypertrophic tonsillar pillars, redundant

folds in the pharyngeal recess, alteration of the longitudinal shape of the airway because of forward head posture, or decreased motor tone because of a comorbid condition, for example. This compromise increases airway resistance and therefore increases the likelihood of airway collapse during sleep, resulting in OSA. Other components of respiratory function that may contribute to mechanical obstruction of the airway will be discussed in Chapter 27 of this text.

REFERENCES

1. Morgenthaler TI, Kapen S, Lee-Chiong L, et al. Sleep apnea. Practice parameters for the medical therapy of obstructive sleep apnea. *Sleep.* 2006;29:1031–1035.
2. Cheyne-Stokes respiration. *WebMD Medical Dictionary.* Available at: http://www.webmd.com/search/search_results/default.aspx?query=Cheyne%20stokes%20respiration. Accessed October 2, 2013.
3. Epstein LJ, Kristo D, Strollo PJ, et al. Clinical guidelines for the evaluation, management and long-term care of obstructive sleep apnea in adults. *J Clin Sleep Med.* 2009;5:263–276.
4. Punjabi NM. The epidemiology of adult obstructive sleep apnea. *Proc Am Thorac Soc.* 2008;5(2):136–143.
5. Jennum P, Piha RL. Epidemiology of sleep apnea/hypopnea syndrome and sleep-disordered breathing. *Eur Respir J.* 2009;33:907–914.
6. Ong KC, Clerk AA. Comparison of the severity of sleep-disordered breathing in Asian and Caucasian patients seen at a sleep disorders center. *Respir Med.* 1998;92:843–848.
7. Lam B, Ip MS, Tench E, Ryan CF. Craniofacial profile in Asian and white subjects with obstructive sleep apnoea. *Thorax.* 2005;60:504–510.
8. Redline S, Tisheler PV, Hans MG, Tosteson TD, Strohl KP, Spry K. Racial differences in sleep-disordered breathing in African-Americans and Caucasians. *Am J Respir Crit Care Med.* 1997;155:186–192.
9. Epworth Sleepiness Scale. Available at: http://www.stanford.edu/~dement/epworth.html. Accessed July 1, 2013.
10. Valko PO, Bassetti CL, Bloch KE, Held U, Baumann CR. Validation of the Fatigue Severity Scale in a Swiss Cohort. *Sleep.* 2008;31(11):1601–1607.
11. Young T, Skatrud J, Peppard PE. Risk factors for obstructive sleep apnea in adults. *JAMA.* 2004;291:2013–2016.
12. Orem J, Osorio I, Brooks E, Dick T. Activity of respiratory neurons during NREM sleep. *J Neurophisol.* 1985;54:1144–1156.
13. Epstein LJ, Kristo D, Strollo PJ, et al. Clinical guideline for evaluation, management and long-term care of obstructive sleep apnea in adults. *J Clin Sleep Med.* 2009;5:263–276.
14. National Sleep Foundation. Drowsy driving fact sheet. Available at: http://www.sleepfoundation.org/article/sleep-topics/drowsy-driving. Accessed March 23, 2012.
15. Pepperell JC, Ramdassingh-Dow S, Crosthwaite N, et al. Ambulatory blood pressure after therapeutic and subtherapeutic nasal continuous positive airway pressure for OSA: a randomized parallel trial. *Lancet.* 2002;359:204–210.
16. Faccenda JF, Mackay TW, Boom NA, Douglas NJ. Randomized placebo-controlled trial of continuous positive airway pressure on blood pressure in the sleep apnea–hypopnea syndrome. *Am J Respir Creit Care Med.* 2001;163:344–348.
17. Bazzano LA, Khan Z, Reynolds K, He J. Effect of nocturnal nasal continuous positive airway pressure on blood pressure in obstructive sleep apnea. *Hypertension.* 2007;50:417–423.

18. Tamisier R, Weiss JW. Cardiovascular effects of obstructive sleep apnea. Available at: http://www.uptodate.com/contents/cardiovascular-effects-of-obstrucitve-sleep-apnea. Accessed October 20, 2011.

19. Pepin JL, Tamisier R, Barone-Rochette G, et al. Comparison of continuous positive airway pressure therapy and valsartan in hypertensive patients with sleep apnea. *Am J Respir Crit Care Med.* 2010;182:954–960.

20. Campos-Rodriguex F, Grilo-Reina A, Perez-Ronchel J, et al. Effect of continuous positive airway pressure on ambulatory BP in patients with sleep apnea and hypertension: a placebo-controlled trial. *Chest.* 2006;129:1459–1467.

21. Giles TL, Lasserson TJ, Smith BJ, White J, Wright J, Cates CJ. Continuous positive airway pressure for obstructive sleep apnea in adults. *Cochrane Database Syst Rev.* 2006;(1):CD001106.

22. Schwab RJ. Sleep apnea is an anatomic disorder. *Am J Respir Crit Care Med.* 2003;168:270–273.

23. Eckert DJ, Malhotra A. Pathophysiology of adult obstructive sleep apnea. *Proc Am Thorac Soc.* 2008;5(2):144–153.

24. Diamond J. *The Third Chimpanzee. The Evolution and Future of the Human Animal.* New York, NY: Harper Perennial; 1991.

25. Schwartz AR, O'Donnell CP, Baron J, et al. The hypotonic upper airway in obstructive sleep apnea: role of structures and neuromuscular activity. *Am J Respir Crit Care Med.* 1998;157(4 pt 1):1051–1057.

26. Patil SP, Schneider H, Schwartz AR, Smith PL. Adult obstructive sleep apnea: pathophysiology and diagnosis. *Chest.* 2007;132:325–337.

27. Isono S. Obstructive sleep apnea of obese adults. Pathophysiology and perioperative airway management. *Anesthesiology.* 2009;110:908-921.

28. Mezzanotte WS, Tangel DJ, White DP. Waking genioglossal electromyogram in sleep apnea patients versus normal controls (a neuromuscular compensatory mechanism). *J Clin Invest.* 1992;89:1571–1579.

29. Trinder J, Whitworth F, Kay A, Wilkin P. Respiratory instability during sleep onset. *J Appl Physiol.* 1992;73:2462–2469.

30. Basner RC, Ringler J, Schwartzstein RM, Weinberger SE, Weiss JW. Phasic electromyographic activity of the genioglossus increases in normals during slow-wave sleep. *Respir Physiol.* 1991;83:189–200.

31. Pillar G, Fogel RB, Malhotra A, et al. Genioglossal inspiratory activation: central respiratory vs mechanoreceptive influences. *Respir Physiol.* 2001;127:23–38.

32. Eckert DJ, McEvoy RD, George KE, Thomson KJ, Catcheside PG. Genioglossus reflex inhibition to upper-airway negative-pressure stimuli during wakefulness and sleep in healthy males. *J Physiol.* 2007;581(pt 3):1193–1205.

33. Malhotra A, Trinder J, Fogel R, et al. Postural effects on pharyngeal protective reflex mechanisms. *Sleep.* 2004;27:1105–1112.

34. Puhan MA, Suarez A, Lo Cascio C, Zahn A, Heitz M, Braendli O. Didgeridoo playing as alternative treatment for obstructive sleep apnoea syndrome: randomised controlled trial. *BMJ.* 2006;332:266–270.

35. Randerath WJ, Galetke W, Domanski U, Weitkunat R, Ruhle KH. Tongue-muscle training by intraoral electrical neurostimulation in patients with obstructive sleep apnea. *Sleep.* 2004;27:254–259.

36. Orem J, Osorio I, Brooks E, Dick T. Activity of respiratory neurons during NREM sleep. *J Neurophisol.* 1985;54:1144–1156.

37. Pierce R, White D, Malhotra A, et al. Upper airway collapsibility, dilator muscle activation and resistance in sleep apnoea. *Eur Respir J.* 2007;30:345–353.

38. Jordan AS, White DP, Lo YL, et al. Airway muscle activity in OSA: airway dilator muscle activity and lung volume during dtable breathing in OSA. *Sleep.* 2009;32:361–668.

39. Kubin L, Davies RO, Pack AI. Control of upper airway motoneurons during REM sleep. *News Physiol Sci.* 1998;13(2):91–97.

40. Ogasa T, Ray AD, Michlin CP, et al. Systemic administration of serotonin 2A/2C agonist improves upper airway stability in Zucker rats. *Am J Respir Crit Care Med.* 2004;170:804–810.

41. Chan E, Steenland HW, Liu H, Horner RL. Endogenous excitatory drive modulating respiratory muscles activity across sleep–wake states. *Am J Respir Crit Care Med.* 2006;174:1264–1273.

42. Mexxanotte WS, Tangel DJ, White DP. Waking genioglossal EMG in sleep apnea versus normal controls: a meuromuscular compensatory mechanism. *J Clin Invest.* 1992;89:1571–1579.

43. Horner RL, Innes JA, Morrell MJ, et al. The effect of sleep on reflex genioglossus muscle activation by stimuli of negative airway pressure in humans. *J Physiol.* 1994;476:141–151.

44. Fogel RB, Trinder J, Malhotra A, et al. Within-breath control of genioglossal muscle activation in humans: effect of sleep–wake state. *J Physiol.* 2003;550(pt 3):899–910.

45. Hudgel DW, Harasick T. Fluctuation in timing of upper airway and chest wall inspiratory muscle activity in obstructive sleep apnea. *J Appl Physiol.* 1990;69:443–450.

46. Leiter JC, Knuth SL, Bartless D. The effect of sleep deprivation on activity of the genioglossus muscle. *Am Rev Respir Dis.* 1985;132:1242–1245.

47. O'Donnell CP, Schaub CD, Haines AS, et al. Leptin prevents respiratory depression in obesity. *Am J Respir Crit Care Med.* 1999;159(5 pt 1):1477–1484.

48. Boyd JH, Petrof BJ, Hamid Q, et al. Upper airway muscle inflammation and denervation changes in OSA. *Am J Respir Crit Care Med.* 2004;170:541–546.

18

Clinical Pharmacology of Sleep

Julie M. Hereford, PT, DPT

Medications that exert their effect on the central nervous system have the possibility of altering the sleep-wake cycle. Some are sedating, while others are excitatory. Some medication may increase the risk of manifestations of sleep disorders. That is, they may cause nightmares, periodic limb movements, or restless leg/legs syndrome. Other medications, such as antidepressants, for example, may exacerbate preexisting sleep apnea. Some medications can cause either excessive daytime sleepiness or insomnia, depending upon the individual or the circumstances in which they are prescribed. Medication can affect sleep as a primary therapeutic effect of the drug, as a symptom of withdrawal from a drug, or as an adverse reaction to a drug.

Sleep architecture can also be altered by a variety of different medications whose primary purpose is not intended to be a central nervous system effect. For example, certain agents used to treat cardiac conditions such as beta-blockers may exert sedative effects, whereas others, such as calcium channel blockers, may induce insomnia.

It is important to understand the effect medication has on sleep, so this can be taken into consideration in a treatment plan (Table 18-1). Timing of medication may also have an impact on a patient's ability to engage in the rehabilitation process or gain the most benefit from an exercise program, for example. This chapter will describe some commonly used agents used to treat sleep disorders and will also describe certain agents used to treat other conditions that often have an impact on sleep.

Each medication has a class-specific and an agent-specific effect on sleep. *Class-specific* refers to medications that are grouped together because of similar chemical structure, mechanism of action, or pharmacological effect.

Agent-specific refers to particular therapeutic aspects unique to an agent within a class. This chapter will discuss certain classes of medications and specific agents used to treat other conditions that may have an impact on sleep architecture or sleep hygiene.

MEDICATIONS THAT AFFECT SLEEP

Often medication, rather than illness, is the culprit behind sleep problems. A number of drugs are common sleep robbers, while others may cause unwanted drowsiness. There are 2 major categories of medications that are used to treat sleep and symptoms of sleep disorder. These include sedatives that induce sleep and stimulants that inhibit sleep or promote wakefulness (Table 18-2).

Sedating Medications

Sedatives are also known as central nervous system depressants or tranquilizers. These medications are used to settle the central nervous system or the autonomic nervous system. They have the effect of calming an individual down, easing agitation, and generally create a nervous system environment that allows sleep. Sedative agents generally work by modulating signals within the central nervous system. They are compounds that cause physiological slowing of bodily functions, including voluntary activity, and allow mental slowing.

Sleep-promoting drugs, or *hypnotics* and *anti-anxiety medications*, are also known as *anxiolytic agents*, produce effects similar to sedative medications. These classes of

- 181 -

Hereford JM. *Sleep and Rehabilitation:*
A Guide for Health Professionals (pp 181-188).
© 2014 Taylor & Francis Group.

Table 18-1.

Effects of Sleep-Promoting Substances on Sleep Architecture

Polysomnographic Measure	Benzodiazepines Barbiturates	Central-Acting Antidepressants	Non-Benzodiazepine Hypnotics	Central-Acting Antihistamines	Sedating Hypnotics	Alcohol
Sleep latency	Markedly decreased	Decreased	Markedly decreased	Decreased	Markedly decreased	Decreased
Total sleep time	Markedly increased	Increased	Markedly increased	Increased	Increased	Unknown
Sleep efficiency	Markedly increased	Increased	Markedly increased	Unknown	Increased	Unknown
Number of awakenings	Markedly decreased	Unknown	Markedly decreased	Unknown	Decreased	Unknown
Wake after sleep onset	Markedly decreased	Unknown	Markedly decreased	Does not affect	Decreased	Decreased
Stage 2 sleep percentage	Markedly increased	Increased	Markedly increased	Does not affect	Does not affect	Unknown
Slow-wave sleep	Decreased	Decreased	Markedly decreased	Does not affect	Does not affect	Unknown
REM sleep percentage	Markedly decreased	Increased	Decreased	Does not affect	Does not affect	Decreased
REM sleep latency	Increased	Unknown	Increased	Unknown	Does not affect	Unknown

drugs can also be used to treat the same types of disorders that sedative medications treat (Table 18-3).

Sedative agents work in the brain by increasing the amount of the neurotransmitter gamma-aminobutyric acid (GABA). Increased GABA levels in the brain decrease neural activity, thus depressing the nervous system. Increased GABA is associated with pain reduction, sleepiness, decreased anxiety, and muscle relaxation.

Sedative medications are often used in conjunction with surgery to reduce anxiety and promote sleep. They are also used to treat pain, anxiety, panic attacks, and insomnia. These agents may also be used to treat convulsions.

Adverse effects of sedative medications include user addiction by increasing the prescribed dose without medical advice, often because there can be a rapid tolerance for these agents. Sedative medications can produce an intoxication that may appear very similar to alcohol intoxication. Sometimes individuals taking these medications can become hostile or aggressive. Sedatives have been associated with mood swings, poor judgment, and inability to function in work, academic, or social settings. Physical withdrawal from sedatives may include slurred speech, lack of coordination, inattention, impaired memory or blackouts, and sluggishness or stupor.

Subcategories of sedative agents used for sleep include benzodiazepines, barbiturates, hypnotics, antihistamines, and antidepressants. These drug subcategories and their effects on sleep will be discussed briefly so the reader may have a general reference point for them. It will not, however, be an exhaustive resource of all medications in the group.

Barbiturates

Widely used during the first half of the 20th century, medications from this class caused significant sedation; however, they alter sleep architecture by decreasing rapid eye movement (REM) and slow-wave sleep. More important, barbiturates also have a high toxic liability—that is, a narrow effective-dose to lethal-dose ratio—and are highly addictive. Because 90% of patients with major depressive disorders also suffer from insomnia and are often treated with sleeping pills, barbiturates represent a tangible hazard because overdose is a real danger with this class of medication. Common barbiturates include amobarbital (Amytal), butabarbital (Butisol), phenobarbital (Nembutal), and secobarbital (Seconal).

Barbiturates have an affinity for $GABA_A$ receptor, which is the primary inhibitory neurotransmitter in the central nervous system. Barbiturates potentiate the effect of

Table 18-2.

Drugs for Sleep Therapy

Sedatives	Stimulants
• Antihistamine (diphenhydramine)	• Eszopiclone
• Choral hydrate	• Hypnostat
• Barbiturates	• Modafinil
• Benzodiazepines (clonazepam, temazepam)	• Sodium oxybate
• Imidazopyridines	• Amphetamine
• Cyclopyrrolones	• Pemoline
• Pyrazolopyrimidine	• Methylphenidate
• Zaleplon (Sonata)	• Cocaine
• Zolpidem tartrate (Ambien)	
• Zopiclone	

Table 18-3.

Drugs Used for Sleep Disorders

Sleep Disorder	Prescribed Drug
Insomnia	• Trazodone
	• Chloral hydrate
	• Melatonin
Hallucinations/nocturnal wandering	• Carbamazepine
	• Clozapine
	• Olanzapine
	• Risperidone
	• Rivastigmine
	• Quetiapine
	• Valproic acid
REM sleep behavior disorder	• Clonazepam
	• Melatonin
Excessive sleepiness	• Modafinil
	• Methylphenidate
Restless leg/legs syndrome	• Pramipexole
	• Ropinirole
	• Gabapentin

GABA at the receptor site. Barbiturates also inhibit the AMPA receptor, which is a subtype of glutamate receptor. Glutamate is the primary excitatory neurotransmitter in the central nervous system. Therefore, barbiturates potentiate inhibitory receptors and inhibit excitatory receptors, creating a central nervous system depressant effect.

Some ultra-short-acting barbiturates, such as thiopental, also known as sodium pentothal, are used for controversial purposes. For example, when administered in high doses, sodium pentothal is used for physician-assisted suicide and for capital punishment by lethal injection. Sodium amytal is an intermediate-acting barbiturate that is used for sedation and to treat insomnia, but has also been used during questioning subjects in criminal cases, for example, because it was thought to decrease inhibitions and cause the person being "interviewed" to provide more truthful answers while under the influence of this drug.[1]

Benzodiazepines

The most widely prescribed and best studied sedatives belong to this group of medications. In the 1960s, the toxic liability of sleeping pills such as barbiturates was drastically reduced when benzodiazepines were introduced as an alternative for the treatment of insomnia. Benzodiazepines, however, are anticonvulsant agents and tend to suppress synchronized electroencephalogram activity, such as delta wave activity seen in slow-wave sleep, and confer some risk of seizure if abruptly withdrawn. Thus, addictive liability was not completely alleviated with benzodiazepines, albeit greatly reduced compared with barbiturates. Additionally, because sleep-stage architecture alterations were produced by benzodiazepines, they are not necessarily ideal for treatment of insomnia. Commonly prescribed benzodiazepines include alprazolam (Xanax), clonazepam (Klonopin),

temazepam (Restoril), lorazepam (Ativan), and diazepam (Valium).

Benzodiazepines act by increasing the frequency of the chloride ion channel opening at the $GABA_A$ receptor increasing the potency of GABA. Barbiturates act at the same receptor, but their action increases the efficacy at the receptor. This is the reason why barbiturates have more toxicity than benzodiazepines in overdose.[1]

Benzodiazepines appear to be safe and effective for short-term treatment of insomnia, although there is a potential for paradoxical effects including disinhibition in some users. They are much less dangerous than their predecessors barbiturates, and usually only problematic when taken with other central nervous system depressants such as alcohol or opiates. Long-term use is often discouraged because of issues with drug tolerance, physical dependence, and withdrawal symptoms.

Non-Benzodiazepine Hypnotics

Non-benzodiazepine hypnotics began to appear in the 1980s and continue to show promise as an alternative to barbiturates and benzodiazepines. This class of hypnotics resembles benzodiazepines with similar pharmacology, side effects, and risks, but have a different chemical structure. They have been introduced for the treatment of certain sleep disorders, and some evidence suggests that they are slower to produce tolerance than barbiturates and benzodiazepines.[2] These newer compounds do not alter sleep architecture when taken at therapeutically recommended doses, although rebound sleeplessness upon cessation of use is known to occur with some medications in this class, except for zaleplon (Sonata).[3] These medications are thought to be less likely to be a source of overdose, and users appear to be less likely to have issues with physical dependence and addiction. This has led to relatively widespread use for the treatment of insomnia particularly in older adults.[4] Disadvantages of this class of medications may include profound amnesia and, rarely, a fugue state in which users have been reported to sleepwalk and even perform complex tasks including eating, cooking, or driving a car while under the influence and have no recollection of the event upon awakening.[5-7] These medications tend to have less next-day sedation because of the shortened elimination half-life. This is especially true with zaleplon, which can be used safely for middle-of-the-night insomnia, due to its ultrashort half-life.[8] These medications have also been associated with a nearly double risk of developing depression; therefore, they are not recommended for use to treat insomnia in depressed patients.[4]

Generally, half-life, duration of action, receptor subtype selectivity, and strength also favor these agents over barbiturates and benzodiazepines. Commonly used non-benzodiazepine hypnotics include zolpidem (Ambien), eszopiclone (Lunesta), zaleplon (Sonata), and buspirone (BuSpar).

Antihistamines

Antihistamines are agents that block the action of histamine at the receptor site or inhibit the action of enzymes that covert histidine into histamine. These medications are commonly taken to relieve cold or allergy symptoms, but they also can cause drowsiness in most people by blocking H-1 receptors in the brain. They are also the active ingredients in most over-the-counter sleep aids and motion sickness pills. While generally prescribed for relief of allergies caused by intolerance to certain proteins, antihistamines also have a powerful hypnotic effect and are often used as nonprescription sleep aids, especially in the form of diphenhydramine citrate. These agents are available over-the-counter under brands such as Benadryl, Unisom, and Tylenol PM. The maximum recommended dose of diphenhydramine mandated by the Food and Drug Administration is 50 mg.[9] When taken for longer than 3 consecutive days, diphenhydramine has been shown to build a tolerance against its sedation side effects.[10] Diphenhydramine has also been documented to cause paradoxical reactions, especially in children, in whom it may cause excitation instead of sedation.[11] Diphenhydramine is also on the Beers list of medications that are potentially inappropriate to use in older adults.[12]

Antidepressant Medications

Antidepressant medications are sometimes used as a treatment to improve sleep. When these medications are used for their sleep and pain-relieving properties, they are generally used in significantly lower doses. The sedating antidepressant medications most commonly used to assist with symptoms of sleep disorders include trazodone (Desyrel), amitriptyline (Elavil), and doxepin (Sinequan). Low-dose antidepressant medications are nonaddictive and also provide some analgesic benefit compared to the hypnotic class of medications, which have no pain-relieving properties. These medications do not produce physical dependence or tolerance and generally have a low incidence of side effects, especially in low doses. Some users report dry mouth, blurred vision, or a hangover effect in the morning.

The selective serotonin re-uptake inhibitors (SSRIs) such as fluoxetine (Prozac), sertraline (Zoloft), and paroxetine (Paxil) disrupt sleep or produce daytime fatigue in about 15% of those who take them. These medications are increasingly used to treat some of the symptoms of narcolepsy, a condition marked by powerful daytime drowsiness, sleep attacks, and a variety of sleep problems, whether or not the person is depressed.

Stimulant Agents

Stimulants are a class of medications that either inhibit sleep or promote wakefulness. Overall, these agents tend to increase alertness and physical activity. Some of these agents temporarily enhance vital function of alertness. For example, caffeine temporarily arouses or accelerates physiological or organic activity by blocking adenosine receptors.

Caffeine and Other Stimulants

Caffeine, which is found in some over-the-counter painkillers and appetite suppressants, is a nervous system stimulant that can induce insomnia. Caffeine makes people feel alert by blocking the action of adenosine, a substance that promotes drowsiness. Caffeine's effects gradually diminish but nonetheless may linger for 6 or 7 hours.

Stimulants counteract sleepiness and symptoms of fatigue in situations in which sleep is not practical or desirable, such as while driving or working. Stimulants are also used to counteract abnormal states of diminished consciousness such as occurs in narcolepsy. They are also sometimes abused to boost endurance and productivity and some stimulant agents may be used to suppress appetite. Patches used to curb smoking deliver small doses of nicotine into the bloodstream around the clock. People who use them often suffer insomnia or experience disturbing dreams.

Stimulants increase the amount of norepinephrine and dopamine in the brain, which acts to increase blood pressure and heart rate, constrict blood vessels, increase blood glucose, and increase respiratory rate. These medications are usually prescribed for individuals with narcolepsy, but are also sometimes prescribed for treatment of symptoms of excessive daytime sleepiness that are not resolved with optimal positive airway pressure therapy, fatigue, and depression. They may be used as therapeutic agents in individuals diagnosed with attentional disruptions such as attention–deficit/hyperactive disorder.

Adverse effects sometimes associated with stimulant agents, particularly the more potent stimulants, include addiction. Some stimulants, taken at high doses repeatedly over a short period of time can lead to feelings of hostility or paranoia. This can also result in dangerously high body temperature and irregular heart rate. Cardiovascular failure or lethal seizure has been reported. Withdrawal symptoms associated with discontinuing stimulant use include fatigue, depression, and disturbance in sleep patterns.

Stimulant agents include caffeine found in beverages such as coffee, soft drinks, and so-called high-energy drinks. They are found in nicotine in tobacco products. They are also found in ephedrine, amphetamines, cocaine, methylphenidate, and modafinil (Provigil). Some of these agents are legally available only by prescription, including methamphetamine (Desoxyn), mixed amphetamine salts (Adderal), Sympathomimetic stimulants—such as dextro-amphetamine (Dexedrine), methamphetamine (Desoxyn), methylphenidate (Ritalin), and pemoline (Cylert)—are powerful central nervous system stimulants that enhance the effect of brain chemicals involved in wakefulness. People taking these agents have difficulty falling asleep; once asleep, they spend less time in REM sleep and non-rapid eye movement (NREM) deep sleep. When the drug is discontinued, extreme sleepiness and a craving for REM sleep may follow. Some stimulants are not legal at all but are abused for recreational purposes including methcathinone. Legal stimulants are often used for recreational purposes and can lead to problems with insomnia. Users may then turn to sedative agents to deal with symptoms of insomnia, thus setting up a cycle of drug-induced levels of consciousness. This scenario has played out in public in the lives of a number of celebrities who have died due to overdosage of these medications.

Chloral hydrate is an older sedative that doctors sometimes prescribe before certain diagnostic tests. It is occasionally used to treat insomnia. Side effects include rash, nausea, stomach pain, dizziness, and headache.

Anti-arrhythmics

These drugs, used to treat heart rhythm problems, may cause daytime fatigue and sleep difficulties at night. Such medications include procainamide (Pronestyl), quinidine, and disopyramide (Norpace).

Beta-Blockers

Beta-blockers are used to treat high blood pressure, arrhythmias, and angina. These drugs can promote insomnia, awakenings in the night, and nightmares. Examples of beta-blockers include propranolol (Inderal), metoprolol tartrate (Lopressor), atenolol (Tenormin), and metoprolol (Toporol).

Medications Containing Alcohol

Cough medicines often contain alcohol, which can suppress REM sleep.

Clonidine

This medication, which acts on nerve cells that respond to the neurotransmitter norepinephrine, is used to treat hypertension and occasionally to curb nicotine craving in people who are quitting smoking. The drug can cause daytime drowsiness and fatigue; it also may interfere with REM sleep. Some people report no problems with clonidine; others note restlessness, early morning awakening, and nightmares.

Corticosteroids

Corticosteroids such as prednisone, which are used to suppress inflammation and asthma, often cause daytime jitters and nighttime insomnia.

Diuretics

Diuretics, which are taken to rid the body of excess sodium and water, can interfere with sleep by inducing urination throughout the night. Potassium deficiency, a common side effect of some diuretics, can cause painful nocturnal cramping of calf muscles during sleep.

Theophylline

This respiratory stimulant used to treat asthma is chemically related to caffeine. Many people who use it require doses that are high enough to disrupt sleep.

Thyroid Hormones

Thyroid hormones, taken to counteract the effects of an underactive gland, may cause sleeping difficulties at higher doses.

Medications for Treating Insomnia

A variety of products including prescription medications and over-the-counter preparations are available for treating insomnia, but their effectiveness varies, and some may carry unpleasant side effects (Table 18-4).

Antihistamines

Antihistamines are the active ingredients in most over-the-counter sleep aids and in motion sickness pills. Many different over-the-counter sleep remedies are available, but these should be used with caution because they may cause dizziness, blurred vision, constipation, nausea, and next-day grogginess.

Table 18-4.

Medications for Insomnia

Medication	Use	Side Effects	Comments
Antihistamines			
Diphenhydramine (Benadryl, Nytol, Sominex, others); doxylamine (Unisom Nighttime Sleep Aid)	Occasional insomnia	Dizziness, blurred vision, nausea, vomiting, constipation, urinary retention; may cause confusion in older people	Available without prescription
Barbiturates			
Pentobarbital (Nembutal); phenobarbital (Barbita, Luminal, Solfoton); secobarbital (Seconal)	Older sleep aid prescribed only occasionally today	Clumsiness or unsteadiness, dizziness, lightheadedness, grogginess, anxiety, constipation, headache, irritability, nausea, vomiting	Should not be used by people with sleep apnea or other breathing difficulties, liver disease, or porphyria; can be fatal if taken in overdose combined with alcohol; abrupt withdrawal may cause delirium or convulsions; habit-forming
Benzodiazepines			
Clonazepam (Klonopin); diazepam (Valium); estazolam (ProSom); flurazepam (Dalmane); lorazepam (Ativan); quazepam (Doral); temazepam (Restoril); triazolam (Halcion)	Short-term treatment of insomnia	Clumsiness or unsteadiness, dizziness, lightheadedness, daytime drowsiness, headache	Should not be used by people with sleep apnea or other breathing difficulties; not to be used with alcohol or other depressants; tolerance may develop; withdrawal symptoms occur if stopped abruptly. Triazolam is a short-acting medication
Imidazopyridines			
Eszopiclone (Lunesta); zaleplon (Sonata); zolpidem (Ambien); non-benzodiazepine hypnotics	Treatment of insomnia	Headache, daytime drowsiness, dizziness, nausea, drugged feeling	Avoid combining these medications with alcohol and certain depressants (including antihistamines, muscle relaxants, and sedatives)
Antidepressants			
Amitriptyline (Elavil, Endep); citalopram (Celexa); doxepin (Sinequan); fluoxetine (Prozac); fluvoxamine (Luvox); mirtazapine (Remeron); paroxetine (Paxil); sertraline (Zoloft); trazodone (Desyrel); trimipramine (Surmontil)	Insomnia, nonrestorative sleep, and depression	May include dizziness, dry mouth, blurred vision, weight gain, constipation, trouble urinating, drowsiness, disturbance of heart rhythm (arrhythmia)	Certain antidepressants should not be used with a monoamine oxidase inhibitor or during immediate recovery from heart attack
Sedative			
Chloral hydrate (Aquachloral Supprettes)	Insomnia	Rash, nausea, stomach pain, dizziness, headache	May be habit-forming; not to be used with alcohol or other depressants

Barbiturates

Drugs in this class have been available for nearly a century and were a common ingredient in sleep medications until benzodiazepines became available in the 1960s. Today, sleep experts prescribe barbiturates only in very rare cases. Because these drugs suppress the activity of the entire central nervous system, barbiturate-induced sleep has a lower level of REM sleep than normal. More important, barbiturates are highly addictive; withdrawal can be painful and difficult, and an overdose can be fatal.

Benzodiazepines

These medications are frequently prescribed as sleeping pills. Drugs of this class work by enhancing the activity of the inhibitory neurotransmitter GABA, which calms brain activity. Many different benzodiazepines are available, although they differ in how quickly they take effect and how long they remain active in the body. Benzodiazepines taken at night can lead to drowsiness and sedation the next day. Depending on the behavior of the insomnia, different medications can be tried. For example, if the primary issue is getting to sleep, a benzodiazepine that works quickly and is short-acting, such as triazolam (Halcion), may be the best choice. If however, the problem is staying asleep, a drug that lasts longer—such as lorazepam (Ativan), estazolam (ProSom), or temazepam (Restoril)—may be necessary. Some drugs in this class also act as muscle relaxants and may be prescribed for this purpose. Additionally, benzodiazepines are used to treat anxiety, so they tend to be useful for patients with anxiety and insomnia that results from it. Many people who use benzodiazepines develop tolerance, in which they need more and more of the drug to obtain the same effect, and after a few weeks, the drugs no longer promote sleep and instead may contribute to rebound insomnia when the medications are stopped. These medications should be discontinued under supervision because withdrawal may lead to muscle tension, restlessness, irritability, or, in rare cases, convulsions.

Imidazopyridines

The class of drugs called imidazopyridines became available in 1992, when the Food and Drug Administration approved zolpidem (Ambien). This medication begins to work after about 30 minutes and leaves the body within 5 hours. Imidazopyridines specifically enhance the sleep-inducing activity of the neurotransmitter GABA. Unlike benzodiazepines, they do not cause muscle relaxation. Treatment seems to promote a normal pattern of sleep. The most common side effects include headache, dizziness, nausea, and grogginess.

Eszopiclone (Lunesta) is approved for use in all types of insomnia. It has been shown to be safe and effective even when used for 6 months. Additional drugs in this class will be released in the near future.

Antidepressants

When depression interferes with sleep, an antidepressant may improve both sleep and mood. If depression is not the problem, an older type of antidepressant medication known as a tricyclic is sometimes used because these drugs reduce the length of time it takes to fall asleep and improve the continuity of sleep. At the low doses used to treat sleep disturbance, tricyclic antidepressants seem to be less habit-forming than benzodiazepines and, therefore, less likely to contribute to rebound insomnia. When the tricyclic drug amitriptyline (Elavil, Endep) is used to treat insomnia in people with rheumatoid arthritis or other painful conditions, improved sleep seems to decrease aches and pains.

Other antidepressants, such as the sedative mirtazapine (Remeron), the serotonin-modulator trazodone (Desyrel), and those in the class known as SSRIs, may also be helpful in treating insomnia. SSRIs include fluoxetine (Prozac), sertraline (Zoloft), fluvoxamine (Luvox), paroxetine (Paxil), and citalopram (Celexa).

SUMMARY

Ironically, though new drug development is advancing, therapeutics may be regressing. Regulatory issues and the lack of information about long-term use of hypnotic medications have encouraged many physicians to use soporific antidepressants to treat chronic insomnia. This practice continues notwithstanding known profound sleep architecture alterations, questionable efficacy, and well-documented side effects. An alternative is the use of centrally acting antihistamines, which may be effective for a few days. Though they do not seem to adversely affect sleep architecture, antihistamines also are not effective when taken chronically. Finally, not treating the insomnia is also common in the face of regulatory issues (most sedative hypnotics are scheduled medications, and package inserts warn against chronic use). Some patients may eventually turn to alcohol, which ultimately does more harm than good.

The next frontier for pharmacological treatment of sleep architecture is to examine the microstructure of sleep in detail, since it may relate more directly than macrofeatures of sleep to the underlying neurologic mechanisms. Electroencephalogram waveforms and patterns may provide the improved sensitivity needed to better understand insomnia and its treatment.

REFERENCES

1. Harrison N, Mendelson WB, de Wit H. Barbiturates. In: Davis KL, Charney D, Coyle JT, Nemeroff C, eds. *Neuropsychopharmacology: The Fifth Generation of Progress.* Philadelphia, PA: Lippincott, Williams & Wilkins; 2002.

2. Wagner J, Wagner ML, Hening WA. Beyond benzodiazepines: alternative pharmacologic agents for the treatment of insomnia. *Ann Pharmacother.* 1998;32:680–691.

3. Lader MH. Implications of hypnotic flexibility on patterns of clinical use. *Int J Clin Pract Suppl.* 2001;116:14–19.

4. Lieberman JA. Update on the safety considerations in the management of insomnia with hypnotics: incorporating modified-release formulations into primary care. *Prim Care Companion J Clin Psychiatry.* 2007;9:25–31.

5. Morgenthaler TI, Silber MH. Amnestic sleep-related eating disorder associated with zolpidem. *Sleep Med.* 2002;3:323–327.

6. Lange CL. Medication-associated somnambulism. *J Am Acad Child Adolesc Psychiatry.* 2005;44:211–212.

7. Liskow B, Pikalov A. Zaleplon overdose associated with sleepwalking and complex behavior. *J Am Acad Child Adolesc Psychiatry.* 2004;43:927–928.

8. Walsh JK, Pollak CP, Scharf MB, Schweitzer PK, Vogel GW. Lack of residual sedation following middle-of-the-night zaleplon administration in sleep maintenance insomnia. *Clin Neuropharmacol.* 2000;23:17–21.

9. Food and Drug Administration, Department of Health and Human Services. Labeling of diphenhydramine-containing drug products for over-the-counter human use. *Fed Regist.* 2002;67:72555–72559. Available at: http://www.fda.gov/OHRMS/DOCKETS/98fr/120602a.htm. Accessed August 2, 2012.

10. Richardson GS, Roehrs TA, Rosenthal L, Koshorek G, Roth T. Tolerance to daytime sedative effects of H1 antihistamines. *J Clin Psychopharmacol.* 2002;22:511–515.

11. de Leon J, Nikoloff DM. Paradoxical excitation on diphenhydramine may be associated with being a CYP2D6 ultrarapid metabolizer: three case reports. *CNS Spectr.* 2008;13(2):133–135.

12. National Committee for Quality Assurance. High risk medications as specified by NCQA's HEDIS measure: use of high risk medications in older adults. Available at: http://www.ncqa.org/Portals/0/Newsroom/SOHC/Drugs_Avoided_Elderly.pdf. Accessed August 2, 2012.

19

Other Therapies Used to Treat Disordered Sleep

Julie M. Hereford, PT, DPT

Because sleep problems are so widespread, a market has developed to provide alternatives to prescription sleep aids and sleep devices. This chapter will provide a survey of some of the products that are available and that patients may be using. This is not intended as an endorsement of any of these items, nor is it an exhaustive list of alternative sleep aids available.

More than 1 in 10 Americans take a prescription or over-the-counter (OTC) sleep aid at least a few nights a month to help them sleep. Approximately 7% use OTC sleep aids while 3% use sleep medications prescribed by a physician. It is reported that nearly 50 million people suffer from chronic sleep problems.[1] This translates into millions of dollars spent on medication and devices to improve sleep and dollars lost on decreased productivity and job-related accidents.

Light Therapy

Some experts recommend exposure to bright light to reset an insomniac's internal clock (Figure 19-1). Researchers from Flinders University in Adelaide, South Australia, successfully used bright light therapy to improve the sleep of 9 insomniacs prone to waking between 3 AM and 5 AM. After 2 evenings of exposure to bright light, the participants slept more than an hour longer.[2] This has been shown to be an effective alternative to medication or behavior modification techniques.

Nonprescription Sleep Aids

The average drugstore carries a bewildering variety of OTC sleep medications from pepper pills to Benadryl to Tylenol PM (Figure 19-2). One small survey of people ages 60 and over found that more than a quarter had taken OTC sleeping aids in the preceding year and that 1 in 12 did so daily.[3] Behind the riot of competing brands, this class of products is surprisingly straightforward. Most OTC sleep aids, including Compoz, Nytol, and Sominex, contain 25 to 50 mg of the antihistamine diphenhydramine. A few, such as Unisom SleepTabs, contain 25 mg of doxylamine, another antihistamine. Others including Aspirin-Free Anacin PM and Extra Strength Tylenol PM combine antihistamines with 500 mg of the pain reliever acetaminophen.

OTC antihistamines have a sedating effect and are generally safe but can cause nausea and, more rarely, fast or irregular heartbeat, blurred vision, or heightened sensitivity to sunlight. Complications are generally more common in children and people over age 60. Alcohol heightens the effect of these medications, which can also interact adversely with some drugs, including central nervous system depressants and monoamine oxidase inhibitors such as phenelzine (Nardil) and tranylcypromine (Parnate).

Dietary Supplements and Alternative Medicines

A 2004 study of alternative medicine use discovered that 36% of adult Americans had used alternative medicines during the last 12 months, including herbal sleep aids.[4] As with other dietary supplements, the Food and Drug Administration (FDA) does not regulate these products, so they are not tested for safety, effectiveness, quality, or

Hereford JM. *Sleep and Rehabilitation:*
A Guide for Health Professionals (pp 189-191).
© 2014 Taylor & Francis Group.

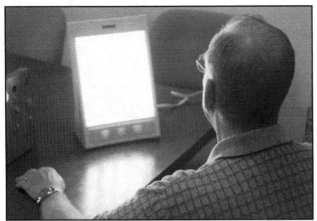

Figure 19-1. Exposure to bright light has been known to help improve sleep especially in those suffering from insomnia and/or depression. This can be accomplished by sitting in the sunlight. During the winter, when daylight is limited, use of a light box that emits full-spectrum light may be a good substitute for exposure to sunlight. Some have recommended brief exposure to a tanning bed as a way to increase light exposure. The risk/benefit of this type of exposure has not been established. (Reprinted with permission from A. Frank.)

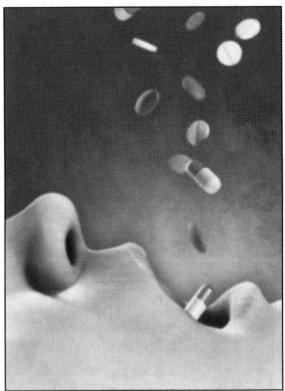

Figure 19-2. There is a seeming endless variety of OTC sleep aids available at any drugstore. (From Fotolia.com)

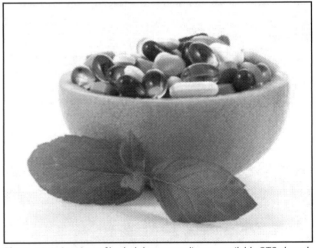

Figure 19-3. A variety of herbal sleep remedies are available OTC, though there is little research on the efficacy of most. (From Fotolia.com)

accuracy of labeling. Although marketed as "natural," these products may contain biologically active substances that can have side effects or can interact with other medications or herbal remedies (Figure 19-3).

Unlike standard OTC sleeping pills, which contain a single antihistamine, many herbal products include a variety of active ingredients. Before using these products, it is important to see if any ingredients might interact with other medications because even a single herb contains multiple chemicals. Scientific understanding of these substances is limited, and studies of them are generally small and short term, making it difficult to extrapolate findings to the general population. Readily available alternative sleep remedies include the following.

Valerian (*Valeriana officinalis*)

Valerian is a popular herbal medicine in the United States, and a few studies suggest that its mildly sedative effect can help people fall asleep and improve sleep quality. Valerian should not be mixed with barbiturates or alcohol. As with other unregulated remedies, the quality of valerian-containing products varies widely. In its July 2001 report, ConsumerLab, a commercial laboratory that periodically tests the quality of herbal remedies, detailed its analysis of 17 valerian-based products. Nearly a quarter appeared to contain no valerian whatsoever, and an equal number had less than half the amount claimed on their labels. Products made with valerian extract proved more trustworthy in this regard than those made with "root powder."[5]

Kava (*Piper methysticum*)

Kava comes from a plant cultivated in the South Pacific islands. The German Commission E, which tests the quality and effectiveness of herbal remedies marketed in Germany, has found it effective in the treatment of anxiety.[6] Although the mechanism is unknown, some studies have reported that it is effective for insomnia. High doses over prolonged periods can cause skin reactions and liver failure, and in 2002, the FDA warned users of the potential risk of liver damage after a previously healthy 45-year-old woman took kava, suddenly developed liver failure, and required a liver transplant.

Melatonin

In the mid-1980s, researchers began to investigate whether oral doses of melatonin, a hormone secreted by the pineal gland, might help reset the biological clocks of travelers, shift workers, and people with insomnia. It seems to be most helpful for people with low levels of naturally occurring melatonin.

In one small study, researchers in Israel tested melatonin as a sleep aid in 12 men and women who had insomnia with an average age of 76. People who took melatonin before going to bed fell asleep faster and slept about 10% longer than those who received a placebo.[7] There were no adverse reactions. Other studies, however, found that melatonin did not have any effect on sleep.[8]

A synthetic form of melatonin is sold in health food stores and pharmacies. In the United States, this product, which is not regulated by the FDA, is considered a nutritional supplement, so there is no guarantee of its purity or efficacy. In Great Britain and Canada, melatonin is now classified as a medicine and is no longer available OTC. To date, there is no reliable information available about its effects during pregnancy or its interactions with other drugs.

Chamomile

Chamomile is a plant in the daisy family, and chamomile tea has long been used as a relaxant and sleep aid. Chamomile is both mild and safe, though rare allergic reactions, including bronchial constriction, can occur. Those who are allergic to plants in the daisy family, which include the ubiquitous ragweed, should probably avoid this herb. There are no scientific studies showing that chamomile is effective in treating insomnia.

Mechanical Devices

Specially designed orthopedic pillows may help people with insomnia sleep better. For people with sleep problems due to snoring or nasal congestion, adhesive-backed nasal strips or devices such as small plastic nasal supports may provide relief. Manufacturers contend that such products help keep nasal passages open, reduce snoring, and increase air flow, thus improving sleep, but little independent research has evaluated these claims.

REFERENCES

1. National Sleep Foundation. Longer work days leave Americans nodding off on the job. Available at: http://www.sleepfoundation.org/article/press-release/longer-work-days-leave-americans-nodding-the-job. Accessed May 12, 2012.
2. Lovato N, Lack L, Wright H. A randomized controlled trial of a combined treatment of cognitive behaviour therapy and evening bright light therapy for insomnia in older adults. *Sleep.* 2011;34:A173–A174.
3. Germain A, Moul DE, Franzen PL, et al. *J Clin Sleep Med.* 2006;2:403–406.
4. Complementary and alternative medicine use among adults and children: United States, 2007. Available at: http://www.cdc.gov/nchs/data/nhsr/nhsr012.pdf. Accessed May 15, 2012.
5. ConsumerLab.com. Many herbal sleep products lack key claimed ingredient. Available at: http://www.consumerlab.com/news/Valerian_Tests/7_9_2001/. Accessed May 15, 2012.
6. Wheatley D. Stress-induced insomnia treated with kava and valerian: singly and in combination. *Hum Psychopharmacol.* 2001;16(4):353-356.
7. Srinivasan V, Maestroni GJ, Cardinali DP, Esquifino AI, Perumal SR, Miller SC. Melatonin, immune function and aging. *Immun Aging.* 2005;2:17.
8. Buscemi N, Vandermeer B, Hooton N, et al. Efficacy and safety of exogenous melatonin for secondary sleep disorders and sleep disorders accompanying sleep restriction: meta-analysis. Available at: www.bmj.com/content/332/7538/385.pdf%2Bhtml. Accessed September 29, 2013.

Section IV

Implications of Sleep in Rehabilitation

Sleep, Pain, and Mood

Julie M. Hereford, PT, DPT

INTRODUCTION TO SLEEP AND PAIN

This chapter will provide a basic review of pain pathways and an overview of current understanding of pain perception, transmission, and modulation, and will attempt to link it to related sleep neural processes. It will discuss the interrelationship between sleep and pain and describe neural pathways that are shared by each system. Though this interrelationship is complex, this chapter will attempt to provide a framework for understanding the complex interaction between sleep and pain. For the purposes of this chapter, the discussion of pain will be primarily limited to chronic pain because it is more likely to be the scenario in a clinical rehabilitation setting. The reciprocal relationship of acute pain and burn pain has been studied but they have their own unique presentations in the clinical setting and are not going to be considered specifically as part of this discussion.

Though an understanding of the basic science of sleep and pain is paramount to this discussion, it is also important to relate this science to a clinical setting. Clinical assessment tools related to sleep and to pain can provide a better understanding of the subjective experience of pain and the impact sleep may have on a patient. With these data, the clinician may gain a better understanding of the patient's experience and therefore be able to provide a more effective treatment program.

Although there is no clinical assessment tool that explores the relationship between sleep and pain in the current literature, this chapter will briefly outline tools that measure self-reported pain, sleepiness, and/or fatigue. The tools offered are readily available and easily administered in the rehabilitation setting. These tools can provide the clinician with a clearer picture of the impact that pain and sleep may have on an individual patient. The instruments described here have been extensively researched and offer reliable and valid methods of gaining insight into a complex patient problem.

In addition to pain rating scales and sleepiness and/or fatigue scales, several tools that measure alterations in mood are discussed. Because chronic pain and dysfunctional sleep have a complex interaction and because they share common neural pathways with systems that affect mood, it is important to consider the impact that an alteration in mood may have on the clinical picture. Though rehabilitation professionals do not specifically evaluate and treat patients for mood disorders, it is important to screen for these and identify individuals who may need referral for further evaluation. It is also important to consider the interaction an underlying mood disorder may have with sleep and pain disorders. Care must be taken to identify mood disorders for what they are and not to over-identify them with the patient. It is important to understand that chronic pain problems and sleep dysfunctions can precipitate a mood disorder or can exacerbate an existing one. It is unfortunate that sometimes a mood disorder can overshadow a pain or sleep disorder and many of the patient's symptoms are blamed on the mood disorder. This may lead to undertreatment of a chronic pain problem and/or underidentification of a sleep dysfunction.

Pain is an enigma. It is an individualized and subjective experience that the International Association for the Study of Pain (IASP) defines as "an unpleasant sensory and emotional experience associated with actual or potential tissue damage and described in terms of such damage." (p. 1).[1] It is important to note that pain is both a physical sensory experience and an emotional experience. The IASP notes "each

Hereford JM. *Sleep and Rehabilitation:*
A Guide for Health Professionals (pp 195-232).
© 2014 Taylor & Francis Group.

individual learns the application of the word [pain] through experiences related to injury in early life."[1] Humans attach different attributes to pain, which can be influenced by the environment in which one is raised and the cultural backdrop of the individual. These attributes of pain can be traced to different areas of the central nervous system that subserve pain, which are known as the *paleospinothalamic system* and the *neospinothalamic system*. The paleospino-thalalmic system is phylogenetically older and carries a motivational–affective component in which the individual identifies the painful experience as something unpleasant or bad that is to be avoided. The neospinothalamic system, which is a more recent evolutionary development, deals with the acquired sensory-discriminative component of pain that allows the individual to localize pain and react in an appropriate fashion. The interaction of these 2 systems combines to result in the complex psychophysiological experience of pain.

Pain, especially chronic pain, frequently interferes with the quality and quantity of sleep. Because components of the neural pathways involved in the initiation and maintenance of sleep are shared, it is reasonable to assume that there is a neurological basis for the interrelationship of sleep and pain. In order to illuminate this relationship, it is important to review these pathways.

EPIDEMIOLOGY OF PAIN AND SLEEP DISORDERS

The IASP defines chronic pain as that which is "...without apparent biological function that has persisted beyond the normal tissue healing time, usually taken to be three months."[2] Using this definition, the World Health Organization conducted a large study in 1998 of primary care settings on 5 continents ($n = 5438$) and revealed a prevalence rate of individual's reporting chronic pain of 21.5%.[3] More recent data, published by Brennan, reported that up to 56 million American adults or 28% of the adult population suffers from chronic pain. These pain problems come from a variety of diagnoses and disease processes, including 48 million with arthritis, 25 million with migraine pain, 20 million with jaw and lower facial pain, 16 million with lower back pain, and 4 million with neuropathic pain.[4,5]

Pain, whether acute or chronic, is a frequent contributor to insomnia. Insomnia is usually defined by either frequency or duration and involves some degree of daytime sleepiness, which is defined as difficulty or inability to maintain wakefulness and dysfunction related to poor sleep quality or quantity. Frequency is usually sleeplessness that occurs at least 3 times per week, and duration is usually recognized as being that which lasts longer than 1 month. It has been described as a persistent difficulty in falling or staying asleep despite adequate opportunity

and circumstance to do so. A nonrestorative quality is also described for the limited sleep that may occur.[6] According to Roth, nearly 30% of the worldwide adult population suffers from some degree of insomnia.[6]

Determining the prevalence of sleep disorders is a daunting task: The *International Classification of Sleep Disorders* has defined more than 80 sleep disorders.[7] However, according to Hossain and Shapiro, problems falling asleep or other symptoms of sleep disorders, including excessive daytime sleepiness, affect approximately 35% to 40% of the adult population in the United States annually. These disorders are a significant contributor to United States morbidity and mortality.[8]

A variety of different chronic pain conditions are known to cause sleep disturbances, including musculoskeletal diseases and disorders; headaches; neurological disorders including neuropathic pain; visceral diseases such as irritable bowel syndrome; chronic orofacial pain; cancer pain; and dysmenorrhea. The prevalence of sleep disturbance in chronic pain conditions has been studied by Ohayon, who surveyed 8989 individuals from Europe and found that 23% of individuals with chronic pain reported at least one symptom of insomnia, such as difficulty initiating sleep, disrupted sleep, early morning awakening, and/or non-refreshing sleep. In this same study, it was found that 40.2% of individuals that reported insomnia symptoms also reported some form of chronic pain.[9] This illustrates the circular nature of the relationship between chronic pain and insomnia.

REVIEW OF PAIN PERCEPTION, TRANSMISSION, AND MODULATION

It is important to review and understand the known concepts of pain perception, pain transmission, and pain modulation when discussing sleep. Pain can influence and sometimes severely disturb sleep and, conversely, sleep deprivation can modify pain sensitivity. Additionally, though both pain and sleep involve very complex neural pathways, they share some common neuronal and neurochemical substrates, although there is much that remains to be determined regarding the specific interaction of these circuits.

CLASSIFICATION OF PAIN: ACUTE VERSUS CHRONIC PAIN

Pain is often classified as acute or chronic in terms of its chronology. With this classification, acute pain is that which lasts 4 to 6 weeks, whereas chronic pain is that which lasts for longer than 6 months.

Acute pain is useful pain that limits body movement following an injury or illness, thereby reducing the risk of further damage. Acute pain can be a signal of underlying disease or dysfunction that requires further evaluation to obtain a diagnosis and in order to develop an effective treatment plan. Although there can certainly be an emotional component to acute pain, it is not generally associated with a significant amount of emotional overlay, nor is there the psychopathology that can sometimes be associated with pain that is more chronic in nature.

Most acute pain is relatively self-limiting and may not require medical intervention. Acute pain episodes may be recurrent and may represent an exacerbation of an underlying disease or dysfunction, but each episode is an acute episode and should not be mislabeled as chronic pain. Pain that outlasts the acute phase may be defined as subacute pain. Subacute pain is usually described as that which lasts between 1 and 6 months.[10]

Using this model, chronic pain is that pain that lasts for 6 months or longer arising from tissue injury, inflammation, nerve damage, tumor growth, or lesion or occlusion of blood vessels. Bonica described chronic pain as "pain that persists one month beyond the usual course of disease or reasonable time for an injury to heal" (p. 18).[10] Chronic pain can sensitize the nervous system, evoking chemical, functional, and even structural changes that increase its sensitivity. It is generally believed that chronic pain has little protective value and is usually associated with changes in mood, memory, attention, concentration, and libido and is frequently accompanied by significant sleep dysfunction. Patients with chronic pain conditions may also experience significant financial and social stresses, and the condition may interfere with their family relationships. Chronic benign pain is distinguished from cancer pain, which may be severe and is related to a malignant process that has its own set of complications. Cancer pain should be treated in the context of the disease and, as such, should not be considered as part of a chronic pain syndrome. Although a lengthy discussion is outside the scope of this text, it is important to note that cancer patients can, and often do, experience exacerbation of an underlying musculoskeletal dysfunction that may cause increased pain. Whereas this pain may not be specifically associated with the individual's malignant process, it must be thoroughly evaluated and appropriately treated. Untreated nonmalignant pain in a cancer patient may be a source of significant stress to the individual; he or she is unable to distinguish what pain is coming from his or her cancer and what is not. This stress can make management of the disease more complex. Untreated pain, no matter the source or classification, can lead to chronicity and disability that might otherwise be avoided with proper management.

Chronic pain usually has a component of suffering that is unrelated to the intensity of the pain. Chronic pain may be described as a constant dull aching pain that limits some functional activity, or it may be reported to be severely debilitating, interfering with the individual's ability to engage in work and perhaps even normal activities of daily living. Chronic pain may so overwhelm the sufferer so as to render him incapacitated and disabled.

Pain, whether acute or chronic, is experienced by the thalamus, sensory cortex, and limbic system. The emotional component to pain is usually experienced as fear, anxiety, depression, or frustration and can increase the overall experience of suffering especially related to chronic pain.

BASIC ANATOMY OF PAIN

When cells are injured, they release chemicals, which include prostaglandins and leucotrienes, that initiate a pain response in the nervous system. Some chemicals cause the sensation of pain to be triggered, whereas others lower the pain threshold to enhance the perception of pain.

An early theory regarding peripheral pain receptors postulated that pain was caused by overstimulation of receptors that carried other modalities. Instead, it has been found that most tissues carry specific pain receptors called nociceptors, which are differentiated by the quality of pain they transmit.

A noxious stimulus is an "actual or potentially tissue damaging event" (p. 473).[11] The stimulus can be a force that deforms tissue (mechanical), a chemical irritant, or an extreme thermal stimulus. Mechanical, thermal, or chemical changes that reach a set threshold initiate activity in free nerve endings or nociceptors. These free nerve endings can be found in the skin, periosteum, joint structures, muscle and organ capsules, as well as other pain-sensitive structures. Nociception is defined by the IASP as "the neural processes of encoding and processing noxious stimuli. (p. 473)"[11] Once noxious information is encoded by the nociceptor, it passes along a nerve fiber to the spinal cord and brain. Along its route, the nociceptor triggers a variety of autonomic responses that create the experience of pain.

There are 3 main nerve fiber types that carry nociceptive information (Table 20-1). Group I fibers, also known as Aβ fibers, make up less than 1% of nociceptors. They are large-diameter, myelinated fibers that predominately respond to nonpainful stimuli. These fibers act at the spinal cord level to inhibit c-fiber information. They are responsible for feelings of tenderness and carry certain neuropathic pain and may be involved in referred pain.

Group III fibers, known as Aδ fibers, are small-diameter, lightly myelinated nerve fibers that propagate rapid pain information and respond to touch and pressure and thermal stimuli.

Group IV fibers are known as c-fibers and are unmyelinated, small-diameter, slow-response fibers that are polymodal. They make up the vast majority of nociceptors in the human skin.[10] They carry a variety of noxious stimuli

Table 20-1.

Pain Fibers		
Fiber Class	**Velocity**	**Effective Stimuli**
Aβ	> 10 and < 40 m/s	Low-threshold mechanical or thermal; high-threshold mechanical or thermal
Aδ	> 40 to 50 m/s	Low-threshold; specialized nerve endings (Pacinian corpuscles)
c-fibers	< 2 m/s	High-threshold thermal, mechanical and chemical; free nerve endings

including mechanical, thermal, and chemical information. These fibers can also be found in muscle, joint structures, periosteum, organ capsules, and viscera.

Aδ nerve fibers have a higher conduction velocity and therefore detect and react to dangerous mechanical and thermal stimuli. They respond to a weaker intensity of stimuli and have a protective function, getting primary pain or first pain information to the central nervous system rapidly in order that the organism can remove itself from further harm. C-fibers, on the other hand, are capable of responding to a much stronger intensity of stimulus. C-fibers are responsible for the slow, more pervasive, and longer-lasting quality of secondary pain. Chemicals released in an inflamed area sensitize c-fibers and act to reinforce Aδ fiber response. It has been suggested that this reinforcement may contribute to protective reactions that are characteristic of the pain response. All nociceptive fibers increase sensitivity following an injury.

C-fiber receptors include multiple nociceptors that are responsible for subtleties involved in the experience of pain. For example, certain c-fiber nociceptors are responsible for secondary burning pain. Other c-fiber warming-specific receptors are responsible for the sensation of warming; ultraslow histamine-selective c-fibers are responsible for the sensation of itch; tactile c-fibers are responsible for sensual touch pain; and c-mechanoreceptors and metaboreceptors in muscle and joints are responsible for muscle exercise burn and cramping pain. This variety of input signals calls for a variety of cortical cells with different modality selectiveness and morphology. These varying neurons are responsible for the variety of sensory experiences and can be classified by their responses to a range of stimuli. The brain uses the integration of these signals to maintain homeostasis in the body.

PAIN TRANSMISSION TO THE CENTRAL NERVOUS SYSTEM

Once a free nerve ending is stimulated by noxious stimuli, it transmits that information to the spinal cord

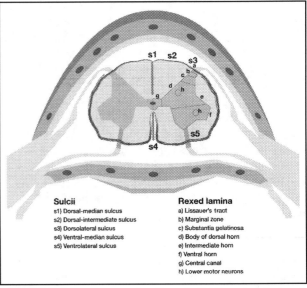

Figure 20-1. A transverse section through the thoracic spinal cord, showing the grey matter and various laminae.

(Figure 20-1). More than half the nerve fibers enter the dorsal horn with the rest entering the ventral horn. Histologically, the gray matter is divided into 10 laminae that are defined by their cellular structure, rather than their location, although location is relatively consistent. Lamina I–V are found in the dorsal horn and receive and process most of the incoming pain fiber information. Up to 40% of sensory fibers enter the ventral horn.[12]

Pain sensation is transmitted to the central nervous system via the spinothalamic tract. The spinothalamic tract is divided into the more lateral neospinothalamic tract and the medial paleospinothalamic tract (Figure 20-2).

The spinothalamic tract enters the spinal cord where it ascends or descends 1 or 2 vertebral levels in the tract of Lissauer and then synapse with second-order neurons in either the substantia gelatinosa or nucleus proprius. The second-order neurons decussate—that is, cross to the contralateral side—in the anterior white commissure and take up a position in the anterolateral part of the spinal cord and travel up the length of the spinal cord to the brain stem.

Different types of pain are carried on different pain fibers and synapse in different lamina of the spinal cord.

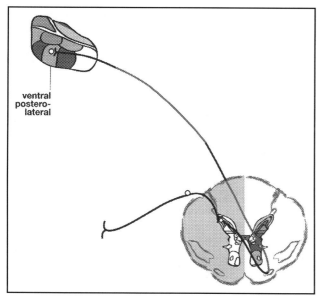

Figure 20-2. Neospinothalamic tract schematic from periphery to thalamus.

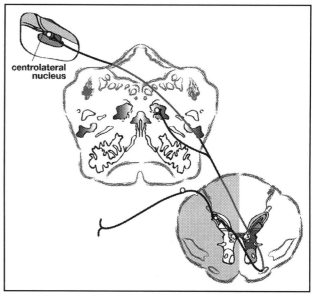

Figure 20-3. Schematic of pain pathway from the periphery to the thalamus.

So-called *fast pain* is carried on Aδ fibers and is characterized by sharply localized sensation. It is transmitted via the neospinothalamic tract and is responsible for immediate awareness of painful stimuli and for discrimination of exact location of that stimulus in order to react in a protective manner. These fibers, the first-order neurons of the system, synapse on the second-order neurons in the Rexed lamina I, also known as the marginal zone, of the dorsal root ganglion. Axons from the marginal zone decussate in the anterior white commissure at approximately the same level they enter the cord and ascend in the contralateral anterolateral quadrant of the spinal cord. Pain fibers from the extremities and body below the neck terminate in third-order neurons at the ventroposterolateral (VPL) and the ventroposteroinferior (VPI) nucleus of the thalamus (Figure 20-3). The VPL is thought to be concerned with discriminatory functions and sends neurons to the primary somatosensory cortex.

The paleospinothalamic tract is responsible for slower, less well-discriminated pain and is generally thought to be responsible for pain that is more chronic in nature. First-order neurons arising from c-fiber input enter the spinal cord dorsal root ganglion and may ascend or descend several levels. These neurons make synaptic contact in the Rexed lamina II, otherwise known as the *substantia gelatinosa*. Second-order neurons synapse within an interneuronal pool in laminae IV–VII where they also receive input from mechanoreceptors and thermoreceptors. These nerve cells are known as wide dynamic range (WDR) nociceptors. Tertiary neurons in this system cross the midline and ascend in the anterior spinal cord as the anterior spinothalamic tract. These fibers contain several tracts that terminate in different locations including the mesencephalic reticular formation (MRF), the periaqueductal gray (PAG),

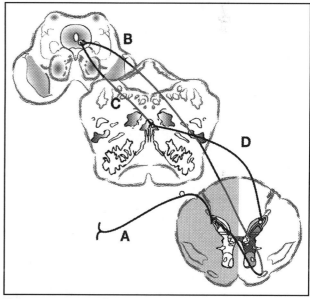

Figure 20-4. Descending serotonergic connections that modulate incoming pain impulses. Incoming painful stimuli are transmitted to (A) the dorsal horn (B) then to the periaqueductal gray, (C) descending impulses pass to the raphe nuclei, (D) and then back to the dorsal horn via reticulospinal fibers.

the tectum, and the interlaminar (IL) nuclei of the thalamus and make up the spinoreticular tract, the spinotectal tract, and the spinothalamic tract. These fibers synapse in the somatosensory cortex.

The paleospinothalamic tract activates brain stem nuclei, which, in turn, make up the descending pain suppression pathway and regulate noxious input at the spinal cord level. The multisynaptic tracts, which course via the reticular formation, also project to the intralaminar nuclei (Figure 20-4). There are extensive interconnections

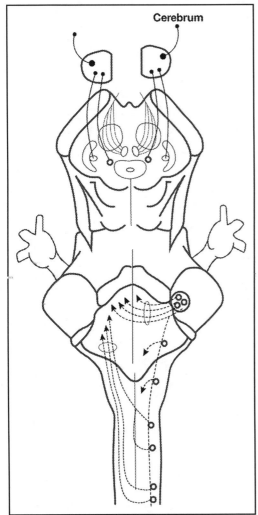

Figure 20-5. Posterior view of the brain stem with the cerebellum removed, illustrating the major ascending pathways of the trigeminal system.

the IL. Third-order neurons ascend to the sensory cortex of the postcentral gyrus and are somatotopically oriented. Affective–motivational information from the trigeminal ganglion sends projections to the reticular formation, midbrain, and midline nuclei of the thalamus. Third-order neurons from the midline nucleus of the thalamus terminal in the cingulate and insular cortex.

The archispinothalamic tract is a diffuse multisynaptic tract that is phylogenetically the oldest pain pathway. First-order neurons synapse in the substantia gelatinosa (lamina II) and project to lamina IV–VII. Second-order neurons ascend and descend the spinal cord via the multisynaptic propriospinal tract and finally synapse in the MRF-PAG areas. These neurons ascend to the intralaminar nuclei of the thalamus and send collaterals to the hypothalamus and limbic nuclei. These fibers serve to mediate visceral, emotional, and autonomic responses to painful stimuli.

PAIN MODULATION

In 1965, Ronald Melzack and Patrick Wall of McGill University presented the gate-control theory of pain.[13] This theory postulates that nonpainful tactile stimulation can "close the gate" to painful input and reduce the amount of painful stimuli that reaches the central nervous system and therefore suppress pain. This theory suggests that large-diameter myelinated sensory nerve fibers (Aβ) exert an inhibitory influence on an interneuronal pool in the dorsal horn of the spinal cord. This interneuronal pool receives excitatory input from c-fiber pain neurons. The sensory fibers inhibit or modulate pain transmission by inhibiting transmission of c-fiber pain at the interneurons level. Therefore, the Aβ produce presynaptic inhibition of c-fiber pain in the dorsal horn of the spinal cord and thereby block incoming noxious information from reaching the cortex for perception.

Aδ and c-fibers reach the dorsal horn of the spinal cord from peripheral sites to innervate the nociceptor neurons in lamina I and II. Cells from lamina II synapse with neurons in lamina IV–VII. These neurons give rise to the ascending spinothalamic tracts. Opiate receptors are located at the presynaptic ends of nociceptive neurons at the interneuronal lamina IV–VII in the dorsal horn. Activation of opiate receptors in the interneuronal pool produces hyperpolarization of neurons, which results in inhibition of the pain transmission neurons.

More centrally, as pain transmission ascends the spinal cord and brain stem, it sends collaterals to multiple regions, including the PAG, the locus coeruleus (LC), the nucleus raphe magnus (NRM), and the nucleus reticularis gigantocellularis (RGC), which, in turn, contribute to a descending pain suppression pathway, which inhibits incoming pain information at the spinal cord level. The primary neurotransmitter in this system is gamma-aminobutyric acid (GABA).

between the IL and the limbic areas including the cingulate gyrus and the insular cortex, which are thought to be involved in the processing of emotional components of pain and help elicit the cognitive components in response to painful stimuli. The limbic structures project to the hypothalamus and initiate visceral responses to pain. The IL also projects to the frontal cortex, which projects to the limbic system where the emotional response to pain is mediated.

Nociceptive information from the head, face, and intraoral structures are carried via the trigeminal ganglion on the anterior trigeminothalamic tract (Figure 20-5). This receives input from the trigeminal nerve, the facial nerve, and glossopharyngeal nerve and the vagus nerve. Trigeminal nerve fibers enter the pons, descend to the medulla and synapse at the spinal trigeminal nucleus, and decussate and ascend at the trigeminothalamic tract. Aδ second-order neurons cross the midline and terminate in the ventroposteromedial (VPM) nucleus of the thalamus and c-fibers terminate in the parafasciculus (PF) and centromedian (CM) thalamus (PF-CM complex) located in

ASSESSING THE INTERACTION BETWEEN PAIN AND SLEEP

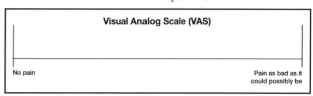

Figure 20-6. Visual analog scale.

A minimal level of consciousness is required in order to be able to express a reaction to pain transmission. Sleep is characterized by a partial isolation from the environment and therefore generally results in a decreased expression of pain. There is, however, a circular relationship between pain and sleep in that reports of decreased quality and quantity of sleep usually result in increased pain reports the following day and increased pain reports during the day frequently result in poor-quality sleep as evidenced by both polysomnographic findings and subjective reports.[14–17] In fact, in one population study,[18] patients with nonmalignant pain were more likely to seek care when it was associated with disrupted sleep or insomnia or self-report of emotional or cognitive components of sleep disruption and when there was a self-reported expectation of improvement.

Because there are confounding factors that may affect sleep disturbance, it is difficult to study the impact of sleep on pain or pain on sleep independent of these factors. Factors such as sleep apnea, abnormal limb movement during sleep, bruxism, and insomnia resulting from psychosocial causes, anxiety, and depression may alter sleep architecture, making it difficult to separate out changes in sleep that are strictly pain related. The use of analgesic medication may alter sleep architecture and present a confounding factor in analyzing the effect of pain on sleep. Unfortunately, there is no universally accepted method of evaluating the comorbidities of sleep and pain, and this can create a significant challenge in balancing adequate pain relief against protection of sleep continuity and the avoidance of daytime sleepiness.

Although there is no single research instrument or clinical tool that assesses the interaction of sleep and pain, it is nonetheless important for the clinician to understand how sleep impacts pain and pain impacts sleep. Because of the dearth of tools presently available, the clinician must rely on individual tools and use the data captured therein to gain some better understanding of the clinical picture. There are a variety of tools that measure self-report of pain, self-report of sleep quality and quantity, and self-report of mood. Some of the tools that are in more common use will be outlined. The instruments were selected for their relative ease of administration and application in the clinical setting and the utility of the data collected.

There are a variety of tools available to measure an individual's pain intensity and/or the symptoms that may accompany pain. Pain scales generally utilize patient self-report, but also may gather behavioral or physiological activity. Known as the *fifth vital sign*, pain scales have been individualized for various populations including infants, children, adolescents, adults, older adults, and individuals with communication impairment. Some commonly used and well-studied clinical pain scales will be outlined.

Visual Analog Scale

The visual analog scale (VAS) is a commonly utilized pain self-report scale (Figure 20-6). It is a psychometric response scale that measures subjective characteristics that cannot be measured objectively. The visual analog scale is made up of a continuous line with descriptor words anchoring either end of the scale. The VAS can be used to measure a number of different qualities including pain, with anchor words being "no pain" at the left end and "pain as bad as it can be" at the right end of the scale. The user indicates a level of agreement with a statement or query by selecting a corresponding position along the analog scale. This type of instrument differs from a Likert scale in which a discrete scale is used. A computer can be used to measure responses indicated on a visual analog scale. The sensitivity and reproducibility of the VAS and other linear scales are similar in a broad sense, but the VAS may outperform the other scales in some cases.[19]

Another common tool used to measure pain in a clinical setting is the numerical scale. It is simple to use and report, although the limitation of this scale is that when compared to the VAS, patients tend to consistently report a higher level of pain, perhaps in an effort to make certain that the clinician takes the pain complaint seriously.

Pain Disability Index

The Pain Disability Index (PDI), developed at Saint Louis University by Tait et al,[20] is a simple, easily administered instrument used for measurement of the interference pain may have on an individual's activities of daily living and the ability to participate in normal activities (Table 20-2). This particular instrument can be used to evaluate the effectiveness of interventions over time. The PDI measures the level of perceived disability related to pain in seven different areas. These areas include family and home responsibilities, recreation and leisure activities, participation in social activities, ability to engage in activities related to work including one's occupation and housework and volunteering, sexual behavior including frequency and quality of the experience, ability to perform self-care activities and, finally, the ability to participate in life-support activities including eating, sleeping, and breathing. The scale is

Table 20-2.

Pain Disability Index

The rating scales below are designed to measure the degree to which aspects of your life are disrupted by chronic pain. In other words, we would like to know how much pain is preventing you from doing what you would normally do or from doing it as well as you normally would. Respond to each category indicating the overall impact of pain in your life, not just when pain is at its worst.

For each of the 7 categories of life activity listed, please circle the number on the scale that describes the level of disability you typically experience. A score of 0 means no disability at all, and a score of 10 signifies that all of the activities in which you would normally be involved have been totally disrupted or prevented by your pain.

Family/Home Responsibilities: This category refers to activities of the home or family. It includes chores or duties performed around the house (eg, yard work) and errands or favors for other family members (eg, driving the children to school).

0	1	2	3	4	5	6	7	8	9	10

Recreation: This disability includes hobbies, sports, and other similar leisure time activities.

0	1	2	3	4	5	6	7	8	9	10

Social Activity: This category refers to activities that involve participation with friends and acquaintances other than family members. It includes parties, theater, concerts, dining out, and other social functions.

0	1	2	3	4	5	6	7	8	9	10

Occupation: This category refers to activities that are part of or directly related to one's job. This includes nonpaying jobs as well, such as that of a housewife or volunteer.

0	1	2	3	4	5	6	7	8	9	10

Sexual Behavior: This category refers to the frequency and quality of one's sex life.

0	1	2	3	4	5	6	7	8	9	10

Self-Care: This category includes activities that involve personal maintenance and independent daily living (eg, taking a shower, driving, getting dressed, etc).

0	1	2	3	4	5	6	7	8	9	10

Life-Support Activities: This category refers to basic life-supporting behaviors such as eating, sleeping, and breathing.

0	1	2	3	4	5	6	7	8	9	10

Reprinted with permission from J. Chibnal.

scored according to the numeric value endorsed on each item with a minimal score of 0 and a maximal score of 70. A higher score on the PDI indicates a greater level of perceived disability due to pain. This instrument shows modest test–retest reliability and offers discrimination between individuals with low and high levels of perceived disability.

McGill Pain Questionnaire

The McGill Pain Questionnaire[21,22] was developed at McGill University by Melzack in 1971. This questionnaire is used to help understand sensory and affective qualities associated with pain. These qualities can include skin color, temperature changes, pressure, tension, or fear. Considered a very valuable tool when assessing chronic pain, this instrument has been shown to be valid, reliable, and consistent. Descriptive terms are categorized into groups and the individual selects descriptive term in each of 20 groups of words. According to Wall and Melzack, "there is a remarkable consistency in the choice of words by patients suffering the same or similar pain syndromes. (p. 94)"[23] This instrument can be used to assist an individual in describing chronic pain and can assist the clinician in ascertaining the source of the pain.

Multidimensional Pain Inventory

The West Haven–Yale Multidimensional Pain Inventory was developed to assist in assessment of chronic pain and the evaluation of treatment approaches. This instrument has a multidimensional quality and strong psychometric properties. It consists of 12 scales in three parts that examine the impact of pain on an individual, the responses of others to that individual's complaints of pain, and the ability of the individual to engage in meaningful activities of daily living. It is recommended that this instrument be utilized in conjunction with behavioral and psychophysiological assessment strategies.[24]

Neuropathic Pain Symptoms Inventory

Neuropathic pain can result from a lesion or injury to a nerve from a variety of different causes, and presents a unique clinical picture, making it important to evaluate this type of pain and its impact on an individual's life in a specific manner. Neuropathic pain has been found to have unique yet commonly described symptoms. The Neuropathic Pain Symptoms Inventory was developed to assess individuals with neuropathic pain syndromes including diabetic peripheral neuropathy, sciatica, trigeminal neuralgia, and postherpetic neuralgia. This instrument has been shown to be an effective tool to measure the unique descriptive components of neuropathic pain and was found to be cross-cultural.[25]

Summary of Clinical Tools Used to Measure Pain

It is important to understand as much as possible about the clinical experience of an individual's pain problem. There are a variety of different instruments available that can be used in order to help better elucidate the quality and quantity of a patient's pain problem. The tools described offer reliable, valid measurements of pain and the impact pain may be having on the life of the individual sufferer. When attempting to gain a complete clinical picture of an individual, it is important to gain an understanding of the impact the pain is exerting on all aspects of the individual's life. Because of the difference in the quality and quantity of pain and the source of a pain syndrome, it is important to choose the instrument that will provide the best clinical information in the most efficient manner possible. Therefore, it is appropriate to choose a standard measurement tool that will be utilized for every individual such as a visual analog scale to help quantify the pain and the PDI to help qualify the impact pain may be having on

the individual's life. Other instruments may be chosen to further delineate the pain problem to better understand the more specific aspects of the problem.

Additionally, in order to gain a complete clinical picture, it is important to understand the quantity and quality of sleep that the individual is getting in a normal 24-hour period. These data can be correlated with pain data to help complete the clinical profile of the individual. To date, there is not a similar instrument that specifically correlates the impact of sleep on pain and pain on sleep, so the clinician may have to rely on several different instruments.

HOW TO MEASURE SLEEP AND SLEEP DYSFUNCTION

It is important to understand not only the amount of sleep that an individual gets in a normal 24-hour period but also the perceived quality of that sleep and potential problems that an underlying sleep dysfunction may be contributing to in the life of the individual. There are a variety of rating scales that help to evaluate different aspects of sleep, which can be incorporated into a clinical setting. These scales can help to clarify components of a complex clinical problem and assist the clinician in determining the impact a sleep dysfunction may be having on a pain problem and vice versa. Various sleep rating scales can help to determine sleepiness versus fatigue, symptoms of apnea, and how comorbid factors such as depression or anxiety may factor into a sleep dysfunction or insomnia versus sleep fragmentation. Sleep rating instruments can assist the clinician in distinguishing various nuances in a sleep problem and help to correlate it with a chronic pain problem to get a more complete profile of a complex clinical picture. Sleep rating scales, especially when used in conjunction with pain rating scales, can also help to track an individual's progress through a treatment program. What follows is a brief description of commonly used sleep rating scales with assets and limitations of each instrument.

Epworth Sleepiness Scale

Murray Johns at the Epworth Hospital in Melbourne, Australia, developed the Epworth Sleepiness Scale (ESS) in 1991.[26] This instrument uses a very short format to measure daytime sleepiness by asking the subject to rate the likelihood of falling asleep, on a scale of 1 to 3, in eight different commonly occurring situations. Scores for each item are added to produce a final score that is compared to a rating scale. A score of 0 to 9 is considered normal, whereas a score of 10 to 24 suggests that the individual should consider further evaluation for a sleep dysfunction. It has been validated with regards to obstructive sleep apnea (OSA).[26] It is frequently administered as part of an initial evaluation for a sleep dysfunction and is usually readministered following initiation of treatment for a sleep disorder such as OSA (eg, continuous positive airway pressure, CPAP) to document improvement in symptoms. Though this scale is widely used, it is limited because it looks at the likelihood of an individual to fall asleep in certain situations, rather than that individual's perceived level of fatigue. Depending on the level of chronicity of the sleep disorder, some individuals do not recognize the impact that sleepiness may be having on their life and may describe their symptoms more in terms of fatigue rather that sleepiness.

Fatigue Severity Scale

Fatigue can be a significant disabling feature reported by patients in a variety of physical and psychological disorders. It is different from sleepiness, and therefore the Fatigue Severity Scale[27] was developed to measure the quantity and quality of fatigue in individuals. This scale can be helpful and is sometimes better at illuminating a potential underlying sleep dysfunction that may require further evaluation, since it asks about levels of fatigue rather than sleepiness. It is sometimes the case that an individual suffering from a long-term chronic sleep disorder may have accommodated to the symptoms of the disorder in such a way as to not recognize their level of excessive daytime sleepiness and merely identify symptoms as fatigue.

The name of the scale is somewhat deceiving because, rather than measure the overall severity of fatigue, this instrument measures the impact that fatigue has on the daily life of an individual. The scale consists of 9 items in which the subject identifies a level of agreement along a 7-point Likert scale. In order to score the instrument, responses are averaged with a score greater than 4 considered indicating a clinically significant level of fatigue.[28-31]

The Fatigue Severity Scale is commonly utilized to measure the impact of fatigue on the daily lives of those with conditions such as multiple sclerosis (MS) and systemic lupus erythematosus (SLE). This scale correlates well with a visual analog scale, is internally consistent and has been shown to be able to detect changes in clinically significant fatigue over time. Research by Krupp et al, using the Fatigue Severity Scale to study fatigue in MS and SLE patients, demonstrated that this scale was able to show that fatigue is a symptom that is independent from self-report of symptoms of depression. The study also suggests that the reported characteristics of fatigue varies somewhat between MS and SLE. Given studies of this nature, it seems clear that fatigue is a separate and distinct symptom. Clinically, it should be distinguished from self-report of pain and from excessive daytime sleepiness.[32]

Pittsburgh Sleep Quality Index

The Pittsburgh Sleep Quality Index[33] (PSQI) was developed to measure the quality of sleep in a psychiatric population. It consists of a self-rated questionnaire that serves to assess sleep quality and sleep disturbances over a given 1-month interval. The instrument scores 19 individual items in 7 different areas of sleep, and the sum of these scores generates a global PSQI score. The areas measured include subjective sleep quality, sleep latency, sleep duration, habitual sleep efficiency, sleep disturbances, use of sleep medication, and daytime dysfunction due to excessive sleepiness or fatigue. This instrument has been shown in a study by Buysse et al to have diagnostic sensitivity and specificity in its ability to distinguish a good versus a poor sleeper in psychiatric practice and research.[34]

Stanford Sleepiness Scale

The Stanford Sleepiness Scale is one of the oldest scales developed to measure subjective sleepiness (Table 20-3). Developed in 1972 by Hoddes et al, this scale asks the subject to indicate his or her level of sleepiness by endorsing descriptors of relative sleepiness that are given a rating of 1 to 7.[35] This scale is simple and very easy to administer and can be used to track the individual's level of sleepiness and wakefulness throughout the day and therefore may give insight into that individual's circadian rhythms. This can be useful in helping to manage sleepiness, especially for a shift worker or others to help them avoid hazardous activities during times of increased sleepiness. This scale has limitations in that it lacks detail and requires the subject to have some awareness of their level of sleepiness and fatigue.

Summary of Tools Used to Assess Sleepiness and Fatigue

There are a wide variety of sleep rating scales available today that can assist the clinician in gaining insight into the relative sleepiness or fatigue of an individual and may indicate one that would benefit from further evaluation of a sleep dysfunction. A few of these rating scales have been outlined here, although there are many others to choose from, including the Toronto Sleepiness Scale,[36] the Canadian Sleep Society Inventory,[37] and others. The scales described here have been chosen because of their relative ease of use and high validity and reliability. It is recommended by the author that a clinician choose a tool to be used regularly in the clinical setting to quantify the quality of a patient's sleep and assist in identifying the individual patient who may need further evaluation.

HOW TO MEASURE MOOD ALTERATIONS

Because an individual who suffers with a chronic pain condition may have an underlying sleep dysfunction that

Table 20-3.

Stanford Sleepiness Scale

"Alertness Test"	
The Stanford Sleepiness Scale is a quick and easy way to assess level of alertness. This scale and chart can identify an individual's pattern of alertness by recording "degree of sleepiness" at different times throughout the day. Using the 7-point scale below choose what best represents level of alertness and note the corresponding number on the chart below.	
Degree of Sleepiness	*Scale Rating*
Feeling active, vital, alert, or wide awake	1
Functioning at high levels but not fully alert	2
Awake, but relaxed; responsive but not fully alert	3
Somewhat foggy, let down	4
Foggy; losing interest in remaining awake; slowed down	5
Sleepy, woozy, fighting sleep; prefer to lie down	6
No longer fighting sleep, sleep onset soon; having dream-like thoughts	7
Asleep	X

may or may not be complicated by a mood disorder, it can be helpful in screening for this. It can be used to develop a better understanding of the interaction of sleep, pain, and depression in developing a treatment program. Though rehabilitation professionals do not directly treat mood disorders, it is important to assist in the identification of an individual with these issues and to be able to refer that individual to the appropriate treating professional. By administering one of the commonly used screening tools, the health care provider can also gain some insight into the interaction of psychological symptoms with a chronic pain condition. A brief description of several commonly utilized rating instruments follows.

Beck Depression Inventory

First published in 1961 by American psychiatrist Aaron T. Beck, the Beck Depression Inventory[38] is one of the most widely used instruments for measuring the severity of depression today. It has been heavily studied and is generally considered to be a reliable and valid instrument.[39] It is a 21-question, multiple-choice self-rating inventory.[40] The current version of the questionnaire is designed for individuals over 13 years of age. The questions relate to symptoms of depression including hopelessness, irritability, and feelings of guilt or being punished and physical symptoms of depression including fatigue, weight loss, or lack of interest in sex.[40]

Medical Outcomes Study Short Form Health Survey

The Medical Outcomes Study Short Form Health Survey[41] was originally developed as part of the Medical

Outcome Study conducted by the RAND Corporation as a health care economics variable in calculations to determine the cost-effectiveness of health treatment. Though a commercial version is available, and a shorter SF-12 version has been developed, the original is now available in the public domain free of license from the RAND Corporation.[42] This tool can be utilized to measure health status and treatment outcomes from a patient point of view. It asks 36 questions that generate 0- to 100-point scales in 8 areas, including vitality (energy/fatigue), physical functioning, bodily pain, general health perceptions, physical role functioning, emotional role functioning, social role functioning, and mental health (psychological distress and psychological well-being). This instrument is useful in evaluating individual patients in clinical practice, as well as a survey tool of general and specific populations to evaluate the cost-effectiveness of treatment and to monitor and compare disease burden. It is a generic measure that does not target specific age, disease, or treatment groups, comparing relative burden of disease and differentiating the health benefits produced by a wide range of different treatments. It may be less useful as an individual measure when evaluating a chronic pain patient or one with a sleep dysfunction, because it does not specifically take into consideration the sleep variable. Another limitation of this tool is that it has a low response rate in individuals over 65 years of age.

The use of certain easily administered clinical screening tools may guide the rehabilitation clinician in recognizing potential patient problems that may become pitfalls in treatment. Any concern regarding the outcome of these tools can be used as a common point of discussion with clinicians from other disciplines, such as mental health professionals. When dealing with a chronic pain population, it is often useful to work with a mental health professional in order to gain an understanding of psychological or psychiatric issues that may interfere with an individual's ability to engage in the rehabilitation process. A mental health provider may administer a variety of evaluation surveys and questionnaires that are pertinent to the rehabilitation process. It is helpful for the rehabilitation professional to have a general understanding of several commonly utilized evaluation tools, even though a rehabilitation provider is unlikely to administer them. These may help to gain a better understanding of an individual's coping strategies and can help to guide the rehabilitation process. These data, taken with pain and sleep data, can help provide a more complete patient profile and ultimately help develop a more effective treatment plan.

Symptom Checklist-90

The Symptom Checklist-90 is a relatively brief self-reporting questionnaire designed to evaluate a broad range of psychological symptoms. It can also be used to measure treatment progress and outcomes of psychiatric and psychological programs. It is designed for individuals over 13 years old and consists of 90 items with 9 scales related to primary psychological symptoms and 3 scales that measure global distress.[43] It provides an overview of symptom severity and intensity, and the instrument can be administered multiple times to determine progress or change in clinical status.

Sickness Impact Profile

The Sickness Impact Profile is a tool that either can be self-administered or can be administered by an interviewer. It is a behaviorally based health status questionnaire of 136 items.[44] It asks the subject to endorse items in 12 categories that include sleep and rest, emotional behavior, body care and movement, work, recreation and pastimes, and eating.

Impact of Events Scale—Revised

The revised version of the Impact of Events Scale is an easily administered 22-item questionnaire utilized to evaluate the degree of distress an individual may feel in response to a trauma.[45] This scale may be particularly important when dealing with the chronic pain population, because the chronic pain condition may be a result of a trauma. Chronic pain conditions may also develop because of a dearth of coping abilities on the part of an individual that may exacerbate a painful condition and result in chronicity. The chronic pain patient may suffer from debilitating anxiety and other physical and psychological symptoms without recognizing that they are in response to a traumatic event. The Impact of Events Scale–Revised provides a structured way for an individual to communicate distress and allows the clinician to identify ways in which a traumatic event may be complicating a chronic pain or sleep dysfunction

or may be creating its own set of psychological symptoms. Studies have shown that this tool is valuable in identifying symptoms of posttraumatic stress disorder (PTSD) and other less intense forms of stress and can help identify the impact such stress is having on an individual.[46,47] The 7 items added to the original Impact of Events Scale are related to the hyperarousal symptoms of PTSD. Subjects are asked to identify a specific stressful or traumatic event and indicate the level of distress they have felt over the past 7 days by each item on the questionnaire. The scale has several subscales to measure intrusion, avoidance, and hyperarousal. The original authors recommended utilizing the data collected from this scale to compare to findings from the SCL.

THE INTERACTION AMONG SLEEP DISTURBANCE, PAIN, AND MOOD DISORDERS

It has been established that pain and sleep have a circular relationship, in that chronic pain may cause sleep fragmentation and sleep fragmentation often leads to increased complaints of pain the following day. Circadian rhythm also may play a role in pain perception and expression, although studies often do not control for circadian patterns. There is some clinical evidence that there is a circadian pattern to some common pain problems. For instance, arthritis pain and certain types of headaches tend to peak in the morning, whereas fibromyalgia and myofascial pain syndromes and neuropathic pain seems to peak mid-afternoon to evening. There are also other types of headaches that occur during sleep.[48–50] Additionally, pain responses that occur in non-rapid eye movement (NREM) versus rapid eye movement (REM) sleep are different in experimental models. Studies have shown that higher pain intensity is needed to disrupt sleep during N3 and N4 sleep and during REM sleep than during N2 sleep.[51] Evidence shows that a loss of N3 and N4 NREM sleep can be associated with increased daytime sleepiness, fatigue, and change in pain perception.[52,53]

Pain research has revealed that pain may be gated in some fashion in normal individuals during sleep. Several studies have shown that when a brief electrical stimulation is applied to a cutaneous nerve, it did not evoke a cortical potential, suggesting that sleep interrupts sensory processing in higher brain centers.[54–56]

Another method that may be considered in an attempt to understand the relationship of sleep, pain, and mood is a diary in which the patient records their time of bedtime, awakenings during the night, time of morning final awakening, daytime naps, time of medication over a 24-hour period, pain levels, exacerbating factors, and related behaviors. Though this method requires diligent patient compliance and appropriate data interpretation, it may offer insight into the relationship between sleep and pain in an individual patient.

HOW PAIN IMPACTS POLYSOMNOGRAPHY

Sleep and pain share a reciprocal relationship and, as such, it can be difficult to sort out components of each in order to create an effective treatment program. Polysomnography (PSG) may offer some additional clues, if the patient is sent for further evaluation by a sleep lab. However, there may be parameters that are macrostructural and microstructural that are measured during a PSG that may be problematic during interpretation regarding the effect pain has on sleep. Okura et al[57] noted that chronic pain patients sleep an average of 1 hour less than age- and gender-matched sleepers. They also noted that those who got less than 6 or greater than 9 hours of sleep per night tended to report increased pain levels the following day. However, care must be taken in interpreting this variable to assure that total sleep time is due to a natural sleep pattern and not to poor sleep habit.

Okura et al[57] also noted that, although normal sleepers cycle from NREM to REM sleep approximately every 90 to 110 minutes for 4 to 7 cycles per night, chronic pain patients seem to have only approximately 3 cycles per night.

A delay in sleep latency greater than 20 to 30 minutes is often seen in patients who suffer from acute and chronic pain and there may be a shorter latency to REM sleep onset. The shorter REM latency is also often seen in depressed patients. Chronic musculoskeletal pain is also associated with a decrease in the duration of N3 and N4 and an increase in N1, which is normally considered a transition stage between wakefulness and sleep. There also seems to be an increasing shifting from one sleep stage to the next in patients with chronic pain, which Okura et al[57] reported to be an indication of decreased sleep stability.

The Okura et al study also found that total sleep efficiency was reduced from 91% in normal controls to approximately 78% in chronic musculoskeletal pain patients, as well as those with other painful conditions including irritable bowel syndrome, fibromyalgia, and rheumatoid arthritis.[57]

The role of microarousals, respiratory disturbances, and movement intrusions can also be significant factors in sleep fragmentation. These factors are the most usually reported in a PSG report and are often used to characterize poor sleep.

A microarousal is defined as an event that lasts from 3 to 10 seconds and is accompanied by increased EMG activity, changes in heart rate, and electroencephalogram (EEG) desynchronization. Normal subjects average 8 to 15 microarousals per hour, but this number may vary with age. These microarousals can be related to respiratory disturbances such as sleep apnea, brief hypopneic–apneic episodes, and upper airway resistance syndrome (UARS) or airway insufficiency. Increased frequency of microarousals is known to be associated with changes in physiological function, but has also been related to increased levels of chronic pain and chronic fatigue. Sleep continuity and sleep architecture are disrupted by periodic body movements, including restless leg/legs syndrome (RLS) or periodic limb movement (PLM), with increased frequency in patients with fibromyalgia or rheumatoid arthritis.[57]

Alpha intrusions seen on EEG have sometimes been reported in patients with fibromyalgia; however, studies have failed to link the association.[58–60] Instead, it appears that women with fibromyalgia present with more cyclic EEG K-complexes and fewer sleep spindles per minute than normal subjects. Sleep spindles, generated in the thalamo-cortex, usually act as a buffer to external influences in an effort to maintain the continuity of sleep. In women with fibromyalgia, the elevated number of K-complexes in the absence of sleep spindles may explain the poor maintenance of sleep. In addition, the rise in sleep arousals tend to occur as cyclic alternating patterns; that is, they cluster together or occur in sequential phases in chronic pain patients, indicating a compromised sleep pattern. This sleep fragmentation leads to reports of increased fatigue and decreased cognitive function.[61–63]

Activation of the brain and the autonomic nervous system may be abnormal during a sleep cycle of a chronic pain patient. During increased activity or during periods of hypervigilance, cardiac and brain activity is elevated, indicating increased levels of sympathetic tone. This increased sympathetic activity is also seen to be elevated during REM sleep, when a sleeper is experiencing muscle hypotonia, as indicated by increased cortical and cardiac activity in a normal sleep pattern. During NREM sleep, however, there is decreased cardiac activity, especially during N3 and N4 sleep, which is associated with the lowest level of sympathetic tone. This phase is characterized by the predominance of parasympathetic tone and maximal power of EEG activity. In chronic pain patients, however, there appears to be a dysfunctional persistence of sympathetic activity during sleep and EEG activity tends to exhibit a higher power than in normal subjects.[64] Other factors that can lead to loss of parasympathetic dominance during sleep include aging and acute stress.

GENETIC MARKERS OF POOR SLEEP AND ITS RELATIONSHIP WITH PAIN

The role of genetics in defining the interaction of sleep and pain is poorly understood but is an area of intense research. Current study suggests that unmodulated stimulation of c-fibers that transmit chronic pain may alter gene expression in the neural pathway and can cause mutation of the coding sequence of genes that process both sleep and pain.[65] This further suggests that chronic pain that is left untreated may cause structural changes in the pain pathways and therefore render central processing more sensitive, which leads to increased pain sensitivity and pain perception. Research also shows that when the source of the c-fiber stimulation is removed and pain processing is reduced, these sensory pathways may eventually return to normal over time and therefore result in decreased pain sensitivity.[65] Sleep fragmentation that is associated with the chronic pain experience seems to magnify these changes. Although research is ongoing in this area, it has been suggested that changes in gene expression may play a role in altered pain perception and may cause or contribute to sleep disorders in chronic pain patients.[65] Current research is aimed at identifying specific genetic markers that may be used as a diagnostic tool to target individuals who may be predisposed to increased pain sensitivity.[66-68]

SLEEP AND FIBROMYALGIA

Fibromyalgia is an idiopathic, chronic, noninflammatory, nonarticular syndrome that is defined by widespread musculoskeletal pain and tender points located throughout the body. The syndrome is often associated with sleep disturbances, fatigue, morning stiffness, headache, tempromandibular joint pain, paresthesias, irritable bowel syndrome, and some psychological symptoms including depression and anxiety.[69-71]

Using the 1990 American College of Rheumatology criteria, the prevalence of fibromyalgia in the United States is reported to be 3.4% in women and 0.5% in men.[72] Fibromyalgia is more common in relatives of patients who have the diagnosis, suggesting both genetic and environmental factors.[73]

Sleep disturbance and fatigue are primary complaints of fibromyalgia, and, therefore, careful evaluation of these complaints must be a part of evaluation for this disorder in order to develop the most effective treatment strategy.[74] The patient should be questioned in some detail about the quantity and the quality of his or her sleep. The nature of fatigue should also be delineated. For instance, there is a difference in mental or central fatigue, physical exhaustion, and sleepiness, but the patient may have difficulty distinguishing among these. Inquiry into these different qualities of fatigue may lead the practitioner to different avenues of treatment based upon a more specific definition of fatigue.[75]

For example, complaints of tiredness may be a central fatigue, which is characterized by mental exhaustion with impaired concentration, difficulty with motivation, and complaints of muddled thinking. A contributing factor in this may be psychological symptoms, including anxiety and depression. It is essential to treat these symptoms as part of an overall treatment program for fibromyalgia.

Physical or bodily exhaustion is characterized by depletion of energy stores as a result of physical effort and occurs in the absence of disease or disorder. In patients with fibromyalgia, however, this energy depletion or physical fatigue may occur with a variable decreased amount of physical effort. Individuals with fibromyalgia may report instead, a profound physical exhaustion that makes it difficult for the patient to engage in normal activities of daily living, much less even a moderate aerobic exercise program.

Central or mental fatigue can occur in the absence of sleepiness. Sleepiness is characterized by an overwhelming urge to sleep, and it is only relieved by sleep. The individual with excessive daytime sleepiness may be unable to stay awake during relatively sedentary activities. Excessive daytime sleepiness is a significant health concern and may pose a threat to safety if he or she attempts to drive or operate machinery.

The precise roles that sleep disturbance and fatigue play in fibromyalgia are unclear but must be accurately identified and effectively treated in order to better manage the disorder. Patient self-rating scales, including the Chalder Fatigue Scale, which separates mental from physical fatigue, may be useful in thoroughly evaluating fatigue in any chronic pain patient, particularly those with fibromyalgia.[76]

Although sleep disturbance is known to play a role, the pathophysiology of fibromyalgia remains unclear, and although a number of studies are available, there does not appear to be a clear consensus. Because of the lack of specific laboratory findings or identifiable pathological changes in the central or the peripheral nervous systems, it is difficult to develop systematic research that can adequately address the many variables seen in the fibromyalgia population. However, research is ongoing that has added to the breadth of knowledge regarding this difficult clinical problem.

A number of studies have demonstrated altered pain thresholds and abnormal responses to repetitive noxious stimuli.[77,78] Other studies suggest that fibromyalgia is a complex disorder that involves an interplay of dysfunction in the musculoskeletal, neuroendocrine, and central nervous systems.[79]

Since a key component of fibromyalgia is unrefreshing sleep, it can be helpful to determine contributing factors to this sleep problem. PSG can be utilized to rule out comorbid sleep disorders including sleep fragmentation, sleep apnea, or sleep-related movement disorders such as RLS or PLM. These sleep disorders may cause nonrestorative sleep and result in increased pain sensitivity and increased pain reports the following day. To date, PSG cannot be used to specifically diagnose fibromyalgia, and even though there have been theories that suggested that alpha intrusions on

EEG are a characteristic of the disorder, studies have been equivocal.

Fibromyalgia is known to be associated with sleep disorders, and a number of studies have been conducted to try to clarify the interaction between sleep and pain. Some studies have suggested that fibromyalgia is a chronic stress disorder that may cause changes in dopaminergic and serotonergic function.[80-83] Van Houdenhove et al,[84] McLean et al,[85] and others[86] have studied the role of hormones and found that human growth hormone (HGH), which is primarily secreted in slow-wave sleep (SWS), and cortisol responses were abnormal compared to normal when subjects with fibromyalgia underwent treadmill stress testing.

Several studies have suggested that the hypothalamic-pituitary-adrenal axis may play a role in fibromyalgia.[85-87] Modifications in immune response have been proposed, but recent studies by Landis et al[88] failed to report any modification in peripheral lymphocyte and natural killer cell activity. Substance P and beta-endorphin levels in serum and cerebrospinal fluid have been investigated, but these studies have shown inconsistent results.[89,90] More recently, oxidative stress and nitric oxide have been studied and seem to be involved in the complex pathogenesis of fibromyalgia.[91]

Finally, the role of psychological stress has been widely studied for its role in the development of and exacerbation of fibromyalgia including changes in pain perception and sleep disruption. In fact, fibromyalgia patients have often reported the onset of or exacerbation of symptoms in relationship to stressful events.[92,93] Care must be taken not to assume that the patient's complaints are solely the result of psychological factors because chronic widespread pain may also create psychological stress.

In summary, the pathophysiology of fibromyalgia is likely a complex interaction between sleep disturbance, altered pain perception, and psychological stress.

Symptoms of fibromyalgia may not improve until the underlying precipitating and perpetuating factors are managed. Because sleep disturbance has been implicated in fibromyalgia, it is important for the clinician to evaluate for this and assist the patient in finding relief for this symptom. Treatment should include sleep hygiene counseling consisting of a discussion of sleep schedule, sleep environment, nutrition, medication use, and alcohol and caffeine use. Adding aerobic fitness activities and improving nutrition may help to improve circadian rhythms. Cognitive behavioral therapy probably has a role with patients with this diagnosis.

There are a number of medications that may be useful to help alleviate the sleep disturbance component of fibromyalgia. Caution should be undertaken with medication management of fibromyalgia because certain hypnotic agents may help initiate and maintain sleep but do not tend to lead to restorative sleep, nor do they decrease pain. However, as has been discussed earlier, because of the circular relationship of sleep and pain, if one of these is managed, it will have a positive impact on the other. Medications used to manage sleep in fibromyalgia patients may include the following.

Tricyclic antidepressants (TCA), particularly amitriptyline in a low dose, have been used to manage both pain and sleep. Selective serotonin re-uptake inhibitors (SSRIs) have shown less efficacy in fibromyalgia, but the newer serotonin–norepinephrine re-uptake inhibitors (SNRIs) such as venlafaxine (Effexor) and duloxetine (Cymbalta) have shown better results than SSRIs. Medications that are dopamine agonists such as pramipexole (Mirapex) normally used to manage Parkinson's disease were efficacious in about 50% of fibromyalgia patients in one study,[94] but this medication is known to cause daytime sleepiness and pathological gambling in higher doses. Benzodiazepines can manage sleep disturbances but are not generally recommended because of concerns about drug dependence and tolerance. Non-benzodiazepines such as eszopiclone (Lunesta) or zolpidem (Ambien) seem to be able to increase sleep efficiency, which in turn may lead to decreased pain in fibromyalgia patients. Chlorpromazine (Thorazine), an antipsychotic medication, has been shown to increase SWS, reduce alpha-delta sleep, and decrease pain and improve mood in patients with fibromyalgia; however, there are considerable side effects to this medication, including sedation and slurred speech. Antiepileptic drugs including pregabalin (Lyrica) have been shown to increase SWS and decrease severity of pain and fatigue while improving sleep quality and do not present significant side effects. Melatonin is often cited in naturopathic treatment of sleep disturbance but has shown less/lower effectiveness in improving sleep quality in fibromyalgia patients. Recombinant growth hormone treatment has shown positive results including decreased sleep disturbance, pain reports, fatigue, and dysthymia. Gamma-hydroxybutyric acid (GHB) has shown increased SWS and increased human growth hormone in women with fibromyalgia; however, this drug has significant known side effects.

In summary, effective management of fibromyalgia requires a multidisciplinary approach that considers thorough evaluation and treatment of the precipitating and perpetuating factors involved. Clearly, sleep disturbance is a major component of this disorder, although the precise nature of the interaction of sleep and pain in this disorder remains to be elucidated. Effective management of sleep disturbance is a very important of any treatment strategy for patients with fibromyalgia.

SLEEP AND HEADACHES

Headache is one of the most common patient complaints seen in clinical practice. Though 2 to 3 per 1000 headaches can be associated with a serious disorder,[95] and therefore require a detailed history and thorough evaluation, most headaches are relatively benign.

Although there is a relationship between sleep and headache, the precise mechanism for this relationship remains open to some debate. As headache sufferers are well aware, sleep is a vital component in arresting some types of headache, particularly migraine. However, paradoxically, other headache sufferers report the onset of headache upon awakening in the morning or from a nap. Still others report headache that comes on particularly at night. It seems clear that headache has some interaction with sleep, and the onset of the headache in relationship to a sleep episode is characteristic of particular headache types. Some of the more common variants of headache will be discussed in more detail with particular attention paid to the relationship of headache pain to sleep.

Migraine

Migraine headache is an intense, recurrent, usually unilateral, and often debilitating headache disorder that is associated with autonomic symptoms. Migraine may be preceded by a prodrome hours or days prior to headache onset in 40% to 60% of sufferers. These symptoms may include altered mood, irritability, fatigue, increased yawning and excessive sleepiness, craving for certain foods, stiffness in the neck, hot ears, increased urination, and other visceral symptoms. Approximately 20% to 30% of those who suffer migraines experience an aura immediately preceding the onset of the head pain. The aura can have sensory or motor features.[96] A visual aura is the most common type and may consist of various disturbances including flashes of light, blurred or cloudy vision, or tunnel vision. Less frequently, the migraine aura may present as a paresthesia in the face or upper extremity on the same side as the headache or may present as auditory, gustatory or olfactory hallucinations, temporary dysphasia, or vertigo. The aura tends to develop gradually a few minutes prior to the migraine pain onset but rarely lasts longer than 60 minutes.

A typical migraine is usually described as a unilateral, throbbing, and moderate-to-severe headache that begins gradually then peaks in pain before subsiding. It usually lasts from 4 to 72 hours and is often accompanied by autonomic symptoms including nausea and sometimes vomiting and sensory hyperexcitability manifested by aversion to light, sound, and smell. Generally, the pain is aggravated by physical activity and usually causes at least some level of temporary disability in which the sufferer may lie down in a quiet, dimly lit room. Other autonomic manifestations can include blurred vision, delirium, nasal stuffiness, tinnitus, pallor, or sweating. Tenderness in the musculature of the jaw and neck is the most common finding in migraine headaches and may be considered a causative and perpetuating factor in this type of headache.[97] Once the acute pain of a migraine has subsided, the sufferer may experience a postdrome in which he or she feels soreness in the head, tiredness, or a feeling of being hungover.[98]

There appear to be certain situations that may trigger a migraine event and may include fatigue, stress, hunger, or altered sleep pattern, either not enough or too much. Migraine onset has also been related to the menstrual cycle. Although the true cause of migraine is not clear, it appears to be a neurovascular disorder. A number of theories have been postulated, including changes in serotonin levels that lead to changes in vascular constriction and dilation. It has also been suggested that an inflammatory response caused by increased release of substance P may cause vascular inflammation that results in the pain characteristic of migraines.[98]

Migraine headaches may have their onset at night, and this variation of migraine headache has been found to occur in association with NREM stage 3 to 4 or with REM sleep.[99] In fact, in susceptible individuals, prolonged SWS appears to be a risk factor in triggering an episode. These individuals will report that if they get too much sleep, they are likely to suffer a migraine episode.

More commonly, however, are the individuals who have some level of sleep deprivation that may precipitate an episode of migraine pain. In these individuals, sleep is a necessity in breaking the cycle of migraine pain. Characteristic of this more common migraine is the requirement to seek a dark, quiet, relatively cool room in which to lie down. Eventually, it seems to be a sleep episode that rescues the migraine sufferer. It has been suggested, although evidence is somewhat controversial, that some migraine attacks are related to serotonin metabolism since 5-hydroxyindoleacetic acid excretions, the main metabolite of serotonin, have been found to be increased in urine following a migraine attack.[100] Additionally, sumatriptan, a 5-HT$_1$ agonist that inhibits receptors found in cerebral arteries, and methysergide, an antagonist that has an excitatory effect on 5-HT$_2$ receptors in temporal arteries, are used to abort migraine headaches.[100]

Other studies have shown that hormone secretion that is related to sleep has been found to be abnormal in individuals suffering from migraine. For instance, there appear to be abnormalities in the nocturnal secretion of various hormones, including a decrease in prolactin, an elevation in cortisol, and a delay and decrease in melatonin concentrations.[101]

Because of the intricate relationship of sleep and migraine attack and cessation, it seems evident that proper sleep hygiene is of paramount importance in dealing with this type of headache.

Headaches Associated With Rapid Eye Movement Sleep

There are several types of headaches that appear to be associated particularly with REM sleep. These include

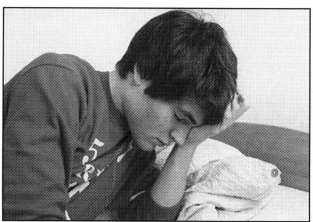

Figure 20-7. Cluster headaches are sometimes called "suicide headaches" because people have taken their lives due to the severity. (From Fotolia.com)

cluster headaches, chronic paroxysmal hemicrania, and hypnic headaches.

Cluster headaches are one of the most severe types of headache with pain from attacks reported as significantly more intense than a typical migraine headache. In fact, cluster headache has been called a "suicide headache" because people have taken their lives during an attack or in anticipation of an attack because of its severity (Figure 20-7).[102] Cluster headache is characterized by an abrupt onset and rapid cessation of perhaps 10 to 30 minutes of severe piercing unilateral head pain, usually in the periorbital, maxillary, or temporal region. Pain is often associated with tearing, rhinorrhea, nasal engorgement, forehead perspiration, and flushing of the cheek. Attacks recur multiple times within a 24-hour period but usually occur at night and have been linked with REM sleep.[103] This type of headache may recur repeatedly over weeks or months and then undergo a spontaneous remission. Though the mechanism of this type of headache is not fully understood, it is known that headaches are associated with a trigeminal-autonomic reflex pathway in the brain stem and are generated by the suprachiasmatic nucleus of the hypothalamus. This may explain the timing of this type of headache because this is where the circadian clock resides.

Cluster headaches are most often triggered in the spring or fall but are not associated with allergies; rather, they are likely results of hypothalamic stimulation related to circadian rhythm. Sleeping late in the morning has also been reported to be a precipitating factor in cluster headache. During a cluster headache period, the individual also seems to be more sensitive to nicotine and alcohol.

Chronic paroxysmal hemicrania is sometimes considered a variant of cluster headache, but attacks are generally of shorter duration and more frequent. This type of headache is characterized by severe unilateral head pain, conjunctival hyperemia, rhinorrhea, and occasionally Horner's syndrome. These headaches usually occur at night and

the individual suffering with this type of headache often reports awakening at the same hour every night with pain. Onset of this headache is usually associated with a REM sleep episode and responds well to indomethacin.

Hypnic headache is a rare idiopathic headache that is observed in older adults, primarily females. Attacks occur exclusively and regularly at night. Head pain from this type of headache is more diffuse and is reported as moderate to severe. Hypnic headache attacks generally last about an hour and usually only occur one time per night. They are not usually associated with autonomic symptoms that are characteristic of migraine, cluster, and paroxysmal hemicrania. Although they have been shown to occur during NREM, onset is usually associated with a REM sleep episode.[104–106]

Headaches Upon Awakening or Morning Headaches

Headaches that occur in the morning or upon awakening are usually reported to be diffuse and are mild to moderate in intensity. These headaches may occur in the early morning and may generally be self-limiting or may develop into or contribute to a tension-type headache or into so-called chronic daily headache. This type of headache may also be reported upon awakening from a nap taken during the day. Some studies suggest that this type of headache is associated with sleep apnea syndrome and report that over half of those identified as having sleep apnea syndrome also report early morning headache.[107] One study reported that successful treatment of sleep apnea syndrome significantly improved this symptom in 30% of patients.[108] A number of mechanisms have been suggested for morning headache associated with sleep apnea including hypoxemia, hypercapnia, changes in cerebral blood flow, and depression. In individuals without sleep apnea syndrome, mechanisms responsible for morning headaches that have been suggested include bruxism, teeth clenching and grinding, temporomandibular dysfunction, systemic hypertension, depression, muscle contraction, alcohol intoxication, and sinus inflammation.[108–110]

Most likely, there are multiple factors that contribute to frequent or chronic morning headache or headache upon awakening (Figure 20-8). Although a number of studies have investigated this type of headache,[111–115] there seems to be no research that has looked at the relationship between cervical dysfunction and headache upon awakening. Even with this dearth of research, it seems worth consideration to investigate the relationship between cervical dysfunction, increased upper cervical muscle tone, and cervical posture during sleep. Because cervicogenic headache is an identified type of headache as classified by the International Headache Society, its potential as a contributory or causative factor in headache upon awakening should receive more attention. Indeed, when one considers the position

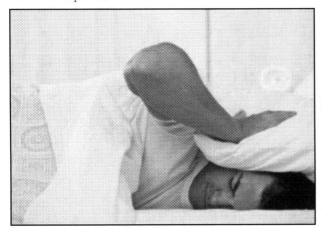

Figure 20-8. Over half of those suffering sleep apnea also report morning headache. (From Fotolia.com)

that the upper cervical spine must be placed in, in order to counteract the collapsibility of the upper airway seen during sleep, particularly during REM sleep, it seems clear that this can cause cervicogenic headache, the symptoms of which one might experience upon awakening.

Cervicogenic headache is one of the most common types of headache and can be a contributing factor in tension-type headache and chronic daily headache. In the author's experience, headaches of cervical origin may also play a role in the precipitation of migraine-like headaches. As such, treatment of this type of headache can significantly improve frequency, intensity, and duration of symptoms in an individual who suffers from headaches. This type of headache also has an intimate relationship with sleep, in that upper cervical dysfunction may exacerbate head and neck pain that may lead to sleep fragmentation. Sleep fragmentation has been shown to be related to increased pain sensitivity and pain perception. In addition, in an individual who has UARS or OSA, cervical posture and positioning may be necessary in an effort to maintain or reestablish an airway during apneic episodes. This posturing, superimposed upon a dysfunctional cervical spine, can lead to increased suboccipital muscle tone, faulty cervical alignment, facet synovitis, and impingement upon upper cervical nerve roots, which supply sensory innervation to the occipital, occipitotemporomaxillary, and supraorbital regions of the head.

In most cases, radiographic imaging studies of the upper cervical spine are found to be normal. Degenerative changes, which may be seen, are often not specifically related to the headache complaints, but may indicate biomechanical dysfunction in the cervical spine. Of greater diagnostic value in determining the existence of cervical involvement in headache is tenderness to palpation. For example, the articular pillars on the affected side are nearly always tender, even when the individual is not suffering an acute headache attack. Prolonged palpation can reproduce the headache referral pattern. Likewise,

compression of the cervical segment will often reproduce the referral pattern, though decompression of that segment will provide relief.

Cervicogenic referral patterns are relatively consistent and are described as occipital, occipitotemporomaxillary, and supraorbital. Occipital headache usually begins in the very top of the neck and back of the head and radiates to the vertex, corresponding with the distribution of the posterior rami of C_2 and C_3. An acute pain episode involving the C_2 nerve root, known as *occipital neuralgia* or *Arnold's neuralgia*, is relatively rare but can be precipitated by forceful or strenuous neck movement. More frequently, occipital headache is associated with dysfunction in the uppermost cervical segments, the occipito-atlantal joints, and the atlanto-axial joint, as well as chronic irritation of the dorsal root ganglion of C_2. This is known to generate a significant cervicogenic headache in the upper neck and occiput. Palpation of the articular pillar on one or both sides is present even when the individual is not experiencing an acute episode. There is also usually tenderness on friction palpation of the posterior scalp, what Maigne described as the "friction sign of the scalp. (p. 3)."[95] There is usually a considerable, often asymmetrical, increase in muscle tone in the suboccipital musculature. Pain is generally exacerbated by upper cervical extension and can often be relieved quickly, but not permanently, by applying distraction to the upper cervical segments.

When one considers the clinical picture seen in occipital headache, it becomes more evident that the prolonged compression or chronic repositioning into cervical extension, as might be seen during sleep apnea or upper airway resistance in order to reestablish the airway, can be a significant factor in cervicogenic headache that manifests itself as headache upon awakening.

Occipitotemporomaxillary headache is a less frequently occurring type of cervicogenic headache characterized by pain located in the retroauricular, mastoid, and parietal region that can radiate into the inferior–posterior mandibular region. This is a region that is innervated by the anterior ramus of C_2 and C_3. Pain is generally mild and often includes tenderness at the angle of the jaw that distinguishes it from trigeminal nerve pain, as the superficial cervical plexus, instead of the trigeminal nerve, innervates this area.

Supraorbital headache is the most frequently occurring cervicogenic-type headache. As the name indicates, pain distribution is usually over the eye socket, but this type of headache is sometimes reported to start in the occipital region and radiate over the top of the head to an area behind the eyes. It also is sometimes reported as retroorbital pain. There is usually a friction sign at the eyebrow on the affected side or it may be positive bilaterally, and there may be similar myofascial restriction and tenderness over the maxilla and anterior temporal region as well. This distribution of pain does not follow a cervical cutaneous distribution; rather, this pain distribution can be attributed to nerve fibers from the trigeminal nucleus, which can descend into the cervical and even upper thoracic spinal cord levels. This type of headache can have a migrainous character, but migraine headache will generally not have these kinds of myofascial signs associated with it. Supraorbital headache may, however, be associated with temporomandibular symptoms, because the pain, tenderness, and friction signs in the face can be misconstrued as muscle spasm in the masseter and temporalis anterior. If the problem is supraorbital cervicogenic headache and there are no true jaw joint problems, successful treatment of the upper cervical spine will often relieve the headache, as well as the temporomandibular symptoms. Supraorbital headache can also have some nasal congestion and occasional unilateral tearing associated with the pain.

Supraorbital headache that is cervicogenic in origin is related to dysfunction in the ipsilateral C_{2-3} vertebral segment. Symptoms are found on the side of segmental involvement, although sometimes pain distribution may be bilateral. Even though this type of headache can have a migrainous character to it, antiserotonin or ergotamine derivatives generally have little effect on pain. An appropriately selected manual therapy maneuver or a facet injection to the C_{2-3} articulation will relieve the pain.

Supraorbital headache can be episodic in nature and can commonly occur upon awakening because of faulty head and neck posture during sleep, possibly as a measure to assist in maintaining a patent airway during sleep. In an individual who has sustained an injury to the upper and/or mid-cervical segments, who has a chronic postural dysfunction or who has a cervical instability or myokinematic dyssynchrony, poor cervical support or upper cervical extension posture at night may precipitate a cervicogenic headache, which will manifest as a classic morning headache. With correction of sustained upper cervical extension posture upon awakening, the symptoms of morning headache are relieved. However, without identification and appropriate treatment, these individuals may continue to suffer and may eventually develop more significant symptoms related to increase myofascial dysfunction and sleep fragmentation.

Cervicogenic headaches are diagnosed based upon mechanical evaluation techniques. Imaging studies are of little use, and findings usually do not correlate with segmental pain distributions. However, a careful history and biomechanical evaluation will help to delineate the problem and direct the clinician to an appropriate intervention.

Given the prevalence of morning headache and the association of a number of different types of headaches with sleep, it is important for the clinician to develop an understanding of this relationship. It is suggested here that there is a mechanical component to many forms of headaches and that this may exacerbate headache pain and may, in fact, mimic symptoms of migraine headache.

This mechanical component can be a factor in the effort to establish or maintain a patent airway during sleep. As such, correction of underlying cervical dysfunction and faulty head and neck posture during sleep may reduce the frequency, intensity, and duration of many different types of headaches and may completely relieve morning headaches.

SLEEP DISORDERS THAT CAN EXACERBATE PAIN

As described earlier, sleep and pain have a circular relationship, in that sleep deprivation or sleep fragmentation can increase pain sensitivity and reduce pain threshold, and increased pain can disrupt sleep and reduce the overall quality of sleep. Both OSA and UARS can be associated with increased pain sensitivity and lowered pain threshold. In some cases, a patient who has classic signs and symptoms of fibromyalgia and later is discovered to have a sleep-related breathing disorder may undergo successful treatment for the sleep disorder and may experience complete remission of his or her musculoskeletal symptoms.

As described in a previous section, headache syndromes often have a relationship to sleep. Cluster headaches may be a consequence of oxygen desaturation that occurs during apnea or hypopnea[117] and have been noted to occur at the same point in the sleep cycle, and this timing may influence the timing of subsequent daytime episodes of cluster headache.[118]

It is unclear what the relationship between sleep apnea and migraine attacks is, but one study by Paiva et al[119] showed that treatment of OSA with nasal CPAP was reported to eliminate migraine headaches.

Rains et al,[116] Idiman et al,[120] and Poceta and Dalessio[114] have all studied the relationship between OSA and so-called morning headache. As described earlier, we postulate here that this type of headache is related to cervical posture adopted in order to assist in overcoming airway resistance or to establish or maintain a patent airway as seen in OSA or UARS. This cervical extension posture increases the tone in the suboccipital musculature, and especially in the presence of rotation of the head, may lead to asymmetrical upper cervical muscle tone and/or faulty segmental alignment, which is a significant contributing factor to cervicogenic headache. Poceta and Dalessio[114] reported that use of CPAP often resolves this type of headache. It stands to reason that CPAP will maintain a patent airway, making upper cervical extension unnecessary to open the airway and thus eliminating the sustained cervical posture in extension, which is a significant causative factor in cervicogenic headache that is reported in the morning.

Treatment for headaches that may have a sleep-related cause have included application of an appropriately titrated CPAP device during sleep or the use of a mandibular repositioning appliance. These treatment options offer some relief but are not universally helpful in reducing symptoms of headaches with a sleep-related component. Weight loss may improve the OAS or UARS. Other treatments are sometimes suggested, including nasopharyngeal or oromandibular surgery, but the efficacy of such procedures is open to significant debate.

For headaches that have a cervicogenic component, treatment of the cervical dysfunction, including manual therapy of articular structures, treatment of muscle imbalance or dysfunction along the polyarticular chain, can offer significant relief of symptoms, when combined with treatment that identifies and correctly treats any underlying sleep-related breathing disorder that may be contributing to a faulty head and neck posture. In addition to manual therapy and therapeutic exercise to improve cervical alignment and stability, therapeutic exercise aimed at restoring and maintaining postural alignment is important. In order to be able to have correct cervical alignment at night, an individual must be able to establish normal head and neck position during the day. Individuals who must adopt an extension posture at night in order to reestablish or maintain a patent airway may develop a habitual extended upper cervical spine. Not only will this compromise articular and neural structures that may contribute to cervicogenic headache, but the extended posture may increase autonomic nervous system tone. This mechanical input into the autonomic system, combined with the sympathetic tone bias that occurs during sleep apneic events, will further elevate sympathetic tone. Increased sympathetic tone, especially when it is chronic, is generally unhealthy and inefficient and can lead to adrenal overdrive and general breakdown of bodily function. Though sympathetic tone and parasympathetic tone tend to reciprocate, in that when sympathetic tone rises, parasympathetic tone tends to drop, this is not always the case. Additionally, though chronically increased sympathetic tone is thought to be generally unhealthy, chronically increased parasympathetic tone is not thought to offer health benefit. In fact, as sympathetic tone rises, there tends to be a rise in the resting tone of the parasympathetic system. In order for the sympathetic and parasympathetic systems to respond effectively, they need to rest somewhere in a mid-range. In fact, it has been suggested that some of the "20th-century diseases" such as chronic fatigue syndrome, fibromyalgia, environmental and food sensitivities, and depression are largely caused by this chronic elevation of both sympathetic and parasympathetic tone.

It seems clear from this discussion that protecting the patency of the airway during sleep is an important consideration when dealing with an individual who suffers from a chronic pain condition. In order to effectively establish and maintain the airway that is somewhat compromised during sleep, one must consider the normal arthrokinematic and myokinematic function of the head and neck. Assessment

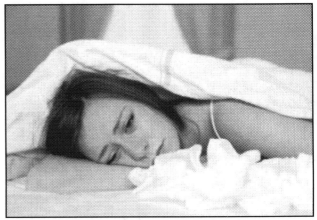

Figure 20-9. Chronic rhinitis may result in sleep fragmentation or sleep-related breathing disorders. (From Fotolia.com)

of cervical alignment, suboccipital tone, muscle balance and stability, and normal movement patterns can be an important component of successful management of headaches that seem to have a sleep-related component.

RHINITIS AND SLEEP

Rhinitis is much more commonly known as a *stuffy nose* and is associated with chronic or acute irritation and inflammation of the mucous membranes that line the nose, which may be due to a virus, bacteria, or irritant. In addition to nasal congestion, there may be excessive nasal mucus and/or a postnasal drip. Rhinitis has been associated with sleeping problems as well as symptoms and problems involving the nose, ears, throat, and eyes.[118] It is caused by increased histamine, which is most often triggered by airborne allergens that irritate the mucosal membranes and increase fluid production.

Chronic rhinitis may disturb respiration during sleep because of increased resistance to nasal breathing (Figure 20-9). These studies suggesting ventilation with oral versus nasal breathing found that ventilation was significantly greater with nasal breathing. The study suggests that there are receptors in the nasopharynx that may have a stimulatory effect on muscle tone in the oropharynx.[122-124] Studies have also shown that the phasic activity of the upper airway muscles is higher with nasal ventilation versus mouth breathing.[123]

Chronic increased nasal resistance has been correlated with increased sleep fragmentation and studies show that increased nasal congestion may worsen sleep-related breathing disorders.[121] Treatment of acute or chronic rhinitis is aimed at decreasing obstruction and may include nasal steroids and other inhalant medications. Other successful treatments may include use of radio frequency to reduce nasal turbinates or other surgical procedures to clear obstruction and normalize nasal breathing.

Chronic rhinitis in children deserves special mention, since decreased or absent nasal breathing during sleep in children can significantly affect craniofacial growth, leading to underdevelopment of the mid-face. It is also possible that genetic underdevelopment of the mid-face is the cause of chronic nasal breathing difficulties. As will be discussed in Chapter 25, this can result in significant changes in the structure and function of the temporomandibular joints, increased prevalence of snoring and development of sleep-disordered breathing, abnormal orthodontics, and bruxism. Sleep disturbance during childhood has been linked to behavioral issues, attention-deficit disorder, memory, concentration and learning problems, and performance deficits.[126]

BRUXISM AND OBSTRUCTIVE SLEEP APNEA

Bruxism literally means gnashing of the teeth. It is characterized by involuntary parafunctional muscle activity in the jaw musculature that results in jaw clenching and tooth grinding during sleep. Clenching that occurs during periods of wakefulness rarely involves teeth grinding, but may include significant jaw clenching and is sometimes termed *rhythmic masticatory muscle activity* (RMMA) or oromandibular myoclonus. Sleep bruxism, which rarely occurs during REM sleep, can be distinguished from jaw clenching during wakefulness. It usually involves rhythmic jaw activity with 3 or more bursts of muscle contraction at a frequency of 1 Hz. Grinding of the teeth is rare in REM sleep, which helps to differentiate sleep bruxism from RMMA or oromandibular myoclonus. Consequences of sleep bruxism can include destruction of teeth, temporomandibular dysfunction, and pain in the jaws, face, or head upon wakening.[127] Clenching and bruxism has been reported in individuals with disordered sleep, as well as in those with normal sleep patterns. Sleep bruxism is more commonly seen in individuals who suffer from increased anxiety and who smoke, and may be diagnosed at any age. Bruxism may also be associated with increased microarousals and is seen with increased frequency in individuals with OSA and UARS, although there remains debate regarding this relationship. In individuals with sleep apnea, it has been suggested that bruxism may help to prevent pharyngeal collapse. Sleep bruxism is usually managed with an oral device, medication, and/or psychological treatment to help manage anxiety disorders. Oral appliances are effective in tooth protection, but debate remains as what specific type of dental device is best for management of bruxism, and there is some discussion regarding the likelihood of these devices actually increasing teeth clenching. Some dental devices have actually been shown to exacerbate sleep-related breathing disorders.[128]

Sleep bruxism in children is reported to occur at twice the rate seen in the adult population. Given the potential relationship to sleep-related breathing disorders and the long-term consequences of sleep fragmentation in children, it is reasonable to have a child with sleep bruxism thoroughly evaluated. Evaluation of the airway is an important part of this and should include examination of the impact of tonsils and adenoids on the patency of the airway. Medication is not usually recommended in the management of childhood sleep bruxism, and oral devices must be evaluated regularly in order to allow for normal growth and development of bone and teeth.

RESTLESS LEG/LEGS SYNDROME AND PERIODIC LIMB MOVEMENT DURING SLEEP

Karl Ekbom first described RLS as a sensorimotor and a sleep disorder.[129] Attempts to clearly describe symptoms of the syndrome have continued to elude clinicians and sufferers alike. It is known to be an ill-defined dysesthesia characterized by an irresistible urge to move in an attempt to assuage uncomfortable sensations, usually in the legs, although the symptoms can occur in the upper extremities, torso, or genitals.[130] RLS is variably described as an aching, an "itch that I can't scratch," a crawling sensation under the skin, or "a snake under my skin." The sensation generally begins or intensifies when the sufferer is sitting quietly or lying down and seems to intensify as bedtime approaches. The timing of the onset or intensification of symptoms seems to indicate a potential circadian component to the disorder.[131] The sensation produces a sense of restlessness and an almost irresistible urge to move. Movement, however, only provides temporary relief from symptoms, and the irritating sensation tends to recur within a few minutes. Sufferers may try a number of other alternate sensory inputs to relieve symptoms, which afford only short-term relief. The degree of symptoms may also vary widely from individual to individual, with some reporting minor annoyances, and others reporting significant and debilitating symptoms with major sleep disruption, depression, and diminishment in quality of life (Figure 20-10).[132]

The prevalence of RLS in the general population is 7% to 10%, with slightly higher prevalence in Caucasians and lower prevalence in those of Asian descent. There appears to be a genetic component to the disorder as there is an autosomal dominant pattern of inheritance, although an autosomal recessive pattern with a high carrier rate has also been suggested.[133–135]

Although a genetic link has been explored, the precise etiology of RLS remains unclear. Research has shown homeostatic dysregulation of iron in the central nervous

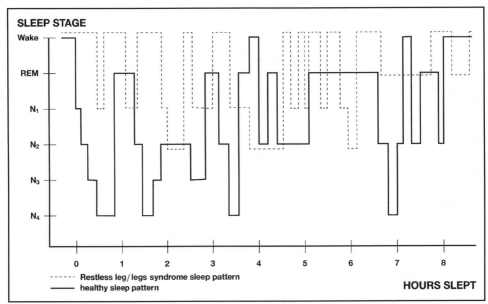

Figure 20-10. Sleep pattern of a restless leg/legs syndrome patient (dotted line) versus a healthy sleep pattern (solid line). X-axis shows hours slept; Y-axis shows stage of sleep.

system. Individuals diagnosed with RLS have shown a decreased level of ferritin in their cerebrospinal fluid and decreased iron stores in the red nucleus and striatum as seen on MRI studies of the brain.[136–138] Iron is necessary for the production of dopamine, and iron depletion has been shown to decrease the number of postsynaptic dopamine receptors.[139] Both iron and levodopa, a dopamine precursor, cross the blood–brain barrier and are metabolized into dopamine and other catecholamines in the brain and have shown usefulness in treatment of symptoms of RLS.[140]

RLS may also to be related to other primary disorders, including any disorder leading to iron deficiency, peripheral neuropathy, diabetes, metabolic disturbances including folate deficiency or magnesium deficiency and hypoglycemia, uremia, varicose vein, thyroid disease, Parkinson's disease, or fibromyalgia. It has been associated with certain autoimmune disorders such as rheumatoid arthritis, Sjogren's syndrome, and celiac disease. It also has been linked to sleep apnea. Some medications have been shown to cause secondary RLS or worsen symptoms including antihistamines, dopaminergic antiemetics, serotonin reuptake inhibitors, antipsychotics, and certain anticonvulsants and dopamine antagonists.

RLS is a clinical diagnosis to be distinguished from periodic limb movement disorder (PLMD), which requires evidence on PSG and is associated with sleep disturbance. PLMD is an involuntary limb movement that occurs at periodic intervals 20 to 40 seconds apart. These episodes disrupt sleep and are generally seen during the first part of a night's sleep. Limb movements do not occur during REM sleep. Patients with PLMD often report excessive daytime sleepiness, trouble falling asleep at night, and difficulty

staying asleep throughout the night. RLS and PLMD are not mutually exclusive.

Treatment for RLS should be based upon symptoms and response to treatment. Underlying and associated disorders should be identified and treated. Individuals who are iron-deficient should receive iron supplementation as appropriate. Dopamine agonists can be effective and the non-ergoline derivatives such as pramipexole (Mirapex) and ropinirole (Requip) are usually selected because of limited side effects. Unfortunately, over time all dopamine agonists become augmented, in which the onset of symptoms shifts earlier, requiring increasing frequency of dosing of medication in order to control symptoms. Rebound and tolerance may also become a problem with this type of medication, and careful pharmacological management is necessary in order to maintain the best symptom control and prevent sleep fragmentation that may be part of these syndromes.

A difficulty arises in effective treatment of RLS in that there may be confusion on the part of the clinician as to cause versus effect. That is, loss of sleep due to RLS could cause weight gain, depression, or symptoms like ADHD, or the medication used to treat these conditions could cause RLS. Considerable care must be taken when evaluating the benefit of treatment for RLS.[141,142]

RLS also occurs in children, although it may be considerably underrecognized. A child may wake up crying and complaining of pain in a leg, but because the child may be unable to fully articulate the dysesthesia that he or she is feeling, the complaint may be called "growing pains" and be dismissed. A parent may notice a pattern of pain complaints, but may not recognize its significance and not report it effectively to the child's pediatrician. However, when a child reports this complaint repeatedly, especially at night or in the evening, a review of family history for RLS is warranted. Walters et al[143] reported that of 138 adults diagnosed with RLS, 43% reported onset of symptoms before the age of 20. RLS in children can be misdiagnosed as ADHD.

INSOMNIA AND PAIN

Insomnia is one of the most common sleep disorders, affecting as many as 27% of the adult population according to a Gallup poll conducted for the National Sleep Foundation (Figure 20-11).[144] Insomnia is defined as poor-quality and usually nonrestorative sleep that is characterized by extended time falling asleep of greater than 30 minutes, difficulty maintaining sleep in which the sufferer awakens during the night and has difficulty falling back to sleep, or short sleep, in which the sufferer awakens in the early morning hours and is unable to return to sleep. Transient insomnia may last 1 to 3 consecutive nights. This type of insomnia is extremely common in adults and can be a result of stressful events in a normal life. Insomnia may be termed short-term insomnia, which may last for up to a month. The far more problematic form of insomnia is the chronic variety, in which the insomnia may last for more than a month.

According to Roth, who helped to write guidelines for the American Academy of Sleep Medicine, the diagnostic criteria for insomnia include "(1) difficulty falling asleep, staying asleep or nonrestorative sleep; (2) this difficulty is present despite adequate opportunity and circumstance to sleep; (3) this impairment in sleep is associated with daytime impairment or distress; and (4) this sleep difficulty occurs at least 3 times per week and has been a problem for at least 1 month."[145]

Risk factors for insomnia include gender, with women affected 1.5 times more than men. Paradoxically, there can be difficulty initiating or maintaining sleep as a consequence of sleep apnea or other sleep-related breathing disorders. Depression may be a factor in insomnia; however, insomnia may also cause or worsen symptoms of depression. The incidence of insomnia also increases with age. Medication that may interfere with sleep onset or sleep maintenance tends to be more prescribed in an aging individual. Comorbidities of aging, including depression, can increase sleep fragmentation with reduced or absent SWS and decreased REM sleep. Several studies suggest that up to 40% of chronic insomnia may be related to psychiatric disorders.[146] Alzheimer's disease and other forms of dementia cause sleep fragmentation in early stages of the disease and may cause frank circadian disorders, with the sleep-wake cycle markedly disturbed as the disease progresses.

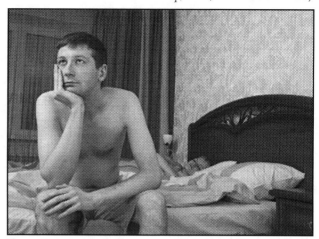

Figure 20-11. Insomnia affects as many as 27% of adults. (From Fotolia.com)

Parkinson's disease is also known to cause problems with initial insomnia and difficulties with sleep maintenance.

The consequences of insomnia are similar to those occurring with other problems of nonrestorative sleep, including daytime fatigue, irritability, decreased memory, and poor concentration. Overall, there is a sense of a nonrestorative nature to sleep.

Comorbid insomnia and depression can have a very significant effect on pain sensitivity, tolerance, and perception. A survey study of pain clinics reported that 50% to 88% of patients who suffer from chronic pain also report impaired sleep.[147] Insomnia has been reported to correlate with higher pain intensity and greater levels of depression and anxiety.[148] However, higher pain levels are also reported in individuals who suffer from insomnia without depression. This is consistent with studies and patient reports of increased pain the day following a night of poor-quality sleep.

Treatment for chronic insomnia requires a careful assessment of the individual, and it may be necessary to institute a multidisciplinary approach that addresses all of the psychophysiological components of the disorder in order to find the approach that is most effective and individualized to the patient.

There have been many studies that have sought to investigate the relationship between sleep and pain, although the precise mechanisms subserving both remain unclear. There is evidence that neurotransmitters and neuropeptides involved in the onset and maintenance of sleep are involved in the modulation of pain, pain perception, and pain tolerance. For example, multiple studies have shown that there is a correlation between pain and serotonin levels, although its role in pain tolerance and pain perception is open to continued study, and the precise mechanisms in pain and sleep are yet to be defined. In addition, analogues of adenosine, which is a sleep promoter, have been administered both systemically and at the spinal cord level and have produced pain suppression in rodents.[149] Other studies correlating the neurochemistry that serves pain pathways and interactions with sleep pathways are ongoing.

Patients suffering from various types of chronic pain conditions may also be suffering from a sleep disorder. Failure to address one side of this equation may result in poor or inadequate control of the other. It has been shown that there is a circular relationship between sleep and pain; therefore, each must be considered in effective patient management. Even though there is a well-known interrelationship between sleep and pain, with the impact of one worsening the symptoms of the other, it is suggested that both pain and sleep disorders be evaluated separately in order to determine whether there is an independent cause of one or the other that may be a contributing factor in the other. Some of the causes of sleep disturbance are more obvious, like OSA or insomnia, but a careful history and physical assessment can help to identify some of the more subtle contributors to the sleep and therefore pain problem.

PEDIATRIC PAIN AND SLEEP

Pain in children may be limited to everyday bumps and bruises that are a natural part of active childhood play or the occasional traumatic event, such as a broken bone as a result of a bicycle mishap. Like acute pain in adults, these events are usually self-limiting and pass without significant disability. Chronic pain in children may occur as the result of systemic disease such as sickle cell anemia or juvenile rheumatoid arthritis. It also may occur without clear etiology, as is the case with chronic pediatric headache syndromes. Chronic pain in children is often associated with mood disorders, functional disability, and pain-related interference in academic performance, peer and social functioning, and parental burden.[150] Chronic pain in children may also interfere with social functioning, leading to isolation and impaired emotional development. It may also result in increased anxiety and depression, which leads to poor quality of life and disability. Studies also indicate that chronic pain that develops in childhood is likely to persist into adulthood.

Although sleep may appear to be a random event occurring sporadically throughout the life of an infant or young child, it is, in fact, a highly complex and well-regulated process. Sleep changes dramatically across infancy and childhood into young adulthood. For example, newborns sleep an average of 16 to 20 hours per 24-hour period with no differentiation between day and night. They show prodigious amounts of REM sleep of up to 50% of the sleep cycle compared to approximately 25% REM in normal adult sleep. During the first year of life, the infant begins to develop a cyclical nature to the sleep pattern, sleeping an average of 14 to 15 hours per 24-hour period by 4 months, but this may decrease to 13 to 14 hours per 24-hour period by 6 months of age. During infancy, it is common for the child to require 2 to 3 naps during the day, with most sleep occurring over night as the child begins to develop circadian rhythms to the sleep cycle. By 9 months of age, 75% of infants are able to sleep through the night. Daytime napping decreases as the child passes from toddler to preschooler. Napping usually disappears altogether by the age of 5 years.[126]

Sleep disturbances are not uncommon in children, as any parent can readily attest, and may occur in 20% to 25% of normal, healthy school-age children.[149] However, when sleep disturbance becomes chronic and the child also has an underlying medical problem that produces chronic pain, the sleep disturbance can significantly complicate the pain problem. Sleep patterns in children must be assessed using both subjective and objective measures. Actigraphy may be a more appropriate objective measure of sleep in a child than PSG because of the sensors and electrodes required for PSG may not allow for a naturalistic valid test. Actigraphy is a relatively noninvasive method of measuring rest–activity cycles. It consists of an actimetry sensor that is usually worn around the wrist and measures gross motor activity. For the most accurate clinical picture of sleep patterns in a child, a number of measures should be undertaken, including subjective retrospective report of sleep, objective report of sleep pattern by a parent or caregiver, prospective sleep diary, and actigraphy. This may help to account for discrepancies in various reporting methods.

Sleep disturbances across childhood are relatively common, as noted earlier, and generally vary according to developmental phase. Newborn sleep issues are usually explained by the discrepancy between the parental desire for sleep and the normal polycyclic nature of infant sleep. Sleep issues may develop if the infant is unable to initiate sleep unless certain conditions are present, such as rocking or feeding, or if the infant is unable to self-soothe in order to return to sleep upon awakening during nighttime sleep. Parents sometimes inadvertently create these conditions by not allowing the infant the opportunity to learn self-soothing by intervening the minute the child begins to stir or cry. It is an important skill for any infant or child to learn to self-soothe in order to initiate sleep or return to sleep if they awaken during the night. For more information about self-soothing and its relationship to sensory integration (see Chapter 23).

Toddlers and preschool age children may develop a sleep-onset problem including limit-setting sleep disorder, in which the parent or caregiver does not set adequate limits regarding bedtime. If the child is allowed to stall or refuse to go to bed or requires increasing numbers of "curtain calls" prior to finally going to sleep, sleep onset can become later and later, resulting in inadequate sleep quantity. Other sleep disorders may begin to make an appearance at this time including sleep walking and sleep terrors. During middle childhood, there can be an increase occurrence of nightmares and anxiety-related sleep onset issues.

As the child reaches adolescence, sleep architecture has developed into that resembling that seen in adulthood. Some research using polysomnographic analysis suggests that healthy youth require approximately 9.25 hours of nighttime sleep to maintain optimal alertness during the day.[151,152] Even though it appears that adolescents generally require more sleep than adults to achieve optimal function, they very often get an insufficient amount of sleep for the substantial physiological demands of puberty. Additionally, there is also a shift in sleep circadian cycle to that resembling a delayed sleep phase syndrome, much to the annoyance of parents and teachers. Other sleep disorders may develop during adolescence including RLS and PLMD. Sleep-related breathing disorders or UARS may become more problematic because of problems with enlarged tonsils and adenoids.

Special populations, including children with developmental disorders, medical conditions, or emotional or behavioral problems, are at increased risk for developing sleep disorders. As in adults, the interrelationship between sleep and pain is a circular one, so it is important to understand the nature of the interference that pain and sleep may produce in the life of the child in order to treat them effectively.

The consequences of poor sleep quality or quantity in children can be substantial, and because of the rapid development of the young nervous system, the adverse effects of sleep disruption or sleep deprivation may be more deleterious than in the adult population. Although research considering consequences of sleep deprivation and sleep disruption in children has lagged behind adult research, there have been some significant findings recently regarding this. Sadeh reported that a consequence of sleep loss in children is a compromise in neurobehavioral functioning, learning, and academic performance.[153] This is especially true if the "neurobiological tasks challenge executive control, attention regulation and working memory."[152] A number of other recent studies support the notion that sleep loss in children is a significant contributor to symptoms of attention-deficit/hyperactivity disorder (ADHD).[154-161] Some of these studies suggest a relationship between sleep-related breathing disorders or PLM and ADHD. Gozal reported that children who were performing in the bottom quarter of their first-grade class who were treated for OSA improved their academic performance by a full letter grade and those who were not treated showed no scholastic improvement.[162] The Tucson Children's Assessment of Sleep Apnea found that of the 1219 children assessed between the ages of 6 and 12 years old who had learning problems were 2.4 times more likely to snore, 2.5 times more likely to have excessive daytime sleepiness, and 5.7 times more likely to have an apneic event observed by a parent.[163] A study conducted by Chervin et al showed

that tonsillectomy and adenoidectomy in children ages 2 to 13 reduced symptoms of sleep-related breathing disorders by 25% and over half of the children no longer met the criteria for ADHD.[164]

Apart from the neurobehavioral problems, children with OSA may have similar consequences as their adult counterparts. Cardiovascular consequences can include hypertension, ventricular hypertrophy, cor pulmonale, and pulmonary hypertension. There are several studies investigating the relationship of hypertension in children with OSA. The conclusion that can be drawn from these studies is that the longer OSA remains untreated, the increased negative effects may be seen on autonomic nervous system function and cardiovascular health.[165-167] Children who develop metabolic syndrome have been found to have an increased incidence of OSA.[168] The study conducted by Redline et al showed that sleep-related breathing disorder caused elevation of blood pressure, increased fasting low-density lipoprotein (LDL), and elevated insulin levels.[168] Pro-inflammatory markers known to be related to the development of atherosclerosis are altered in children with OSA including elevated C-reactive protein (CRP), elevated interleukin 6 (IL-6), and decreased interleukin 10 (IL-10).[169,170] Gozal et al also found that these pro-inflammatory markers returned to normal after tonsillectomy and adenoidectomy.[170]

Gozal et al also looked at obese children before and after tonsillectomy and adenoidectomy and found that though there were significant improvements in sleep fragmentation and apneic–hypopneic index (AHI), there was no change in fasting glucose, but there was improvement in insulin levels and significant improvements in HDL, LDL, and CRP.[170] It appears that OSA has a significant impact on components of metabolic syndrome, except for insulin resistance, which is directly related to body mass index.[171]

In addition to these complications of sleep fragmentation and sleep deprivation, children who have specific medical conditions that result in significant chronic pain problems are further compromised by the circular relationship between sleep and pain. This problem presents additional complications in the developing child, especially with regard to growth and the development of the nervous system. There are also some specific pain conditions that occur in children that require more specific attention.

Some Specific Pediatric Pain Conditions

Recurrent Abdominal Pain

Recurrent abdominal pain (RAP) is defined as paroxysmal abdominal pain in children ages 4 to 16 that persists for more than 3 months and negatively impacts normal activities of daily living (Figure 20-12). It is often called *functional bowel disorder* because no specific structural,

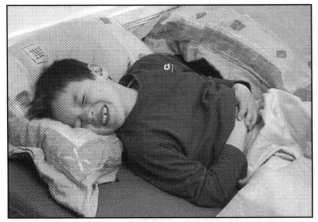

Figure 20-12. Children suffering from recurrent abdominal pain frequently suffer sleep disturbances. (From Fotolia.com)

infectious, inflammatory, or biochemical cause can be found to explain the pain. It is a description of the prominent clinical manifestation of a more precisely defined organic disorder and is often a diagnosis of exclusion. It has been reported to occur in 10% to 15% of children between the ages of 4 to 16.[172] Children with this disorder have increased sleep disturbances because of pain at sleep onset or awakening due to pain. A child who suffers from RAP and has the additional complication of sleep disruption or sleep deprivation, as discussed earlier in this text, may have additional problems with increased pain sensitivity and neurobehavioral concerns and academic and psychosocial issues that may complicate the symptoms of RAP. Effective sleep management is an important component of overall clinical management of recurrent abdominal pain in children.

Headaches

Headaches that occur during childhood and adolescence have characteristics similar to those found in the adult population. A survey study reported a significantly higher occurrence of sleep disturbance, including awakenings, bruxism, and snoring and an increase in reported daytime sleepiness than a population with no complaints of headache population.[173] Just as in the adult population that suffers from headaches, children may have disrupted sleep because of pain or may need additional sleep to help with headache symptoms. The issue of chronic sleep deprivation that may be due to social, athletic, and school functions may play a role in this pain cycle. A careful history and sleep diary may reveal significant aberrations in sleep hygiene in children who suffer from headaches. Improving sleep hygiene, reducing activities in the overscheduled child, and paying close attention to sleep quantity may be an effective step in management of childhood, and especially adolescent, headaches.

Sickle Cell Disease

Sickle cell disease is an autosomal recessive genetic blood disorder that causes a mutation in the hemoglobin gene that is characterized by abnormally shaped red blood cells (RBCs) that are typically rigid and sickle shaped. This abnormality decreases the flexibility of the RBC and results in the manifestations of the disease. Individuals who carry only one sickle cell gene, known as *sickle cell trait*, are afforded better tolerance to infection and are generally less severely involved than those carrying 2 alleles of sickle cell disease. The disease usually presents itself in childhood and occurs more commonly in populations that originate from tropical and subtropical regions where malaria is common. The prevalence of sickle cell disease in the United States is 1:5000. Approximately 1:500 African American children develop sickle cell anemia, a specific form of the disease.[174]

Sickle cell disease may cause a number of acute and chronic anemic conditions. Sickle cell crisis describes acute conditions that can occur and can be lethal. Vaso-occlusive crisis occurs when the abnormally shaped RBCs obstruct capillaries and restrict blood flow to organ systems. This can cause ischemia, pain, and necrosis and often results in organ damage. Treatment involves adequate pain management, hydration, and RBC transfusion. Successfully managed vaso-occlusive crises will resolve in 5 to 7 days. Splenic sequestration crisis results in acute painful enlargement of the spleen because the sinusoids open simultaneously, causing sudden pooling of blood into the spleen, resulting in sudden hypovolemia. This quickly becomes an emergency, and if treatment is not rendered within several hours, the patient can die of circulatory failure. Treatment is supportive and may include blood transfusion. In patients with sickle cell anemia, the spleen is often infarcted during late childhood. In these patients, there is an increased risk of infection from encapsulated organisms. Aplastic crisis is an acute exacerbation of the underlying anemia. This crisis is triggered by the parvovirus B19, which affects RBC production. It invades RBC precursor cells, the reticulocytes, and destroys them and will completely prevent production of RBCs for 2 to 3 days, which is tolerated in a healthy individual. Patients with sickle cell disease, however, have RBCs with a shortened life span, and reticulocytopenia leads to an abrupt and life-threatening drop in hemoglobin. Most patients in aplastic crisis are successfully treated with supportive therapy, though some may require a blood transfusion. Hemolytic crisis occurs in sickle cell patients who also have a glucose-6-phosphate dehydrogenase deficiency (G6PD), which is a metabolic enzyme important in RBC metabolism. Hemolytic crisis causes an increased destruction of RBCs and results in a dramatic and dangerous drop in hemoglobin. Again, treatment is supportive and sometimes includes blood transfusion. Acute chest syndrome, characterized by fever, chest pain, difficulty breathing, and pulmonary infiltrate, can be triggered by a painful crisis, respiratory infection, bone marrow embolization, atelectasis, opioid administration, or surgery.

It is clear from the previous discussion that sickle cell disease can result in a number of painful conditions, and, indeed, pain management is a significant concern in effective management of the disease. Pain from sickle cell disease may be a cause of sleep disruption and therefore may complicate the course of the disease. Children with sickle cell disease have also been shown to have an increased incidence of sleep-related breathing disorders including OSA and UARS.[175,176] Disordered sleep may complicate symptoms of sickle cell disease, and it has been suggested that vaso-occlusive crisis may be triggered by oxygen desaturation that occurs as a result of OSA.[174] For this reason, it is important to evaluate the airway of these children, and Brooks et al have reported that a tonsillectomy and adenoidectomy reduce the risk of vaso-occlusive crisis.[175]

Chronic Musculoskeletal Pain

Chronic musculoskeletal pain in children and adolescents has been reported to coexist with significant sleep fragmentation including significantly prolonged sleep latency, increased arousals and awakenings, decreased REM sleep, increased PLMD, and early morning awakenings, which reduce sleep efficiency.[178-183] This sleep dysfunction is usually accompanied by reports of excessive daytime sleepiness. Chronic musculoskeletal pain may arise from a variety of underlying pathologies including complex regional pain syndrome, juvenile rheumatoid arthritis, and juvenile fibromyalgia syndrome. Poor sleep patterns seen in youth populations associated with chronic pain are often complicated by depressed mood and increased anxiety.[179,184]

A study of adolescent girls with sleep disturbance and chronic musculoskeletal pain conducted by Shao-Yu et al suggested that sleep was not disrupted enough to result in increased pain reports the following day; however, it was also not restorative enough to lead to decreased reported pain the following morning.[185] These studies also hypothesized that youth with chronic musculoskeletal pain who also have increased disruption in sleep are at a greater risk of developing clinically significant psychological symptoms including depression and anxiety. It does also suggest that allowing daytime napping may counteract some of this loss of restorative sleep.[185]

Summary of Sleep, Pain, and Pediatrics

As much as 15% of the pediatric population may suffer from painful conditions that result in increased sleep fragmentation and decreased sleep efficiency. Because of the critical demands of neurocognitive growth and development and later, of puberty, it is imperative that children and

adolescents achieve a normal sleep pattern. When chronic pain conditions interfere with this process, careful consideration must be given to improving the sleep pattern. Some of this is under the control of the parents and the child or especially the adolescent. It is important for parents to encourage the infant and toddler to develop healthy self-soothing habits. These will serve the child well throughout life. When this does not occur, a child may grow into adolescence and even adulthood with specific environmental demands that must be met in order to attain sleep. These can include a specific temperature, certain sounds, and specific light conditions that must exist before the individual is able to fall asleep. These are learned behaviors and can lead to interference with sleep onset or maintenance. If a child is allowed to learn self-soothing without myriad specific conditions and rituals, he or she will have better sleep habits as an adult.

In a child or adolescent who has other factors such as pain that may interfere with sleep onset or sleep maintenance or may cause early morning awakenings, care should be taken to develop good, consistent sleep hygiene and adequately manage pain during the day. This is a particular concern because there is only a limited body of research looking at the efficacy and safety of pharmaceutical agents used for sleep management in children. Additionally, the use of opioids and other analgesic medications has been shown to interfere with sleep. These agents have also received limited research attention in the pediatric population. It is also apparent that chronic pain in children not only leads to sleep disruption but also may be a contributing factor to psychiatric symptoms including depression and anxiety. Each of these symptoms—sleep disruption, chronic pain, and depression and anxiety—must be carefully considered in effective management of the pediatric population.

Because of the circular relationship of pain and sleep disruption, and the potential difficulties associated with use of pharmacotherapy, it is important to consider the value of good basic instruction in proper sleep hygiene. Adolescent populations and their parents and caregivers should also be educated in the importance of normal sleep quantity because there appears to be a significant mismatch in adolescent schedules and activities and the sleep demands for optimal alertness and health.

GERIATRIC PAIN AND SLEEP

As the individual ages, there are normal changes in the sleep pattern, as discussed in an earlier section of this text. In the Established Populations of Epidemiologic Studies of the Elderly (EPESE) report, which studied over 9000 individuals age 65 and older who were living in the community, 43% reported having difficulty initiating sleep, but only 25% reported daytime napping. Increased complaints of sleep disturbance are associated with increased complexities of comorbid medical problems.[186] Pain is often a contributor to sleep disturbance complaints in the older population, with up to 50% of community-dwelling older adults reporting pain problems that interfered with some level of function. Nineteen percent of this population reports pain that results in disrupted sleep.[187,188] Because of the circular relationship between sleep and pain, as described previously, painful conditions experienced in an older population may lead to increased sleep fragmentation, which may, in turn, lead to increased pain sensitivity and decreased pain threshold, resulting in increased pain perception. In addition, changes in normal sleep physiology that occur with aging may render the older adult more vulnerable to subsequent sleep disturbances and the physiological consequences that occur as a result of it. Contrary to some commonly held beliefs, older adults do not seem to have a decreased need for sleep but instead may have difficulty attaining the sleep necessary for optimal alertness and health. Daytime napping may help make up for the decrease in nocturnal sleep.

There are a number of factors that may account for increased sleep fragmentation in an aging population. Normal age-related sleep physiology changes include a decrease in sleep spindle activity, decrease in or even complete loss of SWS, reduction in REM sleep, and decreased arousal thresholds.[189-191] These factors are significantly more pronounced in older adults who reside in institutions or those with increased cognitive impairment in the form of dementia. This is a particular concern in Alzheimer's disease, as is discussed in Chapter 15. Other factors that may contribute to changes in sleep patterns in an older adult include aging of other biological systems, changes in sleep hygiene, increased depression or anxiety, or comorbid medical conditions including chronic pain. Aging of the suprachiasmatic nucleus may account for age-related changes in circadian rhythms, leading to a shift in the sleep–wake cycle known as *advanced phase sleep disorder*. In this situation, the individual will generally be overcome with sleepiness relatively early in the evening and also awaken in the early morning hours. This can be of particular concern for an older individual who does shift work. Older adults with *advanced sleep phase* syndrome will also likely have much more difficulty accommodating to travel between time zones.

Some evidence shows that there are changes in body temperature fluctuation associated with the aging process, in that older adults are more likely to awaken at the point of minimum body temperature, obviously causing increased sleep fragmentation.[192,193] Age-related changes in the urological system contribute to increased sleep fragmentation with increased nocturia.

The older adult may also suffer from increased psychosocial problems, including depression, anxiety, isolation and loneliness, bereavement, and fear of dying. These issues may result in significant sleep fragmentation and decreased sleep efficiency.

Another significant factor contributing to poor sleep quality and quantity in an older adult is comorbid illness, particularly respiratory disease and cardiovascular disease, as well as poorly managed chronic pain conditions. Sleep disturbance in the older adult can be better managed if the underlying comorbidities are well managed.

Chronic pain conditions in the older adult may be the result of a longstanding musculoskeletal condition or because of generalized degenerative changes that occur with aging. Sleep problems related to chronic musculoskeletal dysfunction or degeneration are generally characterized by difficulty initiating sleep, perhaps due to irritation of an inflammatory condition during the day that takes time to settle with rest. Once sleep is established, there may be increased fragmentation as the inflamed joint or muscle is disturbed during position change seen in normal sleep. The individual may awaken early with significant increased stiffness and increased pain because of sleep fragmentation. Additionally, those with degenerative or inflammatory musculoskeletal conditions who also have underlying untreated OSA are likely to have poorer sleep quality, thus leading to increased pain sensitivity and decreased pain tolerance. The overall result is increased pain perception and impaired quality of life.

Headaches tend to decrease in frequency with age, but hypnic headache syndrome occurs particularly in the older adult, as discussed earlier in this chapter. Early morning headaches that occur in the older adult may be related to OSA and are effectively treated with appropriate management of OSA.

Neuropathic pain is known to contribute to sleep disruption in older adults. The most common form of neuropathic pain is postherpetic neuralgia (PHN), with approximately half of the individuals who experience an acute episode of herpes zoster developing this chronic painful condition. These individuals may experience significant pain, which is likely to disrupt sleep. In order to improve sleep disruption, the PHN must be effectively treated. According to a study conducted by Attral et al, medications with well-established efficacy in treatment of postherpetic neuralgia include TCAs, anti-epileptics such as gabapentin and prebabalin, and certain opioids including oxycodone, morphine, and methadone.[191] It is important to treat the underlying pain problem effectively in order to preserve restorative sleep patterns and reduce sequelae of chronic sleep fragmentation.

Sleep dysfunction in the older adult population is frequently treated with administration of sedative–hypnotic medications. These pharmacological agents, however, can be associated with changes in sleep architecture, as will be discussed in the next section. They are known to have a decreased efficacy with chronic usage, and these medications can cause cognitive impairment and are associated with an increased risk of falling. Careful consideration should be given to the use of these medications. In fact, one study indicated that pharmacological treatment of sleep disruption in an older adult tends to lose its efficacy over a longer period of time. However, during the same 2-year follow-up period, a cognitive behavioral approach to sleep disruption showed significant improvements in sleep continuity and efficiency compared to pharmacological therapy.[195]

There is a naturally occurring change in sleep architecture that may impact both sleep quality and sleep quantity as an individual ages. Because of this, comorbid factors that may also lead to sleep fragmentation must be given consideration when implementing a treatment plan for an older adult.

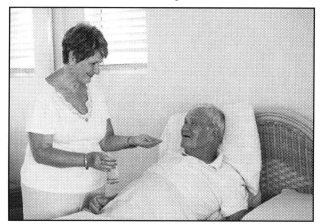

Figure 20-13. Pain medication itself can affect quality of sleep. (From Fotolia.com)

REVIEW OF SLEEP PHARMACOLOGY

As has been discussed, sleep and pain share a circular relationship, in that deficits in quality or quantity of sleep can lead to increased pain sensitivity and increased pain perception. Increased pain perception can further disrupt sleep and a vicious cycle ensues. As an individual ages, they may be more likely to have developed one or more painful conditions, such as are caused by increased degenerative changes in joints and other "wear-and-tear" conditions. This can cause increased pain both during activity and at rest. In fact, a joint that has arthritic changes that has been used all day long may have increased pain at night, thus increasing interference with sleep.

At first consideration and based upon a simple understanding, one may logically conclude that analgesic medication is the answer to the problem of pain-related sleep disturbance; however, there can be an alteration in the quality of sleep produced by administration of pain medication (Figure 20-13). It will be useful to review the pharmacology of sleep in order to gain a better understanding of how pain medication affects sleep quality.

Sleep is normally initiated through NREM, with a cyclical movement through sleep stages of NREM and normally ending with REM sleep. A typical sleep cycle will last 90 to 110 minutes and will contain 75% to 80% NREM and 20% to 25% REM sleep.

The physiological drive for NREM sleep appears to be wake-dependent; that is, the more prolonged the period of wakefulness, the greater the physiological need for NREM sleep. Although the precise mechanism that triggers the onset of sleep remains a subject of study, a naturally occurring change in neurotransmitter tone seems to influence the transition into sleep. One theory suggests that there is a buildup of metabolites in the brain during a period of wakefulness that produces the transition into NREM sleep.[196] Extracellular adenosine, a by-product of adenosine triphosphate metabolism, increases as a result of glycogen

depletion in the cerebral cortex due to prolonged wakefulness. Adenosine suppresses normal neuronal activity in the cortex that occurs during wakefulness and, thus, NREM sleep is initiated. In the real world, this theory is evidenced by the use of caffeine, which promotes wakefulness, since caffeine is an effective adenosine receptor antagonist. Increased adenosine in the central nervous system activates the adenosine A1 receptors, which suppress neuronal activity in structures in the basal forebrain and reticular activating system in the brain stem that are responsible for maintenance of the wakeful state.[197] Suppression of these key structures promotes onset of NREM sleep as GABAergic tone increases in noradrenergic neurons in the locus ceruleus, cholinergic neurons of the parabrachial nuclei of the brain stem reticular activating system, and histaminergic neurons in the tuberomammillary nucleus of the hypothalamus.[198,199] As adenosine release is triggered, neuronal discharge is decreased, resulting in the onset and maintenance of SWS.

SWS activity appears to be affected by the length of prior wakefulness. SWS is homeostatic. It allows for regulation of the internal environment and tends to help maintain a stable, constant condition. Cerebral protein synthesis and glycogen conservation occur during this phase of sleep, and therefore may contribute to metabolic and cognitive recovery related to the prior period of wakeful activity. SWS is also associated with the largest production of human growth hormone, which is responsible for cellular maintenance and various reparative functions. There is decreased synaptic activity during SWS, which may enhance execution in neural circuits because of the change in signal-to-noise ratio with minimized saturation. This may be a factor in enhanced memory across a night's sleep.[200] SWS is generally most prevalent during the first portion of a normal sleep cycle and may be thought of as a recovery mechanism. Because of the restorative function of SWS, there is a prodigious amount of it during infancy and childhood

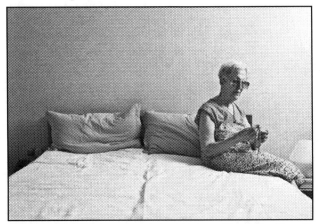

Figure 20-14. REM sleep may decrease in quantity and quality with aging. NREM stage 3 sleep, also known as restorative sleep, may be absent in an older person. In general, sleep quality diminishes and sleep fragmentation increases as an individual ages. (From Fotolia.com)

in response to the great amount of physical and cognitive growth and development.

NREM stage 2 is sometimes thought of as a transition sleep between SWS and REM sleep. NREM2, however, may also facilitate memory processes, particularly sleep spindle activity that occurs during NREM2. This will be discussed in much greater detail in Chapter 21.

REM sleep is characterized by episodic rapid eye movements, muscle atonia, and a desynchronized EEG pattern of low-voltage, high-frequency waveforms. REM sleep is sometimes referred to as *dream sleep* or *circadian sleep* because it is temporally related to circadian rhythms. In the adult, REM sleep is entered into from NREM sleep and the first bout of REM sleep usually occurs 90 to 120 minutes into a normal night's sleep. It may occur earlier in a young adult, and infants are capable of entering into REM sleep directly from a wakeful state. REM sleep density increases during the last third of a normal night's sleep and is concurrent with a decrease in body temperature and blood cortisol level, both of which are under circadian control.

REM sleep is modulated primarily in the brain stem, and transition into REM sleep from NREM sleep is usually associated with a substantial decrease in histaminergic tone and an increase in cholinergic tone. Increase in cholinergic activity influences REM sleep as well as wakefulness; however, during REM sleep, noradrenergic and serotonergic activity is decreased. Pontine cholinergic neuronal activity is facilitated by GABAergic interneurons but inhibited by dopaminergic and norepinephrine input from the pontine-mesencephalic tegmental nuclei and from histaminergic and hypocretinergic neuronal activity in hypothalamic nuclei, turning on REM sleep. There is a reciprocal cycling of pontine cholinergic activity with a monoaminergic neuronal activity during a sleep cycle. This reciprocal activity modulates central nervous system activity and essentially turns REM sleep on while suppressing NREM activity and

allows modulation back into NREM sleep during the cycle. This dynamic balance of inhibitory and excitatory neuronal activity contributes to the cycling of NREM and REM sleep during a normal adult sleep cycle.[199]

REM sleep has been shown to be a state of considerable central nervous system activation as evidenced by increased brain temperature, increased cortical metabolism, and increased cerebral blood flow. REM sleep is thought to be involved in memory enhancement and learning. In addition to increased brain activity, theta wave activity in the hippocampus, which has been shown to be associated with storage of information, is observed to increase during wakefulness and during REM sleep.[201–203] There appears to be a significant correlation between REM sleep and learning, which is seen to occur in prodigious amounts in infancy and youth, which is a time of the most substantial brain development.

Studies suggest that wakefulness is maintained by a combination of cholinergic activity, noradrenergic activity, and dopamine and histamine in the cerebral cortex.[204] Neurons in the lateral hypothalamus containing hypocretin or orexin appear to modulate wakefulness by altering the tone of monoamine neurotransmitters, such as histamine.[205] A decrease in tone in hypocretin or orexin neurotransmitters, which can be a side effect of certain pain medications, can therefore have an effect on wakefulness, experienced as difficulty waking up and excessive drowsiness.

The sleep–wake cycle is also substantially influenced by circadian rhythms, which are largely controlled by the suprachiasmatic nucleus, located in the anterior hypothalamus. This so-called circadian clock receives neuronal and environmental input and is entrained by cyclic changes within the environment, including light–dark cycles and social cues that promote wakefulness or sleep. The suprachiasmatic nucleus utilizes this input to establish the sleep–wake cycle and to allow for coordination of behavioral and physiological responses in a 24-hour cycle. These physiological responses include body temperature, which shows a 24-hour periodicity, reaching its peak at 7 to 10 PM and troughs between 4 and 7 AM. These times correspond to periods of greatest alertness and greatest sleepiness in a normal circadian pattern. There is an additional lesser transient decrease in body temperature, the so-called *circadian dip*, that occurs at approximately 2 to 4 PM and is associated with a well-known afternoon sleepiness experienced by many people.

Aging is associated with increased sleep fragmentation, characterized by increased awakenings, decrease in sleep spindle activity, decreased SWS, and overall decreased REM sleep quantity (Figure 20-14). Sleep efficiency is reduced gradually and generally continuously over the age of 60. This may also be accompanied by a shift in sleep phase, resulting in increased alertness in the early morning and increased sleepiness and sleep drive in the early evening, known as *advanced sleep phase.*

Changes in SWS and the associated reduction in nocturnal release in human growth hormone, especially in males, and reduction in sleep spindle activity may contribute to some of the issues of aging including cognitive decline, truncal obesity, reduction in lean body mass, and impaired exercise response. Decreased REM sleep associated with aging can be accompanied by increased evening cortisol levels, which may contribute to further sleep fragmentation as well as insulin resistance, hippocampal atrophy, and deficits in hippocampal-dependent learning and memory.[196,206]

Neuroregulation of sleep is complex in a normal human adult, but these controls change with aging, changes in environmental cues, illness, introduction of pharmaceutical agents, and pain. Because pain and pharmacological management of pain may have a significant impact on sleep (ie, pain sensitivity and pain tolerance), it is important to understand the effect pharmaceutical agents will have on impact sleep.

The manner in which analgesic medications affect the sleep–wake cycle can be different in a normal adult without an acute or chronic pain condition

Effect of Various Medications on Sleep Architecture

Analgesic agents that are known to have anticholinergic activity logically would promote SWS but inhibit REM sleep. Pain medications that enhance GABAergic tone would be predicted to also promote SWS, and because GABA inhibits cholinergic neurons, this type of pain medication would also be expected to enhance structures that promote REM sleep. Additionally, these medications would be predicted to also inhibit REM sleep.[207–212] Pain medications that selectively enhance monoamine tone, such as SSRIs, would logically be predicted to promote wakefulness and inhibit transition into sleep. In studies of a normal population without acute or chronic pain conditions, this appears to be true. However, in individuals suffering from painful conditions, this does not seem to be the case. It appears difficult to ascertain the precise effect of various medications on sleep architecture and sleep efficiency because of the variety of covariants in studies. However, the following, though not intended to be an exhaustive review of the pharmacology of medications that have an effect on sleep, will give the reader an overview.

Opioids

Opioid medication includes such agents as morphine, codeine, and fentanyl. These medications may be naturally occurring, semisynthetic, or synthetic and are commonly associated with the treatment of moderate-to-severe pain. Opioids bind primarily to 3 classes of opioid receptors in the nervous system, known as mu, kappa, and delta receptors. Mu receptors have 3 important subtypes called mu_1, mu_2, and mu_3. Opioid-receptor-like receptor 1 is another clinically relevant receptor because it is involved in pain responses and plays a major role in tolerance to mu-opioid agonists used in analgesia. These opioids are G-protein-coupled receptors that act on GABAergic neurons. The pharmacodynamic response to an opioid depends upon the receptor site, its affinity for that receptor, and the agonistic or antagonistic character of the opioid. For example, the mu_1 receptor mediates the supraspinal analgesic properties of the opioid agonist morphine, the mu_2 receptor mediates its respiratory depression, constipation, and physical dependence properties, and the kappa-receptor mediates the sedating and spinal analgesia characteristics of the drug.[213] As such, each type and subtype of opioid receptor mediates characteristic and specific neurological responses. Additionally, each opioid has a distinct binding affinity to various types of opioid receptors. These characteristics of opioid receptors provide a mechanism for different opioid agents to exert various effects including variations in duration of action and metabolic breakdown.

Opioids have known sedating characteristics but, in fact, appear to actually disrupt sleep. It is possible that the symptoms of sedation and fatigue associated with opioids may be related to the sleep disruption that they produce. Shaw et al[214] reported that intravenously administered morphine led to decrease in SWS and some decrease in the amount of REM sleep but did not increase sleep arousal or awakenings. Dimsdale et al[215] suggested that even low doses of opioid medications result in an increase in NREM stage 2 sleep and a 30% to 50% decrease in SWS. Moore and Dimsdale[216] found that morphine and morphine-like substances suppress REM sleep and disturb NREM. These studies all evaluated the effects of acutely administered opioids on sleep architecture. Research of opioid medications has been limited and is often carried out in individuals who are currently or previously addicted to opioids. Studies of the effects of opioid use are more difficult because of the obvious difficulty in evaluating it in normal healthy subjects. Long-term opioid use has been shown to be associated with increased sleep-related breathing disorders.[217] It is difficult to make broad-reaching conclusions on the available research across a wide variety of patient populations because of the inherent difficulty and limitation of the available literature and the uncertainty as to whether one can conclude that the effect on sleep is drug related or pain related. Even so, use of opioid agents must be considered in light of sleep disruption issues.

Nonsteroidal Anti-Inflammatory Drugs and Acetaminophen

Nonsteroidal anti-inflammatory drugs (NSAIDs) include medications such as aspirin, ibuprofen, and naproxen. These medications act as nonselective inhibitors of the cyclooxygenase (COX) enzyme. COX inhibits arachidonic acid from converting to prostaglandins and leukotrienes that produce a protective response to cellular injury and mediate inflammation and pain at the site of tissue injury. NSAIDs also have an effect on centrally active prostaglandins that promote arousal by enhancing central histaminergic tone. Other centrally acting prostaglandins may increase adenosine levels, which is known to promote sleep, and it has been suggested that certain prostaglandins may be part of a molecular cascade that triggers the transition from wakefulness to SWS.[218]

Multiple studies of both experimentally induced arthritic conditions in animals and studies of healthy and arthritic adults have been conducted to observe the effect of NSAIDs on sleep architecture. It is known that individuals with arthritis are likely to have fragmented sleep characterized by disrupted SWS and decreased REM sleep. Though it was evident that the NSAIDs were effective in reduction of arthritic pain, there appears to be no evidence that NSAIDs alter the pain-related changes in sleep architecture. It is postulated that COX inhibition decreases centrally active prostaglandins, which may account for the lack of improvement in sleep architecture with use of NSAIDs.[219]

Acetaminophen is a widely used over-the-counter pain medication and antipyretic. The main mechanism of action of acetaminophen is that it reduces the oxidized form of the COX enzyme in the central nervous system, preventing it from forming pro-inflammatory chemicals. It also modulates the endogenous cannabinoid system, thus reducing pain. Even though it has more specific central action, acetaminophen also has little effect on sleep architecture.

Antidepressants

Antidepressant medications are psychiatric drugs that may be prescribed to treat a variety of mood disorders including major depression, dysthymic disorders, and anxiety disorders. These types of medications include several different classes of drugs including monoamine oxidase inhibitors (MAOIs), TCAs, SSRIs, and SNRIs. Though it is well outside the scope of this work to discuss the proposed mechanisms of action of these various medications, it should be noted that they are the subjects of myriad studies with often controversial claims regarding efficacy, risk, and use. A proposed theory for the pathophysiology of depression, described in general terms, states that depression may be caused by an increased sensitivity of the postsynaptic receptor for amine neurotransmitters including norepinephrine and serotonin. Antidepressant medications act in a variety of ways to increase amine transmission, which, in turn, work to overstimulate postsynaptic receptors. This overstimulation leads to a compensatory downregulation and therefore decreased sensitivity of the postsynaptic receptors. As receptor sensitivity decreases, symptoms of depression are relieved.[206] Serotonin may play a permissive role in this downregulation.

Most antidepressants have a delayed onset of action and are usually administered for months to years. In addition to the obvious use of these medications, they have been prescribed for off-label applications including anxiety disorders, obsessive–compulsive disorders, eating disorders, chronic pain disorders, and dysmenorrhea. Taken in conjunction with anticonvulsant medications, antidepressants have been used in treatment of attention-deficit disorder and substance abuse issues by addressing the underlying depression.

Disordered sleep is a symptom in a major percentage of individuals who suffer from depression, with 60% to 80% reporting fragmented sleep, including initial insomnia or early morning awakenings, and 15% to 20% reporting hypersomnia.[220] Studies utilizing PSG to analyze sleep in depressed patients have shown that up to 90% of those studies have changes in sleep architecture including decreased REM sleep latency, increased intensity of REM bouts, and decrease in SWS.[219] It should also be noted that improvements in sleep architecture as seen on PSG often occur with administration of antidepressant medication and these changes are associated with reports of sustained clinical remission. It appears that when sleep abnormalities persist even with reported improvement in clinical symptoms of depression, there is an increased likelihood of clinical relapse.[221] Individuals with a history of insomnia are 4 times more likely to develop a major depressive disorder than those with no history of insomnia.[219]

Agents from this class of medications affect some of the same neurotransmitters that are part of the systems that control and modulate sleep and wakefulness; therefore, it stands to reason that antidepressants will have an impact on sleep and wakefulness. Antidepressant medications are also regularly used in treatment of chronic pain conditions. Though the precise mechanism of action of antidepressants, particularly TCAs, in modulation of chronic pain remains speculative, studies show that it is an effective adjunctive treatment.[206,222–224] Some studies suggest that depression is a part of chronic pain conditions and therefore treatment of the former will help in treatment of the later. However, TCAs have been very effectively utilized in patients with chronic pain conditions without depression. Because of the shared central pathways of the pain modulation system, the affective system, and the systems controlling sleep and wakefulness, it is likely that action on monoamine transmission in one system will exert some influence along critical brain pathways in the other systems.

TCAs act to block presynaptic reuptake of norepinephrine and serotonin to varying degrees and therefore make more norepinephrine or more serotonin available to act on the postsynaptic receptors. Generally, TCAs inhibit histamine H_1 receptors and muscarinic cholinergic receptors, which can cause increased sleepiness, promote sleep onset, and lead to increased daytime sleepiness. TCAs have also been shown to suppress REM sleep. TCAs that are more noradrenergic have a tendency to prolong sleep latency and create more sleep fragmentation, resulting in decreased sleep efficiency. TCAs that have more of a serotonergic action tend to be more sedating and may cause increased daytime sleepiness.

Trazodone is a TCA that has been shown to be particularly effective in the treatment of disordered sleep. Trazodone has a modulatory action on serotonin by exerting an inhibitory effect on 5-HT_{1A}, 5-HT_{1C}, and 5-HT_2 receptors. Additional sleep-promoting effects are likely produced via the medication's inhibitory effects on alpha_1 adrenoreceptors and histamine H_1 receptors. Trazodone also produces weak inhibition of presynaptic serotonin reuptake and blocks 5-HT_2 receptors, which results in minimal, if any, suppression of REM sleep.

MAOIs, as their name suggests, act by inhibiting the MAO enzyme, which in turn, increases presynaptic concentrations of norepinephrine, dopamine, and serotonin. MAOIs disrupt sleep continuity by stimulation of catecholaminergic receptors.

SSRIs may disrupt sleep in some cases but may be responsible for increased daytime sleepiness in other cases, depending upon the agent being employed. These diverse sleep-related effects of SSRIs appear to be related to an increase in serotonin because of the potent presynaptic reuptake inhibition, which results in greater availability of the neurotransmitter to act in shared serotonergic pathways and in pathways that have been linked with sleep regulation. Experiments have shown that administration of serotonin precursors L-tryptophan and 5-hydroxytryptophan has led to a more rapid sleep onset, though application of reserpine or electrolytic or neurotoxic lesions along this pathway have led to a profound state of insomnia.[28-34] Different SSRI medications exert various effects because of the activation of different 5-HT receptor subtypes. These are associated with inhibition of specific sleep stages. For example, some SSRIs may decrease REM sleep while increasing wakefulness. SSRIs that have primary action at another receptor site may inhibit SWS, though others may show a profound increase in SWS. Because SSRIs produce an increase in 5-HT concentrations at different serotonin receptor subtypes, they can produce significant and variable effects on nighttime sleep and daytime sleepiness. For example, nefazodone (Serzone) has been shown to preserve sleep architecture and, unlike some SSRIs, to also preserve REM sleep. Nefazodone acts as a weak presynaptic reuptake inhibitor of 5-HT and a potent inhibitor of postsynaptic 5-HT_2 receptor sites.[22] Bupropion (Wellbutrin) has been shown to increase REM sleep but has been clinically associated with insomnia. Bupropion does not appear to affect 5-HT transmission. Rather, it selectively inhibits presynaptic reuptake of catecholamine, dopamine, and norepinephrine, even though the inhibition is weak. This increase in dopamine and norepinephrine concentration appears to explain complaints of insomnia without suppression of REM sleep. Mirtazapine (Remeron) has been reported to produce improved sleep latency and improvements in total sleep time.

SUMMARY

Sleep and pain are intricately intertwined. Sleep deprivation increases pain sensitivity and increased pain sensitivity may interfere with sleep, thus creating a vicious cycle. Both sleep deprivation and pain can affect mood. It is important to screen patients for sleep, pain, and mood, which can be done using easily administered clinical tools such as the Epworth Sleepiness Scale, the PDI, and the Becks Depression Inventory or similar tools. This information can offer insight into the manner in which sleep, pain, and mood may be impacting one another. It can also point to areas that may require further evaluation by a specialist.

REFERENCES

1. International Association for the Study of Pain. Pain definition. Available at: http://www.iasp-pain.org/AM/Template.cfm?Section=Pain_Defi...isplay.cfm&ContentID=1728#Pain. Accessed March 7, 2011.
2. Merskey H, Bogduk N. *Classification of Chronic Pain: Descriptions of Chronic Pain Syndromes and Definitions of Pain Terms.* 2nd ed. Seattle, WA: IASP Press; 1993.
3. Gureje O, Von Korff M, Simon GE, Gater R. Persistent pain and well-being: a World Health Organization study in primary care. *JAMA.* 1998;280(2):147–151.
4. Brennan F, Carr DB, Cousins M. Pain management: a fundamental human right. *Anesth Analg.* 2007;105:205–221.
5. Pain balance. Available at: http://www.naddi.org/aws/NADDI/asset_manager/get_. October 2, 2013.
6. Roth T. Insomnia: definition, prevalence, etiology, and consequences. *J Clin Sleep Med.* 2007;3(5 suppl):S7–S10.
7. American Academy of Sleep Medicine. *International Classification of Sleep Disorders, Revised: Diagnostic and Coding Manual.* Chicago, Illinois: American Academy of Sleep Medicine, 2001.
8. Hossain JL, Shapiro CM. The prevalence, cost implications, and management of sleep disorders: an overview. *Sleep Breath.* 2002;6(2):85–102.
9. Ohayon MM. The relationship between chronic painful physical condition and insomnia. *J Psychiatr Res.* 2005;39(2):151–159.
10. Fishman SM, Ballantyne JC, Rathmel JP. *Bonica's Management of Pain.* 4th ed. Philadelphia, PA: Lippincott Williams & Wilkins; 2009.
11. Loeser JD, Treede RD. The Kyoto Protocol of IASP basic pain terminology. *Pain.* 2008;137:473–477.
12. Basbaum AI, Jessell TM. The Perception of Pain. In: Kandel E, Schwartz J. *Principles of Neural Science.* St. Louis, MO: The McGraw Hill Company; 2000:472–491.
13. Melzak R, Wall PD. Pain Mechanisms: A New Theory. *Science.* 1965;150(3699):971–979.
14. Smith MT, Perlis ML, Smith MS, Giles DE, Carmody TP. Sleep quality and pre sleep arousal in chronic pain. *J Behav Med Rev.* 2000;23(1):1–13.
15. Craig AD. Interoception: the sense of the physiological condition of the body. *Curr Opin Neurobiol.* 2003;13:500–505.

16. Raymond I, Nielsen TA, Lavigne GJ, Manzini C, Choiniere M. Quality of sleep and its daily relationship to pain intensity in hospitalized adult burn patients. *Pain.* 2001;92:381–388.

17. Nicassio PM, Moxham EG, Schuman CE, Gevirtz RN. The contributions of pain, reported sleep quality, and depressive symptoms to fatigue and fibromyalgia. *Pain.* 2002;100:271–279.

18. Papas RK, Riley JL, Robinson ME. Multidimensional associations with health care use for pain in the community. In: Flor H, Kalso E, Dostrovsky JO, eds. *Proceedings of the 11th World Congress on Pain.* Seattle, WA: IASP Press; 2006:745–759.

19. Grant S, Aitchison T, Henderson E, et al. A comparison of the reproducibility and the sensitivity to change of visual analogue scales, Borg scales, and Likert scales in normal subjects during submaximal exercise. *Chest.* 1999;116:1208–1217.

20. Tait RC, Chibnall JT, Krause S. The pain disability index: psychometric properties. *Pain.* 1990;40:171–182.

21. Melzack R. Short form McGill pain questionnaire. *Pain.* 1987;30:191–197. Available at: http://www.ncbi.nlm.nih.gov/pubmed/3670870. Accessed October 2, 2013.

22. Melzack R. McGill pain questionnaire. *Pain.* 1975;1:277–299. Available at: http://www.cebp.nl/vault_public/filesystem/?ID=1400. Accessed April 19, 2011.

23. Wall PD, Melzack R. *Textbook of Pain.* New York, NY: Churchhill Livingstone; 1994:339–345.

24. Kerns RD, Turk DC, Ruby TE. West-Haven Yale Multidimensional Pain Inventory. *Pain.* 1985;23:345–356. http://www.midss.ie/content/west-haven-yale-multidimensional-pain-inventory-whym-pimpi. Accessed October 2, 2013.

25. Crawford B, Bouhassira D, Wong A, Dukes E. Conceptual adequacy of the neuropathic pain symptom inventory in six countries. *Health Qual Life Outcomes.* 2008;6:62–70.

26. Johns MW. A new method for measuring daytime sleepiness: the Epworth sleepiness scale. *Sleep.* 1991;14:540–545.

27. Fatigue Severity Scale. Available at: http://www.healthywomen.org/sites/default/. Accessed October 2, 2013.

28. Dittner AJ, Wessely SC, Brown RG. The assessment of fatigue: a practical guide for clinicians and researchers. *J Psychosom Res.* 2004;56:157–170.

29. Schwid SR, Covington M, Segal BM, Goodman AD. Fatigue in multiple sclerosis: current understanding and future directions. *J Rehabil Res Dev.* 2002;39:211–224.

30. Mathiowetz V. Test–retest reliability and convergent validity of the fatigue impact scale for persons with multiple sclerosis. *Am J Occup Ther.* 2003;57:389–395.

31. Egner A, Phillips VL, Vora R, Wiggers E. Depression, fatigue, and health-related quality of life among people with advanced multiple sclerosis: results from an exploratory telerehabilitation study. *Neuro Rehabilitation.* 2003;18(2):125–133.

32. Krupp LB, LaRocca NG, Muir-Nash J, Steinberg AD. The fatigue severity scale. Application to patients with multiple sclerosis and systemic lupus erythematosus. *Arch Neurol.* 1989;46:1121–1123.

33. Buysse DJ. Pittsburgh sleep quality index. Available at: http://www.sleep.pitt.edu/content.asp?id=1484&subid=2316. Accessed April 19, 2011.

34. Buysse DJ, Reynolds CF, Monk TH, Berman SR, Kupfer DJ. The Pittsburgh sleep quality index: a new instrument for psychiatric practice and research. *Psychiatry Res.* 1989;28:193–213.

35. Hoddes E, Zarcone V, Smythe H, Phillips R, Dement WC. Quantification of sleepiness: a new approach. *Psychophysiology.* 1973;10:431–436.

36. Toronto Sleepiness Scale: Shahid A, Shen J, Shapiro CM. Measurements of sleepiness and fatigue. J Psychosom Res. 2010;69(1):81–89.

37. Anch AM, Lue FA, LacLean AW, Moldofsky H. Canadian Sleep Society Inventory: sleep physiology and psychological aspects of the fibrositis (fibromyalgia) syndrome. *Can J Psychol Rev.* 1991;45(2):179–184.

38. Beck AT. *Beck Depression Inventory.* Available at: http://academicdepartments.musc.edu/family_medicine/rcmar/beck.htm. Accessed October 2, 2013.

39. Beck A. Psychometric properties of the Beck depression inventory: twenty-five years of evaluation. *Clin Psychol Rev.* 1988;8:77–100.

40. Beck AT, Ward CH, Mendelson M, Mock J, Erbraugh J. An inventory for measuring depression. *Arch Gen Psychiatry.* 1961;4:561–571.

41. Rand Health. SF-36. Available at: http://www.rand.org/health/surveys_tools/mos/mos_core_36item_survey.html. Accessed April 19, 2011.

42. Rand Health. Medical outcomes study: 36-Item short form survey. Available at: http://www.rand.org/health/surveys_tools/mos/mos_core_36item.html. Accessed April 18, 2011.

43. Derogatis LR, Savitz KL. The SCL-90-R and the brief symptom inventory (BSI) in primary care. In: Maruish ME, ed. *Handbook of Psychological Assessment in Primary Care Settings.* Vol 236. Mahwah, NJ: Lawrence Erlbaum Associates; 2000:297–334.

44. Bergner M, Bobbitt RA, Carter WB, Gilson BS. The Sickness Impact Profile: development and final revision of a health status measure. *Med Care.* 1981;19:787–805.

45. Weiss DS, Marmar CR. Impact of events scale. Available at: http://www.ptsd.va.gov/professional/pages/assessments/ies-r.asp. Accessed April 18, 2011.

46. Horowitz M, Wilner N, Alvarez W. Impact of event scale: a measure of subjective stress. *Psychosom Med.* 1979;41:209–218.

47. Weiss DS, Marmar CR. The Impact of Event Scale–Revised. In: Wilson JP, Keane TM, eds. *Assessing Psychological Trauma and PTSD.* New York, NY: Guilford; 1997:399–411.

48. Cutolo M, Sulli A, Pizzorni C, et al. Circadian rhythms: glucocorticoids and arthritis. *Ann NY Acad Sci.* 2006;1069:289–299.

49. Odrcich M, Bailey JM, Cahill CM, Giltron I. Chronobiological characteristics of painful diabetic neuropathy and postherpetic neuralgia: diurnal pain variations and effects of analgesic therapy. *Pain.* 2006;120:207–212.

50. Koltyn KF, Focht BC, Ancker JM, Pasley J. Experimentally induced pain perception in men and women in the morning and evening. *Int J Neurosci.* 1999;98:1–11.

51. Bentley A, Newton S, Zio CD. Sensitivity of sleep stages to painful thermal stimuli. *J Sleep Res.* 2003;12:143–158.

52. Moldofsky H, Scarisbrick P. Induction of neurasthenic musculoskeletal pain syndrome by selective sleep stage deprivation. *Psychosomatic Med.* 1976;38:35–44.

53. Older SA, Battafarano DF, Danning CL, et al. The effects of delta wave sleep interruption on pain thresholds and fibromyalgia like symptoms in healthy subjects, correlations with insulin like growth factor I. *J Rheumatol.* 1998;25:1180–1186.

54. Beydoun A, Morrow TJ, Shen J. Variability of laser-evoked potentials: attention, arousal and lateralized differences. *Electroencephalogr Clin Neurophysiol.* 1993;88(3):173–181.

55. Wang X, Inui K, Qiu Y, Hoshiyama M, Tran TD, Kakigi R. Effects of sleep on pain related somatosensory evoked potentials in humans. *Neurosci Res.* 2003;45:53–57.

56. Lavigne GJ, Okura K, Smith MT. Pain perception–nociception during sleep. In: Bushnell MC, Smith DV, Beauchamp GK, et al. (Eds). *The Senses: A Comprehensive Reference.* Vol 5. San Diego, CA: Academic Press; 2007:783–794.

57. Okura K, Pompre S, Manzini C, et al. Sleep duration and quality in chronic pain patients in comparison to the sleep of fibromyalgia, insomnia, RLS and control subjects. *Sleep.* 2004;27(suppl):A329, 736.

58. Mahowald ML, Mahowald MW. Nighttime sleep and daytime functioning (sleepiness and fatigue) in less well-defined chronic rheumatic disease with particular reference to the "alpha-delta NREM sleep anomaly." *Sleep Med.* 2000;1(3):195–207.

59. Rains JC, Penzien DB. Sleep and chronic pain challenges to the alpha-EEG sleep pattern as a pain specific sleep anomaly. *J Psychosom Res.* 2003;54:77–83.

60. Menefee LA, Cohen M, Anderson WR, et al. Sleep disturbance and nonmalignant chronic pain: a comprehensive review of the literature. *Pain Med.* 2000;1:156–172.

61. Staedt J, Windt H, Hajak G, et al. Cluster arousal analysis in chronic pain-disturbed sleep. *J Sleep Res.* 1993;2(3):134–137.

62. Rizzi M, Sarzi-Puttini P, Atzeni F, et al. Cyclic alternating pattern: a new marker of sleep alteration in patients with fibromyalgia? *J Rheumatol.* 2004;31:1193–1199.

63. Moldofsky H. Sleep and pain: clinical review. *Sleep Med Rev.* 2001;5:387–398.

64. Okura K, Lavigne GJ, Nomtplaisir JY, et al. Slow wave activity and heart rate variation are less dominate in fibromyalgia and chronic pain patients than in controls. *Sleep.* 2005;28(suppl):A302, 0894.

65. Mogil JS, ed. *The Genetics of Pain: Progress in Pain Research and Management.* Vol 28. Seattle, WA: IASP Press; 2004.

66. Seltzer Z, Dorfman R. Identifying genetic and environment risk factors for chronic orofascial pain syndromes: human models. *J Orofac Pain.* 2004;18:311–317.

67. Solovieva S, Leino-Arjas P, Saarela J, et al. Possible association of interleukin 1 gene locus polymorphisms with low back pain. *Pain.* 2004;109(1–2):8–19.

68. Tafti M, Maret S, Dauvilliers Y. Genes for normal sleep and sleep disorders. *Annals Med.* 2005;37:580–589.

69. Inanici F, Yunus MB. History of fibromyalgia: past to present. *Curr Pain Headache Rep.* 2004;8:369–378.

70. Wolfe F, Smythe HA, Yunus MB, et al. The American College of Rheumatology 1990 criteria for the classification of fibromyalgia. Report of the Multicenter Criteria Committee. *Arthritis Rheum.* 1990;33:160–172.

71. Weir PT, Harlan GA, Nkoy FL, et al. The incidence of fibromyalgia and its associated comorbidities: a population-based retrospective cohort study based on *International Classification of Diseases*, 9th revision codes. *J Clin Rheumatol.* 2006;12(3):124–128.

72. Wolfe F, Ross K, Anderson J, Russell IJ, Hebert L. The prevalence and characteristics of fibromyalgia in the general population. *Arthritis Rheum.* 1995;38:19–28.

73. Neumann L, Buskila D. Epidemiology of fibromyalgia. *Curr Pain Headache Rep.* 2003;7:362–368.

74. CFIDS Association of America. Selecting a fatigue rating scale. Available at: http://www.cfids.org/archives/2002rr/2002-rr4-article02.asp. Accessed May 3, 2011.

75. Chalder T, Berelowitz G, Pawlikowska T, et al. Development of a fatigue scale. *J Psychosom Res.* 1993;37:147–153.

76. Shahid A, Wilkinson K, Marcu S, Shapiro CM. Chalder fatigue scale. Stop that and one hundred other sleep scales. Available at: http://link.springer.com/chapter/10.1007/978-1-4419-9893-4_17#. Accessed July 5, 2013.

77. Kosek E, Hansson P. Modulatory influence on somatosensory perception from vibration and heterotopic conditioning stimulation in fibromyalgia patients and healthy subjects. *Pain.* 1997;70:41–51.

78. Lautenbacher S, Rollman GB. Possible deficiencies of pain modulation in fibromyalgia. *Clin J Pain.* 1997;13(3):189–196.

79. Al-Allaf AW, Dunbar KL, Hallum NS, Nosratzadeh B, Templeton KD, Pullar T. A case-control study examining the role of physical trauma in the onset of fibromyalgia syndrome. *Rheumatology.* 2002;41:450–453.

80. Wood P. Stress and dopamine: implications for the pathophysiology of chronic widespread pain. *Med Hypotheses.* 2004;62:420–424.

81. Wood P. Mesolimbic dopaminergic mechanisms and pain control. *Pain.* 2006;120:230–234.

82. Wikner J, Hirsch U, Wetterberg L, Rojdmark S. Fibromyalgia: a syndrome associated with decreased nocturnal melatonin secretion. *Clin Endocrinol.* 1998;49:179–183.

83. Alnigenis MN, Barland P. Fibromyalgia syndrome and serotonin. *Clin Exp Rheumatol.* 2001;19:205–210.

84. Van Houdenhove B, Egle UT. Fibromyalgia: a stress disorder? Piecing the biopsychosocial puzzle together. *Psychother Psychosom.* 2004;73:267–275.

85. McLean SA, Williams DA, Harris RE, et al. Momentary relationship between cortisol secretion and symptoms in patients with fibromyalgia. *Arthritis Rheum.* 2005;52:3660–3669.

86. Paiva ES, Deodhar A, Jones KD, Bennett R. Impaired growth hormone secretion in fibromyalgia patients: evidence for augmented hypothalamic somatostatin tone. *Arthritis Rheum.* 2002;46:1344–1350.

87. Bennett RM, Clark SR, Walczyk J. A randomized, double-blind, placebo-controlled study of growth hormone in the treatment of fibromyalgia. *Am J Med.* 1998;104:227–231.

88. Landis CA, Lentz MJ, Rothermel J, Buchwald D, Shaver JL. Decreased sleep spindles and spindle activity in midlife women and fibromyalgia and pain. *Sleep.* 2004;27:741–750.

89. Vaeroy H, Qiao Z, Morkrid L, Forre O. Altered sympathetic nervous system response in patients with fibromyalgia (fibrositis syndrome). *J Rheumatol.* 1989;16:1460–1465.

90. Evengard B, Nilsson C, Lindh G, et al. Chronic fatigue syndrome differs from fibromyalgia. No evidence for elevated substance P levels in cerebrospinal fluid of patients with chronic fatigue syndrome. *Pain.* 1998;78:153–155.

91. Ozgocmen S, Ozyurt H, Sogut S, Akyol O. Current concepts in the pathophysiology of fibromyalgia: the potential role of oxidative stress and nitric oxide. *Rheumatol Int.* 2006;26:585–597.

92. Payne TC, Leavitt F, Garron DC, et al. Fibrositis and psychologic disturbance. *Arthritis Rheum.* 1982;25:213–217.

93. Yunus MB, Ahles TA, Aldag JC, Masi AT. Relationship of clinical features with psychological status in primary fibromyalgia. *Arthritis Rheum.* 1991;34:15–21.

94. Holman AJ, Myers PR. A randomized, double-blind, placebo-controlled trial of pramipexole, a dopamine agonist, in patients with fibromyalgia receiving concomitant medications. *Arthritis Rheum.* 2005;52:2495–2505.

95. Maigne R. Cervicogenic headache. Available at: http://www.sofm-moo.com/english_section/1_cephalalgia/rm_cervical_headache. Accessed May 10, 2011.

96. Levy D, Strassman AM, Burstein R. A critical view on the role of migraine triggers in the genesis of migraine pain. *Headache.* 2009;49:953–957.

97. Tfelt-Hansen P, Lous I, Olesen J. Prevalence and significance of muscle tenderness during common migraine attacks. *Headache.* 1981;21(2):49–54.

98. Robbins MS, Lipton RB. The epidemiology of primary headache disorders. *Semin Neurol.* 2010;30:107–119.

99. Dahmen N, Querings K, Grun B, Bierbrauer J. Increased frequency of migraine in narcoleptic patients. *Neurology.* 1999;52:1291–1293.

100. Sicuteri F, Testi A, Anselmi B. Biomedical investigations in headache: increase in hydroxyindoleacetic acid excretion during migraine attacks. *Int Arch Allergy.* 1961;19:55–58.

101. Pérez MF, Sánchez del Río M, Seabra ML, et al. Hypothalamic involvement in chronic migraine. *J Neurol Neurosurg Psychiatry.* 2001;71:747–751.

102. Torelli P, Manzoni GC. Pain and behavior in cluster headache. A prospective study and review of the literature. *Funct Neurol.* 2003;18(4):205–210.

103. Kudrow L. *Cluster Headache: Mechanisms and Management.* New York, NY: Oxford University Press; 1980.

104. Russell D. Cluster headache: severity and temporal profile of attacks and patient activity prior to and during attacks. *Cephalalgia.* 1981;1(4):209–216.

105. Evers S, Goadsby PJ. Hypnic headache. Clinical features, patho-physiology, and treatment. *Neurology.* 2003;60:905–909.

106. Liang JF, Fuh JL, Yu HY, et al. Clinical features, polysomnography and outcome in patients with hypnic headache. *Cephalalgia.* 2008;28:209–215.

107. Aldrich MS, Chauncey JB. Are morning headaches part of obstructive sleep apnea syndrome? *Arch Intern Med.* 1990;150:1265–1267.

108. Poceta JS, Dalessio DJ. Identification and treatment of sleep apnea in patients with chronic headache. *Headache.* 1995;35:586–589.

109. Lavigne GJ, Montplaisir JY. Restless leg/legs syndrome and sleep bruxism: prevalence and association among Canadians. *Sleep.* 1994;17:739–743.

110. Laberge L, Tremblay RE, Vitaro F, Montplaisir JY. Development of parasomnias from childhood to early adolescence. *Pediatrics.* 2000;106(1 pt 1):67–74.

111. Boutros N. Headaches in sleep apnea. *Tex Med.* 1989;85(4):34–35.

112. Gold A, Marcus C, Dipalo F, et al. Upper airway collapsibility during sleep in upper airway resistance syndrome. *Chest.* 2002;121:1531–1540.

113. Gold AR, Dipalo F, Gold MS, et al. Symptoms and signs of upper airway resistance syndrome: a link to the functional somatic syndromes. *Chest.* 2003;123:87–95.

114. Poceta J, Dalessio D. Identification and treatment of sleep apnea in patients with chronic headache. *Headache.* 1995;35:586–589.

115. Rains J, Penzien D, Mohammed Y. Sleep and headache: morning headache associated with sleep disordered breathing. [abstract] *Cephalalgia.* 2001;21:520.

116. Leone M, D'Amico D, Grazzi L, Attanasio A, Busone G. Cervicogenic headache: a critical review of the current diagnostic criteria. *Pain.* 1998;78(1):1–5.

117. Nobre M, Leal A, Filho P. Investigation into sleep disturbance of patients suffering from cluster headache. *Cephalagia.* 2005;25:488–492.

118. Chevrin R, Zallek S, Lin X, et al. Timing patterns of cluster headaches and association with symptoms of obstructive sleep apnea. *Sleep Res Online.* 2000;3(3):107–112.

119. Pavia T, Farinha A, Martins A, et al. Chronic headaches and sleep disorders. *Arch Intern Med.* 1997;157:1701–1705.

120. Idiman F, Oztura I, Baklan B, et al. Headache in sleep apnea syndrome. *Headache.* 2004;44:603–606.

121. Centers for Chronic Nasal and Sinus Dysfunction. Rhinitis. Available at: http://www.ncbi.nlm.nih.gov/pubmed/19663122. Accessed October 2, 2013.

122. White D, Cadieux R, Lomard R, et al. The effects of nasal anesthersia on breathing during sleep. *Am Rev Respir Dis.* 1985;132:972–975.

123. McNicholas W, Tarlo S, Cole P, et al. Obstructive sleep apnea during sleep in patients with seasonal allergic rhinitis. *Am Rev Respir Dis.* 1982;126:625–628.

124. McNicholas W, Coffey M, Boyle T. Effects of nasal airflow on breathing during sleep in normal humans. *Am Rev Respir Dis.* 1993;147:620–623.

125. Basner R, Simon P, Shcwartzstein R, et al. Breathing route influences upper airway muscle activity in awake normal adults. *J Appl Physiol.* 1989;66:1766–1771.

126. Weissbluth M. *Healthy Sleep Habits, Happy Child.* New York, NY: Ballantine Books; 1999.

127. Lavigine GJ, Manzini C, Kato T. Sleep bruxism. In: Kryger MH, Roth T, Dement WC, eds. *Principles and Practice of Sleep Medicine.* Philadelphia, PA: Elsevier-Saunders; 2005:946–959.

128. Gagnon Y, Mayer P, Morisoson F, Rompre PH, Lavigne GJ. Aggravation of respiratory disturbance by the use of an occlusal splint in apneic patients: a pilot study. *Int J Prosthodont.* 2004;17:447–453.

129. Earley CJ. Restless leg/legs syndrome. *N Engl J Med.* 2003;348:2103–2109.

130. Skidmore FM, Drago V, Foster PS, Heilman KM. Bilateral restless legs affecting a phantom limb, treated with dopamine agonists. *J Neurol Neurosurg Psychiatry.* 2009;80:569–570.

131. Allen R, Picchietti D, Hening WA, Trenkwalder C, Walters AS, Montplaisi J. Restless leg/legs syndrome: diagnostic criteria, special considerations, and epidemiology. A report from the Restless Leg/Legs Syndrome Diagnosis and Epidemiology Workshop at the National Institutes of Health. *Sleep Med.* 2003;4(2):101–119.

132. Earley CJ, Silber MH. Restless leg/legs syndrome: understanding its consequences and the need for better treatment. *Sleep Med.* 2010;11:807–815.

133. Winkelmann J, Muller-Myhsok B, Wittchen H, et al. Complex segregation analysis of restless leg syndrome provides evidence for an autosomal dominant mode of inheritance in early age at onset families. *Ann Neurol.* 2002;52:207–302.

134. Botani M, Strambi F, Aridon P, et al. Autosomal dominant restless leg/legs syndrome maps on chromosome 14q. *Brain.* 2003;126(pt 6):1485–1492.

135. Desautels A, Turecki G, Monplaisir J, et al. Identification of a major susceptibility locus for restless leg/legs syndrome on chromosome 12q. *Am J Hum Genet.* 2001;69:1266–1270.

136. Allen R. Dopamine and iron in the pathophysiology of restless leg/legs syndrome (RLS). *Sleep Med.* 2004;5:385–391.

137. Earley CJ, B Barker P, Horska A, Allen R. MRI-determined regional brain iron concentrations in early- and late-onset restless leg/legs syndrome. *Sleep Med.* 2006;7:458–461.

138. Allen RP, Connor JR, Hyland K, Earley CJ. Abnormally increased CSF 3-ortho-methyldopa (3-OMD) in untreated restless leg/legs syndrome (RLS) patients indicates more severe disease and possibly abnormally increased dopamine synthesis. *Sleep Med.* 2009;10:123–128.

139. Chen G, Guilleminault C. Sleep disorders that can exacerbate pain. In: Lavigne G, Sessle BJ, Choiniere M, Soja PJ, eds. *Sleep and Pain.* Seattle, WA: IASP Press; 2007:311–339.

140. Clemens S, Rye D, Hochman S. Restless leg/legs syndrome: revisiting the dopamine hypothesis from the spinal cord perspective. *Neurology.* 2006;67:125–130.

141. Lavigne GJ, Montplaisir JY. Restless leg/legs syndrome and sleep bruxism: prevalence and association among Canadians. *Sleep.* 1994;17:739–743.

142. Simon H, Zieve D. Attention deficit hyperactivity disorder—other disorders associated with it. Available at: http://www.umm.edu/patiented/articles/other_disorders_associated_with_attention-deficit_disorder_000030_5.htm. Accessed June 20, 2011.

143. Walters AS, Hickey K, Maltzman J, et al. A questionnaire study of 138 patients with restless leg/legs syndrome: the "night-walkers" survey. *Neurology.* 1996;46:92–95.

144. Ascoli-Isreal S, Roth T. Characteristics of insomnia in the United States: results of the 1991 National Sleep Foundation Survey. *Sleep.* 1999;22(suppl 2):S347–S353.

145. Roth T. Insomnia: definitions, prevalence, etiology and consequences. *J Clin Sleep Med.* 2007;3(5 suppl): S7.

146. Sateia M, Hauri P. *The International Classification of Sleep Disorders.* 2nd ed. Westbrook, IL: American Academy of Sleep Medicine; 2005.

147. Pilowsky I, Crettenden I, Townley M. Sleep disturbance in pain clinic patients. *Pain.* 1985;23:27–33.

148. Menefee L, Frank E, Doghramji K, et al. Self-reported sleep quality and quality of life for individuals with chronic pain conditions. *Clin J Pain.* 2000;16:290–297.

149. Sawynok J. Adenosine receptor activation and nociception. *Eur J Pharmacol.* 1998;347:1–11.

150. Palermo TM, Kiska R. Subjective sleep disturbances in adolescents with chronic pain: relationship to daily functioning and quality of life. *J Pain.* 2006;6:201–207.

151. Carskadon MA, Harvey K, Duke P, Anders TF, Litt IF, Dement WC. Pubertal changes in daytime sleepiness. *Sleep.* 1980;2:453–460.

152. Carskadon MA, Wolfson AR, Acebo C, Tzischinsky O, Seifer R. Adolescent sleep patterns, circadian timing, and sleepiness at a transition to early school days. *Sleep.* 1998;21:871–881.

153. Sadeh A. Consequences of sleep loss or sleep disruption in children. *Sleep Med Clin.* 2007;2:513–520.

154. Sadeh A, Raviv A, Gruber R. Sleep patterns and sleep disruptions in school age children. *Dev Psychol.* 2000;36:291–301.

155. Carskadon MA, Dement WC. Effects of total sleep loss on sleep tendency. *Percept Motor Skills.* 1979;48:495–506.

156. Sadeh A, Gruber R, Raviv A. Sleep, neurobehavioral functioning and behavior problems in school-age children. *Child Dev.* 2002;73:405–417.

157. Sadeh A, Gruber R, Raviv A. The effects of sleep restriction and extension on school-age children: what a difference an hour makes. *Child Dev.* 2003;74:444–455.

158. Durmer JS, Dinges DF. Neurocognitive consequences of sleep deprivation. *Semin Neurobiol.* 2005;25:117–129.

159. Corkum P, Tannock R, Moldofsky H, Hoff-Johnson S, Humphries T. Actigraphy and parental ratings of sleep in children with attention-deficit/hyperactivity disorder (ADHD). *Sleep.* 2001;24:303–312.

160. Dahl RE. The consequences of insufficient sleep for adolescents: links between sleep and emotional regulation. *Phi Delta Kappan.* 1999;80:354–359.

161. Obrien LM, Gozal D. Neurocognitive dysfunction and sleep in children: from human to rodent. *Pediatr Clin North Am.* 2004;51:187–202.

162. Gozal D. Sleep disordered breathing and school performance in children. *Pediatrics.* 1998;102:616–620.

163. Goodwin JL, Babar SL, Kaemingk KL, et al. Symptoms related to sleep disordered breathing in white and Hispanic children: the Tucson Children's Assessment of Sleep Apnea study. *Chest.* 2003;124:196–203.

164. Chervic RD, Ruzicka D, Archbold KH, Dillon JE. Snoring predicts hyperactivity four years later. *Sleep.* 2005;28:885–890.

165. Sofer S, Weinhouse E, Tal A, et al. Cor pulmonale due to adenoidal or tonsillar hypertrophy or both in children: noninvasive diagnosis and follow-up. *Chest.* 1998;93:119–122.

166. Amin R, Somers VK, McConnell K, et al. Activity adjusted 24-hour ambulatory blood pressure and cardiac remodeling in children with sleep disordered breathing. *Hypertension.* 2008;51:84–91.

167. Bixler EO, Vgontzas AN, Lin HM, et al. Blood pressure associated with sleep-disordered breathing in a population sample of children. *Hypertension.* 2008;52:841–846.

168. Redline S, Storfer-Isser A, Rosen CL, et al. Association between metabolic syndrome and sleep disordered breathing in adolescents. *Am J Respir Crit Care Med.* 2007;176:401–408.

169. Tauman R, O'Brien LM, Gozal D. Hypoxemia and obesity modulate plasma C reactive protein and interleukin-6 levels in sleep disordered breathing. *Sleep Breath.* 2007;11(2):77–84.

170. Gozal D, Capdevila OS, Kheirandish-Gozal L. Metabolic alterations and systemic inflammation in obstructive sleep apnea among non-obese and obese prepubertal children. *Am J Respir Crit Care Med.* 2008;177(10):1142–1149.

171. Steinberger J, Daniels SR. Obesity, insulin resistance, diabetes, and cardiovascular risk in children. *Circulation.* 2003;107:1448–1453.

172. Boyle JT. Recurrent Abdominal pain: an update. *Pediatr Rev.* 1997;18:310–321.

173. Miller VA, Palermo TM, Powers SW, Scher MS, Hershey AD. Migraine headaches and sleep disturbance in children. *Headache.* 2003;43:362–368.

174. Centers for Disease Control and Prevention. Sickle cell awareness month. Available at: http://www.cdc.gov/Features/SickleCellAwareness. Accessed July 2, 2011.

175. Spivey JF, Uong EC, Strunk R, Boslaugh SE, DeBraun MR. Low daytime pulse oximetry reading is associated with nocturnal desaturation and obstructive sleep apnea in children with sickle cell anemia. *Pediatr Blood Cancer.* 2008;50:359–362.

176. Siddiqui AK, Ahmed S. Pulmonary manifestations of sickle cell disease. *Postgrad Med J.* 2003;79:384–390.

177. Brooks LJ, Koziol SM, Chiarucci KM, Berman BW. Dose sleep-disordered breathing contribute to the clinical severity of sickle cell anemia? *J Pediatr Hematol Oncol.* 1996;18:135–139.

178. Roizenblatt S, Tufik S, Goldenberg J, Pinto LR, Hilario MO, Feldman D. Juvenile fibromyalgia: clinical and polysomnographic aspects. *J Rheumatol.* 1997;24:579–585.

179. Tayag-Kier CE, Keenan GF, Scalzi LV, et al. Sleep and periodic limb movement in sleep in juvenile fibromyalgia. *Pediatrics.* 2000;106(5):E70.

180. Bloom BJ, Owens JA, McGuinn M, Nobile C, Schaeffer L, Alario AJ. Sleep and its relationship to pain, dysfunction, and disease activity in juvenile rheumatoid arthritis. *J Rheumatol.* 2002;29:169–173.

181. Labyak SE, Bourguignon C, Docherty S. Sleep quality in children with juvenile rheumatoid arthritis. *Holist Nurs Pract.* 2003;17(4):193–200.

182. Passarelli CM, Roizenblatt S, Len CA, et al. A case-control sleep study in children with polyarticular juvenile rheumatoid arthritis. *J Rheumatol.* 2006;33:796–802.

183. Meltzer LJ, Logan DE, Mindell JA. Sleep patterns in female adolescents with chronic musculoskeletal pain. *Behav Sleep Med.* 2005;3(4):193–208.

184. Palermo TM, Kiska R. Subjective sleep disturbances in adolescents with chronic pain: relationship to daily functioning and quality of life. *J Pain.* 2005;6:201–207.

185. Shao-Yu T, Labyak SE, Richardson LP, et al. Brief report: actigraphic aleep and daytime naps in adolescent girls with chronic musculoskeletal pain. *J Pediatri Psychol.* 2008;33:307–391.

186. Foley DJ, Monjan AA, Brown SL, et al. Sleep complaints among elderly persons: an epidemiologic study of three communities. *Sleep.* 1995;18:425–432.

187. Latham J, Davis BD. The socioeconomic impact of chronic pain. *Disabil Rehabil.* 1994;16:39–44.

188. Helme RD, Katz B, Gibsom SJ, et al. Multidisciplinary pain clinics for older people. Do they have a role? *Clin Geriatr Med.* 1996;12:563–582.

189. Ohayon MM, Carskadon MA, Guilleminault C, Vitiello MV. Meta-analysis of quantitative sleep parameters from childhood to old age in healthy individuals: developing normative sleep values across the human lifespan. *Sleep.* 2004;27:1255–1273.

190. Van Cauter E, Leproult R, Plat L. Age-related changes in slow wave sleep and relationship with growth hormone and cortisol levels in healthy men. *JAMA.* 2000;284:861–868.

191. Nicolas A, Petit D, Rompre S, Montplaisir J. Sleep spindle characteristics in healthy subjects of different age groups. *Clin Neurophysiol.* 2001;112:521–527.

192. Monk TH. Sleep and circadian rhythms. *Exp Gerontol.* 1991;26:233–243.

193. Monk TH. Aging human circadian rhythms: conventional wisdom may not always be right. *J Bio Rhythms.* 2005;20:366–374.

194. Attal N, Cruccu G, Haanpaa M, et al. EFNS guidelines on pharmacological treatment of neuropathic pain. *Euro J Neurol.* 2006;13:1153–1169.

195. Morin CM, Colecchi C, Stone J, Sood R, Brink D. Behavioral and pharmacological therapies for late-life insomnia: a randomized controlled trial. *JAMA.* 1999;281:991–999.

196. Siegel J. Brain mechanisms that control sleep and waking. *Naturwissenschaften.* 2004;91:355–365.

197. Vaz Fragoso CA, Gill TM. Sleep complaints in community-living older persons: a multifactorial geriatric syndrome. *J Am Geriatr Soc.* 2007;55:1853–1866.

198. Gottesman C. Brain inhibitory mechanisms involved in basic and higher integrated sleep processes. *Brain Res Rev.* 2004;45:230–249.

199. Nelson LE, Guo TZ, Lu J, et al. The sedative component of anesthesia is mediated by GABA(A) receptors in the endogenous sleep pathway. *Nat Neurosci.* 2002;5:979–984.

200. Carskadon MA, Dement WC. Normal human sleep: an overview. In: Kryger M, Roth T, Dement WC, eds. *Principles and Practice of Sleep Medicine.* 5th ed. Philadelphia, PA: Elsevier-Saunders; 2011:16–25.

201. Roehrs T, Roth T. Sleep–wake states and memory function. *Sleep.* 2000;23(suppl 3):S64–S68.

202. Rausch G, Bertran F, Guillery-Girard B, et al. Consolidation of strictly episodic memories mainly requires rapid eye movement sleep. *Sleep.* 2004;27:395–401.

203. Rauchs G, Desgranges B, Foret J, Eustache F. The relationships between memory systems and sleep stages. *J Sleep Res.* 2005;14:123–140.

204. Saper CB, Scammell TE, Lu J. Hypothalamic regulation of sleep and circadian rhythms. *Nature.* 2005;437:1257–1263.

205. Mignot E, Taheri S, Nishino S. Sleeping with the hypothalamus: emerging therapeutic targets for sleep disorders. *Nat Neurosci.* 2002;5(suppl):1071–1075.

206. Marshal L, Born J. The contribution of sleep to hippocampus-dependent memory consolidation. *Trends Cogn Sci.* 2007;11:443–450.

207. Watson CJ, Baghdovan HA, Lydic R. Neuropharmacology of sleep and wakefulness. *Sleep Med Clin.* 2010;5(4):513–528.

208. Thorpy M. Therapeutic advances in narcolepsy. *Sleep Med.* 2007;8(4):427–440.

209. Barot N, Barot I. Optimal sleep habits in middle-aged adults. In: Kushida C (ed). *Encyclopedia of Sleep.* San Diego, CA: Academic Press; 2013;88–94

210. Nishino S. Neurotransmitters and neuropharmacology of sleep/wake regulations. *Sleep Med Clin.* 2010;5(4):513–528.

211. Aronson MD. Nonsteroidal anti-inflammatory drugs, traditional opioids, and tramadol: constrasting therapies for the treatment of chronic pain. *Clin Therapeutics.* 1997;19(3):420–432.

212. Schnitzer TJ. Non-NSAID pharmacologic treatment options for the management of chronic pain. *Am J Med.* 1998;105(1):45S-52S.

213. Ciccone CD. *Pharmacology in Rehabilitation.* 3rd ed. Philadelphia, PA: FA Davis Company; 2002.

214. Shaw IR, Lavigne G, Mayer P, Choiniere M. Acute intravenous administration of morphine perturbed sleep architecture in healthy pain-free young adults: a preliminary study. *Sleep.* 2005;28:677–682.

215. Dimsdale JE, Norman D, DeJardin D, Wallace MS. The effect of opioids on sleep architecture. *J Clin Sleep Med.* 2007;3:33–36.

216. Moor P, Dimsdale JE. Opioids, sleep and cancer-related fatigue. *Med Hypotheses.* 2002;58:77–82.

217. Farney RJ, Walker JM, Cloward TV, Rhondeau S. Sleep-disordered breathing associated with long-term opioid therapy. *Chest.* 2003;123:632–639.

218. Hayaishi O, Urade Y. Prostaglandin D2 in sleep–wake regulation: recent progress and perspectives. *Neuroscientist.* 2001;8:12–15.

219. Murphy PJ, Badia P, Myers BL, et al. Non-steroidal anti-inflammatory drugs affect normal sleep patterns in humans. *Physiol Behav.* 1994;55:1063–1066.

220. DeMartinis NA, Winokur A. Effects of psychiatric medications on sleep and sleep disorders. *CNS Neurolog Disord Drug Targets.* 2007;6:17–29.

221. Thase ME, Fsiczka AL, Berman SR, Simons AD, Reynolds CF. Electroencephalographic sleep profiles before and after cognitive behavior therapy of depression. *Arch Gen Psychiatry.* 1998;55:138–144.

222. Bryson HM, Wilde MI. Amitriptyline: a review of its pharmacological properties and therapeutic use in chronic pain states. *Drugs Aging.* 1996;8:459.

223. Godfrey RG. A guide to the understanding and use of tricyclic antidepressants in the overall management of fibromyalgia and other chronic pain syndromes. *Arch Intern Med.* 1996;156:1047–1052.

224. McQuay HJ, Carroll D, Glynn CJ. Low dose amitriptyline in the treatment of chronic pain. *Anaesthesia.* 1992;47:646–652.

21

Sleep, Memory, and Motor Learning

Catherine Siengsukon, PT, PhD and Julie M. Hereford, PT, DPT

INTRODUCTION TO MEMORY SYSTEMS

Sleep impacts memory, learning, and motor behavior and therefore is an important factor in rehabilitation from injury or disease. Sleep affects all types of memory and is involved in how memory is consolidated, stored, organized, retrieved, and reconsolidated. Motor learning and motor memory follow a similar process of encoding, storage, and retrieval and generally interact with components of memory and learning.

Motor learning, which involves nondeclarative memory, is of primary concern to the rehabilitation professional in developing and progressing in a treatment plan designed to improve motor function. It is also important to realize that problems with declarative memory, which is that memory for consciously recalled facts and knowledge, can create difficulties in the rehabilitation process. For example, if a patient is unable to effectively store memory regarding their illness or injury, they may not be able to follow treatment precautions. Problems with declarative memory may also interfere with successful implementation of a therapeutic exercise program. Understanding how sleep and sleep disorders impact this process is essential in order to maximize rehabilitation outcomes. Because of the importance of declarative, nondeclarative, and procedural memory in the rehabilitation process, this chapter will give an overall review of memory and will discuss in some detail the processes by which both declarative and nondeclarative memory are encoded, consolidated, and recalled. The

current understanding of the role of sleep in these memory processes will also be presented.

Memory is described as a cognitive process by which an experience is retained, reactivated, and reconstructed, independent of internal representation and usually as it pertains to a current situation. Internal representation is the expression of memory at the behavioral or conscious level and the neural changes that accompany that memory encoding process.[1] Memory may be utilized to relate a current event to like situations in one's past in order to compare the events and plan responses to particular situations. It may be used to have a complete understanding about a current situation or may be used to apply knowledge in an immediate circumstance in order to solve problems or engage in a task.

Memory is integral to personal identity and processes of memory retrieval and integration help to animate an individual's personal history. Memory is different from perception. Perception is a process in which an organism gains awareness or understanding of the environment by interpreting and organizing incoming sensory information or imagination. It involves the ability to form images and sensations that are not the result of physical sensory input. Although there is a close relationship among the components of memory and perception, the neurobiological processes by which they occur differ and yet they help to provide fundamental meaning to an experience and an understanding to knowledge that is gained.

Memory is often suffused with emotion as seen in situations of grief or commemoration. It may be a source of information and is essential for reasoning and decision making. Memory can shape one's moral and social life

Hereford JM. *Sleep and Rehabilitation: A Guide for Health Professionals* (pp 233-252).
© 2014 Taylor & Francis Group.

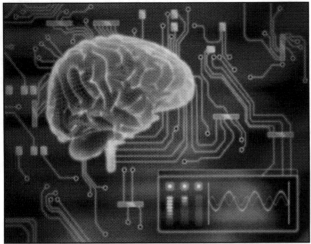

Figure 21-1. Memory involves 3 major processes: encoding, storage, and retrieval of information. (From Fotolia.com)

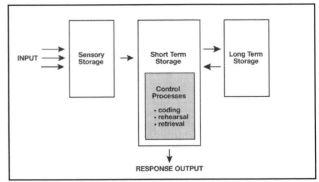

Figure 21-2. Atkinson and Shiffrin memory model.

depending on the particular way in which an individual memory is embedded in time. It is not absolute or complete and, in fact, can be faulty in mundane and minor ways or in dramatic and disastrous ways. Accusation, trial, and conviction of some individuals have been based largely on the memory of another person. In some cases, these memories have later proven to be inaccurate. Thus, memory is important to experience and learning but remains an imperfect representation of reality.

The study of human memory has been the subject of neurobiology, medicine, and cognitive psychology. Interestingly, the study of memory and its role in human life has been a major interest in the field of philosophy for thousands of years, and theories of memory development and meaning began with the ancient philosophers including Plato and Aristotle.

What is human memory? For the purposes of this text, human memory will be defined as the processes by which information is acquired, stored, retained, and later retrieved. In very simple terms, there are 3 major processes involved in development of memory, that include encoding, storage, and retrieval (Figure 21-1). For instance, when a human interacts with the environment, information is processed by the brain and changed into a usable form through a process known as encoding. Once encoded, the information must be stored for later use. Stored memory is generally outside conscious awareness until such time as it is needed. At this point, memory can be retrieved and restored to conscious awareness in order to be acted upon in a given situation. This interaction may change the memory, and the process of encoding and storage is repeated. In this way, memory will undergo remodeling and reconsolidation, which may solidify the memory, or this process may change the content recall of the original memory.

Philosophical models of memory helped to form the basis of psychological models. These models have since served as a platform upon which neurobiological models

of memory have been studied and tested. If memory is defined as a method by which storage of learned information is retrieved for further use, several key questions come to mind. First, how does information get into memory, second, how is information maintained in memory, and, finally, how is information retrieved from memory for further use? These questions lead then to the question of what happens when memory does not work or what happens when one forgets.

A commonly referenced theoretical framework for memory is the information processing theory proposed by Atkinson and Shiffrin in 1968 upon which computers are modeled (Figure 21-2). According to this model, there are 3 separate stages of memory including sensory memory, short-term memory, and long-term memory. If information is going to be stored, it must pass through the first 2 stages that act as temporary storage buffers before it can be retained in more permanent storage for retrieval at a later time. It should be noted that not all incoming sensory information is processed into short- or long-term memory. In fact, Sperling demonstrated that the capacity of sensory memory is approximately 12 items, but that memory degrades within a few hundred milliseconds. He also suggested that because this memory decays so quickly, this type of perceived memory cannot be prolonged with rehearsal.[2]

Sensory memory refers to the sensory information gathered from interaction with the environment. This may include visual, auditory, tactile, proprioceptive, or kinesthetic information. This information is stored for a very brief period ranging from 0.5 seconds for visual information to 3 to 4 seconds for auditory information. The brain is only able to and only needs to attend to certain aspects of sensory memory as it passes into short-term memory.

According to this model, short-term memory, referred to by Atkinson and Shiffrin[3] as "active memory" or "working memory," gathers information from the initial sensory memory stage and brings it to conscious awareness relative to other information that is currently in conscious awareness or being thought about. Attending to sensory memory assists in generating short-term memory. This information

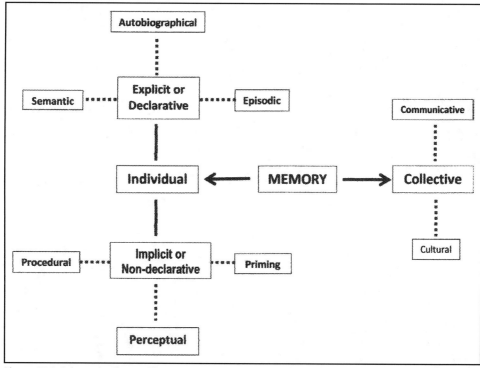

Figure 21-3. Schematic of types of memory. (From Fotolia.com)

will be kept in active memory for 20 to 30 seconds but will quickly be forgotten unless it is allowed to continue on to long-term memory. This active, short-term memory capacity can be stretched by using memory strategies such as "chunking" in which related information is grouped into chunks.

Long-term memory, according to the Atkinson and Shiffrin model, refers to memory that, having passed from sensory information and reached conscious awareness, is attended to sufficiently to generate a process that will continue the storage of this information. Freud referred to this memory as preconscious or unconscious memory and this memory remains largely outside awareness until such time as the situation or environmental cues require its recall. Some information stored in long-term memory is easily recalled, whereas other information is far more difficult to access. There are a number of psychological theories proposed regarding the ease, or more importantly, the difficulty with which it may be to recall certain memories. Once a memory stored in long-term memory is accessed, however, it becomes working memory and is acted upon and modified and will once again undergo the process of memory storage.

Types of Memory

The classification of different types of memory helps to understand the different functions of memory and how memory and memory deficits may be encountered in a rehabilitation setting. Clearly, rehabilitation is very

involved in identifying and correcting faulty movement patterns whether the patient is a child with a developmental problem, an adolescent with an athletic injury, an adult with long-term consequences of abnormal posture, or an older adult who has suffered a stroke. Regardless of the patient type and the specific approach or techniques that are utilized, motor learning and motor memory will play a part in the rehabilitation process. Additionally, patient education and communication is a vital component of any rehabilitation program. Both of these functions require memory processes, but those processes are different.

Memory may involve recognition or recall. An individual may recognize information to which he or she has previously been exposed. On the contrary, recall requires an individual to retrieve previously stored information. For example, a patient may be asked whether she has certain medical conditions when presented with a list, an example of recognition, or she may be asked to recall whether she has had any surgeries or illnesses, an example of recall.

Researchers usually divide memory into explicit, or declarative, and implicit, or nondeclarative, memory (Figure 21-3). Explicit memory is conscious, intentional recollection of previous experiences and information. An example of explicit memory can be seen in a patient who remembered their appointment time, or was able to give a concise history of an accident that occurred years ago. Explicit memory is further divided into episodic memory and semantic memory. Episodic memory consists of recollection of events in the life of the individual and autobiographical memory is a component of episodic memory.

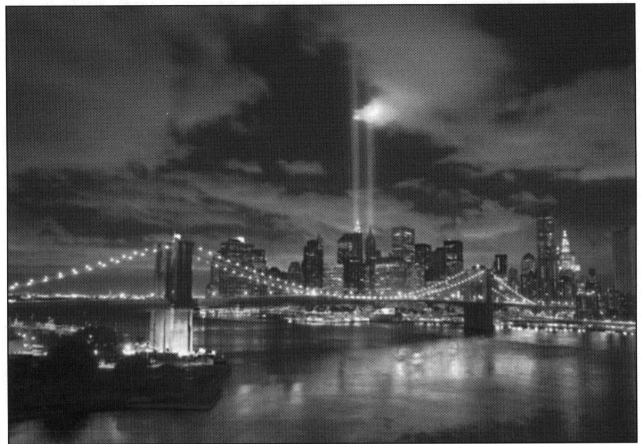

Figure 21-4. Autobiographical memory is a type of episodic memory. These tend to have strong emotional content; for many Americans, an example is the memory of where you were when you learned of the attack on the World Trade Center on 9/11. (From Fotolia.com)

These memories are usually unique and may include significant emotional content. For example, remembering where you were when you first heard about the terrorist attacks on 9/11 is an example of episodic memory (Figure 21-4).

Semantic memory consists of all explicit memory that is not autobiographical or the memory that contains information that an individual "knows." For example, recollection of historical facts is semantic memory. Visual memory involves preserving information related to visual experience. Initial exposure to a visual memory can prime it for additional exposures. For example, if an individual sees an incomplete picture that he or she is unable to identify and then is shown more of the picture, the individual's memory is said to be primed and he or she will be able to recognize the incomplete picture when shown later. This is also thought to be the mechanism by which an individual is able to produce a mental image. An example of semantic memory occurs when a patient recognizes his or her therapist from appointment to appointment.

Though explicit memory involves conscious, intentional recollection of previous experiences and learned information, implicit memory is unconscious and unintentional. Riding a bike is often used as an example of implicit memory; however, recalling a lesson of a specific biking skill is an example of explicit memory, although performing the skill years later is an example of implicit memory.

Implicit memory is also known as nondeclarative memory that does not require conscious recall of information but rather on implicit learning. It includes procedural memory and perceptual memory. Procedural memory is the memory of how to do things and is primarily employed in learning new motor skills. Procedural memory is automatically retrieved and utilized without conscious control or attention. Repeated performance of a task allows all of the relevant neural systems to work together to automatically produce the activity. Nondeclarative procedural learning is essential for the development or refinement of a motor skill or cognitive activity.

Procedural memory has explicit and implicit components that refer to awareness of the sequential nature of a task to be learned. For example, when evaluating a patient, the therapist may note a faulty movement pattern and determine that a particular exercise will improve the movement deficit. The patient does not know how to perform the exercise. Implicit procedural learning is employed in this situation as the patient learns how. If the therapist provides detailed instruction regarding the sequence of movements involved in the exercise, or the patient is given a copy of an exercise and becomes aware of the sequence while he or she is practicing the task, this is an example of explicit procedural memory.

Rehabilitation clinicians are primarily accessing and modifying the nondeclarative procedural memory of the patient as they teach perform therapeutic exercise, gait training, or neuromuscular reeducation as part of a treatment plan.

Organization of Memory

Declarative and nondeclarative memory is organized, consolidated, and accessed differently. The ability to access information from declarative memory allows an individual to utilize this information in order to interact with others, make decisions, and solve problems. Although the process by which one accesses long-term memory is not well understood, a number of theories have been developed to describe organization of memory. It is believed that declarative memory information is clustered into similar content and stored according to that content. For instance, emotionally charged memories are stored according to emotional content rather than stored chronologically. This may explain why a particular emotional experience will cause recall of memories with similar emotional context. This model of memory organization is known as the *hierarchical network model of semantic memory*. It states that information is stored in categories that are logically related to each other in a hierarchy. For example, broad categories of information, like "animal," are subdivided into narrower categories such as "snake" or "bird," which is further subdivided into a narrower category such as "copperhead" or "blue jay." Information stored at one level of the hierarchy is not repeated at other levels. Data are stored at the highest level in a particular category in this cognitive economy model.

During the process of recall, information is retrieved from a logical hierarchy and may include a kind of reasoning in which facts are put together logically to make an assumption, as opposed to simply recalling facts. This retrieval process is a form of logical deduction called a *syllogism*, which, for example, offers a general principle like "no reptiles have fur," followed by a more specific premise like "all snakes are reptiles" followed by the conclusion that "no snakes have fur." This is an example of the logical fact recall from the hierarchy of stored facts and processing that takes place in the process of information retrieval from long-term memory. The speed of this process will vary according to familiarity of information and direct concept property associations.

Memory Retrieval

In order to access stored memories, various cues are used to impact how information is retrieved. These cues prompt different methods by which memory is retrieved from long-term memory. Types of cuing include recall, recollection, recognition, and relearning. The type of cue that is selected depends upon the demand upon which the retrieved memory will be used. These types of memory retrieval strategies are exemplified in a scholastic examination. When an instructor wants to test whether a student has learned and retained the information imparted during a class, a written examination is a typical method of testing. Recall is a method of memory retrieval that can be accessed without cuing. Completing a fill-in-the-blank question requires recall. Recollection requires reconstruction of a memory using logical sequences, narratives, or clues. Writing an essay answer requires this more complex method of memory retrieval because it requires not only retrieval of facts but also reconstruction of the facts into a logical, sequential narrative. Recognition is another type of memory retrieval that requires identification of information after it is experienced. Multiple-choice testing requires recognition of the correct answer selected from a group of possible choices. Relearning is a memory retrieval strategy that involves re-exposure to information that has already been stored. This method often makes it easier to retrieve the information in the future and seems to improve the strength of the memory.

Memory, memory retrieval, and retrieval failure have been the subject of study for hundreds of years. In fact, in 1885, Hermann Ebbinghaus engaged in an experiment to evaluate memory and forgetting, the findings of which he published in a paper entitled "Memory: A Contribution to Experimental Psychology."[4] His results, plotted in what has come to be known as the Ebbinghaus forgetting curve, showed the relationship between time and lost information or forgetting. He showed that information may be quickly forgotten after initially learning, but the "forgetting curve" does not continue to decline until all memory is lost. In fact, the degree of forgetting levels off, which seems to indicate that information stored in long-term memory is surprisingly stable.

Retrieval Failure

Retrieval of declarative memory is not flawless. In fact, retrieval errors are fairly common according to Schacter et al, who noted in their work, "The Seven Sins of Memory," that normal adults experience memory retrieval failure at least once a week, and this failure increases with aging and may occur 2 to 4 times per week, in older adults.[5]

Memory retrieval failure or forgetting can occur for a number of reasons. Elizabeth Loftus identified 4 reasons for forgetting, namely, retrieval failure, interference, failure to store memory, and motivated forgetting.[6] Retrieval failure or the inability to retrieve a memory is one of the most common causes of forgetting. Given that a new memory trace is created every time a new memory is formed, this theory suggests that, over time, these traces begin to disappear or decay, and information that is not retrieved or rehearsed will eventually be lost. The problem with this theory is that research has shown that even memory that has not been retrieved or rehearsed can remain stable in long-term memory.

The interference theory suggests that some memories compete with others and interfere with memory encoding into long-term memory. This is particularly likely to occur with memories that are similar to the memory in question. Proactive interference refers to an old memory that makes it more difficult to remember a newer memory. Retroactive interference occurs when new information interferes with the ability to remember previously created memory or learned information.

Sometimes forgetting has more to do with a failure to effectively store the memory, as opposed to a retrieval failure. This failure to encode will prevent information from being stored into long-term memory. An experiment conducted by Nickerson and Adams exemplifies this theory. In the experiment, subjects were asked to identify the correct penny from a series of penny designs. Because most individuals only store enough information to distinguish pennies from other coins, many were unable to identify subtle variations in the penny design. This is a situation of a failure to store a memory.[7] Another memory retrieval problem may occur when an individual actively works to suppress or repress a memory. This may be a conscious or an unconscious form of forgetting. Because one of the ways a memory is strengthened is by being retrieved or rehearsed, and painful or traumatic memories may not be, they may be more subject to failure of retrieval problems. The concept of repression, however, is a subject of significant controversy in the field of psychology.

Summary of Memory

Short-term memory is known as primary or active memory and contains the information that one is currently aware of or thinking about. This memory is often a result of information that comes from various sensory stimuli, visual, auditory, tactile, etc. Information is kept in short-term memory for approximately 20 to 30 seconds but may be less if active maintenance of the information, by way of rehearsing it or paying attention to it, is not performed in order to prevent loss of the memory and progression of the information into long-term memory. The amount of information that can be maintained in short-term memory varies.

In his paper titled, "The Magic Number Seven, Plus or Minus Two,"[8] George Miller suggested that a normal human can store 5 to 9 items in short-term memory at any given time, although more recent research suggests that short-term memory is likely grouped into related data as chunks of data and an individual is probably capable of storing approximately 4 chunks of information in short-term memory. Once information has been rehearsed or attended to, it may move on to be stored as long-term memory. Long-term memory is data that are stored, but can be recalled into working memory in order to be acted upon or manipulated for the task at hand. Long-term memory is generally stored outside conscious awareness until such time that it is required for recall. Some of these memories are easily accessed, whereas others are much more difficult to recall, depending upon the amount of rehearsal and association of the information with other memories. Long-term memory can last for days to decades, depending upon the type of memory, its associations with other information, and the manner in which it was stored.

The Role of the Hippocampus in Memory

The hippocampus, a part of the limbic system, is a bilateral system in the basilar brain that is associated with consolidating declarative but not necessarily nondeclarative information from short-term into long-term memory. Because of its association with the limbic system, the hippocampus is involved in a complex process of forming, organizing, and storing declarative memories and the emotional content of those memories. Because it is a bilateral system, it appears that damage to one side of the hippocampus would cause minimal change in memory function. Damage to both sides of the structure appears to result in anterograde amnesia or an impediment to the ability to form new declarative memories. Individuals with bilateral hippocampal damage can, however, still learn new motor skills. Hippocampus function begins to decline with age, and it is thought that by the time an individual reaches the 80s, they may have lost as much as 20% of the neural connections in the hippocampus. This loss of neurons may be a contributing factor in decreased performance in declarative memory tests, although there are other factors that contribute to decreased performance, including depression and sleep loss.

Being tested on information can help memory storage because the act of studying is rehearsing the information (Figure 21-5). Interestingly, research has shown that students who studied in preparation of being tested on material had better long-term recall of the information, even if the information was not actually included in testing. However, students who studied, but were not tested, had less long-term recall than their tested counterparts. It appears that rehearsing the information as part of studying and then being tested upon the material enhanced recall, although the mechanism for this is not clear.[9] Amnesia, the complete inability to recall declarative memories has 2 basic forms. Anterograde amnesia is characterized by the loss of the ability to form new memories. Retrograde amnesia is characterized by the loss of ability to recollect past memories, although the capacity to create new memories may

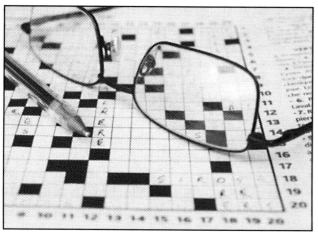

Figure 21-5. Testing information can actually help long-term memory storage and recall. (From Fotolia.com)

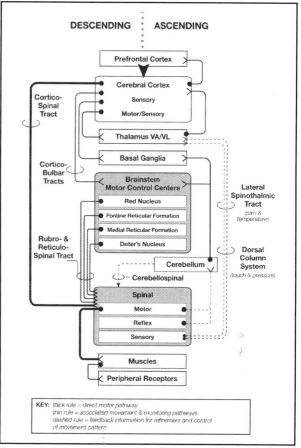

Figure 21-6. Simplified schematic of the motor pathway.

remain intact. Movies and television shows depict amnesia as a fairly common occurrence, but in reality these depictions are generally wildly inaccurate. In fact, retrograde amnesia with loss of memory of one's past and identity is extremely rare. Anterograde amnesia, or the ability to lay down new memory, is more common and much of what is known about it has been drawn from the famous case of a patient known as H.M. In 1953, H.M. underwent brain surgery to help control severe epileptic seizure activity.[10] During the surgery, bilateral hippocampi were removed and, as a result, H.M. was no longer able to create new declarative memories; however, he was able to learn new motor tasks.

MOTOR LEARNING AND NONDECLARATIVE MEMORY

A Review of the Production of Motor Output

A review of the production of motor output will remind the reader of the pathways and neural activity involved in motor processing. It is also important to review the systems that are involved in the production of motor output in order to better understand the process of motor learning and motor memory. This review will remind the reader of how systems interact, particularly as this interaction relates to the generation and maintenance of sleep and wakefulness.

A model of motor output using a schematic description of events that occur in the motor system to initiate, correct, and execute a movement will be presented to facilitate understanding of the connection between neural pathways involved in motor learning and in production and maintenance of sleep (Figure 21-6). For this discussion, voluntary flexion of the elbow of the upper extremity will be used as a simple movement model.

Initially, the idea for elbow flexion occurs in the prefrontal cortex. A motor command is sent from the prefrontal cortex to the motor cortices of the cerebrum, including the primary motor cortex, the premotor region, and the primary sensory cortex, which is involved in processing incoming sensory information from the muscle and joint as the movement command progresses. The primary motor cortex, where the corticospinal tract originates, produces a "go" signal for movement. A motor command is sent from the cerebral motor cortex to the basal ganglia, a structure that modulates the initiation of movement. The basal ganglia send collateral neurons to the ventrolateral and ventroanterior nuclei of the thalamus for monitoring of the movement command. A motor command is also sent from the cerebral motor cortex to the brain stem motor centers of the red nucleus, pontine reticular formation, medial reticular formation, and Deter's nucleus via the rubrospinal tract and the reticulospinal tracts to the ventral horn of the spinal cord for associated postural adjustments and axial stabilization, which will be necessary to accompany the primary movement command. A motor command is sent from the cerebral motor cortex via the corticospinal tract to the spinal motor centers in the ventral horn of the spinal cord

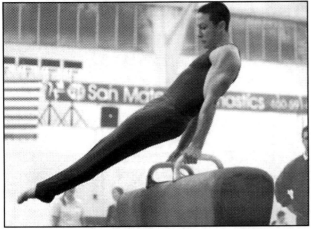

Figure 21-7. Motor learning requires consolidation of motor memory and reconsolidation of that memory as the task is practiced. Sleep appears to be a necessary step for this consolidation and reconsolidation. Some motor tasks can be performed relatively by rote. More complex tasks that have unexpected variables require increased attention. (From Fotolia.com)

to synapse on the second-order neurons in the anterior horn cell column. The motor command sends collateral information to the spinal relay nuclei (pontine, lateral reticular, and inferior olive) so that these nuclei can monitor the movement command. The second-order neuron of the corticospinal nerve fiber, called the *alpha motor neuron* and is a lower motor neuron, sends a motor command to the neuromuscular junction in the upper extremity flexion muscles with information to contract. Prior to muscle contraction, receptors in the primary and secondary endings of the muscles, Golgi tendon organ, and skin and joint proprioceptors provide sensory information from the muscle and process information regarding joint preparedness for movement including relative tension in the muscle, position of the joint, muscle length, blood flow, and temperature. This sensory information will ascend via the spinothalamic and dorsal column pathways to the sensory cortex to be processed so that information regarding the amount of muscle tension and joint position, for example, can be incorporated into a precise, controlled movement. Receptor information is also fed into the spinal relay nuclei, including the lateral reticular and inferior olive nuclei, which process information for precision of movement. Spinal relay nuclei feed sensory information from the joint into the spinocerebellum, the part of the cerebellum that processes proprioception information from the joints of the ipsilateral limbs. This information comes from both motor command monitors and receptor feedback and is combined and sent to the spinocerebellum for correction of the rate of movement, the range through which the muscle is prepared to move and the rhythm of that movement. Spinocerebellum combines information regarding the requested motor command and the actual movement being programmed, via feedback and monitor mechanisms, and issues a correction to the thalamus, red

nucleus, and cerebral motor cortex. Ventrolateral nuclei relay command corrections to the cerebral motor cortex for execution of the requested movement. Spinocerebellar nuclei also send command correction information to the red nuclei to suppress aberrant reflex activity associated with movement. A new, corrected command is issued by the cerebral motor cortex and the loop repeats itself. The time required to complete the circuit is approximately 100 ns. The bulk of that time is required by the muscle and muscle receptor functions. The thalamus-to-cortex-to-brain stem relay to cerebellum part of the circuit requires only 20 ns. This system monitoring and command correction system allows a motor command to be corrected approximately 5 times before evidence of muscle activity is present.

Motor Learning and Memory

Motor learning is a form of procedural memory in which a specific motor task is performed repeatedly and the memory of that task performance is consolidated into a long-term memory (Figure 21-7). As the movement is repeated over time, a long-term memory for that procedure is created, allowing the task to be performed with minimal or no conscious effort. As the task is repeated over and over, there is a decrease in the need for attention and an increase in the efficiency of the neuronal processing within the motor and memory systems. In this manner, everyday activities become automatic and improve with practice.

The acquisition of motor skills was an important component of human evolution as increasingly complex movements allowed use of tools, development of shelter, and other survival skills. Although most motor learning is acquired over a lifetime, there is evidence that some motor memory is genetically determined. This was hypothesized after the observation that facial expressions can actually be observed in children who are blind.[11]

Edward Thorndike observed that motor learning can occur without conscious awareness and memory can be retained for extended periods of time even without regular practice. This explains the adage "you never forget how to ride a bike."[12] These tasks seem to be effortlessly and unconsciously executed skills even without repeated skill practice. When a motor task is first learned, the movement is slow and deliberate. Performance of the skill is easily disrupted unless one pays close attention. Multiple areas of the brain are activated when a novel task is being learned. As the skill becomes well learned, areas of brain activation become more consolidated and there is less brain activity associated with attention and less working memory is required (Figure 21-8). With practice, a neurological pathway is developed and the execution becomes smoother, and less and less conscious effort is required to complete the task.[13] As a motor memory pathway is repeated, there is less need for conscious attention to the memory. This process is also known as procedural memory, and with practice, some of these procedural or motor memories can be performed efficiently without attention as might be the case in a piece of music that is practiced and "learned by heart."

The neuroanatomy of memory is widespread but is localized according to the type of memory that is encoded. For instance, the pathways for motor memory are separate from those pathways associated with declarative memory. Motor learning, like declarative memory, includes short-term encoding, which is fragile, and long-term motor memory consolidation, which is more stable and less susceptible to damage.[14,15] During the initial stages of motor learning, motor and somatosensory cortices are active, but as the motor pathway is practiced and refined, there is decreased activity in these areas. During initial learning, prefrontal and frontal cortices are active, as there is an increased need for attention to the task at hand.[9] The cerebellum is a primary structure involved in motor learning. Models of cerebellar-dependent motor learning, particularly the Marr-Albus model, suggest that a single plasticity mechanism is involved, in which there is a long-term depression of parallel fiber synapses onto Purkinje cells. This modification of the synaptic activity mediates motor output critical to inducing motor learning.[16] Other evidence suggests that the single plasticity mechanism is not sufficient to account for the multiple motor memories over time. Regardless, studies of cerebellar-dependent motor tasks show that cerebral cortical plasticity is crucial for motor learning even if it is not necessary for storage of these motor memories.[17]

The basal ganglia play an important role in motor memory and learning, particularly regarding stimulus–response associations and the formation of habits. The basal ganglia–cerebellar connections increase as a novel motor task is practiced.[18] Consolidation of novel motor memory continues to be modified even after practice of the motor task has ceased. Although the precise mechanism of motor memory consolidation remains an area of study, Hebb's rule states that synaptic connectivity changes as a function of repetitive firing.[19] This indicates that the higher amount of synaptic activity that would accompany practicing of a novel motor task would result in increased firing rates in certain motor pathways. This would thereby increase the efficiency of these pathways over time.[14]

Studies suggest that motor memory involves interregional brain connections that improve motor memory consolidation rather than decreasing overall regional activity. That is, production of a well-learned task will produce activation of small, specific regions of the brain. It appears that as the motor memory pathway becomes more efficient and consolidated, there is a weakened connection from the cerebellum to the primary motor cortex. However, the connection between the basal ganglia and the primary motor cortex is strengthened, suggesting that the basal ganglia play an important role in motor memory consolidation.

When an individual learns a complex task, such as a new skill on the soccer field, movement combinations are

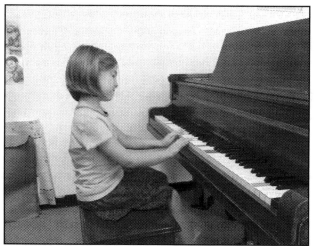

Figure 21-8. With motor memory, a specific activity requires multiple areas of the brain at first, but with practice, there is less need for conscious attention to the activity. Performing artists such as musicians often develop such integration of motor and auditory pathways for performance of a piece of music that they need little conscious control of the motor task and can use more attention to add to the artistic expression of the piece. (Reprinted with permission from V. Mebruer.)

frequently used and repeated. These movement sequences may require strength, endurance, and skill. The initial fast-learning phase in which the optimal motor pattern for performance of a task is established is influenced by changes in neural circuitry rather than by changes in muscle size. In addition to improvement in neural firing patterns, slow-phase motor learning eventually results in structural modifications to the musculature itself, including muscle hypertrophy.[20] Therefore, though some of motor learning involves neurological changes, there are also local changes that occur in muscle tissue in order to support the acquisition of skill. Increase in strength occurs well before physiological muscular adaptation or muscle hypertrophy, and conversely, decrease in strength occurs due to detraining precede muscle atrophy.[21] Endurance training involves angiogenesis in the motor cortex and an upregulation of neurotrophic factors within the cortex in response to endurance training in order to promote and preserve changes in neural mapping that develop as a result of skill acquisition training.[16]

According to Kleim and Hogg,[22] in a mouse model, motor learning leads to rapid formation of dendritic spines in the motor cortex contralateral to the reaching forelimb. The reorganization of the motor cortex in response to motor learning does not occur at a consistent rate across the learning period, however. The eventual changes in synapses and motor pathway following a training session represent the consolidation effort rather than the specific acquisition of the motor skill.[16,22]

Fine motor skill, such as those involved in using tools, vary in the neurological processes required when compared with gross motor tasks. Fine motor tasks become programmed in the premotor cortex, which, when triggered, activates the motor cortex and results in characteristic movement patterns. These are learned movement patterns that become rote and are stored as a motor program. It is important to note that though a motor program may exist for a fine motor task; for example, that a motor program can be adapted based upon specific task characteristics or particular environmental constraints. Studies of fine motor tasks such as sequential fingering, which are learned and stored, can be disrupted if the individual is distracted or if another task interferes with the execution of the task. Rather than unlearning the task, a novel motor pattern appears to supersede a previously encoded memory. The degree to which the new memory will interfere with the older memory depends upon how ingrained the original motor program is, how much the new task is performed, and how quickly after learning the first task the second task is practiced. In other words, it depends upon how stable the original task memory has become. This disruption of motor memory can be restored fairly readily with repetition of the original movement pattern, leading researchers to conclude that learning a motor task back to back may cause memory B to interfere with retention of memory A. However, memory B can be fragile and may be more prone to difficulty in permanently encoding and consolidating that memory.[23]

Of particular interest when reviewing fine motor skill is the motor learning and memory process that occurs when an individual learns to play a musical instrument (Figure 21-9). As a musical piece is learned, the motor patterns required to produce the notes and tongue and facial muscles required to move air through a wind instrument must be combined with bi-manual coordinated fingering skills needed to produce specific note patterns. These complex movement patterns must also be paired with auditory memory. This requires a very complex interconnection of neural networks in which information must be transmitted across multiple brain areas. Studies have shown that functional imaging of professional musicians is different from their non-musician counterparts.[24] Professional musicians appear to have increased efficiency in recall and execution of motor memory. In fact, one study found that when a pianist hears a very familiarly played piece of music, patterned fingering can be automatically triggered, indicating that motor memory is initiated with an auditory queue. This degree of training and motor memory development allows the complex action of patterned fingering to occur at a lower neurological level, thus allowing the musician to attend to the artistic aspects of execution of a piece rather than attending to motor pattern selection, attention, and timing.[25]

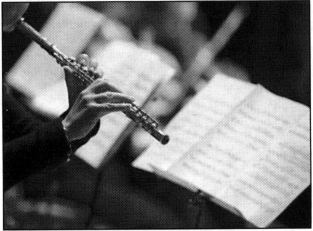

Figure 21-9. Musicians appear to have more efficient recall and execution of motor memory. (From Fotolia.com)

Gross Motor Memory

Gross motor learning and memory usually refers to movements that involve large muscle groups or major body movements. During growth and development, a child gains gross motor skills before he or she is able to refine these into finer motor skills. Examples of gross motor memory are those movement patterns involved in walking, kicking, and large arm movements. Gross motor skills can be refined and trained to improve the degree of precision of the skill. This is largely dependent upon muscle tone and strength, as well as neuromuscular and proprioceptive adaptation.

Impairment of motor memory is difficult to study and identify specifically because of the widespread nature of the systems that subserve motor memory. In diseases commonly associated with motor deficits, such as Parkinson's disease or Huntington disease, symptoms are variable and areas of damage are widespread, making precise localization of the impact on memory difficult to assess.

It is apparent that motor memory consolidates in a different manner than declarative memory. Procedural memory of a well-learned skill is demonstrated through recall of that skill that is consolidated over several trials of learning, whereas declarative learning involves recall of information that occurs once. This was demonstrated in the case of Clive Wearing,[26] a British musicologist and keyboardist who suffered significant damage to temporal lobes, frontal lobes, and the hippocampi. He has severe anterograde and retrograde amnesia and is not able to store any new memories, has little perception of time, and is only aware of the present moment. However, he continues to have access to procedural memories, particularly those that allowed him to play the keyboard. This suggests that lesions in certain areas of the brain normally associated with declarative memory will not affect motor memory for a well-learned skill.

SLEEP-DEPENDENT MOTOR LEARNING, SKILL DEVELOPMENT, AND BRAIN PLASTICITY

Once information has been acquired, it is initially encoded, but further processing is necessary in order for that information to pass from sensory memory to short-term memory to long-term memory. Although the precise mechanisms of declarative and nondeclarative memory continue to be areas of significant research, it is increasingly clear that sleep is an important component of memory consolidation, although the process of memory consolidation for declarative and nondeclarative memory occurs by different pathways.

For a memory to become relatively permanent, it must be consolidated, integrated into a memory representation, and translocated. If the information is deemed unnecessary for storage, it is usually erased at this point. Following later recall of the memory, it is believed that the memory becomes unstable once again and then must be reconsolidated. After this post encoding reconsolidation, the memory is thought to be more stable.[27]

It is now clear that sleep plays an important role in memory consolidation, although the manner in which declarative and nondeclarative memory are consolidated is different and is subserved by different processes and systems (Figure 21-10). In this way, memory consolidation, erasure, and reconsolidation occur outside of awareness and without necessarily any additional training or exposure to the original stimuli.

Studies suggest that slow-wave sleep (SWS) and rapid eye movement (REM) sleep are involved in the processing of human declarative memory.

Motor learning, which involves nondeclarative memory, of which procedural memory is a subcategory, has been shown to be deficient with experimentally induced non-rapid eye movement (NREM) stage 2 sleep.[28] Sleep has been shown to improve speed and accuracy in performance of certain sequential finger-tapping tasks, but there is no improvement in these tasks during equivalent periods of wakefulness.[29]

Sleep is a critical component for motor skill learning and memory consolidation. Participants who sleep following practice of a motor skill perform the task faster, with fewer errors, or more efficiently following sleep, compared to a similar length period of being awake. Sleep has been shown to be involved in the consolidation of various types of simple motor skills, including a finger opposition task,[29-34] a finger-tapping task,[35-38] the Serial Reaction Time (SRT) task,[39-43] a continuous tracking task,[44,45] a pursuit rotor task,[29,46] and a motor adaptation task.[47] The variety of tasks utilized to assess sleep-dependent off-line learning of motor skills makes comparison between studies

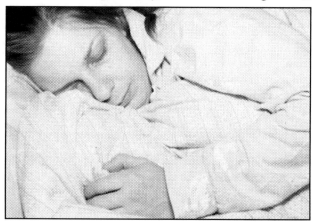

Figure 21-10. Sleep plays an important role in memory consolidation, particularly in the SWS and REM stages. (From Fotolia.com)

difficult, and the specific task characteristics (ie, implicit vs explicit motor skill learning, continuous vs discrete motor skill learning, motor skill learning vs motor adaptation) likely influence the relative degree of sleep-dependent consolidation. However, the overall finding of these studies is sleep produces the consolidation of these motor skills.

One factor that appears to impact the influence of sleep on motor skill learning is participant awareness of the regularities of the task. Explicit motor skill learning refers to conscious awareness of the regularities of the task to be learned.[48-51] For example, when learning the SRT task, participants can be given explicit instruction on the nature of the sequence to be learned or become aware of the presence of the sequence during practice. Implicit motor skill learning refers to learning a skill without conscious awareness of the task regularities. For example, the SRT task is learned implicitly when the participants are unaware of the presence of the sequence to be learned. Studies demonstrate that explicit motor skill learning is enhanced following sleep,[47,52,53] though evidence is conflicting on whether or not implicitly learned motor tasks benefit from sleep to promote learning.[54-56]

Another factor that may impact sleep-dependent motor skill learning is the type of task utilized, including a continuous task with no clear beginning or end (such as swimming or running) or a discrete task with a definite beginning or end (such as kicking a ball or pressing a key on the computer). Evidence suggests sleep may impact discrete and continuous tasks differently.[57] Furthermore, sleep may impact motor adaptation tasks that involve a strong perceptual component to adjust motor behavior due to environmental perturbations differently, compared to motor sequencing tasks that involve learning a novel movement.[58] Different mechanisms appear to be involved in the consolidation of probabilistic motor tasks compared to deterministic motor tasks.[59] Taken together, there are many factors to consider when assessing the role of sleep in the consolidation of motor memories. More research is needed to determine specifically how each of these factors impact sleep-dependent motor skill learning.

Although the aforementioned studies demonstrate that sleep promotes motor skill learning, these studies all utilized computer-based, relatively simple motor tasks. Of particular interest to the rehabilitation provider is whether or not sleep promotes learning functionally relevant motor tasks, such as the exercises of a home exercise program or how to walk with a prosthesis following a lower extremity amputation. Studies are currently underway to determine whether sleep consolidates learning of more functionally relevant tasks.

Recent studies have demonstrated that more complex computer-based tasks appear to have a greater benefit from sleep to promote learning. Kuriyama et al found that a longer bi-manual finger sequencing task showed a greater improvement in speed following sleep, compared to a shorter unimanual version.[60] Brawn et al found that performance on a video game was stabilized following sleep but not following a period of being awake.[61] These 2 studies suggest that more complex tasks benefit from sleep to produce memory consolidation of these more complex motor tasks. Future studies will shed light on the role sleep plays in promoting learning and memory consolidation of functionally relevant complex tasks.

Although much research demonstrates that sleep promotes learning of motor skills, sleep also promotes learning of other types of nondeclarative memories, including a visual discrimination perceptual task.[62-64] In these studies, participants are asked to correctly identify a letter and the orientation of figures among distraction figures. Similar to the motor skill tasks, participants who slept following practice of the visual discrimination task were faster in correctly identifying the figures compared to those participants who stayed awake.[45-47] This research shows that sleep is critical for the consolidation of nondeclarative motor skills and perceptual tasks.

Information learned while awake is thought to be "replayed" during sleep so the functional neural connections supporting the memory are strengthened,[29,65,66] and the neural connections that are not critical for supporting the memory are pruned.[67,68] Imaging studies in humans show changes in neural activity due to sleep-dependent learning result in more efficient neural organization.[29,69,70] Fischer et al used functional magnetic resonance imaging (fMRI) to determine brain areas active during practice of a finger-to-thumb opposition task using the left hand, which were reactivated during retention testing 48 hours later.[71] As expected, they found improved performance at retention in the sleep group compared to the sleep-deprived group. Interestingly, they found a *reduction* in brain activation in the left prefrontal cortex and the right lateral premotor cortex in the sleep group from training to retention. The authors suggest that this indicates a decreased need to consciously regulate and monitor continued finger movements.

The area of *increased* activity was found in the left superior parietal lobe, which they concluded indicates that this area is involved in automated performance. The decrease in brain activation following sleep supports the synaptic homeostasis hypothesis by Tononi and Cirelli, which proposes that the role of sleep (SWS in particular) is to globally downscale the synaptic strength of brain circuits that were increased during learning back to baseline to save energy and gray matter space.[72]

In a similar study using fMRI, Walker et al found different activation patterns but arrived at a similar conclusion.[70] These researchers determined that participants who practiced a sequential finger-tapping task using the left hand and slept following training exhibited an *increased* activation in the right primary motor cortex, right prefrontal lobe, right hippocampus, right ventral striatum, and left cerebellum compared to participants who stayed awake following training. They suggest that increases in activation support faster, more efficient output and optimize transitions. The increase in hippocampal activation is likely due to the explicit nature of this task due to the hippocampus having a role in explicit memory formation.[73] Walker et al found a *decrease* in bilateral parietal cortices, the left insular cortex, the left temporal pole, and the left inferior front-polar cortex.[70] They attribute this decrease in activation to a reduction in need to monitor performance and a decrease in emotional burden. The discrepancy between the findings these two studies may be because Walker et al[70] used a paced task vs an unpaced task in the Fischer et al[71] study as well as because of the slightly different task used. However, these 2 studies provide the first glimpse into the consolidation of motor memory following sleep.

SLEEP AND MOTOR LEARNING

Sleep has been shown to produce off-line improvements on a variety of tasks. Researchers have frequently used simple discrete computer-based tasks to assess sleep-dependent off-line motor skill learning. One such task is a sequential finger-tapping task. Walker et al have consistently demonstrated that people who sleep following practice of the sequential finger-tapping task are able to perform the task with increased speed and accuracy.[74-76] On a similar task, a finger-to-thumb opposition task, participants demonstrated faster performance and produced the sequence with fewer errors following a period of sleep.[77,78]

Several factors appear to influence sleep-dependent off-line learning. One of these factors is the level of awareness the participants have of the skill they are trying to learn. Robertson et al demonstrated that participants who were explicitly aware of the sequence they were practicing experienced significantly faster response times after sleep compared to a period of being awake.[79] However, those participants who were unaware of the sequence being practiced (implicit awareness) demonstrated significantly faster response times both after a period of sleep and a period of being awake.[79] Studies utilizing an implicitly learned probabilistic sequencing task found mixed results when assessing whether sleep or passage of time enhances general compared to sequence-specific skill performance.[80,81] The variation in the findings of these studies may be related to sleep's differential effect on fixed compared to probabilistic tasks, as well as general compared to sequence-specific skill learning.

Another factor to consider is whether the task is a discrete or a continuous task. A discrete task is a task with an obvious beginning and an end, such as kicking or throwing a ball, whereas a continuous task does not have an obvious beginning or an end, such as swimming or walking.[82] One study utilized both an explicitly learned discrete task and an explicitly learned continuous task and found that participants demonstrated significantly faster response times following sleep on the discrete task, but did not demonstrate significantly reduced tracking error on the continuous task.[83]

The level of task complexity also appears to influence sleep-dependent off-line learning. A study by Kuriyama et al demonstrated that participants who practiced a more complex version of a finger-tapping task and slept following practice demonstrated a higher percentage improvement in speed compared to participants who practiced a simpler version of the task.[84] Another study demonstrated that individuals who practiced a video game showed less deterioration in performance on the game if they slept following practice compared to those individuals who stayed awake.[85] These studies suggest that more complex motor skills benefit from sleep for consolidation in young healthy individuals.

Taken together, the impact of sleep on motor skill learning is influenced by the following factors: whether the task is implicitly or explicitly learned, whether the task is fixed or probabilistic, whether the outcome assessed is general skill learning or sequence-specific learning, whether the task is discrete or continuous, and task complexity.

Studies have demonstrated that variable lengths of time between motor skill practice and the sleep episode produces off-line motor learning. Typically, participants practice the motor skill and then sleep either following practice[54,56,58,62] or about 12 hours later.[54] However, multiple nights of sleep have been shown to produce even greater improvements in speed on a finger-tapping task compared to one night of sleep.[55] Other studies have assessed skill performance following 3 nights of sleep[86] or after 1 week.[87,88]

Which specific stage of sleep is associated with sleep-dependent off-line motor skill learning remains in debate, although studies have demonstrated that NREM stage 2 sleep,[54] and in particular sleep spindles,[66,67,89–91] is associated with sleep-dependent motor skill learning. Walker et al demonstrated that an overnight improvement in speed on a finger-tapping task was significantly

correlated with NREM stage 2 sleep.[74] Multiple studies have demonstrated that an improvement in overnight skill performance is associated with an increase in spindle density or spindle frequency.[66–70]

Others have demonstrated that REM sleep is associated with improved task performance.[56] The discrepancy between whether NREM stage 2 and/or REM sleep is involved in sleep-dependent off-line motor skill learning may be due to the cognitive requirements of the task as well as the novelty of the task. NREM stage 2 has been associated with the overnight improvement on a less cognitively involved pursuit rotor task, whereas improvements on a more cognitively involved mirror tracing task was associated with REM sleep.[69] Furthermore, NREM stage 2 sleep is associated with off-line learning of a pursuit rotor task if the subject has high initial skill levels, but REM sleep is associated with off-line learning if the subject has low initial skill levels.[66]

The amount of practice required to produce off-line motor skill learning remains in debate and the amount of practice participants undergo varies considerably between studies. Walker et al found that doubling the amount of practice did not significantly impact the degree of off-line improvement on a finger-tapping task.[75] In addition, Walker et al found no correlation between the degree of improvement in speed or accuracy during practice and the degree of overnight improvement in these variables.[55] There is presumably a critical amount of practice required to produce off-line improvements in motor skill performance, but what that critical amount is remains to be determined.

Daytime Naps and Skill Learning

Naps of 60 to 90 minutes have been demonstrated to produce off-line improvements in performance on procedural memory tasks, including motor[92–94] and perceptual tasks,[71,95] as well as declarative memory tasks[71] (Figure 21-11). Backhaus and Junghanns found that a nap of 45 minutes improved performance on a procedural mirror tracing task but not on 2 declarative memory tasks.[93] The discrepancy in findings between studies may depend on the length of nap, composition of sleep stages within the nap period, and the type of task utilized. Evidence suggests that SWS combined with REM sleep is critical for producing off-line learning over a nap period,[74] whereas others suggest that off-line learning over a nap period is reliant on NREM stage 2 sleep,[72,73] and sleep spindles in particular.[73] Milner et al suggested that napping enhances off-line motor learning of a ball-n-cup task, but only for individuals who frequently take naps, and that sleep spindles density is associated with improved performance on the task.[96] Wamsley et al demonstrated that individuals who practiced a spatial maze navigation task and took a 90-minute nap showed improved performance on the task compared to those who stayed awake.[97] Furthermore, they found those individuals

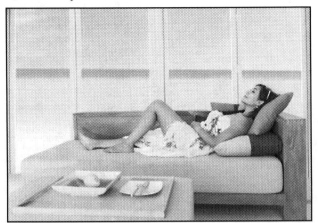

Figure 21-11. Naps have shown to improve procedural memory performance. (From Fotolia.com)

who dreamed about the task during the nap period demonstrated significant improvement on the task compared to those who napped but did not dream about the task.[76] One study looked at the effect of naps in individuals with schizophrenia and individuals with depression and found a nap of 40 minutes improved performance on a declarative memory task for individuals with schizophrenia and individuals with depression, but only those individuals with depression demonstrated off-line learning of a procedural mirror-tracing task.[98] Although some discrepancy persists, these studies demonstrate a nap is sufficient to produce off-line learning of a variety of memories and tasks.

SLEEP AND ATHLETIC PERFORMANCE

The amount of sleep an athlete gets appears to have a significant impact on performance. Sleep deprivation can hinder athletic performance. It has been shown that sleep deprivation can impair glucose metabolism as much as 30% to 40%. Spiegel et al studied induced sleep deprivation in subjects over time.[99] Subjects were allowed to sleep 8 hours for 3 nights, and then only allowed 4 hours of sleep for the next 6 nights. They were then allowed 12 hours per night for the last 7 nights. Results of the study showed impairment in glucose metabolism immediately during the sleep deprivation period. The stress hormone cortisol was also elevated during the sleep deprivation period. This study showed that even after only 1 week of sleep restriction, young healthy subjects showed impairment in glucose metabolism and glycogen synthesis and impairment in processes needed for tissue repair and recovery. Impairment of glucose metabolism in these sleep-deprived subjects was similar to that found in elderly subjects. Studies have also linked sleep deprivation with decreased aerobic endurance and increased perceived exertion ratings.

It is the alternation of adaptation and recovery that allows an athlete to achieve a higher level of fitness and performance. Glucose and glycogen are the primary sources of energy for athletes, and the ability to store glucose in muscle and the liver is particularly important for endurance athletes. Sleep deprivation impairs glucose storage for endurance events beyond 90 minutes. Elevated cortisol levels may interfere with tissue repair and muscle recovery. Over time, this may interfere with effective training and lead to overtraining injury. Sleep deprivation appears to be particularly damaging for endurance athletes.[100]

Although a number of studies have looked at the effects of sleep deprivation on athletic performance, other research has begun to look at the effect of increased sleep on athletic performance. A study by Mah et al, at the Stanford Sleep Disorders Clinic and Research Lab, has shown that basketball players at the elite college level were able to improve their on-the-court performance by increasing their amount of total sleep time (Figure 21-12).[101] The study suggested that sleep is an important factor in peak athletic performance. Athletes may be able to optimize training and competition outcomes by identifying strategies to maximize the benefits of sleep. It is widely understood that sleep deprivation has negative consequences on cognitive function, mood, and physical performance, but this study showed that improved sleep, including sleep extension, can improve physical performance.

Athletes understand that nutrition and physical training must be part of the daily regime for a good competitive edge, but they do not typically take into consideration the importance of optimizing sleep and recovery. Very often, players and coaches allow sleep to be sacrificed, not understanding the consequences. Healthy and adequate sleep is not understood to be as important to peak performance as other aspects of training.

A study of undergraduate students has shown that sleep extension improves cognitive function[102] (Figure 21-13). Several participants in the study were also collegiate swimmers and reported that they had set personal swim records during portions of the study in which they got more sleep than normal. These findings led researchers to investigate the effects of sleep extension on athletic performance.

In another study, collegiate basketball players were followed over the course of 2 basketball seasons, and the effects of sleep extension on reaction time, mood, and daytime sleepiness were measured. Players maintained normal nighttime sleep schedule consisting of 6 to 9 hours of sleep per night for 2 to 4 weeks, then increased sleep to 10 hours per night for the next 5 to 7 weeks. They took daytime naps when travel prohibited 10 hours of nighttime sleep. During the study period, players abstained from caffeine and alcohol. At the end of the sleep extension period, players were evaluated on a number of athletic performance parameters. Compared to baseline data, they ran faster in sprints, improved free throw and 3-point field goal shooting by more than 9%, and reported decreased fatigue and improved practices and games. Although this study did

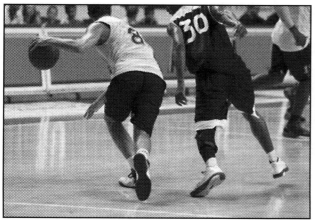

Figure 21-12. A Stanford study of basketball players showed improved performance. (From Fotolia.com)

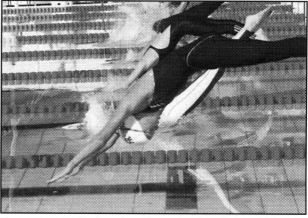

Figure 21-13. Studies have shown increasing sleep time to 10 hours per night can improve athletic performance. (From Fotolia.com)

not measure in-game performance differences, it is likely that improvements made with proper sleep can be extrapolated to improvements in athletic performance during competition.

Prior to the study, daytime sleepiness was measured by questionnaire, and it was found that most of the athletes reported a moderate to high level of daytime sleepiness, indicating significant chronic sleep deprivation. This finding suggests that it is important to recognize that sleep deprivation and its consequences are cumulative and proper sleep must be maintained on a regular basis, not just the night before game day. The importance of good quality and quantity of sleep to peak athletic performance has only recently been recognized but is likely a critical factor in achieving peak performance not only in collegiate and professional athletes but also for those in high school and recreational athletes alike. The overall message is that more sleep can lead to better performance. Sports teams and coaches need to integrate optimal sleep into the athletic training and competition schedule and to consider sleep needs when planning travel to competitions.

In earlier studies, Mah et al found that extending sleep over several weeks improved performance, mood, and alertness in athletes. Further research has shown that extending sleep can improve athletic performance in specific aspects of a sport and help the athlete achieve peak performance. One study showed that extending sleep in collegiate tennis athletes can lead to specific improvement in tennis performance (Figure 21-14).[103] Athletic performance of collegiate tennis players was measured during normal routine and after they extended sleep to 10 hours per night. Results showed that they had improved hitting accuracy up to 23%. They also showed more valid serves, faster sprint times, better hitting depth drill performance, and reports of improved vigor and less fatigue. Studies have also shown that extended sleep improves mood and performance in collegiate football, collegiate swimming, and other athletic

performances.[102,104,105] Some of the athletes who participated in these studies set new personal records and broke longstanding records while participating in these studies. Stanford University, where the studies were conducted, has also made changes to practice and travel schedules to accommodate the athlete's need for more sleep. Research shows that as little as 20 hours of sleep deprivation can have a negative impact on athletic performance, particularly for power sports and skill sports.[106–108]

Researchers speculate that deep sleep helps improve athletic performance because this is when human growth hormone is released (Figure 21-15). Human growth hormone is involved in muscle growth and tissue repair, bone health, and fat burning and in recovery from the vigorous physical performance that is part of training and athletic competition. NREM stage 2 sleep is also important for encoding new motor memories and consolidating motor skills training that are involved in athletic training. This stage of sleep may be critical in motor learning that is part of athletic performance.

Athletes can easily fail to get regular consistent sleep, and the accumulating sleep debt can have a negative impact on athletic performance as well as on cognitive function, mood, and reaction time. Therefore, keeping a regular sleep schedule and accommodating for sleep loss that may occur as a result of traveling to competitions by incorporating naps into the schedule can help maintain adequate sleep. It is apparent that maintaining a regular, adequate sleep schedule is as important to athletic performance as proper nutrition and training. Athletes should make sleep a priority in the training schedule by going to bed and waking up at the same time every day. They should incorporate a daytime nap into their schedule when travel or competition may interfere with a normal length of a night's sleep. They should also consider trying to increase sleep time several weeks before a major competition in order to maximize athletic performance.

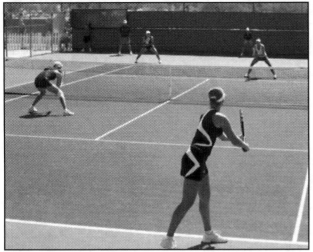

Figure 21-14. In addition to improved mood, tennis players tested with normal sleep and with extended 10 hours' sleep showed marked improvement in speed, accuracy, and endurance. (From Fotolia.com)

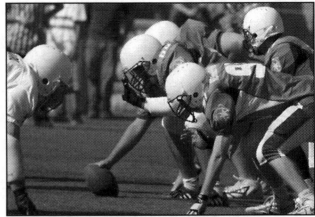

Figure 21-15. Deep sleep may improve athletic performance because it is when human growth hormone is released. (From Fotolia.com)

Jet Lag in Athletes

Travel for competition, especially international competition that involves long-distance air travel and changing time zones can present a particular problem for athletes. Long-distance flights can cause disruption in circadian rhythms and interfere with sleep–wake cycles (Figure 21-16). Sleep loss caused by this jet lag can also cause headaches, dizziness, fatigue, and decreased energy and affect alertness, cognitive function, and mood. Circadian rhythms are internally driven variations in the biological clock that is primarily influenced by the light–dark cycle but can also be modified by melatonin and exercise.

Although there is no clear evidence regarding jet lag and athletic performance, it seems likely that symptoms of jet lag will result in a decline in performance because of both physiological and emotional factors. Many athletes choose to reset their circadian clocks to match the time zone of the destination city prior to a major competition.

Circadian rhythms can be modified by exposure to bright light and darkness, taking low-dose melatonin supplements, and exercising at certain times of the day. Exposure to bright light and darkness has the most significant influence on improving jet lag symptoms. Bright light has the most direct impact on shifting circadian rhythms. The intensity, duration, and timing of the light are also important. Exposure to bright light just before the lowest body temperature, which occurs at approximately 5:00 AM delays the circadian cycle. Exposure to bright light after that time speeds up the circadian cycle.[109]

Melatonin may also influence the circadian cycle. It may be delayed by taking a low dose of 0.5 mg of melatonin between morning and mid-afternoon hours and that cycle can be advanced by taking melatonin between mid-afternoon and bedtime.

It appears that exercising for 1 to 3 hours may induce significant circadian phase shifts. For example, early morning exercise performed before body temperature is at its lowest has consistently been associated with circadian phase delays. Early evening exercise can result in circadian rhythm advances.

It is apparent that the timing of these interventions used to deal with the symptoms of jet lag is critical, otherwise the efforts may have the opposite effect on the sleep–wake cycle. There are other techniques that can help improve symptoms of jet lag and adjustment of the circadian clock to the destination venue.[110] These include reducing stress by good planning and avoiding sleep deprivation prior to the trip. The athlete can also gradually shift the sleep schedule toward the destination time zone starting a few days prior to departure. Using timed bright light and dark cycles, melatonin, or exercise to shift circadian rhythms can also help.

During the flight, it is important for the athlete to drink plenty of water and limit alcohol and caffeine intake in order to reduce dehydration from dry airplane air. Stretching, performing mild isometric exercise, and walking at least every hour can help minimize muscle stiffness and reduce the risk for thrombosis associated with prolonged inactivity.

Upon arrival, the athlete should avoid heavy, exotic, or spicy meals. Exercise should be performed at a low intensity to reduce muscle stiffness. Exercising indoors depending upon the time of day may help in making the desired circadian phase shift. Heavy training should be avoided for the first few days after a long flight. Using bright light, melatonin, and exercise may help make the shift in circadian rhythm.

When traveling eastward, it may be helpful to advance the body clock to adjust to the new time zone by maximizing light exposure in the morning after awakening and minimizing light exposure at night before bedtime. Beginning a few days before travel, athletes can gradually advance wake time and bedtime about 30 minutes per day.

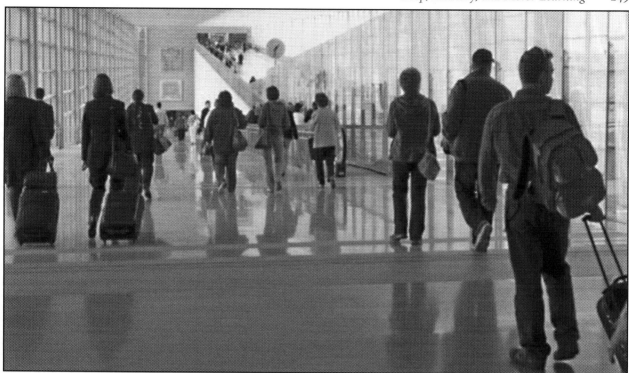

Figure 21-16. Travel and especially jet lag can disrupt circadian rhythms and negatively impact athletic performance. There are a number of steps that can be taken to mitigate the impact. (From Fotolia.com)

After arrival, using the point of origin should be considered to determine when to plan light exposure. Maximum light exposure should occur from 5:00 to 10:00 AM and minimum light exposure from midnight to 4:00 AM.

When traveling westward, it is helpful before departure to maximize light exposure during the 4 hours before bedtime and minimize light exposure during the 4 hours after awakening. In other words, the athlete should delay bedtime and waking time, 30 to 60 minutes later per day, for a few days prior to travel. After arrival, using the point of origin as a reference and maximize light exposure from midnight to 4:00 AM and minimize light from 5:00 to 9:00 AM will help to ameliorate jet lag-induced performance problems.

Circadian rhythms may also provide clues as to the best time of day to exercise. Generally, when one can fit exercise activity into a busy schedule is best, but research shows that there are some times of day that are most optimal for peak athletic performance. Late afternoon, when the body temperature is at its highest, which for most people is between 4 and 5 PM, appears to be the optimal time to exercise. Strength is greater in the afternoon, with one study showing that strength output is 5% higher at midday and anaerobic performance in activities such as sprinting improves by 5% in the late afternoon. Aerobic capacity and endurance is approximately 4% higher in the afternoon.[111] Injuries are less likely in the afternoon because the athlete is usually the most alert and body temperature is highest so muscles are warm and flexible and strength is highest. These 3 factors reduce the incidence of injury.

Even though late afternoon exercise appears to be most effective from a physiological standpoint, morning exercisers tend to be more consistent with an exercise program compared to those who wait until the late afternoon to exercise.[112] Most research shows that exercise can improve the quality of sleep; however, exercising too late in the evening has been linked to sleep-onset insomnia.[113]

SUMMARY

It has become abundantly evident that sleep is critical for consolidation of motor memory. Sleep has also been shown to produce off-line improvements in motor performance in simple and complex tasks. Sleep deprivation adversely affects motor skill as well as neurocognitive function. Given these facts, rehabilitation professionals need to understand sleep and the manifestations and consequences of sleep deprivation.

Additionally, it seems clear that sleep should be an important consideration in developing and implementing a therapeutic exercise program. Although the relationship appears clear, research is needed to provide evidence of the link between sleep and therapeutic exercise performance. It would be of interest to study the effect of the timing of a sleep episode relative to the performance of a therapeutic exercise program to determine whether there is an optimal time to maximize performance improvements.

REFERENCES

1. Dudai Y. Memory: it's all about representations. In: Roediger HL, Dudai Y, Fitzpatrick SM, eds. *Science of Memory Concepts*. New York, NY: Oxford University Press; 2007:13–16.
2. Sperling G. A model for visual memory tasks. *Hum Factors*. 1963;5:19–31.
3. Atkinson RC, Shiffrin RM. Human memory: A proposed system and its control processes. In: Spence KW, Spence JT. *The Psychology of Learning and Motivation* (Volume 2). New York, NY: Academic Press. 1968;89–195.
4. Green CD. Memory: a contribution to experimental psychology. Available at: http://psychclassics.yorku.ca/Ebbinghaus/index.htm. Accessed December 19, 2011.
5. Schacter DL, Chiao JY, Mitchell JP. Seven sins of memory: implications of self. *Ann N Y Acad Science*. 2003;1001:226–239.
6. Loftus EF, Loftus GR. On the permanence of stored information in the human brain. *Am Psychol*. 1980;35:409–420.
7. Nickerson RS, Adams JJ. Long-term memory for a common object. *Cogn Psychol*. 1979;11:287–307.
8. Miller GA. The magical number seven, plus or minus two: some limits on our capacity for processing information. *Psychol Rev*. 1956;63:343–355.
9. Cherry K. Study finds that testing improves recall. Available at: http://psychology.about.com/b/2006/11/21/study-finds-that-testing-improves-recall.htm. Accessed December 19, 2011.
10. Neylan TC. Memory and the medial temporal lobe: patient H.M. neuropsychiatric classics. *J Neruopsych Clin Neurosci*. 2000;12(1):103.
11. Shanks DR, St. John MF. Characteristics of dissociable human learning systems. *Behav Brain Sci*. 1994;17:367–447.
12. Thorndike EL, Rock RT. Learning without awareness of what is being learned or intent to learn it. [abstract] *J Experimental Psychol*. 1934;17(1):1.
13. Shadmehr R, Holcomb HH. Neural correlates of motor memory consolidation. *Science*. 1997;227:821–825.
14. Atwell P, Cooke S, Yeo C. Cerebellar function in consolidation of motor memory. *Neuron*. 2002;34:1011–1020.
15. Boyden E, Katoh A, Raymond J. Cerebellum-dependent learning: the role of multiple plasticity mechanisms. *Annu Rev Neurosci*. 2004;27:581–609.
16. Ma L, Wang B, Naravana S, Haszeltine E, Chen X, Robin DA, Fox PT, Xiong J. Changes in regional activity are accompanied with changes in inter-regional connectivity during 4 weeks motor learning. *Brain Res*. 2010;1318:64–76.
17. Packard M, Knowlton B. Learning and memory functions of the basal ganglia. *Annu Rev Neurosci*. 2002;25:563–593.
18. Adkins DL, Boychuck J. Motor training induces experience specific patterns of plasticity across motor cortex and spinal cord. *J Appl Physiol*. 2006;101:1776–1782.
19. Hebb DO. *The Organization of Behavior*. New York, NY: Wiley & Sons; 1949:107–139.
20. Karni A, Meyer G. The acquisition of skilled motor performance: fast and slow experience-driven changes in primary motor cortex. *Proc Natl Acad Sci U S A*. 1998;95:861–868.
21. Deschenes MR, Giles JA. Neural factors account for strength decrements observed after short-term muscle unloading. *Am J Physiol Regul Integr Comp Physiol*. 2002;282:R578–R583.
22. Kleim JL, Hogg TM. Cortical synaptogenesis and motor map reorganization occur during late, but not early, phase of motor skill learning. *J Neurosci*. 2004;24:628–633.
23. Dowell LR, Mahone EM, Mostofsky SH. Associations of postural knowledge and basic motor skill with dyspraxia in autism: implications for abnormalities in distributed connectivity and motor learning. *Neuropsychology*. 2009;23:563–570.
24. Kim D, Shin M, Lee K, Chu K, et al. Musical training induced functional re-organization of the adult brain: functional magnetic imaging and transcranial magnetic stimulation study on amateur string players. *Hum Brain Mapp*. 2004;23:188–199.
25. Haslinger B, Erhard P, Altenmüller E, Hennenlotter A, et al. Reduced recruitment of motor association areas during bimanual coordination in concert pianists. *Hum Brain Mapp*. 2004;22:206–215.
26. Sacks O. *Musicophilia: Tales of Music and the Brain*. New York, NY: Vintage Books; 2007.
27. Walker MP, Stickgold R. Sleep-dependent learning and memory consolidation. *Neuron*. 2004;44:121–133.
28. Smith C, MacNeill C. Impaired motor memory for a pursuit rotor task following stage 2 sleep loss in college students. *J Sleep Res*. 1994;3:206–213.
29. Walker MP, Brakefield T, Morgan A, Hobson JA, Stickgold R. Practice with sleep makes perfect: sleep-dependent motor skill learning. *Neuron*. 2002;35:205–211.
30. Fischer S, Hallschmid M, Elsner AL, Born J. Sleep forms memory for finger skills. *Proc Natl Acad Sci U S A*. 2002;99:11987–11991.
31. Fischer S, Drosopoulos S, Tsen J, Born J. Implicit learning—explicit knowing: a role for sleep in memory system interaction. *J Cogn Neurosci*. 2006;18:311–319.
32. Walker MP, Brakefield T, Seidman J, Morgan A, Hobson JA, Stickgold R. Sleep and the time course of motor skill learning. *Learn Mem*. 2003;10:275–284.
33. Walker MP, Brakefield T, Hobson JA, Stickgold R. Dissociable stages of human memory consolidation and reconsolidation. *Nature*. 2003;425:616–620.
34. Walker MP, Stickgold R, Alsop D, Gaab N, Schlaug G. Sleep-dependent motor memory plasticity in the human brain. *Neuroscience*. 2005;133:911–917.
35. Robertson EM, Pascual-Leone A, Press DZ. Awareness modifies the skill-learning benefits of sleep. *Curr Biol*. 2004;14:208–212.
36. Maquet P, Schwartz S, Passingham R, Frith C. Sleep-related consolidation of a visuomotor skill: brain mechanisms as assessed by functional magnetic resonance imaging. *J Neurosci*. 2003;23:1432–1440.
37. Schmidt RA, Lee TD. *Motor Control and Learning: A Behavioral Emphasis*. 3rd ed. Champaign, IL: Human Kinetics; 1999.
38. Pew RW. Levels of analysis in motor control. *Brain Res*. 1974;71:393–400.
39. Wulf G, Schmidt RA. Variability of practice and implicit motor learning. *J Exp Psychol Learn Mem Cogn*. 1997;23:987–1006.
40. Shea CH, Wulf G, Whitacre CA, Park JH. Surfing the implicit wave. *Q J Exp Psychol A*. 2001;54:841–862.
41. Boyd LA, Winstein CJ. Explicit information interferes with implicit motor learning of both continuous and discrete movement tasks after stroke. *J Neurol Phys Ther*. 2006;30(2):46–57.
42. Boyd LA, Winstein CJ. Cerebellar stroke impairs temporal but not spatial accuracy during implicit motor learning. *Neurorehabil Neural Repair*. 2004;18(3):134–143.
43. Boyd LA, Winstein CJ. Providing explicit information disrupts implicit motor learning after basal ganglia stroke. *Learn Mem*. 2004;11(4):388–396.
44. Siengsukon CF, Boyd LA. Sleep to learn after stroke: implicit and explicit off-line motor learning. *Neurosci Lett*. 2009;451:1–5.
45. Siengsukon C, Boyd LA. Sleep enhances off-line spatial and temporal motor learning after stroke. *Neurorehabil Neural Repair*. 2009;23:327–335.
46. Smith C, MacNeill C. Impaired motor memory for a pursuit rotor task following Stage 2 sleep loss in college students. *J Sleep Res*. 1994;3:206–213.
47. Huber R, Ghilardi MF, Massimini M, Tononi G. Local sleep and learning. *Nature*. 2004;430:78–81.
48. Yordanova J, Kolev V, Verleger R. Awareness of knowledge or awareness of processing? Implications for sleep-related memory consolidation. *Front Hum Neurosci*. 2009;3(40);1–13.

49. Diekelmann S, Born J. The memory function of sleep. *Nat Rev Neurosci.* 2010;11:114–126.

50. Robertson EM, Pascual-Leone A, Press DZ. Awareness modifies the skill-learning benefits of sleep. *Curr Biol.* 2004;14:208–212.

51. Yordanova J, Kolev V, Verleger R, Bataghva Z, Born J, Wagner U. Shifting from implicit to explicit knowledge: different roles of early- and late-night sleep. *Learn Mem.* 2008;15:508–515.

52. Drosopoulos S, Wagner U, Born J. Sleep enhances explicit recollection in recognition memory. *Learn Mem.* 2005;12:44–51.

53. Fischer S, Drosopoulos S, Tsen J, Born J. Implicit learning—explicit knowing: a role for sleep in memory system interaction. *J Cogn Neurosci.* 2006;18:311–319.

54. Rieth CA, Cai DJ, McDevitt EA, Mednick SC. The role of sleep and practice in implicit and explicit motor learning. *Behav Brain Res.* 2010;214:470–474.

55. Nemeth D, Janacsek K, Londe Z, Ullman MT, Howard DV, Howard JH Jr. Sleep has no critical role in implicit motor sequence learning in young and old adults. *Exp Brain Res.* 2010;201:351–358.

56. Debas K, Carrier J, Orban P, et al. Brain plasticity related to the consolidation of motor sequence learning and motor adaptation. *Proc Natl Acad Sci U S A.* 2010;107:17839–17844.

57. Siengsukon CF, Al-Sharman A. Sleep promotes offline enhancement of an explicitly learned discrete but not an explicitly learned continuous task. *Nat Sci Sleep.* 2011;3:39–46.

58. Doyon J, Korman M, Morin A, et al. Contribution of night and day sleep vs simple passage of time to the consolidation of motor sequence and visuomotor adaptation learning. *Exp Brain Res.* 2009;195:15–26.

59. Song S, Howard JH Jr, Howard DV. Sleep does not benefit probabilistic motor sequence learning. *J Neurosci.* 2007;27(46):12475–12483.

60. Kuriyama K, Stickgold R, Walker MP. Sleep-dependent learning and motor-skill complexity. *Learn Mem.* 2004;11:705–713.

61. Brawn TP, Fenn KM, Nusbaum HC, Margoliash D. Consolidation of sensorimotor learning during sleep. *Learn Mem.* 2009;15:815–819.

62. Stickgold R, Whidbee D, Schirmer B, Patel V, Hobson JA. Visual discrimination task improvement: a multi-step process occurring during sleep. *J Cogn Neurosci.* 2000;12:246–254.

63. Stickgold R, James L, Hobson JA. Visual discrimination learning requires sleep after training. *Nat Neurosci.* 2000;3:1237–1238.

64. Gais S, Plihal W, Wagner U, Born J. Early sleep triggers memory for early visual discrimination skills. *Nat Neurosci.* 2000;3:1335–1339.

65. Peigneux P, Laureys S, Fuchs S, et al. Learned material content and acquisition level modulate cerebral reactivation during posttraining rapid-eye-movements sleep. *NeuroImage.* 2003;20:125–134.

66. Laureys S, Peigneux P, Phillips C, et al. Experience-dependent changes in cerebral functional connectivity during human rapid eye movement sleep. *Neuroscience.* 2001;105:521–525.

67. Tononi G, Cirelli C. Sleep function and synaptic homeostasis. *Sleep Med Rev.* 2006;10:49–62.

68. Bushey D, Tononi G, Cirelli C. Sleep and synaptic homeostasis: structural evidence in *Drosophila. Science.* 2011;332:1576–1581.

69. Fischer S, Nitschke MF, Melchert UH, Erdmann C, Born J. Motor memory consolidation in sleep shapes more effective neuronal representations. *J Neurosci.* 2005;25:11248–11255.

70. Walker MP, Stickgold R, Alsop D, Gaab N, Schlaug G. Sleep-dependent motor memory plasticity in the human brain. *Neuroscience.* 2005;133:911–917.

71. Fischer S, Nitschke MF, Melchert UH, Erdmann C, Born J. Motor memory consolidation in sleep shapes more effective neuronal representations. *J Neurosci.* 2005;25:11248–11255.

72. Tononi G, Cirelli C. Sleep function and synaptic homeostasis. *Sleep Med Rev.* 2006;10:49–62.

73. Squire LR, Stark CE, Clark RE. The medial temporal lobe. *Annu Rev Neurosci.* 2004;27:279–306.

74. Walker MP, Brakefield T, Hobson JA, Stickgold R. Dissociable stages of human memory consolidation and reconsolidation. *Nature.* 2003;425:616–620.

75. Walker MP, Brakefield T, Morgan A, Hobson JA, Stickgold R. Practice with sleep makes perfect: sleep-dependent motor skill learning. *Neuron.* 2002;35:205–211.

76. Walker MP, Brakefield T, Seidman J, Morgan A, Hobson JA, Stickgold R. Sleep and the time course of motor skill learning. *Learn Mem.* 2003;10:275–284.

77. Fischer S, Hallschmid M, Elsner AL, Born J. Sleep forms memory for finger skills. *Proc Natl Acad Sci U S A.* 2002;99:11987–11991.

78. Fischer S, Nitschke MF, Melchert UH, Erdmann C, Born J. Motor memory consolidation in sleep shapes more effective neuronal representations. *J Neurosci.* 2005;25:11248–11255.

79. Robertson EM, Pascual-Leone A, Press DZ. Awareness modifies the skill-learning benefits of sleep. *Curr Biol.* 2004;14:208–212.

80. Song S, Howard JH, Howard DV. Sleep does not benefit probabilistic motor sequence learning. *J Neurosci.* 2007;27:12475–12483.

81. Nemeth D, Janacsek K, Londe Z, Ullman MT, Howard DV, Howard JH Jr. Sleep has no critical role in implicit motor sequence learning in young and old adults. *Exp Brain Res.* 2010;201:351–358.

82. Schmidt RA, Lee TD. *Motor Control and Learning: A Behavioral Emphasis.* 3rd ed. Champaign, IL: Human Kinetics; 1999.

83. Siengsukon CF, Al-Sharman A. Sleep promotes offline enhancement of an explicitly learned discrete but not an explicitly learned continuous task. *Nat Sci Sleep.* 2011;3:39–46.

84. Kuriyama K, Stickgold R, Walker MP. Sleep-dependent learning and motor-skill complexity. *Learn Mem.* 2004;11:705–713.

85. Brawn TP, Fenn KM, Nusbaum HC, Margoliash D. Consolidation of sensorimotor learning during sleep. *Learn Mem.* 2009;15:815–819.

86. Maquet P, Schwartz S, Passingham R, Frith C. Sleep-related consolidation of a visuomotor skill: brain mechanisms as assessed by functional magnetic resonance imaging. *J Neurosci.* 2003;23:1432–1440.

87. Peters KR, Smith V, Smith CT. Changes in sleep architecture following motor learning depend on initial skill level. *J Cogn Neurosci.* 2007;19:817–829.

88. Peters KR, Ray L, Smith V, Smith C. Changes in the density of stage 2 sleep spindles following motor learning in young and older adults. *J Sleep Res.* 2008;17:23–33.

89. Nishida M, Walker MP. Daytime naps, motor memory consolidation and regionally specific sleep spindles. *PLoS ONE.* 2007;2:e341.

90. Fogel SM, Smith CT. Learning-dependent changes in sleep spindles and stage 2 sleep. *J Sleep Res.* 2006;15:250–255.

91. Fogel SM, Smith CT, Cote KA. Dissociable learning-dependent changes in REM and non-REM sleep in declarative and procedural memory systems. *Behav Brain Res.* 2007;180:48–61.

92. Mednick SC, Cai DJ, Kanady J, Drummond SP. Comparing the benefits of caffeine, naps and placebo on verbal, motor and perceptual memory. *Behav Brain Res.* 2008;193:79–86.

93. Backhaus J, Junghanns K. Daytime naps improve procedural motor memory. *Sleep Med.* 2006;7:508–512.

94. Nishida M, Walker MP. Daytime naps, motor memory consolidation and regionally specific sleep spindles. *PLoS ONE.* 2007;2:e341.

95. Mednick S, Nakayama K, Stickgold R. Sleep-dependent learning: a nap is as good as a night. *Nat Neurosci.* 2003;6:697–698.

96. Milner CE, Fogel SM, Cote KA. Habitual napping moderates motor performance improvements following a short daytime nap. *Biol Psychol.* 2006;73:141–156.

97. Wamsley EJ, Tucker M, Payne JD, Benavides JA, Stickgold R. Dreaming of a learning task is associated with enhanced sleep-dependent memory consolidation. *Curr Biol.* 2010;20:850–855.

98. Seeck-Hirschner M, Baier PC, Sever S, Buschbacher A, Aldenhoff JB, Goder R. Effects of daytime naps on procedural and declarative memory in patients with schizophrenia. *J Psychiatr Res.* 2010;44:42–47.

99. Spiegel K, Leproult R, Van Cauter E. Impact of sleep debt on metabolic and endocrine function. *Lancet.* 1999;354:1435–1439.

100. Lamberg L. Sleep may be athletes' best performance booster. *Psychiatr News.* 2005;40(16):21.

101. Mah CD, Mah KE, Kezirian EJ, Dement WC. The effects of sleep extension on the athletic performance of collegiate basketball players. *Sleep.* 2011;34:943–950.

102. Mah C, Mah K, Dement W. The effect of extra sleep on mood and athletic performance amongst collegiate athletes. *Sleep.* 2007;30(suppl):A151.

103. Mah CD, Mah KE, Dement WC. Athletic performance improvements and sleep extension in collegiate tennis players. *Sleep.* 2009;32(suppl):A155.

104. Mah CD, Mah KE, Dement WC. Sleep extension and athletic performance in collegiate football. *Sleep.* 2010;33(suppl):A105.

105. Mah CD, Mah KE, Dement WC. Extended sleep and the effects on mood and athletic performance in collegiate swimmers. *Sleep.* 2008;31(suppl):A128.

106. Mah C. Study shows sleep extension improves athletic performance and mood. Paper presented at: Annual Meeting of the Associated Professional Sleep Societies; Seattle, WA: June 8, 2009.

107. Mah C. Extra sleep improves athletes' performance. Paper presented at: Annual Meeting of the Associated Professional Sleep Societies; Minnesota, MN: June 14, 2007.

108. Samuels C. Sleep, recovery, and performance: the new frontier in high-performance athletics. *Phys Med Rehabil Clin N Am.* 2009;20:149–159.

109. Parry BL. Jet lag: minimizing its effect with critically timed bright light and melatonin administration. *J Mol Microbiol Biotechnol.* 2002;4(5):463-466.

110. O'Connor PJ, Youngstedt SD, Buxton OM, Breus M. International federation of sports medicine (FIMS) position statement: air travel and performance in sports. 2004. Available at: http://www.fims.org/en/position-statements/previously-published/. Accessed July 5, 2013.

111. Medarov BI. Hour-to-hour variation of FEV1/FVC. *Chest.* 2004;126(4):744-745.

112. Hill DW, Cureton KJ, Collins MA. Circadian specificity in exercise training. *Ergonomics.* 1989;32:79–92.

113. Youngstedt SD, Kripke DF, Elliott JA. Is sleep disturbed by vigorous late-night exercise? *Med Sci Sports Exerc.* 1999;31:864–869.

22

Dentistry's Role in Sleep Medicine

Michael D. Hoefs, DDS, DABCP

Dentists are in a position to contribute to the overall health of their patients by screening for the possibility of sleep-related breathing disorder (SRBD). This screening can be done by having the patient complete a health history. The dentist should also have a solid knowledge of the basics of SRBD in order to recognize the symptoms and use of oral appliances. This requires dentists to receive adequate training to manage the patient and work together with the sleep medicine physicians and other health care providers.

The role of the dentist in treating the overall health of the patient has expanded rapidly in recent times. The dentist and dental hygienist may see the patient as often as the patient's primary care physician. With suitable training, they are as likely as the well-trained physician to detect SRBD symptoms.

SCREENING OF DENTAL PATIENTS

The screening of the patient can be done by adding some basic and simple questions to the existing health history. This may include a questionnaire like the Epworth Sleepiness Scale (ESS), which is commonly used to evaluate the patient's risk for daytime sleepiness and other factors.[1]

The addition of 5 basic questions to a health history currently in use by the dentist may help detect a sleep disorder.

1. Do you have difficulty falling asleep or staying asleep?
2. Do you snore?

3. Are you frequently tired during the day?
4. Are you aware of or have you been told you stop breathing during sleep?
5. Do you wake up feeling refreshed in the morning?

A positive response to these questions would warrant further evaluation.

Another set of basic questions has the acronym STOP/BANG[2]:

- S for *snoring*: Does the patient snore loudly?
- T for *tired*: Does the patient often feel tired?
- O for *observed*: Has someone observed that the patient's breathing stops during sleep?
- P for *pressure*: Does the patient have high blood pressure?
- B is for *Body mass index* > 35
- A is for *Age* > 50
- N is for *Neck* size > 17
- G is for *Gender* = male

The dentist needs to be acquainted with clinical observations that may indicate the risk for SRBD in addition to using questionnaires for relevant health history. Recognizing these clinical observations should prompt the dentist to have a detailed discussion with the patient about the risks of SRBD. This may also lead to a more extensive examination of the oropharyngeal area as well as the oral cavity. Table 22-1 presents an easy way to connect some clinical observations.

Hereford JM. *Sleep and Rehabilitation:*
A Guide for Health Professionals (pp 253-264).
© 2014 Taylor & Francis Group.

Table 22-1.

Clinical Finds That May Indicate a Risk for Sleep-Disordered Breathing

Clinical Observation	Potential Relationship
Tongue	
Coated	Risk for GERD, mouth breathing
Enlarged	Increased tongue activity, possible OSA
Scalloping (at lateral borders)	Increased risk for sleep apnea
Blocks view of oropharynx	Mallampati scores of I and II: low risk of OSA
Tongue grooved at midline	Mallampati scores of III and IV: increased risk of OSA
	Mouth breathing
Teeth and Periodontal Structures	
Gingival inflammation	Mouth breathing, poor oral hygiene
Gingival bleeding upon probing	Risk for periodontal disease
Dry mouth	Mouth breathing, can be related to medications
Gingival recession	Possibly clenching/parafunction
Abfraction (cervical erosions)	Increased clenching/parafunction
Tooth wear	Sleep bruxism suspected
Extraoral	
Cracking at the corners of the mouth	Inability for nasal respiration
Poor lip seal	Chronic mouth breathing
Mandibular retrognathia	Increased risk of OSA/snoring
Long face (doliocephalic)	Consequence of chronic mouth breathing
Enlarged masseter muscle	Sleep bruxism/clenching/parafunction
Bone deposition at gonial angle	Response to parafunction
Airway	
Long sloping soft palate	Risk for OSA
Swollen or elongated uvula	Risk for OSA/snoring
Nasal Airway	
Increased difficulty for nasal breathing	Small nostrils
Alar rim collapses with forced inhalation	Risk for OSA/sleep breathing disorder
Head and Neck Posture	
Forward head posture	Compensation for airway restriction
Loss of lordotic curve	Chronic mouth breathing

(Reprinted with permission from Johns Dental Lab, Terre Haute, IN.)

THE HISTORY AND CHIEF COMPLAINTS

A history of SRBD symptoms and complaints can be collected from a question-and-answer format about the symptoms and concerns of the patient. Questions should relate to commonly found symptoms of sleep disorders. This could include the presence of poor or disturbed sleep, daytime sleepiness or tiredness, observed apneas, snoring, headaches, tooth grinding, gastroesophageal reflux disease (GERD), low energy, poor concentration, irritability, and depression. A review of a sleep study should be included if patient has had one done.

The patient's medical history may be indicative of an underlying sleep problem (Figure 22-1). Medical conditions that may suggest an increased risk for obstructive sleep apnea (OSA) are the following:

- Hypertension
- Cardiovascular disease
- Headaches

G. Photographs ☐ **Not Performed**

Full Face: ☐ with tongue blade ☐ without tongue blade ☐ both

Facial asymmetry ☐   Occlusal cant up to left ☐   Occulusal cant up to right ☐
Ear left externally rotated ☐   Ear left internally rotated ☐
Ear right externally rotated ☐   Ear right internally rotated ☐

Standing Posture: ☐ Frontal ☐ Saggital ☐ Back   **Revealed the following:**

Forward head posture: ☐   Head tilt: left ☐ right ☐   Shoulder cant: up to left ☐ up to right ☐
Shoulder rolled forward: left ☐ right ☐ both ☐   Hip cant: up to left ☐ up to right ☐   Feet Divergent: left ☐ right ☐ both ☐
Other: _____

TM Joint Vibration Analysis (Hard and Soft Tissue Evaluation in Function)
Taken ☐   Printed ☐

II. Doctor's Evaluation

A. Limited Opening Evaluation ☐ **Not Performed**

Soft end feel ☐   Hard end feel ☐

B. TM Joint Vibration Analysis *(Hard and soft tissue evaluation in function)*

☐ Within normal limits, both soft and hard tissue
☐ Low energy ratio of vibrations >300 HZ/<300 HZ is <0.3, consistent with inflammation, right ☐, left ☐
☐ Medium energy ratio of vibrations >300 HZ/<300 HZ is <0.5, consistent with early osseous changes, right ☐, left ☐
☐ High energy ratio of vibrations >300 HZ/<300 HZ is <1.0, consistent with significant osseous changes, right ☐, left ☐
☐ **Right** TMJ evaluation revealed significant volume vibration of _____ HZ, which is consistent with ☐ partial - ☐ complete disc displacement with reduction that is (select one) ☐ early ☐ middle or ☐ late and in an (select one) ☐ anterior ☐ medial or ☐ anterior medial direction
☐ **Left** TMJ evaluation revealed significant volume vibration of _____ HZ, which is consistent with ☐ partial - ☐ complete disc displacement with reduction that is (select one) ☐ early ☐ middle or ☐ late and in an (select one) ☐ anterior ☐ medial or ☐ anterior medial direction

C. Sleeping and Airway Evaluation ☐ **Not Performed**

Epworth rating _____

Can the patient get to sleep easily? Yes ☐ No ☐
Can the patient stay asleep throughout the night? Yes ☐ No ☐
Does the patient wake rested? Yes ☐ No ☐
What is the patient's sleeping position? Back ☐ Side ☐ Stomach ☐ Varies ☐
Tonsils Absent ☐ Purulent ☐

Hypertrophied pharyngeal tonsils:
Left-category 1 ☐, 2 ☐ 3 ☐ 4 ☐
Right-category 1 ☐, 2 ☐ 3 ☐ 4 ☐

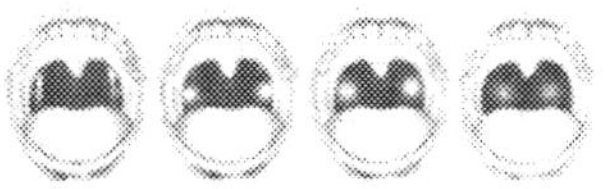

Adenoids ☐ Present ☐ Purulent / ☐ Absent ☐ Within normal limits / ☐ Obstructive

Palato-glossus & Palato-pharyngeal walls:
Left-category 1 ☐, 2 ☐ 3 ☐ 4 ☐
Right-category 1 ☐, 2 ☐ 3 ☐ 4 ☐

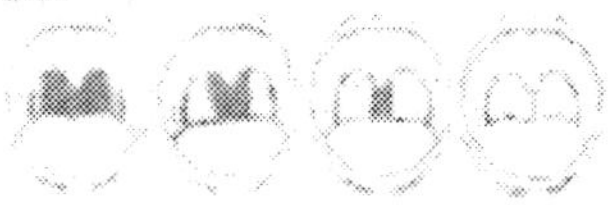

Uvula ☐ Elongated ☐ Within normal limits / ☐ Absent / ☐ Edematous / ☐ Enlarged / ☐ Obstructs airway

Mallampati *(tongue height)*
☐ Class 1
☐ Class 2
☐ Class 3
☐ Class 4

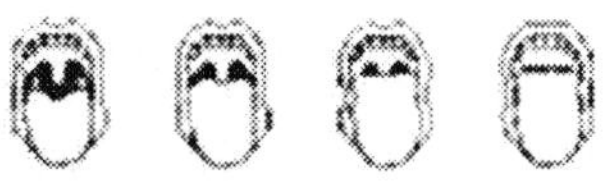

Soft Palate ☐ Firm ☐ Low draping / ☐ Loss of tone ☐ Within normal limits / ☐ Appears to obstruct airway

Gag Reflex ☐ Firm ☐ Within normal limits / ☐ Exaggerated

Additiona Findings: _____

2

Figure 22-1. A typical form for recording oropharyngeal evaluation. (Reprinted with permission from Johns Dental Lab, Terre Haute, IN.)

- Asthma and other respiratory conditions
- Diabetes
- GERD
- Hypothyroidism
- Allergy

A review of current medications should include prescription medications that are being used for management of existing medical conditions as well as over-the-counter medicines. Though the patient's medical condition may be related to a sleep disorder, it should be noted that many medications have an impact on the patient's sleep.

Medications associated with insomnia include the following:

- Amphetamines
- Caffeine
- Nicotine
- Corticosteroids
- Theophylline

Medications and other substances associated with sleepiness (as reported in clinical trials and case reports) include the following:

- Antihistamines
- Skeletal muscle relaxers
- Alcohol
- Opiate agonists
- Anti-parkinson an agents

Natural or alternative agents associated with sleepiness include the following:

- Vitamin C
- Dehydroepiandrosterone (DHEA)
- Ginseng
- St. John's wort
- Ephedra
- Valerian

Medications for treatment of insomnia include the following:

- Zaleplon (Sonata)
- Zolpidem (Ambien)
- Eszopiclone (Lunesta)
- Flurazepam (Dalmane)
- Temazepam (Restoril)
- Estazolam (ProSom)
- Triazolam (Halcion)

- Ramelteon (Rozerem)

Medications that depress breathing include the following:

- Benzodiazepines
- Barbiturates
- Narcotics
- Topamax

Medications that increase slow-wave sleep include the following:

- Tiagabine (Gabitril)
- Gabapentin (Neurontin)
- Pregabalin (Lyrica)
- Trazodone (Desyrel)
- Mirtazapine (Remeron)
- Valdoxan (Agomelatine)

TEMPOROMANDIBULAR DISORDERS EVALUATION

An evaluation for temporomandibular joint disorder (TMD) should be included for all dental patients, but particularly for the SRBD patient. The SRBD patient will often present with TMD and, conversely, the TMD patient often has an underlying SRBD. The dentist should also keep in mind the symptoms that can be associated with both conditions, such as headaches, jaw pain, and cervical muscle pain. The TMD issues will need to be addressed prior to the oral appliance therapy (OAT) or concomitantly when considering OAT for OSA.

Evaluation of temporomandibular joint dysfunction (TMJD) includes the following:

- Range of motion (opening, protrusion, lateral excursions)
- Joint sounds (clicking, popping, crepitus)
- Joint palpation for tenderness (capsulitis, retrodiscitis)
- Previous treatment for TMD or OSA

Masticatory and Cervical Muscles

Palpation of the head and neck musculature should be performed to determine referred pain patterns and areas of local tenderness. The dentist then needs to determine whether treatment is necessary prior to starting OAT. These findings should be recorded for future reference if it is determined that immediate treatment is not warranted.

ORAL AIRWAY EVALUATION

- Uvula: normal, enlarged or swollen, elongated
- Soft palate: normal, enlarged or swollen, long or draping into oropharynx
- Gag reflex: normal, diminished, absent, exaggerated
- Tonsils grade: 0, I, II, III, IV

Dentition and Periodontium

- Angle classification of occlusion: I, II, Div. 1 or 2, III
- Deep bite
- Cross-bite
- Wear facets
- Periodontal status (important for tooth stability to support oral appliances)
- Hard palate: high, narrow, normal
- Incisors: tipping forward or back, crowding
- Lip posture: are lips resting apart or together, creating a seal

Tongue Evaluation

- Size: large, small, normal
- Coated: may indicate GERD and mouth breathing
- Scalloping: tongue pressing against teeth leaving impressions
- Fissured: midline groove may indicate mouth breathing
- Tongue-tied: attachment of lingual frenum may restrict movement
- Mallampati score: I, II, III, IV

PARAFUNCTIONAL ACTIVITY

An intra-oral evaluation should pay close attention to the parafunctional activities of sleep bruxism and clenching. These activities are associated with SRBD and may be factors in the development of TMD. Worn teeth, palatal and mandibular tori (bony exostosis), and abfraction lesions (notching in roots along gingiva) are signs of parafunctional activity and may be a sign of development of SRBD.

NASAL AIRWAY EVALUATION

Nasal respiration is preferred over oral respiration (mouth breathing). Nasal airway obstruction can lead to chronic mouth breathing. This increases the risk for SRBD in adults.[3] In children, it can influence the growth of the craniofacial complex.

Nasal airway evaluation would include the following:

- Nasal airway: open, obstructed, stuffy, septal deviation
- Inferior turbinates, right and left: normal, enlarged
- Columella: normal, wide
- Nasal valve, right and left: open, narrow, blocked
- Cottle Test (effect of nasal dilation): no effect, improved nasal breathing

Airway Testing

Subjective testing of the airway can be accomplished by having the patient position mandible forward during inspiration. To stabilize the mandible's position, the patient can rest on cotton rolls, bite wax, or other bite registration materials. The patient is asked to make a snoring sound while breathing through the nose prior to repositioning. Various positions of the mandible in both the anterior and vertical directions can then be tried to eliminate snoring sound. This exercise can demonstrate to both the patient and the dentist that OAT could be effective in treating snoring/OSA.

TREATMENT PLANNING AND PATIENT MANAGEMENT

Utilizing the findings from the initial assessment of the patient, a plan of further action can be made and presented to the patient. This will then depend on the need for further testing, imaging, or referral. These options may include the following:

- Scheduling: Consultation with the dentist for a more detailed evaluation
- Referral: For a sleep study or to a sleep physician
- Obtain sleep study results if the patient has had a sleep study
- Determine whether continuous positive airway pressure or surgical options have been ruled in or out—if out, then OAT can be considered
- Schedule OAT if patient is ready to proceed or obtain additional records, if needed, such as: panoramic, cephalometric, cone beam computed tomography (CBCT), or TMJD tomographic images
- Refer to an ear, nose, and throat physician, physical therapy, or other provider as indicated
- Make other recommendations for over-the-counter or other home management techniques

Imaging for Sleep-Related Breathing Disorders

It is important to evaluate patterns of respiration to determine the status of the airway and determine where obstruction may be occurring.

Imaging can play a role in anatomic assessment of the airway and related structures. However, though SRBD is not diagnosed with imaging, imaging can be used to evaluate anatomic characteristics that may contribute to SRBD in certain patients. With CBCT, now used widely in dentistry, the airway can be visualized and even measured with appropriate software. The skeletal support for the airway can be seen as well as adjacent structures. Common airway encroachments include turbinates, adenoids, long soft palate, large tongue, and pharyngeal/lingual tonsils. Less common airway encroachments could include polyps and tumors.

Cephlometric Imaging

The hyoid bone position is known to have a relationship with tongue position. As the Go (gonion)-Gn (gnathion) angle to the superior aspect of the hyoid increases, the hyoid assumes a lower and more posterior position (Figure 22-2). This can allow the tongue to be positioned posteriorly in the pharyngeal airway. Also measuring the distance from the hyoid to the Go-Gn line can also be an indication of lower hyoid position. A distance of less than 20 mm is more ideal.[4]

Volumetric Imaging

Volumetric imaging can be used to look at the airway in three dimensions. In the software, it is possible to take a virtual tour of the airway looking at areas that may be contributing to restrictions (Figure 22-3).

Tomographic images of the TMJD combined with range of motion measurements taken in the clinical examination can aid the dentist in evaluation of the integrity of the TMJD. It is the experience of this author and other clinicians treating SRBD that TMD is a common finding of the SRBD patient.

Pharyngometry and Rhinometry

The use of acoustic reflection technology is often used by dentists to assess the airway. Pharyngometry allows a noninvasive method of looking at the changes when different mandibular positions are tried. This helps with the screening process to determine whether OAT is a viable

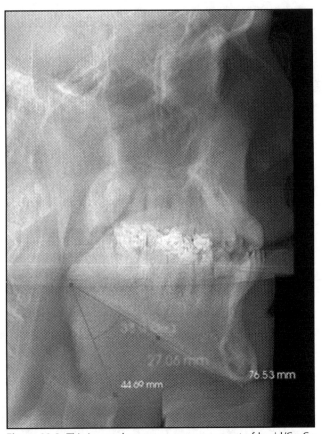

Figure 22-2. This image demonstrates measurement of hyoid/Go-Gn line angle and distance of hyoid to same line. A commonly accepted norm is less than 20 mm from hyoid to Go-Gn line. (Reprinted with permission from Johns Dental Lab, Terre Haute, IN.)

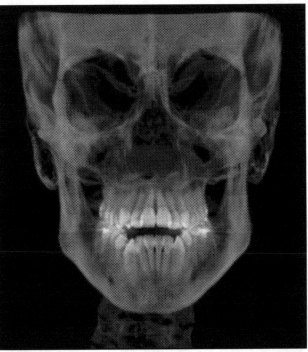

Figure 22-3. Volumetric imaging allows the dentist or orthodontist to evaluate facial form and symmetry/asymmetry. (Reprinted with permission from Johns Dental Lab, Terre Haute, IN.)

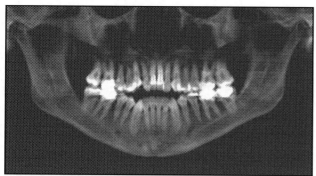

Figure 22-4. Panoramic imaging is useful to the dentist in evaluating the general condition of the dentition and its supporting structures. (Reprinted with permission from Johns Dental Lab, Terre Haute, IN.)

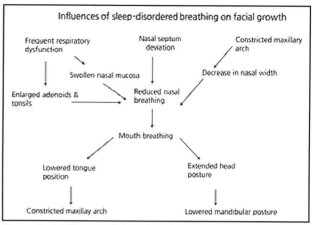

Figure 22-5. Influences of sleep-disordered breathing on facial growth. (Reprinted with permission from Johns Dental Lab, Terre Haute, IN.)

option for the patient. If it is demonstrated that mandibular positioning is effective, then the most suitable position can be found. This position is a guideline because there are more variables to be considered. Rhinometry can allow the dentist to assess the nasal airway patency. Recommendations on home therapies or physician referral can be advised.

TEMPOROMANDIBULAR DISORDERS AND SLEEP-RELATED BREATHING DISORDERS

The interrelationship of pain and sleep must not be overlooked. The clinician treating only orofacial pain and the clinician treating only sleep disorders must realize there is a complex relationship between these 2 comorbidities. The interaction between pain and sleep may be (1) disturbed sleep leads to pain, (2) pain may disturb normal sleep, and (3) these 2 conditions may exacerbate each other. Studies have also shown that patients with both pain and sleep problems had a greater psychiatric morbidity in the form of anxiety and depression. This, in turn, can lead to a negative response to pain and treatment.[5]

Headaches may be associated with snoring and sleep apnea. The comorbidity of headache and orofacial pain has been reported in the literature. The reports show that 72.7% of patients coming to an orofacial pain clinic had headache, whereas 32% of patients coming to the general dentistry clinic reported headache.[6]

TMJD disorders may be categorized as (1) internal derangements of the TMJD, (2) pain in the muscle of mastication associated with the TMJD, and (3) arthrides of the TMJD. Sleep position can aggravate the muscles and the TMJDs. Parafunctional activities of bruxism and clenching are associated with SRBD and can be a source of microtrauma to the masticatory system; that is, the dentition and its supporting structures, the TMJD, and muscles (Figure 22-4). The nociception produced by this activity

may be associated with sleep disturbance. The relationship of bruxism and pain, however, is still not clearly understood. Not all patients who are bruxers have pain and sleep disturbances.

The relationship between orofacial pain and sleep disorders is well documented. The orofacial pain specialists are advised to evaluate pain patients for sleep disorders as they are comorbid with orofacial pain. Proper evaluation and treatment of both disorders will be necessary for treatment success.

FACIAL GROWTH AND THE AIRWAY

Many factors influence the shape and function of the airway. These factors change over time with aging in addition to changes in musculature and physical condition. Facial form determined during growing years, starting at birth, can have profound effects on the airway in childhood and adult years. The largest increase in facial growth occurs within the first 4 years of life and is 90% complete by 12 years of age (Figure 22-5).[7]

Oral Breathing Versus Nasal Breathing

Mouth breathing has long been known to have a strong influence on the facial form when it occurs during childhood. Causes of mouth breathing are multiple, with nasal obstruction being the most common. Enlarged tonsilar and adenoidal tissues are another common finding. Tongue size and positioning may also influence an open mouth posture for breathing.

Retamoso et al discovered that end-tidal CO_2 concentrations were higher during nose breathing than during oral breathing. This research study revealed that a group of healthy volunteers had an average CO_2 of about 43.7 mm Hg for nose breathing and only around 40.6 mm Hg for oral breathing. Hence, mouth breathing reduces oxygenation of the whole body.[8]

Effects of Mouth Breathing Related to CO_2

- Reduced CO_2 content in alveoli of the lungs (hypocapnia).

- Hypocapnic vasoconstriction (constrictions of blood vessels due to CO_2 deficiency).

- Suppressed Bohr effect (physicist Niels Bohr): hemoglobin's oxygen-binding affinity is inversely related to acidity and inversely related to the concentration of CO_2.

- Reduced oxygenation of cells and tissues of all vital organs of the human body.

- Biochemical stress due to cold, dry air entering into the lungs.

- Biochemical stress due to dirty air (viruses, bacteria, toxic, and harmful chemicals) entering into the lungs.

- Possible infections due to absence of the autoimmunization effect.

- Pathological effects due to suppressed nitric oxide (NO) utilization.

Mouth breathers have an increased risk of OSA and airway collapsibility determined.[9] Lowering the mandible and hyoid bone allows the tongue to retrude into the oropharynx, increasing the risk of SRBD. Mouth breathing dries oral and pharyngeal tissues, which increases the resistance for inspiration and expiration and therefore increases the risk for SRBD.

Mammals are nasal breathers by nature. Nasal respiration is beneficial to mammalian health because it allows for production of NO in the sinuses. This production has the following effects:

1. Destruction of viruses, parasitic organisms, and malignant cells in the airways and lungs by inactivating their respiratory chain enzymes.

2. Regulation of binding–release of O_2 to hemoglobin. This effect is similar to the CO_2 function (the Bohr effect).

3. Vasodilation of arteries and arterioles (regulation of blood flow or perfusion of tissues).

4. Inhibitory effects of inflammation in blood vessels.

5. Hormonal effects. NO influences secretion of hormones from several glands (adrenaline, pancreatic enzymes, and gonadotropin-releasing hormone).

6. Neurotransmission. Memory, sleeping, learning, feeling pain, and many other processes are possible only with NO present (for transmission of neuronal signals).

During mouth breathing, it is not possible to utilize NO produced in the sinuses. The mouth was created for eating, drinking, and speaking; at other times, it should be closed.

Numerous studies have shown that mouth breathers will develop longer and narrower faces than nasal breathers. Described as a doliocephalic face in cepholometric terms, this is a result of several factors, including mandibular rest position, tongue posture, and lip posture. All of these are necessary for air to pass through the mouth. Abnormal tongue posture and mouth breathing during facial growth may lead to the following structural variances:

1. Lips (and buccal musculature) overpower the tongue and the maxilla fails to develop in sagittal and transverse planes.

2. The premaxilla fails to develop.

3. Maxillary incisors are pulled palatally and inferiorly during eruption along with clockwise rotating maxilla.

4. The tongue takes a lower position in the mouth during swallowing; that is, it does not go into the palate to support both transverse and sagittal development.

5. The nasal cavity fails to reach full dimension, further encouraging mouth breathing and poor oral posture.

All of these factors combine to create a maxillary and mandibular relationship that grows with an increased inferior vertical vector relative to the cranial base. This lengthens and narrows the face and represents a clockwise growth. It lowers the hyoid bone position and narrows the pharynx, thus reducing the size of the airway.

In early growth, breastfeeding has been shown to increase jaw development. Reduced use of oral pacifiers and elimination of digital sucking habits also increases the possibility of normal facial growth. Allergies and pollutants that increase nasal congestion are factors that can be removed with proper treatment and can aid normal development. Myofunctional therapy in children can also have great benefits and prevent or diminish the need for surgical and orthodontic correction at a later date.

Studies have shown that orthopedic development of the jaws in both the transverse and sagittal planes can improve the volume of the area. Traditional orthodontics, however, fails to achieve this development.[10–13] This would lead to the conclusion that dentistry should take on a more active role in identifying children at risk for development of SRBD. This can be done by looking at jaw, tongue, and lip posture at regular dental visits. If facial changes are noted, proper referrals can be made to the medical and dental specialists to improve nasal respiration. Referrals may involve surgical intervention to remove airway obstruction and functional orthopedics in mixed dentition to redirect facial growth.

Early treatment has been indicated to be more effective because, as previously mentioned, facial growth is nearly complete by the age of 12. More studies need to address the effectiveness of later treatment; however, anecdotal evidence exists that suggests later treatment can still have good benefits. Work being done in epigenetics and orthodontics indicates improvement in nasal respiration and increased oral volume through maxillary morphogenesis can help the non-growing patient.[14] It is this author's experience that many patients have airways improved from these types of orthopedic treatments, even though the treatment was directed toward orthodontic and TMJD issues. Resolving structural orthopedic incompatibilities can lead to soft tissues changes as well. Many TMD, SRBD, and malocclusion problems develop concomitantly. They may manifest themselves in different ways and at different times in the patient's life, but it is likely they all started from dysfunctional postures at an earlier point in life.

Dentists are in a good position to screen for these problems and treat or refer. There is growing evidence that dental and orthodontic professionals may be able to prevent the development of OSA with early facial growth guidance that can put nature back on her intended course and not allow facial deformity to be part of SRBD at any time in a patient's lifetime. However, this may take a paradigm shift in the current philosophies of treatment of malocclusions from an orthodontic, tooth movement solution to an orthopedic resolution. There is still much controversy in the dental profession on treatment timing. Perhaps looking at the total patient and not just the occlusion and face is the new standard of care.

SOME COMMONLY USED FUNCTIONAL ORTHOPEDIC APPLIANCES FOR FACIAL GROWTH GUIDANCE

Surgical Interventions

Beyond the scope of this chapter, but certainly worth mentioning, are surgical procedures that have been used to improve airways with various degrees of success. The list would include the following:

- Uvulopalatopharyngoplasty (UPPP): indicated when the soft palate occludes the airway.
- Hyoid bone suspension: bring the base of the tongue forward.
- Genioglossus advancement: a "window" of bone where the genioglossus attachment on the mandible is cut and

moved forward and fixed anteriorly to aid in moving the tongue out of the pharyngeal airway.

- Maxillomandibular advancement: the maxilla and mandible are both advanced with osteotomies in a counterclockwise direction to open pharyngeal airway.

Oral Appliance Therapy

Oral appliance therapy has become a well-recognized method of treating OSA. OAT can be a primary treatment method for mild-to-moderate sleep apnea or an alternative to continuous positive airway pressure or surgery (Figures 22-6 and 22-7). Oral appliance therapy to treat OSA has been available for over three decades. Since the beginning, appliances have become increasingly popular due to ease of use and reported reversibility. There are now over 90 appliances marketed for snoring and OSA treatment. The training of dentists in sleep medicine and the co-treatment of snoring and OSA has increased dramatically in the past decade.

There are 2 types of OAT appliances used today. The tongue-retaining device holds the tongue forward, whereas the mandibular-advancement device holds the mandible forward. The exact mechanism of action for OAT may not be completely understood, but dilating the airway is the main objective. These appliances typically fit on both dental arches and then reposition the mandible forward. By repositioning the mandible, the tongue and other oropharyngeal structures are thought to be modified to open the airway. This prevents the mandible, and therefore the tongue, from collapsing back into the airway during sleep. It is thought that the increased tension in the pharyngeal muscles can also help stabilize and support the airway to prevent further collapse.

After diagnosis and once the treatment plan is completed, impressions of the upper and lower dental arches are taken, and a bite registration of the two arches is recorded. The dentist should note the amount of protrusion for each individual patient. Care should be taken not to exceed 50% of the protrusion for the initial position. Dental midlines should be maintained with the appliance. Another method of determining initial position is using wax or cotton rolls to have the patient bite on while protruding in a potential position and then have the patient attempt to make a snoring sound. When the patient cannot make a snoring sound, that is a good potential starting point for the oral appliance. After delivery, the appliances can be adjusted to advance mandibular position by either mechanical adjustment of positioning mechanism or changing the length of elastics. This is typically done in 1-mm increments and is stopped when the patient reports better sleep quality. Typically, a follow-up sleep study is done 3 to 6 months after placement to confirm effectiveness. This may be a polysomnogram or home sleep study depending on the working relationship with the sleep physician.

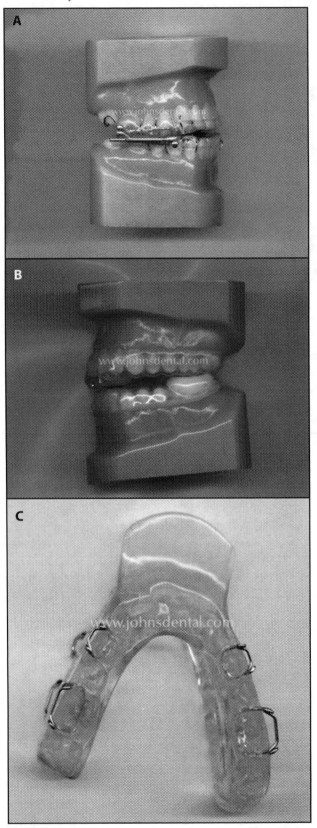

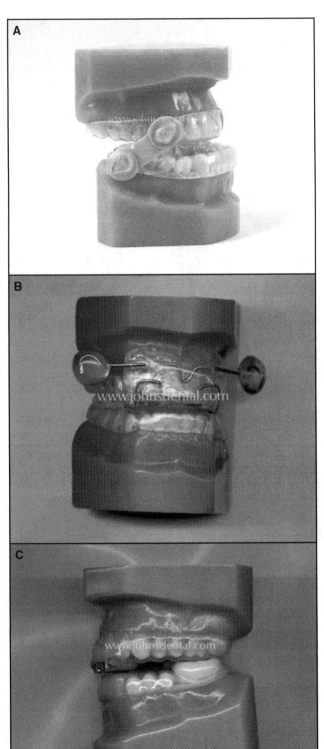

Figures 22-6. Commonly used appliances for sagittal development (mandibular advancement). (A) Herbst, (B) Tap 3, and (C) NAPA. Appliances commonly used to develop the transverse arch (not pictured) are the Crozat, Advanced Lightwire Functional, and the Rapid Maxillary Expander. Another option is the Biobloc system, which accentuates the need for control of anterior and vertical developmental vectors of facial growth. (Reprinted with permission from Johns Dental Lab, Terre Haute, IN.)

Figure 22-7. These devices are basically of 2 types: those that retain the tongue and those that advance the mandible. (A) Pictured is the Elastic Mandibular Advancement (EMA) appliance; (B) the Silencer appliance; and (C) the OASYS appliance. The "buttons" of the maxillary portion of the OASYS appliance goes under the lip to support opening of the nares to increase nasal respiration and the lower portion can be advanced. (Reprinted with permission from Johns Dental Lab, Terre Haute, IN.)

The type of appliances used today has components that fit on both upper and lower dental arches. Between the arches is either rigid or elastic fixation that keeps the mandible positioned forward. The tongue-retaining device is not widely used, but it can be an alternative for edentulous patients. Selection of the proper appliance is determined by the nature of the patient and the experience of the dentist. This author prefers appliances that will not intrude on the space needed for the tongue to reposition anteriorly. With this in mind, appliances that have their mechanisms on the cheek side are usually preferable. However, some patients with strong musculature and a history of bruxism may need appliances that are more rigid and durable and have the mechanism for advancement in the anterior part of the appliance. Finding a dentist who has experience in treating both the OSA patient and orofacial pain patient becomes helpful in long-term success in managing the use of OAT. Studies have shown that OAT does not lead to TMJD changes or dental changes in most patients. But proper appliance selection and supervision is required along with long-term follow-up with these patients.

Summary

Dentistry is in a unique position to both screen and treat SRBD in conjunction with other health care providers, and specifically sleep physicians. By increasing knowledge of SRBD and understanding the anatomic features and signs of SRBD, earlier detection of this disorder can be accomplished. Patients are more likely to have more frequent dental visits than visits to physicians. By taking a current health history and careful review of that history, the dentist can identify many potential health risks for their patients and make the proper referral for further evaluation.

For dentists who have an interest and training in treating SRBD and who also have adequate training in the area of orofacial pain, expanding the dental practice to include treatment of these disorders can be a rewarding experience. Patients can benefit from earlier detection and treatment. This can save countless future dollars spent on the consequences of SRBD, not to mention increased quality of life. Decreased mortality in the form of accidents and cardiovascular disease, among other things, can also be a great benefit to families and our society. OSA still continues to be underdiagnosed and untreated at this time. Decreased time of sleep is a common finding in our society, though increased pain and psychological consequences are on the rise. Improving the quality of sleep to improve the quality of life and health should become a priority in the health care community.

References

1. Johns MW. A new method for measuring daytime sleepiness: the Epworth Sleepiness Scale. *Sleep.* 1991;14:540–545.
2. Bailey DR. Dentistry's role in sleep medicine. *The Clinics.com.* 2010;5(1). Available at: http://download.journals.elsevierhealth.com/pdfs/journals/1556-407X/PIIS1556407X09001313.pdf. Accessed July 7, 2013.
3. Harari D, Redlich M, Miri S, Hamud T, Gross M. The effect of mouth breathing versus nasal breathing on dentofacial and craniofacial development in orthodontic patients. *Laryngoscope.* 2010;120:2089–2093.
4. Vieira BB, Itikawa CE, de Almeida LA, et al. Cephalometric evaluation of facial pattern and hyoid bone position in children with obstructive sleep apnea syndrome. *Int J Pediatr Otorhinolaryngol.* 2011;75:383–386.
5. Lavigne GJ, Sessle B, Choiniere M, Soja P, eds. *Sleep and Pain.* Seattle, WA: IASP Press; 2007.
6. Bailey DR. Tension headache and bruxism in the sleep disordered patient. *Cranio.* 1990;8:174–182.
7. Shepard J, et al. Evaluation of the upper airway in patients with OSA. *Sleep.* 1991;14:361–371.
8. Retamoso LB, Knop LA, Guariza Filho O, Tanaka OM. Facial and dental alterations according to the breathing pattern. *J Appl Oral Sci.* 2011;19:175–181.
9. Choi JH, Kim EJ, Choi J, et al. The effect of adenotonsillectomy on changes of position during sleep in pediatric obstructive sleep apnea syndrome. *Am J Rhinol Allergy.* 2009;23(6):e56–e58.
10. Stellzig-Eisenhauer A, Meyer-Marcotty P. Interaction between otorhinolaryngology and orthodontics: correlation between the nasopharyngeal airway and the craniofacial complex. *GMS Curr Top Otorhinolaryngol Head Neck Surg.* 2010;9:Doc04.
11. Baik UB, Suzuki M, Ikeda K, Sugawara J, Mitani H. Relationship between cephalometric characteristics and obstructive sites in obstructive sleep apnea syndrome. *Angle Orthod.* 2002;72(2):124–134.
12. Jefferson Y. Mouth breathing: adverse effects on facial growth, health, academics, and behavior. *Gen Dent.* 2010;58:18–25.
13. Page DC, Mahony D. The airway, breathing and orthodontics. *Today's FDA.* 2010;22(2):43–47.
14. Singh GD, Krumholtz JA. *Epigenetic Orthodontics in Adults.* Chatsworth, CA: SMILE Foundation, The Appliance Therapy Group; 2009.

Suggested Readings

Battagel JM, Johal A, L'Estrange PR, Croft CB, Kotecha B. Changes in airway and hyoid position in response to mandibular protrusion in subjects with obstructive sleep apnoea (OSA). *Eur J Orthod.* 1999;21:363–376.

Burris JL, Evans DR, Carlson CR. Psychological correlates of medical comorbidities in patients with temporomandibular disorders. *J Am Dent Assoc.* 2010;141:22–31.

Cistulli PA, Palmisano RG, Poole MD. Treatment of obstructive sleep apnea syndrome by rapid maxillary expansion. *Sleep.* 1998;15;21:831–835.

Cistulli PA, Richards GN, Palmisano RG, Unger G, Berthon-Jones M, Sullivan CE. Influence of maxillary constriction on nasal resistance and sleep apnea severity in patients with Marfan's syndrome. *Chest.* 1996;110:1184–1188.

Cunali PA, Almeida FR, Santos CD, et al. Prevalence of temporomandibular disorders in obstructive sleep apnea patients referred for oral appliance therapy. *J Orofac Pain.* 2009;23:339–344.

Gagnon Y, Mayer P, Morisson F, Rompré PH, Lavigne GJ. Aggravation of respiratory disturbances by the use of an occlusal splint in apneic patients: a pilot study. *Int J Prosthodont.* 2004;17:447–453.

Giannasi LC, Almeida FR, Magini M, et al. Systematic assessment of the impact of oral appliance therapy on the temporomandibular joint during treatment of obstructive sleep apnea: long-term evaluation. *Sleep Breath.* 2009;13:375–381.

Göder R, Friege L, Fritzer G, Strenge H, Aldenhoff JB, Hinze-Selch D. Morning headaches in patients with sleep disorders: a systematic polysomnographic study. *Sleep Med.* 2003;4:385–391.

Hoekema A. *Oral Appliance Therapy in Obstructive Sleep Apnea-Hypopnea Syndrome, a Clinical Study on Therapeutic Outcomes* [thesis]. 2008. University Medical Centre Groningen, Department of Oral and Maxillofacial Surgery.

Katz ES, D'Ambrosio CM. Pathophysiology of pediatric obstructive sleep apnea. *Proc Am Thorac Soc.* 2008;15;5:253–262.

Mahony D, Karsten A, Linder-Aronson S. Effects of adenoidectomy and changed mode of breathing on incisor and molar dentoalveolar heights and anterior face heights. *Aust Orthod J.* 2004;20(2):93–98.

Schwab RJ. Imaging for the snoring and sleep apnea patient. *Dent Clin North Am.* 2001;45:759–796.

Schwab RJ, Goldberg AN. Upper airway assessment: radiographic and other imaging techniques. *Otolaryngol Clin North Am.* 1998;31:931–968.

Schwab RJ, Gupta KB, Gefter WB, Metzger LJ, Hoffman EA, Pack AI. Upper airway and soft tissue anatomy in normal subjects and patients with sleep-disordered breathing. Significance of the lateral pharyngeal walls. *Am J Respir Crit Care Med.* 1995;52(5 pt 1):1673–1689.

Sharav Y, Benoliel R. *Orofacial Pain & Headache.* St Louis, MO: Mosby; 2008.

Smith AM, Battagel JM. Non-apneic snoring and the orthodontist: radiographic pharyngeal dimension changes with supine posture and mandibular protrusion. *J Orthod.* 2004;31:124–131.

Vieira BB, Itikawa CE, de Almeida LA, et al. Cephalometric evaluation of facial pattern and hyoid bone position in children with obstructive sleep apnea syndrome. *Int J Pediatr Otorhinolaryngol.* 2011;75:383–386.

Yucel A, Unlu M, Haktanir A, Acar M, Fidan F. Evaluation of the upper airway cross-sectional area changes in different degrees of severity of obstructive sleep apnea syndrome: cephalometric and dynamic CT study. *AJNR Am J Neuroradiol.* 2005;26:2624–2629.

Sleep, Occupation, and Dysfunction in Sensory Integration

Lauren E. Milton, OTD, OTR/L and Bridget E. Lovett, OTR/L, CEAS

All people need to be able or enabled to engage in the occupations of their need and choice, to grow through what they do, to experience independence or interdependence, equality, participation, security, health, and well-being.[1]

INTRODUCTION

Defined as "a state of complete physical, mental and social well-being and not merely the absence of disease or infirmity (p. 2)," health is measured by the World Health Organization (WHO) based on an individual's ability to participate in life, using the *International Classification of Functioning, Disability, and Health* (ICF) model.[2] The Centers for Disease Control and Prevention (CDC) asserted that the general lack of restorative sleep among Americans qualifies as a health crisis, given the resulting consequences of lower performance and participation across various occupations.[3] Even the youngest members of society are vulnerable to sleep issues. In fact, an estimated 20% to 30% of infants and toddlers regularly experience sleep problems.[4–6] The result? Parents and children with compromised daily functioning due to sleep deprivation.

In its Healthy People 2010 initiative, the United States Department of Health and Human Services emphasized health promotion and disease prevention in order to improve the quality of life of all Americans, as well as overall health and well-being. The United States Department of Health and Human Services' more recent initiative, Healthy People 2020, includes the new topics of Health-Related Quality of Life and Well-Being (HRQoL), encompassing physical, mental, emotional and social functioning, and sleep health. This federal initiative arose as a result of research into the negative effects of sleep deprivation and the recognition that sleep dysfunction is rampant in the general population and is poorly recognized by many, including health professionals.[7]

REST AND SLEEP AS AN OCCUPATION

The American Occupational Therapy Association (AOTA) *Occupational Therapy's Practice Framework: Domain & Process*, 2nd edition, is an official document intended to define and guide the practice of occupational therapy. In this revised edition, rest and sleep (Table 23-1) are specifically included and defined as an area of occupation addressed by occupational therapy practitioners. Noted as areas of occupation, rest and sleep "include activities related to obtaining restorative rest and sleep that supports health active engagement in other areas of occupation (p. 632)."[8] Though recognition by the AOTA of rest and sleep as an occupation is a step forward, perhaps considering sleep as not just any occupation but rather a *foundation for* other occupations or a *foundational* occupation needed for survival, much like respiration, nutritional intake, and physical activity, is plausible. As suggested in the introductory chapter of this book, it is not enough for today's health care professional, including occupational therapists, to know that sleep is vital to the health of our clients. Such professionals must understand the complexities of sleep, confidently articulating the positive impact of healthy sleep and the adverse effect of dysfunctional sleep

Hereford JM. *Sleep and Rehabilitation: A Guide for Health Professionals* (pp 265-277).

Table 23-1.

Summary of Rest and Sleep as Defined by the American Occupational Therapy Association in *Occupational Therapy's Practice Framework: Domain & Process*, 2nd Edition

Rest	Sleep	Sleep Preparation	Sleep Participation
• Identify need for sleep • Reducing involvement in physical, mental, and/or social activities • Relaxation/restoration of energy • Calm state • Renewed interest in engagement	Series of activities resulting in: • Going to sleep • Staying asleep • Health and safety through participation in sleep (involves physical and social environments)	Preparatory routines: • Grooming, dressing, reading, etc • Determining time of day/length of sleep/duration of time needed to wake • Establish pattern of sleep to support growth and health (personally and culturally influenced) Environmental preparation: • Preparing the sleep space (ie, bed) • Setting alarm • Securing home • Turning off lights, etc	• Taking care of need for sleep such as promoting onset of sleep by concluding activities • Napping • Dreaming • Sleeping without interruption • Care of toileting/hydration needs • Negotiating social environment demands • Interacting with others (ie, children, partners) • Providing care at night (ie, breastfeeding) • Monitoring comfort/safety of others during sleep (ie, children, partner)

Adapted from the American Occupational Therapy Association. Occupational therapy practice framework: domain and process, 2nd ed. *Am J Occ Ther.* 2008;62:625–683.

have on an individual's performance and participation in everyday life or on one's daily occupations. Once knowledge and understanding are established, then one can then apply such principles to practice to better service diverse patient populations, including children and adults with dysfunction of sensory integration (DSI).

THE SLEEP/SENSORY INTEGRATION CONNECTION

Dr. A. Jean Ayres, in her 1972 publication *Sensory Integration and Learning Disorders*, first identified common threads among children with learning disabilities who appeared to have difficulties with day-to-day functioning across environments (home, school, and community).[9] She went on to describe the process of sensory integration as the organization of sensation for use, required for a child to effectively interact with his or her environment. A child's ability to produce an appropriate response to environmental stimuli requires the successful integration of received information.[10] Sensory integration theory is commonly

used in occupational therapy practice, as it takes into account the individual's neurobiological ability to process and integrate information, then considers how that ability either helps or inhibits participation across environments.[11] Occupational therapy using a sensory integrative approach (OT/SI) is one of the most used and researched approaches within occupational therapy.[12,13]

Despite this, current research in the field of sensory integration lacks in identifying sleep as an occupation that may be negatively impacted by DSI. Instead, current available literature focuses on other daily occupations of individuals with sensory difficulties and the use of a sensory integrative approach to improve participation in everyday life activities. Measures of sensory difficulties, such as Ayres's Sensory Integration and Praxis Test, Parham & Ecker's Sensory Processing Measure Home Form, Dunn's Sensory Profile, and the DeGangi-Berk Test of Sensory Integration (TSI), measure important aspects of sensory function but do not include any sections specifically related to sleep function.[14-17] Given the importance of sleep health and the negative impact sleep dysfunction has on everyday occupations, the question arises: Does sleep dysfunction and difficulties with sensory integration work hand-in-hand?

Which came first—Is it dysfunction of sleep that manifests as sensory dysfunction, or is it sensory dysfunction that leads to poor sleep patterns?

This chapter explores an ever-emerging and widely accepted area of occupational therapy practice that could perhaps be integral in addressing sleep dysfunction. In addition, healthy sleep should be considered a factor in addressing sensory integration dysfunction. Occupational therapists, among other health professionals, are encouraged to consider these factors in practice and contribute to research in the field. Given that current available literature is limited in how a sensory integrative approach is used to address the vital occupation of sleep, in this chapter, we will explain sensory integration theory as defined by Ayres, as well as the nervous system as it relates to sensory integration. Specifically, the tactile, vestibular, proprioceptive, and sleep difficulties as they relate to DSI will be explored.

SENSORY INTEGRATION

As discussed earlier in this book (Chapter 2), sleep is dependent upon a person's ability to remain still, be less sensitive to sensory input, and assume a stereotypical posture (such as lying down). If a person's neurological system is not working functionally, calming the nervous system and/or creating the motor plan to be able to assume a necessary sleep posture may be very challenging and can make the daily occupation of sleep difficult to manage.

Sensory integration is a normal neural process that allows a person to develop effective motor plans and to be able to assume the appropriate arousal level (eg, drowsy, excited, calm, alert, terrified) for the moment they are in. Smith and Gouze, in their book, *The Sensory-Sensitive Child: Practical Solutions for Out-of-Bounds Behavior*, explained:

> …the delicate interaction between the brain and body known as sensory integration is nothing short of marvelous. It allows us to move purposefully through the world without being driven to distraction by the cacophony of sensory experience that bombards us each moment we are awake. When brain–body connections are intact, the lower brain constantly interprets input from sensory receptors all over the body and responds with motor reactions. Those actions create more sensory feedback, which provides more self-correcting information to the brain in a never-ending cycle. Thankfully, this occurs outside of our awareness in most instances. We are free to focus on conscious thoughts while our subcortical brain and its agents literally keep us from bumping into walls (pp. 15–16).[18]

If there is a dysfunction in this normal neural process, completing daily occupations, including sleep, may be very difficult for a person. To understand how sensory integration and DSI may impact a person's ability to sleep, it is necessary to have a basic understanding of the nervous system and understand the theory and history of Ayres' Sensory Integration. According to Fisher and Murray, this theory primarily focuses on children; however, it is applicable to adults who demonstrate a continuation of sensory integration issues that were evident during childhood.[19] In an article by Champagne and Frederick, the authors concluded following their review of current literature that, "Sensory integration approaches, however, can be modified and used in a client-centered manner by occupational therapy practitioners working with individuals with a variety of issues across the life course, for the purposes of enhancing occupational performance and increasing participation (p. 7)."[20]

THE NERVOUS SYSTEM AS IT RELATES TO SENSORY INTEGRATION

The nervous system is made up of a *peripheral nervous system* (sensory receptors and nerves) and *the central nervous system* (CNS; the spinal cord, brain stem, cerebellum, and cerebral hemispheres). There are many senses that receive information about a person's environment into the sensory receptor. The senses that will be discussed more in depth later in this chapter are the tactile (touch), proprioceptive (joint position), vestibular (movement), and vision (sight) senses.

When an individual experiences a sensation such as touch, the touch receptors of the skin change the energy of the touch into an electrical impulse, which flows through a *neuron*. The neuron is the most basic unit of the nervous system. Each neuron consists of a cell body and a nerve fiber that divides into many other smaller twig-like structures, allowing each neuron to communicate with many other neurons throughout the entire nervous system. This is how a simple smell can bring back a physical response or a childhood memory. The fibers carry signals/impulses that only travel in one direction—the nerve fibers toward the CNS. The electrical energy that flows from the sensory receptors to the CNS is called *sensory input*.

The neurons that carry sensory input from the 7 senses to the CNS are called *sensory neurons*. Thousands upon thousands of different types of input are carried by the sensory neurons to the CNS at any given time. When the sensory input from our touch receptor is brought to the CNS, the information is then organized with the input from our other sensory receptors so that the CNS then knows what to do with the information from the environment. This organizational process is called *sensory integration*. Sensory integration was defined by Dr. Ayres as, "The organization of sensory input for use" or "the neurological process that organizes sensation from one's own body and from the environment and makes it possible to use the body effectively within the environment.[10] The spatial and temporal aspects of inputs from different sensory modalities are interpreted, associated, and unified."[21] The "use" Ayres refers to is the CNS's reaction to the sensory input. The sensory input from the touch receptor is integrated in the CNS to tell the brain, "danger/get away" or "this feels nice/move closer" or "do nothing," or thousands of other responses. The reaction that results from the integrated sensory input in the CNS is then sent through the motor neurons back to the body so that the person can produce an appropriate behavioral response to the information from the environment.

An appropriate behavioral response is also dependent upon the nervous system's ability to modulate the information received from the senses in a manner that is fitting for the situation the person is in. *Modulation* is the nervous system's ability to facilitate some neural messages and inhibit other neural messages dependent upon the situation.[10] Stackhouse and Wilbarger defined sensory modulation as "the intake of sensation via typical sensory processing mechanisms such that the degree, intensity and quality of response is graded to match environmental demand and so that a range of optimal performance/adaptation is maintained."[22] Ultimately, sensory integration therapy provides specific stimulation that addresses certain brain levels (primarily sub-cortical), "enabling them to mature [or function more normally], and thereby assisting the brain to work as an integrated whole (p. 200)."[23]

A Functional Review of the Senses

The nervous system is composed of several different structures that communicate with one another as described in detail in Chapter 6 and Chapter 7. The overview of the nervous system presented in Section I of this book provides an exploration of how the nervous system functions in relation to the integration of sensations and the functional occupation of sleep.

Each and every sensation that comes into the body (sensory input) is information regarding the surrounding environment. The neurological system requires a wide variety of sensory inputs/stimuli in order to develop and function. A person must be able to integrate each of the following types of information into the CNS and process and modulate the input with other types of input in order to create accurate motor plans and maintain an appropriate arousal level for the environment he or she is in.[10]

This overview of the types of sensory input provides a very basic introduction into each of the senses. Each sense is highly specified, and the manner in which they are integrated into the CNS is a very technical process; however, a simplified introduction to the senses will be discussed here. For the purposes of this chapter, "higher levels of the brain" refers to the cerebral hemispheres and the cerebral

cortex, and "lower levels of the brain" refers to the brain stem, vestibular nuclei, and cerebellum. Though all of the senses play an integral part in the sensory integration process, this chapter will focus on the following: the sense of proprioception, the tactile (touch) sense, and the vestibular (movement) sense.

Sense of Proprioception

The proprioceptive sense is the sense that provides information to the brain about changes in joint position and muscle length. Proprioceptive sensations occur mostly with movement (changes in length of the muscle and joint space).[10] Lifting heavy objects, pushing, pulling, jumping, climbing, and crashing all send proprioceptive input into the brain.

The body also continues to receive proprioceptive input when a person is standing still. Most of the input from the joints and muscles is processed in the lower level of the brain, and therefore a person is likely not aware of the input unless he or she is specifically thinking about the position of his or her joints and muscles. When a person integrates proprioception adequately, he is able to button his jacket, walk downstairs, etc, without looking directly at what he is doing. When a person is not processing proprioceptive input effectively, he tends to need to compensate for this deficit with his vision.[10] When integrated accurately with other types of sensory stimulation, proprioceptive input is one of the most powerful types of input the nervous system can receive to maintain a calm–alert arousal level.[24]

Touch/Tactile Sense

The skin has many different types of receptors that take in information about touch, pressure, heat, cold, pain, and movement of the hairs on the skin. This information is processed in the lower levels of the brain, and most of the time does not even reach the higher level of the brain that makes us aware of the sensation. This lower level processing of tactile input can affect a person's arousal state, attention, and emotions without that person ever being aware of the sensation in the first place.[10] Typically, deep touch provides a calming effect on the nervous system, and light tickle touch puts the nervous system on high alert (Figure 23-1). The same is shown in various pediatric populations as well as animal models.[25] Temple Grandin described this calming effect in her book, *Thinking in Pictures*, where she explained her personal account of deep pressure input calming her and, thus, reducing her anxiety.[26]

Vestibular/Movement Sense

Within the inner ear, there is a structure called a *labyrinth*, which contains receptors for hearing and 2 types of receptors for movement. One type of movement receptors is calcium carbonate crystals, which are the gravity receptors.

Any change in head position causes a change in the pull of the crystals, which tells the brain where a person is in relationship to gravity. The other type of receptor is the semicircular canal, and there are 3 pairs of liquid-filled tubes that lay in different spatial relationships to one another (one lying front to back, one lying right to left, and one lying up and down). Any rapid movement of the head produces a backup of liquid inside of the tubes, which sends a signal to the nervous system, which alerts the brain to changes in direction and acceleration/deceleration. The input received by both of these types of receptors is integrated together to provide accurate information about whether a person is moving or still, where she is in relation to gravity, and how fast she is moving and in which direction. The vestibular system is closely related to the visual system to provide accurate information about where a person is in space. The vestibular system is extremely sensitive and begins to develop very early in utero.[10] For most individuals, rotary (spinning) or fast movements have an excitatory/alerting effect on the nervous system, whereas slow/rhythmic, linear movements have a calming effect on the nervous system.[27] Based on available literature and research, much like the calming effect of deep pressure input vs the alerting effect of light touch, it is also widely accepted in clinical practice that linear/slow/rhythmic movement elicits a calming effect on the nervous system vs rotary/fast movement, which results in an alerting effect.

DYSFUNCTION OF SENSORY INTEGRATION AND DISRUPTION OF SENSORY MODULATION

An individual must be able to receive the input from her senses into her nervous system and then integrate that information with all of the other information/input she receives from her environment in order to create an appropriate reaction or adaptive response to the situation she is in at that moment.

If a person is not able to integrate the information she receives from her environment in an effective manner, then she is not able to respond in an appropriate, functional manner. This is called *sensory integrative dysfunction* (or DSI). Ayres defined DSI as "an irregularity or disorder in the brain function that makes it difficult to integrate sensory input."[10] DSI affects a person's ability to create effective motor responses as well as her ability to maintain a functional, calm–alert arousal level.

An individual's nervous system must also be able to facilitate some neural messages while inhibiting other neural messages dependent upon the situation the person is in. This process is called *sensory modulation*. Ayres defined *modulation* as the "brain's regulation of its own activity."[10] If a person has difficulty modulating sensory input, then she may react in a manner that is not appropriate for the situation she is in (ie, a child who defensively pushes his

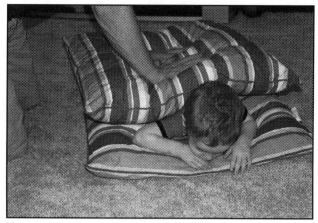

Figure 23-1. A child lies prone between 2 large pillows to engage in deep pressure tactile input by a caregiver gently "squishing" the child between pillows. Prompting the child to crawl out, proprioceptive input is added to the activity. (Reprinted with permission from L. Milton.)

grandma away when she gives him a kiss). This type of inappropriate reaction is defined as a disruption of sensory modulation (historically called *sensory modulation dysfunction*).[22] Disruption of sensory modulation is just one of the clusters of symptoms categorized under DSI; however, it is one that greatly impacts a person's ability to participate functionally in the occupation of sleep. In a 2007 study by Davies and Gavin, the concept of sensory gating was explored by providing subjects with a repeated, irrelevant clicking stimulus. Children with sensory modulation difficulties did not demonstrate the ability to inhibit, or "gate," the second click, implying that children with a hyperresponsive type of sensory modulation disorder neurologically may not have the ability to inhibit the second stimulus despite exposure to the condition stimulus first.[28]

SLEEP DIFFICULTIES AND DYSFUNCTION IN SENSORY INTEGRATION

In order to better understand why an individual with DSI may also experience sleep difficulties, it is important to first review the neurology of sleep. As discussed in Chapter 2, sleep is defined by meeting the following specific criteria:

1. Sleep consists of very little movement.

2. Individuals achieve a stereotypic posture (ie, lying down).

3. Individuals typically become gradually less responsive to sensory input as they fall asleep (or enter into the progressive stages of sleep).

4. Sleep is reversible, meaning that one can be readily awakened as distinguished from coma or death.

In order to meet sleep criteria 1 to 3, it is essential to accurately integrate sensory information. When sleep is

Table 23-2.

Case Examples of Dysfunction in Sensory Integration as It Relates to Sleep Problems

An individual who integrates the touch stimulus he or she receives from the sheet or blanket on his or her bed to mean "danger/get away" may be alerted as a result of the touch simulation, keeping him or her awake. Or, he or she may resist lying in bed, particularly under the covers.

An individual who does not accurately integrate information as to where his or her body is in space may have difficulty navigating a new, unfamiliar comforter or a different bed, such as when on vacation.

An individual who does not receive accurate information about his or her body position in space may be at risk for falling out of bed or may be fearful of falling out of bed; therefore, he or she will not achieve deep, comprehensive sleep. He or she may "pay attention" to where his or her body is in the bed while trying to sleep, maintaining a lighter sleep state.

An individual unable to integrate the calming input he or she gets from the surrounding environment (such as a deep-massage-type touch or slow rocking movement) with the alerting input (such as voices in another room, the annoying tag in pajamas) will have difficulty becoming less and less responsive to alerting sensory input as he or she falls asleep.

desired, intact sensory modulation allows an individual to facilitate neural messages that will help to calm his or her nervous system. Simultaneously and unconsciously, neural messages that would otherwise arouse the nervous system are inhibited. An individual with impaired sensory modulation may have difficulty regulating his arousal level and therefore calming his body. Laying still in an effort to achieve sleep may be difficult. In that instance, the brain may be sending a signal to the body to remain in motion or to sit up in bed, which is counter-intuitive to the very basic criteria for sleep. An individual with difficulty neurologically integrating calming input along with arousing sensory input may be overly sensitive to stimuli such as touch, sound, or light. The brain may be tuned into these types of arousing inputs in much the same way that a nursing mother is tuned into the sound of her own crying infant. This makes the third criterion especially difficult to meet for a person who is not able to modulate sensory information. Similarly, an individual's sensitivity to a tag on his clothing or to the noise of the television or voices in another room may prevent, delay, or slow him from progressing through the typical stages of sleep. Such symptoms of DSI prevent a person from achieving the essential criteria necessary for sleep (Table 23-2).

STRATEGIES TO ASSIST WITH DYSFUNCTION OF SENSORY INTEGRATION

In general, the body uses the information it receives from each of the 7 senses (vision, hearing, taste, smell, touch, proprioception, movement) for 2 different purposes: to (1) teach the individual how his or her body moves in space and provide accurate body scheme and motor plans

and (2) help the individual to regulate his or her arousal level, depending upon his or her situation or environment.

An individual exhibiting difficulty with motor planning or self-regulation should be evaluated to determine whether he has a DSI. Because this is not a formal diagnosis recognized by the *Diagnostic and Statistical Manual of Mental Disorders*, fourth edition text edition (DSM-IV-TR),[29] or the *International Classification of Diseases* (ICD-10th revision),[30] DSI is not able to be formally diagnosed by a physician. An occupational therapist, physical therapist, or speech and language pathologist who is highly trained in the theory and treatment of Ayres Sensory Integration is able to determine whether a person exhibits clusters of symptoms that are indicative of a DSI. The qualified professional can then individualize a treatment plan that can specifically meet that person's needs. If one of the major functional complaints a person has reacted to his or her DSI is in regards to his or her sleep or other daily living activities, it would be appropriate to discuss intervention with a qualified occupational therapist.

If a DSI is identified, the main goal of an occupational therapist is to improve a person's ability to participate in his or her daily living skills (occupations) by developing his or her ability to integrate sensory information effectively and also adapting their environment (or the external demands) so that the person is more likely to be able to complete his or her daily occupations in a functional manner.

An occupational therapist may use several different treatment approaches to encourage improved occupational performance. It is important that the underlying cause of the functional (occupational) deficit is addressed in order to support the occupational goals. For example, it is important that sensory integration deficits such as difficulty modulating sensory input and/or difficulty with motor planning is addressed in order to support more functional sleep. The following is a brief overview of a few popular treatment approaches used with an individual exhibiting symptoms of a DSI.

Table 23-3.

Ayres Sensory Integration Principles

✓	Service is provided by a qualified professional (ie, occupational therapist, occupational therapy assistant, physical therapist, or speech and language pathologist).
✓	Intervention plan is family centered.
✓	Therapy takes place in a safe environment that provides opportunity for vestibular, proprioceptive, and tactile sensations and opportunities for praxis (motor planning).
✓	Activities are rich in sensation.
✓	Activities promote regulation of alertness.
✓	Activities promote optimal postural control in the body.
✓	Activities promote praxis (motor planning).
✓	Intervention strategies promote "the just right challenge."
✓	Opportunities exist for the client to make adaptive responses, especially whole-body responses in a 3-dimensional space.
✓	Intrinsic motivation and drive are used to interact through pleasurable activities.
✓	The therapist develops an environment of trust and respect. Activities are not preplanned; therefore, the therapist is responsive to altering the task, interaction, and environment based upon the client's responses.
✓	The activities are their own reward and the therapist ensures the client's success by altering the activities to meet the client's abilities.

Adapted from Ayres AJ. *Sensory Integration and Learning Disorders.* Los Angeles, CA: Western Psychological Services; 1972.

Ayres Sensory Integration Treatment Approach

A traditional Ayres Sensory Integration Treatment Approach (Table 23-3) is typically used with a pediatric population. This treatment strategy is used to promote a person's ability to integrate sensory information more effectively in order to be able to achieve an adaptive response or, in other words, a functional goal. Typical outcome expectations of this approach is that a child would better be able to organize his or her arousal system in order to be at an optimal arousal level in order to meet his or her

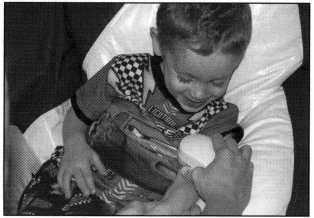

Figure 23-2. The Wilbarger deep pressure and proprioceptive technique is performed on a young child using the deep pressure device. For added deep pressure input, the child sits in a large bean bag chair while the protocol is performed. Following the use of the deep pressure device, joint compressions are performed. (Reprinted with permission from L. Milton.)

occupational demands and/or that a child will demonstrate improved body awareness and motor planning in order to be able to meet his or her occupational demands.[31]

Other Sensory-Based Strategies

Other strategies used to promote similar functional outcomes as the Ayres Sensory Integration Treatment Approach (see Table 23-3) are complementary methods used in a therapeutic approach to treating individuals with sensory integration difficulties but do not follow the strict fidelity measures of the traditional Ayres Sensory Integration Treatment Approach.

The Wilbarger deep pressure and proprioceptive technique, otherwise known as the *Wilbarger brushing protocol,* is a strategy in which a specifically designed deep pressure device, or "brush," is used in a strategic manner and in conjunction with joint compressions to effect a specific neurological changes, such as increasing body awareness, decreasing oversensitivities, etc (Figure 23-2). According to the protocol creators, Patricia and Julie Wilbarger, the process is to be repeated every 90 minutes to 2 hours during waking hours for maximum benefit.[32]

The Alert Program for Self-Regulation works to encourage a cognitive awareness of a person's arousal level and uses sensory-based strategies to help a person to better regulate their arousal level. This program encourages a person to be aware of their arousal state and make adaptations and or use strategies to change their arousal state. Language such as "How Does Your Engine Run?" is commonly used and this allows children to have an active role in determining their arousal state.[33]

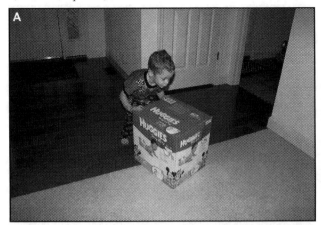

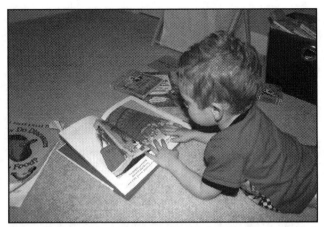

Figure 23-4. A child engages in reading books with mom or dad just prior to going to sleep in his bed. By lying prone on elbows, his body receives added organizing inputs through his skin (tactile/deep pressure), joints, and muscles (proprioceptive/heavy work). Sitting in a bean bag chair to read books adds deep pressure input, and a rocking chair adds vestibular (movement) input. Books replace screen time before bed. (Reprinted with permission from L. Milton.)

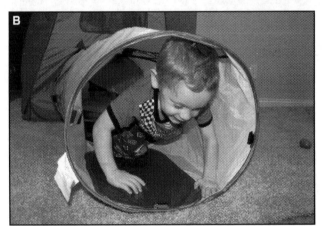

Figures 23-3. (A) As part of his nightly bedtime routine, a young child accesses weighted items in his environment to receive calming, proprioceptive input. Pushing/pulling weighted boxes or laundry baskets or stacking/knocking down weighted boxes or blocks is an effective way to facilitate proprioceptive input within a child's natural environment. Using a carpeted surface versus smooth, hard flooring, provides additional input to the joints and muscles. (B) A child crawls through a tunnel for deep pressure and proprioceptive input. The intensity of such inputs can be increased by adding pillows to the tunnel for the child to crawl over. (Reprinted with permission from L. Milton.)

STRATEGIES TO HELP PROMOTE SLEEP ACROSS THE LIFE SPAN

It's All About Routine … and Not Just at Night

Daily routines, not just bedtime routines, for children are directly related to improved daytime behaviors and lower mental distress in mothers, in addition to less stressful environments overall.[33–36] One study noted that over 90% of pediatricians recommended a bedtime routine to address sleep concerns voiced by parents.[37] Research strongly supports the use of a nightly bedtime routine as part of a treatment program for addressing sleep issues in children.[36] Such routines are known to result in children falling asleep faster as well as overall improvement

of bedtime behaviors.[35] Though considered a behavioral approach, establishing a consistent, predictable routine at bedtime is a crucial piece of healthy sleep (Figure 23-3). It is through this behavioral routine the sensory system is prepared for the onset and maintenance of sleep.

Decrease Visual and Auditory Stimulation

It is essential that television, computer, e-reader, cell phone, or any other device with a lighted screen is removed from the bedtime routine or use is discontinued at least 1 hour before bedtime to promote healthy sleep. Increased amounts of television watching, watching television close to bedtime, and having a television in a child's room have all been linked to poor sleep habits, such as bedtime resistance, sleep-onset delay, anxiety around sleep, and shortened sleep duration.[38]

A report from WebMD stated that the "blue light" emitted from television and other screens (cell phones, computers, etc) causes sleep disruption and should be avoided before bedtime.[39] Michelle Garrison, PhD, a research scientist at Seattle Children's Research Institute, reported in a *Pediatrics* research study that the light from screen time disrupts a person's melatonin levels from rising naturally. Melatonin is a hormone that is essential for a healthy sleep-wake cycle.[40] If the light from the screen tells the brain that it is daytime, a person cannot make the amount of melatonin necessary for sleep. Parents may think their child is melatonin deficient or has behavioral problems when going to sleep when in actuality turning off the television or other screens (eg, iPad [Apple Inc], iPhone [Apple Inc], LeapPad [LeapFrog Enterprises Inc]) 1 hour before bedtime may suffice (Figure 23-4).

Negative content in television programming (ie, programming including violence) can impact bedtime routines as well.[40] Fast-paced television programming impairs a child's ability to complete high-level brain functioning such as controlling impulses and problem solving, whereas slow-paced programming such as *Calliou* does not.[41] For these reasons, it is recommended that the television is turned off and other types of screen time are ended 1 hour before bedtime and that the programming/activities are limited to slow-paced, nonviolent programs to prevent behavioral difficulties around bedtime. Providing dim light during the transition to bedtime as well as a quiet environment with soft background music, gentle white noise, or other soft sound machine will cue the neurological system that sleep is approaching and assist in initiating the sleep process. Setting up the environment to promote sleep is essential in preparing the individual for the onset and progression of sleep.

Appropriate Bedtimes and Necessary Amount of Sleep Each Night

When a child goes to sleep can often impact how much sleep he or she gets. Dr. Marc Weisbluth, pediatrician and founder of the Sleep Disorders Center at Children's Memorial Hospital in Chicago, suggested that earlier bedtimes can often lead to later wake times, and for younger children, the more consistent the child's napping routine becomes, the better the child will sleep at night. In his book *Healthy Sleep Habits, Happy Child*, Weisbluth explained, "the most common cause for waking up too early...after four months of age is a too late bedtime (p. 119)."[42]

Often parents misread their child's drowsy cues and/or the parent's busy work schedules do not allow for an early bedtime for their children. The parents may report that their child does not "seem tired" in the evening. This may be due to increased arousal caused by extreme fatigue. Weisbluth stated, "Fatigue causes increased arousal. Therefore, the more tired your child, the harder it is for him to fall asleep, stay asleep or both (p. 292)."[42] This suggests that children have a regular, relatively early bedtime to ensure an optimal level of arousal for successfully meeting all 4 criteria for sleep as mentioned earlier, particularly number 3, progressing through the stages of sleep. The onset of sleep begins in a linear fashion, so to skip a stage of sleep or to have a shortened stage due to engagement in stimulation (eg, screen time, playing, not yet in crib/bed) is detrimental to the sleep process and results in sleep dysfunction and negative behaviors associated with the bedtime routine and sleep in general. The National Sleep Foundation[43] suggested the guidelines shown in Table 23-4 for determining an appropriate amount of sleep for an individual based on age.

Table 23-4.

National Sleep Foundation's Recommendations for Sleep Quantities Based on Age

Newborns (0–2 months)	Needs 12–18 hours
Infants (3–11 months)	Needs 14–15 hours
Toddlers (1–3 years)	Needs 12–14 hours
Preschoolers (3–5 years)	Needs 11–13 hours
School-aged children (5–10 years)	Needs 10–11 hours
Teens (10–17 years)	Needs 8½–9¼ hours
Adults (18 years+)	Needs 7–9 hours

Adapted from the National Sleep Foundation. Available at www.sleepfoundation.org. Accessed October 14, 2013.

Sensory-Based Strategies to Promote Sleep

Strategies based on the sensory integration principles discussed in previous sections of this chapter help a person to regulate his arousal level and improve his body awareness so that he is better able to fall asleep and stay asleep. Sensory-based strategies used to calm a baby—that is, swaddling (deep pressure and proprioceptive input), shushing/shhhing (constant "white" noise), swinging (rocking/linear input), such as described as part of the "5 S's" by Dr. Harvey Karp in his book, *Happiest Baby on the Block*[44]—can be adapted to the older child or adult to help them to calm their system and fall asleep. For a crying or colicky infant, Dr. Karp described the concept of the "calming reflex" and using the "5 S's" (swaddling, side/stomach position, shhhing, swinging, and sucking) in combination and simultaneously to trigger a calming reflex, soothing the nervous system. In essence, Dr. Karp suggested bombarding the nervous system with a variety of calming, organizing sensory inputs, similar to the experience of a baby still in utero.[44]

The strategies suggested are meant to be a guide, not a "to-do" list, and should be adapted to each individual as the treating therapist deems necessary. When addressing sleep difficulties with a child, it is important that the sensory activities are child-directed and that the adult listens to and respects the wishes of the child with each activity. Each individual is different and may not respond in a typical fashion to these types of inputs so it is important to get feedback from the person and monitor his/her arousal state after input is provided. Always keep in mind general principles of sensory input while engaging in such tasks (Table 23-5).

Table 23-5.
Important Points to Remember While Providing Various Types of Sensory Inputs in an Effort to Promote Sleep

Heavy work = Calming
Deep pressure = Calming
Light touch = Alerting
Linear (back and forth), slow, rhythmic movement = Calming
Rotary (spinning), fast, erratic, uneven movement = Alerting

Table 23-6.
Ideas for Heavy Work Activities at Home as Part of a Nightly Bedtime Routine

Carry books upstairs for bedtime.
Carry/push a laundry basket full of blankets or a weighted box into room (see Figure 23-3A).
Play blanket tug of war.
Tunnel play. May put books, pajamas, etc, in the tunnel for child to retrieve as part of the bedtime routine (see Figure 23-3B).
Countertop push-ups before and after brushing teeth.
Wheelbarrow walk from room to room during evening bedtime routine.

Proprioceptive (Heavy Work) Input

In general, proprioceptive input provides information to the CNS about changes to the joint space and muscle length. When a person pulls, pushes, carries heavy objects, receives traction or compression to joints, jumps, or crashes, the proprioceptive receptors send this information to the CNS (Table 23-6). For most individuals, this input has a regulatory effect on other types of input coming into the nervous system and has a general calming effect to the entire system. This aids in the process of becoming less and less aware of sensory input, which enables the person to fall asleep. Table 23-6 provides activities that may be implemented in a child's natural environment to transition to/prepare for the sleep process. Such input may be replicated in a more age-appropriate manner for older children and adults.

Tactile (Deep Pressure) Input

For most people, deep touch/pressure to the skin has a calming effect, whereas a light/tickle touch or unexpected/

Table 23-7.
Ideas for Tactile/Deep Pressure Input as Part of the Bedtime Routine

Massage with lotion, such as following bath time. If bath time appears to alert the individual, consider moving to the morning routine.
Deep pressure and proprioceptive technique ("brushing" protocol) using deep pressure device, followed by joint compressions.
Burrito game: Wrap/roll up in a blanket and push firmly with palms on child's back, arms, and legs.
"Squishing" the child under pillows and blankets. Important to note: NEVER cover the child's face. For added proprioceptive input, encourage the child to crawl out from under the pillow while providing gentle pressure (see Figure 23-4).
Use a lightly weighted lap pad or weighted blanket, such as while reading books while prone on elbows. Avoid weight on the chest and remove once asleep.

surprise touch has an alerting effect on the nervous system. Tickle or surprise activities should be avoided before bedtime. Table 23-7 provides activities to facilitate deep pressure input. Just like proprioceptive (heavy work) input, tactile (deep pressure) input can be replicated and adjusted for older children and adults.

Vestibular (Movement) Input

Rocking or swinging back and forth in a linear, slow, rhythmical fashion may help a person to calm (Figures 23-5 to 23-7). Fast, changing, or spinning (rotary) movement can alert the nervous system and should be avoided. Specifically, rotary input is contraindicated in certain special populations, such as individuals with seizure disorder. Refer to Table 23-8 for vestibular-based activities.

An Image of a "Perfect" Evening

To illustrate how calming strategies can be used throughout the evening, it is important to see what an ideal evening routine would look like (Table 23-9). This illustration walks through the after-school routine for a family of a toddler/school-aged child. As mentioned earlier, it is important that routine is used throughout the day and not just at bedtime. Strategies can be adapted for younger or older children and even teenagers and adults.

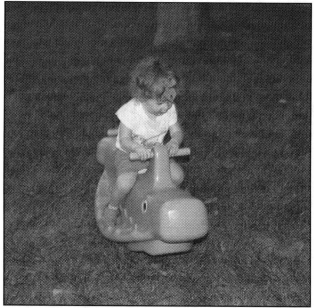

Figure 23-5. A child participates in linear vestibular input in her natural environment as part of her evening routine. (Reprinted with permission from T. Rothgangel.)

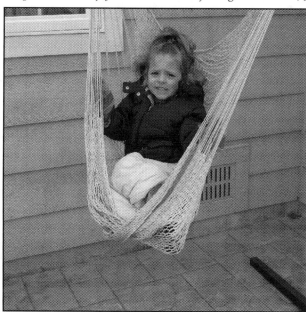

Figure 23-6. A child participates in linear vestibular movement via a hammock swing. Adding a weighted doll, backpack, lap pad, or blanket provides deep pressure input as well. (Reprinted with permission from B. Lovett.)

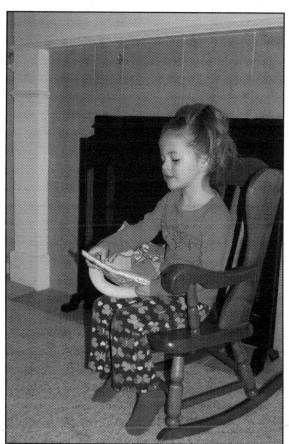

Figure 23-7. Another linear vestibular movement activity before bedtime. (Reprinted with permission from B. Lovett.)

Table 23-8.
Ideas for Calming Movement Activities as Part of the Bedtime Routine

Rocking in a rocking chair (perhaps while reading books with caregiver or softly singing familiar, rhythmic songs).
Sitting on caregiver's lap and rocking. For added deep pressure, wrap the child in a blanket tightly or add a heavy book or weighted lap pad.
Sit on floor facing child at arm's length apart. Hold hands and rock back and forth, quietly singing, "Row, Row, Row Your Boat."
Gently swinging in a hammock or door swing.
Swinging with 2 caregivers holding ends of blanket.

Table 23-9.

Sample Evening and Bedtime Schedule

Sam's Evening Routine	
3:45 PM	Sam is picked up from day care/school.
4:00 PM	Family heads to the park and ensures that Sam gets intense amounts of heavy work from climbing and jumping and linear movement from swinging on the swings.
5:00 PM	Family arrives home. Dinner includes crunchy and chewy foods and a drink that requires sucking through a straw. While dinner is prepared, Sam reads a book or plays with other parent or by himself. If television is allowed in the home, a slow-paced, nonviolent, half-hour program may be watched. This may also be a good time for homework, if applicable.
5:15 PM	Family dinner with calm conversation. Be conscious of surrounding environmental stimulants such as background noise including voices, dishes clanking, etc. Turn off the TV and play soft music.
6:00 PM	Playtime packed with calming strategies (as discussed previously). Blanket burritos, swinging in a hammock, getting "squished" with deep pressure, tunnel play, deep pressure, and proprioceptive technique/joint compressions.
6:30 PM	Mom and Dad explain to Sam that he has 5 more minutes to play and then it is time to take a bath.
6:35 PM	Bath time! Warm water and deep touch pressure are used to help Sam wash up before bedtime.
6:45 PM	Mom or Dad provides Sam with a deep pressure massage while drying him with a towel and applying lotion.
6:47 PM	Time to brush teeth. Sam is encouraged to do 20 counter top push-ups before and after brushing teeth. Sam uses the toilet. Mom or Dad explains that this is the last time to use the toilet this evening. Wheelbarrow walking from the bathroom to bedroom.
6:50 PM	Sam gets dressed in comfortable (possibly tagless) pajamas. While getting dressed, Mom or Dad prepares Sam for the next day by explaining the morning routine.
6:55 PM	Dim lights if possible. Read books. Sam chooses 3 books to read. He may choose to have them read while lying on the floor (prone) or in his child-size rocker or in bed.
7:00 PM	Sam gets in bed.
7:02 PM	Mom or Dad puts firm pressure with the use of a pillow on top of Sam's legs (if tolerated) to get his "wiggles out."
7:07 PM	Lights out. Mom or Dad sings 2 routine songs (same songs every night) in a soft, calm voice and does "waterfall" massage down his back.
7:10 PM	Routine "sign-off." Having a familiar way to say good night cues Sam that it is time to go to sleep. (eg, "Night-Night. Sleep tight. I'll see you in the morning!")
7:15 PM	Mom and Dad close the door. Soft music or white noise may be played.

REFERENCES

1. Wilcock AA, Townsend EA. Occupational justice. In: Crepeau EB, Cohn ES, Schell BB, eds. *Willard and Spackman's Occupational Therapy*. 11th ed. Baltimore, MD: Lippincott Williams & Wilkins; 2008:198.

2. World Health Organization. Preamble to the Constitution of the World Health Organization. Available at: http://whqlibdoc.who.int/hist/official_records/constitution.pdf. Accessed June 17, 2012.

3. Centers for Disease Control and Prevention. Perceived insufficient rest or sleep—four states, 2006. *MMWR Morb Mortal Wkly Rep.* 2008;57:200–203.

4. Mindell JA, Kuhn BR, Lewin DS, et al. Behavioral treatment of bedtime problems and night wakings in infants and young children. *Sleep.* 2006;29:1263–1276.

5. Sadeh A, Mindell J, Luedtke K, Wiegand B. Sleep and sleep ecology in the first 3 years: a Web-based study. *J Sleep Res.* 2009;18:60–73.

6. Midell JA, Telofski LS, Wiegand B, Kurtz ES. A nightly bedtime routine: impact on sleep in young children and maternal mood. *Sleep.* 2009;32:599–606.

7. HealthyPeople.gov. Sleep health. Available at: http://www.healthypeople.gov/2020/topicsobjectives2020/overview.aspx?topicid=38. Accessed July 10, 2012.

8. American Occupational Therapy Association. Occupational therapy practice framework: domain and process. 2nd ed. *American Journal of Occupational Therapy.* 2008;62:625–683.

9. Ayres AJ. *Sensory Integration and Learning Disorders.* Los Angeles, CA: Western Psychological Services; 1972.

10. Ayres AJ. *Sensory Integration and the Child.* Los Angeles, CA: Western Psychological Services; 1979.

11. Mailloux Z, Roley SS. Sensory integration. In: Miller-Kuhaneck H, ed. *Autism.* 2nd ed. Bethesda, MD: AOTA Press; 2004:215–244.

12. American Occupational Therapy Association. *Member Survey Data.* Rockville, MD: American Occupational Therapy Association; 1996.

13. Mulligan S. Advances in sensory integration research. In: Bundy AC, Lane SJ, Murray EA, eds. *Sensory Integration Theory and Practice.* 2nd ed. Philadelphia, PA: FA Davis; 2002:397–411.

14. Ayres AJ. *Sensory Integration and Praxis Tests Manual.* Los Angeles, CA: Western Psychological Services; 1989.

15. Parham LD, Ecker C. *Sensory Processing Measure Manual.* Los Angeles, CA: Western Psychological Services; 2007.

16. Dunn W. *Sensory Profile Manual.* San Antonio, TX: Psychological Corporation; 1999.

17. Berk RA, DeGangi GA. *DeGangi-Berk Test of Sensory Integration Manual.* Los Angeles, CA: Western Psychological Services; 1983.

18. Smith KA, Gouze KR. *The Sensory-Sensitive Child: Practical Solutions for Out-of-Bounds Behavior.* New York, NY: HarperCollins Publisher; 1994.

19. Fisher AG, Murray EA. Introduction to sensory integration theory. In: Fisher AG, Murray EA, Bundy AC, eds. *Sensory Integration: Theory and Practice.* Philadelphia, PA: FA Davis; 1991:3–26.

20. Champagne T, Frederick D. Sensory processing research advances in mental health: implications for occupational therapy. *OT Practice.* 2011;16(10):7–12.

21. Ayres AJ. *Sensory Integration and Praxis Tests.* Los Angeles, CA: Western Psychological Services; 1989.

22. Wilbarger J, Stackhouse T. Sensory modulation: a review of the literature. Available at: http://www.ot-innovations.com/content/view/29/58/. Accessed July 20, 2012.

23. Short-Degraff AA. *Human Development for Occupational and Physical Therapists.* Baltimore, MD: Williams & Wilkins; 1988.

24. Smith Roley S, Imperatore BE, Schaaf RC. *Understanding the Nature of Sensory Integration With Diverse Populations.* San Antonio, TX: Therapy Skill Builders; 2001.

25. Grandin T. Calming effects of deep touch pressure in patients with autistic disorder, college students, and animals. *J Child Adolesc Psychopharmacol.* 1992;2:63–72.

26. Grandin T. *Thinking in Pictures.* New York, NY: Doubleday; 1995.

27. Biel L, Peske N. *Raising a Sensory Smart Child: The Definitive Handbook for Helping Your Child With Sensory Integration Issues.* London, UK: Penguin Books; 2005.

28. Davies PL, Gavin WJ. Validating the diagnosis of sensory processing disorders using EEG technology. *Am J Occup Ther.* 2007;61:176–189.

29. American Psychiatric Association. *Diagnostic and Statistical Manual of Mental Disorders.* 4th rev. ed. Washington, DC: American Psychiatric Association; 2000.

30. World Health Organization. *ICD-10: International Statistical Classification of Diseases and Related Health Problems.* 10th rev. ed. New York, NY: World Health Organization; 2008.

31. Smith Roley S, Mailloux Z, Miller-Kuhaneck H, Glennon T. Understanding Ayres Sensory Integration. *OT Practice.* 2007;12(17):CE-1–CE-8.

32. Williams S, Shellenberger MS. *How Does Your Engine Run?: A Leader's Program to the Alert Program for Self-regulation.* Albuquerque, NM: Therapy Works; 1996.

33. Fiese BH, Tomcho TJ, Douglas M, Josephs K, Poltrock S, Baker T. A review of 50 years of research on naturally occurring family routines and rituals: cause for celebration? *J Fam Psychol.* 2002;16:381–390.

34. Gordon BN. Parenting practices. In: Ollendick TH, Schroeder TS, eds. *Encyclopedia of Clinical Child and Pediatric Psychology.* New York, NY: Kluwer Academic/Plenum; 2003:447–451.

35. Leiferman JA, Ollendick TH, Kunkel D, Christie IC. Mothers' mental distress and parenting practices with infants and toddlers. *Arch Womens Ment Health.* 2005;8:243–247.

36. Midell JA, Telofski LS, Wiegand B, Kurtz ES. A nightly bedtime routine: impact on sleep in young children and maternal mood. *Sleep.* 2009;32:599–606.

37. Mindell JA, Moline ML, Zendell SM, Brown LW, Fry JM. Pediatricians and sleep disorders: training and practice. *Pediatrics.* 1994;94:194–200.

38. Owens J, Maxim R, McGuinn M, Nobile C, Msall M, Alario A. Television-viewing habits and sleep disturbance in school children. *Pediatrics.* 1999;104(3):e27.

39. WebMD. The benefits of a good night's sleep. Available at: http://www.webmd.com/sleep-disorders/sleep-benefits-10/slideshow-sleep-tips. Accessed July 10, 2012.

40. Garrison MM, Liekweg K, Christakis DA. Media use and child sleep: the impact of content, timing, and environment. *Pediatrics.* 2011;128:29–35.

41. Lillard AS, Peterson J. The immediate impact of different types of television on young children's executive function. *Pediatrics.* 2011;128:772–774.

42. Weisbluth M. *Healthy Sleep Habits, Happy Child.* 3rd ed. New York, NY: Ballantine Books; 2003.

43. National Sleep Foundation. Available at: http://www.sleepfoundation.org/article/how-sleep-works/how-much-sleep-do-we-really-need. Accessed July 19, 2012.

44. Karp H. *Happiest Baby on the Block: The New Way to Calm Crying and Help Your Newborn Sleep Longer.* New York, NY: Bantam Dell; 2003.

24

Sleep and Specific Populations

Julie M. Hereford, PT, DPT

SLEEP IN INFANTS AND CHILDREN

Sleep in premature infants, newborns, and infants is characteristically different from sleep in children and certainly different from sleep in adults (Figures 24-1 and 24-2). Physiology, regulation, organization, architecture, and distribution of sleep vary from one age group to the next throughout the life span (Table 24-1).

Sleep among newborns is polyphasic; that is, sleep episodes occur regularly and are distributed relatively equally over a 24-hour period (Table 24-2). Newborn infants sleep approximately 70% of the time, whereas adults normally sleep for about 30% of a 24-hour period. As the infant grows to childhood, sleep takes on a more predictable schedule, with naps occurring at relatively regular intervals. Daytime napping diminishes with age and usually disappears at about 5 years; however, some individuals naturally continue to prefer a bi-phasic sleep pattern with an afternoon nap and a major nocturnal sleep period.

In the first 6 months of life, sleep is divided into active sleep, intermediate sleep, transition sleep, and quiet sleep. Active sleep is equivalent to rapid eye movement (REM) sleep but contains frequent body and facial twitches and jerks. It can include limb movements, sucking, grimacing, vocalization, and tremors. This is the first behavioral sleep state to appear and is the predominant sleep state in the newborn. It accounts for 60% of newborn sleep, 30% of sleep in infancy, and 20% of sleep in childhood. Quiet sleep is equivalent to non-rapid eye movement (NREM) sleep and is characterized by minimal or no body movements and by a regular breathing pattern. Electroencephalogram (EEG) shows high-voltage, slow-wave activity. Intermediate sleep is defined as that which does not fully meet the criteria for either active or quiet sleep. Transitional sleep is that which occurs in the transition between active, quiet, and intermediate sleep.

Sleep is often entered into as REM sleep in the infant (Figure 24-3). This is normal in the infant and child but is considered disordered sleep in the adult. REM sleep and NREM sleep occur in equal amounts in infancy, but the proportion of REM sleep declines as the child grows older. In infancy, REM sleep occupies about 50% of total sleep time but decreases to approximately 20% to 25% of total sleep time in the adult. NREM stages 3 and 4 sleep are the greatest in early childhood and gradually decrease in amount as the child gets older.

The NREM and REM sleep cycle alternates approximately every 50 minutes in the infant, but that cycle time gradually increases with age. In the normal adult sleeper, the NREM to REM cycle lasts approximately 90 to 110 minutes. Slow-wave sleep occurs in greater proportion in the early part of sleep and REM sleep increases later in a normal sleep cycle.

Characteristics of the EEG change as the infant grows and develops. In fact, characteristic EEG patterns can be seen in gestational life. A trace alternate pattern is defined as an "EEG pattern of the sleeping newborn, 32 to 34 weeks' gestation, characterized by bursts of slow waves, at times intermixed with sharp waves and intervening periods of relative quiescence with extremely low-amplitude activity."[1] Sleep spindles begin to appear as early as 4 weeks of age, and K-complexes appear at 6 months of age. Slow-wave sleep appears between 8 and 12 weeks of age, and the

Hereford JM. *Sleep and Rehabilitation:*
A Guide for Health Professionals (pp 279-294).
© 2014 Taylor & Francis Group.

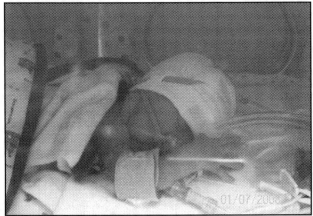

Figure 24-1. Infants born prematurely have very high percentages of REM sleep, up to 80%. This is thought to be essential for continued brain development. (Reprinted with permission from B. Roetheli.)

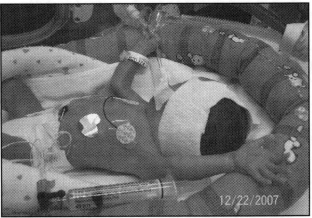

Figure 24-2. Infants born prematurely are exposed to sensory input to which they would not usually be exposed until normal term birth. It has been speculated that this abnormal exposure to sensory input (lights, sounds, and smells of the neonatal ICU) may change sensory integration in these infants. Studies that look at the incidence of sensory integration issues versus level of exposure in this population may shed light on this. (Reprinted with permission from B. Roetheli.)

distinct EEG features that allow differentiation of NREM sleep into 4 specific stages begin at approximately 3 to 6 months of age.

Regulation of sleep homeostasis is present early in life. The suprachiasmatic nuclei, which controls circadian processes, is functional in utero, and rhythmic fluctuations in body temperature become apparent as early as 1 month of age. Nocturnal consolidation of sleep tends to develop shortly after the onset of body temperature rhythms.

Developmental milestones that occur in the sleep pattern of infants and children include specific sleep behaviors that are considered typical for the age, although depending upon cultural perceptions and parental expectations can be considered problematic. During the first 6 weeks of life, the newborn sleeps up to 70% of the time, with sleep distributed relatively equally throughout the 24-hour period. After approximately 6 weeks of age, sleep begins to take on a pattern, and the longest sleep period occurs at night. Some infants have the neurological maturity to begin to sleep through the night at this stage.

At 3 months of age, the infant is able to consolidate daytime sleep into discrete naps. By this time the parent or caregiver can begin to mold sleep–wake patterns by establishing specific daytime napping times and routines. Generally, the infant will take 2 to 3 naps during the daytime. The first nap occurs within a few hours of morning wakening and is relatively short. The second daytime nap occurs in the early afternoon, usually after lunch, and coincides with the normal circadian dip. This nap is longer and may last for 2 to 3 hours. The last daytime nap is often very short, lasting as briefly as 15 to 20 minutes and may occur around dinner time. A general rule of thumb is that the infant should not be kept awake for longer than 2 to 3 hours at a time.

Between 6 and 9 months of age, nocturnal sleep is consolidated, and the infant has developed the ability to sleep through the night. Daytime naps may remain the same, or

the infant may show a decreased need for the third nap. It is important to establish a regular bedtime routine that includes a particular time that the child is put to bed.

By the time the child is 1 year old and until approximately 3 years of age, the toddler may experience an increase in the frequency of nighttime awakenings. At this time it is important for the child to learn self-soothing skills in order to return to sleep on his or her own. This is a normal developmental stage, and self-soothing should be encouraged. It is at this stage when some parents or caregivers may begin to interfere with this process and insist upon intervening and not allowing the child to learn this important life skill. Lack of ability to self-soothe may be linked to other problems of sensory integration (see Chapter 23).

At this age, it is not uncommon for the parents or caregivers to make the mistake of allowing the infant child to stay up later in the evening. Sometimes this is done for social reasons because the parents may work and have not been able to see and play with their infant during the day. As the child is becoming more social and active, this is a tempting habit to get into; however, it is usually done at the expense of the child's sleep requirement. Another common mistake made in establishing early sleep patterns is that of having the child stay up later in an attempt to get him to sleep later in the morning. Paradoxically, this creates problems with sleep onset and sets the child up for a sleep debt situation. The overtired child is one with an irritated, overactive brain (Figure 24-4). It has been postulated that if the child cannot experience the fluctuations in brain chemistry that are necessary to allow normal brain development, which can lead to behavioral and emotional problems. Parents and caregivers should work to establish a good sleep routine for their child and safeguard their sleep

Table 24-1.

Sleep Distribution From Premature Infant to Adolescent

Age	Sleep Characteristic	Common Sleep Disorders
Premature infant	• At 24 to 26 weeks, there is no clearly definable sleep states present • Active sleep present 28 to 30 weeks and constitutes most of sleep • At same conceptual age, premature and full-term infants have similar EEG pattern • Premature infant has sleep spindles sooner than full-term infant	• Irregular sleep patterns
Neonate (0 to 2 months)	• Sleeps 12 to 18 hours per day • No clear day/night sleep pattern • Breast-fed infants sleep 2 to 3 hours at a time; bottle-fed infants sleep 3 to 5 hours at a time • Frequent awakenings	• Irregular sleep pattern • Day/night reversal
Infant (3 to 11 months)	• Sleeps 14 to 15 hours per day • Progressive increase in night sleep • Quiet sleep becomes dominant • Increased use of transition objects (pacifier) • Most infants sleep through the night by 6 to 9 months except for brief arousals • May develop separation anxiety at this time	• Difficulty with sleep onset • Bedtime resistance • Sleep-onset association disorder • Rhythmic movement disorder • Problematic night awakenings
Toddler (1 to 3 years)	• Sleeps 12 to 14 hours/day • Progressive decrease in duration of nighttime sleep and frequency of daytime napping • One nap per day by 18 months • Increasing mobility and independence	• Difficulty with sleep onset • Bedtime resistance • Sleep-onset association disorder • Rhythmic movement disorder • Problematic night awakenings
Preschool (3 to 5 years)	• Sleeps 11 to 13 hours per 24-hour period • Most children stop napping between 3 and 5 years • Gradual decrease in percentage of REM sleep	• OSA • Bedtime resistance • Limit-setting sleep disorder • Sleep-onset association disorder • Rhythmic movement disorder • Problematic night awakenings • Nighttime fears/nightmares
Preadolescent (5 to 14 years)	• Sleeps 10 to 11 hours per 24-hour period	• Snoring • OSA • Disorders of arousal • Insufficient sleep syndrome • Inadequate sleep hygiene • Bruxism

(continued)

Table 24-1 (continued).

Sleep Distribution from Premature Infant to Adolescent

	Sleep Characteristic	Common Sleep Disorders
Adolescent (14–18 years)	• 8½ to 9¼ hours of sleep per 24-hour period • Increase in daytime sleepiness at puberty • Phase delay in circadian sleep–wake rhythms usually occurs during puberty	• Snoring • OSA • Delayed-phase sleep syndrome • Excessive daytime sleepiness • Narcolepsy • Inadequate sleep hygiene • Insomnia

Table 24-2.

Sleep Distribution Across Infancy

Age	Distribution of Sleep and Sleep Behavior	Sleep Classification	Sleep Stages
Newborn (<6 to 9 months)	Distributed equally across a 24-hour period	Active or quiet sleep	Active, quiet, intermediate, and transitional sleep
Infant (>6 to 9 months)	Consolidation of sleep to night	REM or NREM sleep	NREM stages 1 to 4 and REM sleep
1 to 6 years of age	Increase frequency of wakings during the night	Same	Same

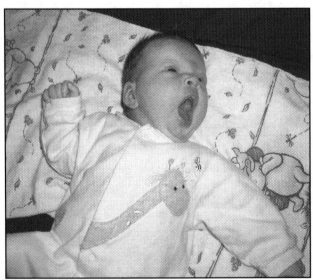

Figure 24-3. In the infant, sleep is often entered into at the REM stage. (Reprinted with permission from J. Hoskins.)

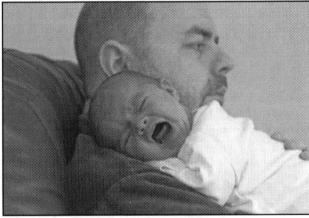

Figure 24-4. Sleep problems infants are sometimes aggravated by parents' and caregivers' attempts to soothe the child or overstimulate the child in an attempt to "wear him or her out." (From Fotolia.com)

habits for the first years of life. Once well established, good sleep habits are usually lifelong contributors to good health.

Between the ages of 3 and 5 years old, the child will decrease daytime napping, and usually by the time the child is 5, daytime napping disappears altogether. Between the ages of 6 and 12 years, the child tends to develop the tendency toward a particular circadian sleep phase, that is being a "morning lark" or a "night owl." Between the ages of 12 and 18, also known as adolescence, the individuals will develop the tendency toward a delayed sleep phase. This is a normal developmental stage of sleep, although it is often allowed to reach an extreme and can then become disruptive to normal function.

CHARACTERISTICS OF SLEEP PATTERNS—PREMATURE INFANT TO THE ADOLESCENT

This section is not intended to be a guide to identifying and solving infant and childhood sleep problems but to give a general outline of normal developmental stages of sleep and common sleep problems associated with each age. Generally, treatments of behavioral sleep disorders that do not include a specific neurological component are similar. They include parental education, maintenance of consistent bedtimes and appropriate nighttime activities, establishment of optimal sleep environment extinction procedures, faded bedtime, positive bedtime routines, scheduled awakenings, and cognitive behavioral therapy.

Chapter 23 will offer some insight into treatment techniques that can be utilized with particular sleep problems. This author also recommends *Healthy Sleep Habits, Happy Child* by Marc Weissbluth as an excellent guide to identifying sleep problems in children and developing good strategies to improve infant, childhood, and adolescent sleep.[2]

Sleep is identifiable as early as the 24th week of gestation. Though EEG patterns consistent with sleep are apparent, there is no clearly definable sleep states present at that age. Active sleep, characterized by the presence of eye movements, body movements, and irregular respiration, can be identified by 28 to 30 weeks of gestation. Active sleep, analogous to REM sleep in the adult, constitutes the majority of sleep. Quiet sleep, with EEG patterns of trace discontinue, which is a burst of medium to high amp, mixed frequency waves that are random and paroxysmal against an almost flat background, are normally seen at 30 weeks of gestation, and trace alternant, which are bursts of a shorter duration, can be seen at 36 weeks of gestation. Premature and full-term infants attain similar EEG sleep patterns at the same conceptual age, although development of sleep spindles is advanced in premature infants compared to full-term infants. This may be related to motor cortex maturation that continues during sleep in the premature infant. Sleep disorders are uncommon at this age, although usually manifest themselves as irregular sleep patterns.

The neonate, considered to be newborn to 2 months of age, has a high total amount of sleep time, usually 16 to 18 hours per 24-hour period, but may be higher in the premature infant. Sleep periods occurring throughout the 24-hour period do not have a clear diurnal–nocturnal pattern and range from 2 to 3 hours among breast-fed infants and 3 to 5 hours among bottle-fed infants. Sleep periods are usually separated by wake periods of 1 to 3 hours. Awakenings from sleep are more likely to occur during active sleep than from quiet sleep. Sleep disorders during this age usually include a day–night reversal and irregular sleep patterns.

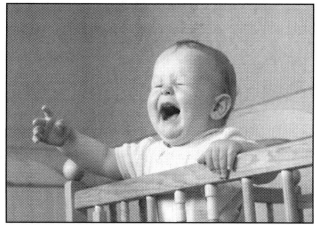

Figure 24-5. Bedtime resistance is a challenge most parents experience. (From Fotolia.com)

During the first year of life, the total sleep time is usually 12 to 16 hours of sleep per 24-hour period but includes several daytime nap periods. There is a progressive decrease in the duration of nocturnal sleep, and daytime napping becomes less frequent as the infant gets older. Quiet sleep becomes the dominant sleep stage by 3 months of age. Except for brief arousals, usually occurring 4 to 5 times per night, most infants are able to sleep through the night by 6 to 9 months of age. Many infants older than 6 months do not require night feedings, although there is a greater frequency of nighttime awakenings for feeding in breast-fed infants compared to bottle-fed infants. It is at this age that the infant may show signs of separation anxiety at bedtime. The child may also show increasing use of a transitional object during bedtime, such as a pacifier, blanket, or stuffed animal. Sleep problems at this age include difficulties with sleep onset, bedtime resistance, sleep onset association disorder, rhythmic movement disorder, and problematic night awakenings. Some of these behavioral disorders of sleep onset develop naturally with the toddler's increased sense of independence and autonomy (Figure 24-5).

During the toddler stage of 1 to 3 years old, the total amount of sleep time decreases to 11 to 12 hours per 24-hour period. There is a progressive decrease in the duration of nighttime sleep and in daytime napping as the child gets older. Daytime naps tend to occur once per day by 18 months of age. The child is also developing increased mobility and independence during this time. Sleep problems can become more prevalent as a function of the child's fledgling independence. These may include difficulties with sleep onset, bedtime resistance, limit-setting sleep disorder, sleep-onset association disorder, rhythmic movement disorder, and problematic nighttime awakenings.

During the preschool years, from ages 3 to 5, the total sleep time is usually 10 to 12 hours per 24-hour period (Figure 24-6). The younger child may continue to take a daytime nap, but these tend to disappear completely by the age of 5. There is also a reduction of the percentage of REM

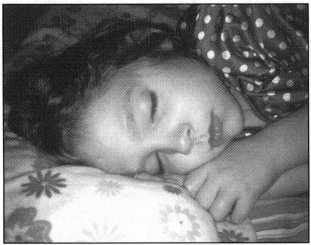

Figure 24-6. Children ages 3 to 5 sleep an average of 10 to 12 hours per 24-hour period. (Reprinted with permission from M. Mebruer.)

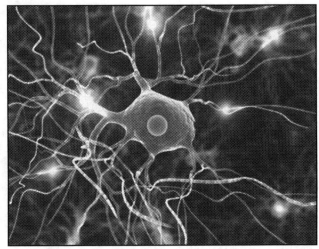

Figure 24-7. Sleep plays an important role in neural pathway development in infants and children. (From Fotolia.com)

sleep in children of this age. Sleep problems often consist of behavioral problems including bedtime resistance, limit-setting sleep disorder, and sleep-onset association disorder. Nighttime fears and nightmares can begin to occur at this age; however, the toddler usually does not have the cognitive maturity to be able to make sense of "bad dreams," so management of them can be a bit more complex than in the older child or adult. Other more complex sleep problems can begin at this age as well. These can include night terrors, confusional arousals, and sleepwalking. Obstructive sleep apnea (OSA) may become a problem in this age group because of the frequency of upper respiratory infections, the development of the airway, and enlargement of the lymphatic tissue that may narrow the upper airway including tonsils and adenoids.

During the preadolescent years, generally from age 5 to 14, the total sleep time is 8 to 11 hours, with a progressive decrease in the duration of nighttime sleep. Daytime sleepiness is less common than in adolescence. Circadian sleep-wake rhythm preferences begin to manifest themselves. Sleep problems in this age group include snoring, OSA, disorders of arousal, insufficient sleep syndrome, inadequate sleep hygiene, and bruxism.

During adolescence, from age 14 to 18, the sleep requirement is slightly higher than in the preadolescent years, although adolescents are notorious for not getting enough sleep. This increased in sleep requirement is consistent with the increased in energy demands of puberty. Daytime sleepiness is also a manifestation of puberty. Adolescents have a naturally occurring shift in sleep-wake cycle to a delayed phase circadian rhythm, which is often in conflict with the demands of school and family life. Common sleep problems of adolescence include snoring, OSA, delayed phase sleep disorder, excessive daytime sleepiness, narcolepsy, inadequate sleep hygiene, and insomnia.

The Function of Sleep in Infants and Children

During the first few years of life, there are a number of developmental changes that occur in the sleep–wake cycle that ultimately mature into the characteristic adult sleep pattern. There is growing evidence that sleep and sleep cycles are essential for the development of neural circuitry of primary sensory systems and for maturation of various sensory systems in the fetal, newborn, and infant life[3] (Figure 24-7). Sleep is also known to be important for brain plasticity and for encoding of long-term memory and learning. Sleep deprivation in young life has been shown to have a profound impact on early sensory development.[4]

These early neural connections are established by cell generation through successive cell division and cell differentiation. As cells are differentiated, axons develop and travel to specific target regions along specific pathways. This axonal guidance is genetically driven by specified molecular cues to target areas to develop a functional sensory system. During this process, billions of neurons are developing and make up to a thousand synapses in order to form a precise system of neural circuits, designed for a specific sensory modality. The initial rendering of this neural pathway, with its multiple interconnections, is imprecise. In order to develop the precision needed in neural circuitry, a series of elaborations, retractions, and remodeling of the neural connections must take place within the target area. This activity is thought to be activity dependent rather than genetically driven. This is evidenced by the ability of the neural pathway development to be disrupted by blocking of neuronal activity. This may be an important role of sleep and sleep cycle in the developing brain.[5]

According to Graven and Browne, REM sleep in particular is required for the development of multiple sensory systems in fetal and infant life.[6] Included in these systems are somatesthesia, kinesthesia, proprioception, chemosensory systems, the auditory and visual systems, the limbic system, social learning, and the hippocampus and its involvement in memory formation and consolidation. The impact of sleep on the development of the human brain makes clear how important it is to facilitate and protect sleep in early life.

The development of REM sleep at 28 to 30 weeks' gestation is part of the endogenous stimulation necessary for development of neural circuits, which form the "basic architecture of the sensory cortex and brain stem nuclei that relay the signal from the sensory organ to the appropriate site in the neocortex. (p. 1133)"[5] Immature, irregular electrical activity of ganglionic cells that are required for axonal growth and interconnection in the sensory systems begins to develop a more regular and synchronous pattern during this same time. This synchronicity is associated with the development of distinct sleep stages and sleep cycles in fetal life. REM and NREM sleep cycles are established between weeks 36 and 38 of gestation.[5]

In utero, REM sleep dominates the sleep cycle, and NREM sleep may be completely absent. At normal term birth of 40 weeks, REM and NREM usually comprise equal proportions of the sleep cycle. At approximately 9 months of age, REM sleep has been reduced to 20% to 30% of the sleep cycle. This is the normal ratio of REM to NREM sleep that will be present into and throughout adulthood. As in the adult, wakefulness must be actively maintained by aminergic activity in the brain stem, and sleep is a function of cholinergic activity.

During REM sleep, specific EEG waveforms are associated with development of specific modalities in the sensory system. Disruption of the normal amount of REM sleep from approximately 30 weeks' gestation until 4 to 5 months of age may result in developmental delay in somatosensory function. Disruption of normal sleep may occur because of premature birth or significant or persistent alteration of the sensory environment in utero or in neonatal life.

Normal REM/NREM sleep cycling is also critical for the capacity of the brain to adapt and learn in response to environmental needs. This brain plasticity involves activation and preservation of nerve growth factor, brain-derived neurotrophic factor, and ubiquitin, which is a small regulatory protein found in almost all tissues of eukaryotic organisms, which among other functions directs protein recycling.[5] It has been postulated as well that the activation of certain parts of the nervous system, including the autonomic nervous system, during REM sleep contributes to functional maturation of the brain.

MATURATION OF SLEEP ARCHITECTURE

Healthy full-term newborn infants display distinct sleep patterns compared to older infants and children. Newborns sleep longer, up to 16 to 20 hours per 24-hour period. REM sleep can occur at the onset of sleep compared to the older sleeper, in which REM sleep is only entered into from NREM sleep. The newborn has proportionately more REM sleep, usually comprising 50% of total sleep time and the sleep cycle. In addition, the NREM/REM cycle is of a much shorter duration, usually 45 to 60 minutes in the newborn, than it is in the adult, which is usually 90 to 110 minutes. As the newborn infant matures out of newborn status into the first 8 to 9 months of infancy, there is a gradual decrease in total sleep time. Maturation of the central nervous system is marked by a decreased proportion of REM sleep, a gradual increase in the length of the REM/NREM cycle, and a shift to the adult pattern of entering REM from NREM sleep stages.

As the individual continues to grow and develop through childhood and into adolescence, sleep is characterized by an increase in NREM sleep, now comprising approximately 75% of total sleep time. REM sleep, after infancy is entered into from a NREM sleep stage, and the NREM/REM sleep cycle alternates throughout the night approximately every 90 to 100 minutes, with progressive lengthening of REM sleep bouts in the final one third of the night's sleep. Contrary to a perhaps firmly held belief by many adolescents, this age group actually requires slightly more sleep than the younger child of 5 to 10 years of age (Figure 24-8). Because of the significant metabolic and hormonal demands of puberty, the average adolescent requires 8.5 to 9.25 hours of sleep per 24-hour period. They generally experience a decrease in the total amount of slow-wave sleep, which continues into adulthood. In addition, there is a physiological shift in sleep onset to a later time, a fact that may annoy parents but is part of a normal maturation.

A normal child experiences a relatively brief latency to sleep onset and breathes quietly and comfortably with high sleep efficiency. The child may waken briefly, but a healthy sleeper is able to self-soothe and return to sleep quickly and then awaken in the morning refreshed and able to engage with the environment and learn effectively. The well-rested child will be able to function well and generally will not be sleepy, except during normally scheduled nap times.

Children may develop disordered sleep for a variety of reasons. If a child snores, he or she should be assessed for an upper airway problem. During normal sleep, as in the adult, the child will experience some upper airway resistance and therefore a decrease in nocturnal ventilation. During normal sleep, a child may experience O_2 desaturation of up to

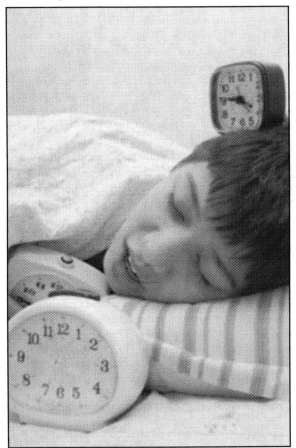

Figure 24-8. Adolescents require more sleep than children ages 5 to 10 and experience a shift in sleep hours. These often run contrary to the demands of school and social life. (from Fotolia.com)

7% and a rise in PCO_2 of 13 mm Hg. There may be brief apneas associated with movement, but OSA is never normal in a child. If a child snores or has apneic episodes during sleep, he or she should be evaluated.

CONSEQUENCES OF SLEEP-RELATED BREATHING DISORDERS IN CHILDREN

A child with a sleep-related breathing disorder will have exaggerated upper airway resistance, which will lead to increased mechanical work required for breathing and may cause snoring, OSA, and/or sleep hypoventilation. This situation will cause sleep disruption and may result in decreased oxygen saturation and increased end-tidal PCO_2.

The physiological consequences of apneic sleep in children can be substantial. Current literature describes a spectrum of these consequences that may include growth impairment, systemic or pulmonary hypertension, and myocardial remodeling.[7-10] Neurocognitive and behavioral problems that have recently been linked with disordered sleep in children include attention-deficit/hyperactivity disorder (ADHD), behavioral or mood-related problems, and poor school performance.[7,11,12]

Disordered sleep in children can take many forms. Some children may have problems with sleep onset and maintenance. Insomnia in children may be part of a conditioned response; it may have behavioral components or social or environmental components. It may involve a problem with circadian rhythm, or it may have a medical basis.

Obstructive Sleep Apnea and Obstructive Hypoventilation

OSA or sleep hypoventilation is caused by a complete or partial collapse of part of the upper airway that occurs during sleep. This may be due to an anatomically small upper airway and/or decreased neuromuscular tone in the pharyngeal dilators during sleep. Studies have shown that the cross-sectional area of the upper airways of children with OSA are significantly smaller than those of normal controls.[13] The lateral dimensions of the normal child sleeper are consistently larger than the anteroposterior dimension, and there is very little change in the size and shape of the airway between inspiration and expiration. In the child with a sleep-related breathing disorder, the upper airway is generally smaller along the entire length from the nasopharynx to the epiglottis. The AP dimension is consistently larger than the lateral dimension, and there is a change in airway size most significantly in the nasopharynx when comparing inspiration and expiration.[14,15]

The consequences of OSA in adults include cognitive dysfunction such as alteration in attention, concentration, problem solving, and recall. Children with OSA experience similar symptoms as adults, but the consequences of OSA in children are less well studied. Because of the rapid development of the brain in children, it stands to reason that the consequences of OSA in children are more damaging. Studies show that OSA in children can have neurobehavioral, cardiovascular, and metabolic effects.[16]

A number of significant studies have shown that children with learning problems are more likely to have sleep-related breathing disorders. In fact, the Tucson Children's Assessment of Sleep Apnea (TuCASA), which studied a large number of children, found that children with learning problems were 2.4 times more likely to snore and 2.5 times more likely to report excessive daytime sleepiness.[16] Another study linked snoring to an increased incidence of hyperactivity.[17] A study by Gozal reported that 30% of children who were rated as having loud snoring also had a significant increase in hyperactivity and inattentiveness.[18]

As reported earlier, a relatively common reason for snoring in children is the presence of enlarged tonsils and/or adenoids (Figure 24-9). Studies of children diagnosed with ADHD who were treated with tonsillectomy/

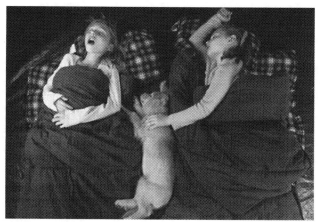

Figure 24-9. Snoring in children may be linked to enlarged tonsils and/or adenoids. (From Fotolia.com)

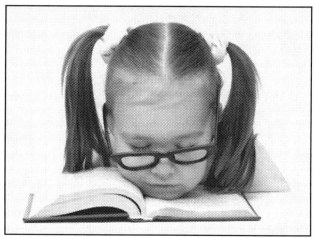

Figure 24-10. It is important to be vigilant if sleep apnea is a possibility in children. Early identification can prevent a number of physical and psychological consequences. (From Fotolia.com)

adenoidectomy showed a significant decrease in symptoms of sleep-related breathing disorders. Over half of the children treated on one study of 229 children ages 2 to 13 no longer qualified for the diagnosis of ADHD.[17] Similar findings were seen in adolescents who were poor performers in school. One study showed that snoring was extremely highly correlated with learning problems in sleep-related breathing disorders. It appears that learning problems is a specific and sensitive indicator of children who have sleep-related breathing disorders.[19]

Children and adolescents with sleep-related breathing disorders have an increased incidence of cardiac consequences. These include hypertension, ventricular hypertrophy, cor pulmonale, and pulmonary hypertension. Studies of blood pressure in children with sleep-related breathing disorders with an apnea–hypopnea index (AHI) of less than 5 showed an increase in morning blood pressure surges, blood pressure load, and mean nocturnal and diurnal blood pressure.[20,21] Children with severe OSA, defined as an AHI greater than 5 in children, were found to have a significant elevation of systolic blood pressure. Children with an AHI greater than 1 were shown to have elevated heart rate both at night and during the day. Children with severe OSA were also at a significantly increased risk of relative heart muscle thickness in the presence of hypertension. This evidence suggests that children with untreated OSA likely have elevated autonomic tone and are at increased risk for cardiovascular disease.

Children with severe OSA have a greater risk of developing metabolic syndrome, even if other factors that are known to contribute to development of the syndrome are eliminated.[22] OSA is related to elevated blood pressure, elevated fasting low-density lipoprotein, and elevated insulin levels. Pro-inflammatory markers including C-reactive protein are also elevated in children with OSA. Effective treatment of childhood OSA has been shown to reverse cardiovascular risk and most aspects of metabolic syndrome.[23]

Sleep disordered breathing has been shown to have numerous consequences including neurobehavioral, cardiovascular and metabolic. It can have an overall negative impact on the quality of life of a child. Because children are not routinely assessed for sleep apnea, the majority probably are undiagnosed and untreated. The risks to general health are substantial. Clinicians should be aware of some of the manifestations of sleep-related breathing disorders in children and be able to educate the parent or caregiver in order to find effective treatment for the at-risk child (Figure 24-10).

SLEEP IN ADOLESCENTS

Studies show that teenagers need more sleep than they usually get, apparently because they tend to sacrifice sleep time when making choices about time management. School often begins relatively early and teenagers are notorious for keeping late hours, which complicates the situation. In addition, this age group has an increased sleep requirement because of the enormous energy demands of puberty. Teenagers should receive more than 9 hours of sleep every night.[24] One difficulty with adolescents experiencing puberty is that the internal time clock can be just a little different during the teenage years. There is a natural drift in circadian rhythm to what appears to be a delayed-phase sleep syndrome. This causes teenagers to want to stay up later and sleep later in the morning. However, most school schedules do not take this into account. The result is a chronic sleep deprivation that manifests as difficulty concentrating in school, especially in early morning classes. The phase shift to later sleep-onset time is also driven by psychosocial factors including social activities, sports, academic pressure, evening jobs, and social media. Recent studies have also linked chronic sleep deprivation in

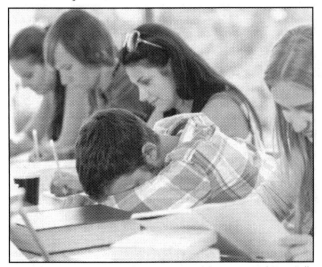

Figure 24-11. Chronic sleep deprivation in adolescents may be partially explained by the shift in their circadian clocks. (From Fotolia.com)

teenagers to diminished academic success.[25-27] Adolescents tend to sleep less on school nights, with one study reporting that 26% of these sleepers average only 6.5 hours of sleep on school nights.[22] They often increase sleep on the weekends by sleeping in, and this can lead to habitual poor-quality sleep.

The ability to remember is related to the ability to learn. Sleep is vital in processing, encoding, and consolidating memory and therefore is important in learning and retention. This suggests that good sleep habits are important to good study habits. For example, one study showed that when learning a different language, which requires a particular type of perceptual memory, studying just prior to sleep promotes retention.[28] Other studies show that sleep strengthens information consolidated into memory so that it becomes resistant to decay and interferences from other incoming information.[29,30]

Chronic sleep deprivation is a significant problem and appears to put some adolescents at risk for cognitive and emotional problems, decreased academic performance, and increased incidence of motor vehicle accidents. It has also been related to increased incidence of psychopathology, including depression.

Improving adolescent sleep patterns has been shown to improve some of these consequences. For example, a study conducted by Wolfson and Carskadon found that students who had poor academic performance reported getting an average of 25 to 40 minutes less sleep than their better-performing counterparts.[31] More recent evidence has shown that taking steps to adjust the school day to the needs of adolescent sleep habits can pay significant dividends. For example, school districts that have changed school start time from 7:15 AM to 8:40 AM have reported less sleepy students who are performing better and improved school attendance. They also report fewer behavior problems, and

survey information indicates fewer feelings of depression in students.[32]

Studies show that as adolescents mature, melatonin production tapers off later than it does in less mature teenagers, suggesting that circadian timing switches on later at night as pubescent development progresses. Changes in circadian timing complicated by early morning awakenings demanded by school schedules can produce a potentially damaging situation in which teenagers suffer from excessive daytime sleepiness, sometimes falling asleep during early classes, and displaying markedly decreased REM sleep latency. One study showed an average of only 3.4 minutes of REM sleep latency, a pattern similar to that which is seen in individuals with narcolepsy.[33] Chronic sleep deprivation in adolescents has also been associated with depression and ADHD.

The chronic sleep deprivation seen in many adolescents is partially explained by the shift in the circadian clock to a later phase that appears to occur at the start of puberty (Figure 24-11). Crowley et al suggested that the adolescent brain changes its sensitivity to light at the onset of puberty.[33] In the evening, exposure to even very dim light delayed melatonin secretion for participants who were in the middle or late puberty but not for prepubertal participants.[34]

Adolescent alcohol use may affect brain mechanisms that regulate sleep. Research is ongoing to discover the effects that alcohol may have on the developing brain and the mechanisms that control and regulate sleep in these individuals. It has been noted that changes in sleep patterns in the adolescent can influence emotional regulation and behavior. Research has noted that sleep-deprived teenagers appear to be especially vulnerable to depression and symptoms of ADHD and have increased difficulties controlling emotions and impulses.

It is difficult to untangle the cause and effect of these issues, but sleep deprivation and problems controlling impulses and emotions have been shown to exacerbate one another, leading to a negative spiral of fatigue and sleepiness, labile emotions, poor decision making, and risky behavior.[35,36]

Despite the evidence that insufficient sleep affects adolescent thinking, emotional balance, and behavior, the long-term effects of chronic sleep deprivation on learning, emotion, social relationships, and overall systemic health are uncertain. Although research has demonstrated that sleep problems affect adolescent cognitive skills, behavior, and temperament in the short term, it is not clear whether these effects are long lasting.

The National Sleep Foundation suggests that adolescents 10 to 18 years of age need between 8.5 and 9.25 hours of sleep each night. It is suggested that in order to optimize sleep and health in this age group, regular sleep schedules should be enforced and teenagers should keep appropriate sleep–wake schedules until they mature. Teenagers should understand the importance of recognizing how their level of tiredness and sleep–wake schedule affect their overall health. They should understand how commitments to extracurricular activities and after-school jobs should be adjusted in order to optimize health. Attending to a regular sleep–wake cycle is a vital component of good overall health habits.

SLEEP IN OLDER ADULTS

The requirements for sleep do not decrease with aging, but the ability to sleep and the quality of sleep may decline significantly (Figure 24-12). Approximately 50% of older adults complain of some sort of sleep disturbances. They generally take longer to fall asleep, have lower sleep efficiency, and experience increased sleep fragmentation with increased frequency of arousal and awakenings during the night. They also report increased incidence of excessive daytime sleepiness than younger sleepers. Men are reported to have more sleep problems than women.

Some changes in sleep patterns associated with older adulthood may be attributed to age-related changes in circadian rhythms or changes in brain chemistry. More likely, however, sleep disorders in the older adult are related to comorbid medical, neurological, and psychiatric conditions. They may also be exacerbations of a primary sleep disorder and not simply a consequence of aging.

There are a number of other factors that may contribute to sleep disturbance in an older individual. Chronic pain may cause sleep-onset insomnia because the sleeper has difficulty finding a comfortable position in order to relax and fall asleep. This is likely related to disorders of an aging musculoskeletal system. They may have difficulty maintaining sleep because they change positions and move into a position that is painful enough to awaken them. Decreased mobility as a consequence of aging may cause pain from prolonged positioning and result in awakening, or the effort required to change positions may be excessive and cause awakening. Of greater concern is deep, unrelenting pain that awakens the sleeper and is severe enough to not allow them to return to sleep. This is a sign of serious disease and requires more careful evaluation.

Menopause may disrupt the sleep of women, especially if they experience significant hot flashes. Menopause is associated with sleep-onset insomnia, increased sleep latency, decreased sleep efficiency, decreased total sleep time, and increased wakening after sleep onset. There is an increased prevalence in OSA associated with postmenopausal women. This is thought to be due to decreasing levels in estrogen and progesterone. Hormone replacement therapy has been shown to decrease the prevalence of OSA.

Nocturia, or frequent voiding during the night, can cause significant sleep disruption. It may be due to age-related physiological changes including decreased capacity

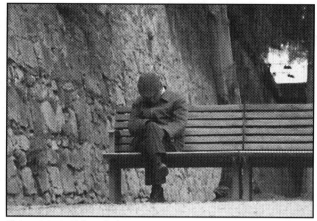

Figure 24-12. Although the stereotype is that the older adult sleeps all of the time, sleep quality tends to decrease with age, resulting in more daytime sleepiness. (From Fotolia.com)

of the urinary bladder, increased urine production because of decreased ability to concentrate urine, prostatic enlargement, and overactivity of the detrusor muscle.

Stress may play a significant role in sleep disturbance in the older adult. These individuals are more likely to suffer significant life changes and grief such as retirement or the death of a spouse.

Finally, the older adult is more prone to advance phase sleep disorder. This is an age-related reduction in the amplitude of circadian rhythms and a decrease in melatonin production and core body temperature. There is a decrease or even a complete cessation in production of human growth hormone and an increase in the circadian nadir of cortisol production. This can lead to increased sleepiness during the day and decreased nighttime sleep efficiency. Sleep phase advancement may be related to degeneration of the suprachiasmatic nucleus that controls circadian rhythm. Weakening eyesight may cause decreased retinal sensitivity to light, which may lead to dysfunction in the entrainment mechanism for circadian rhythms. This causes increased sleep drive earlier in the evening and earlier awakening in the morning. The phase advancement in body temperature also contributes to the earlier morning awakening.

Insomnia in the Older Adult

Insomnia is the most common sleep complaint in the older adult. The prevalence is estimated to be between 20% and 40% and is higher in elderly women than in men. Younger sleepers are more likely to complain of sleep-onset insomnia, whereas the older sleeper is more likely to complain of difficulty maintaining sleep. The older sleeper may also complain of early morning awakenings.

Insomnia in the older adult is often caused by age-related changes in circadian rhythm, including phase advancement, and dampening of circadian amplitude. Insomnia is also more likely caused by underlying medical, neurological, or psychiatric disorders. It is also a side effect of a number of medications that the older adults use in treatment in comorbid conditions. Rarely is insomnia in an older adult due exclusively to aging itself.

Consequences of insomnia in the older adult are similar to those in anyone else. They include diminished quality of life, excessive daytime sleepiness, changes in mood, and decrease in neurocognitive function. Balance may also be affected, and therefore the older adult with insomnia may be at increased risk for falls.

Use of hypnotics in older adults with insomnia may produce increased daytime somnolence or hangover effect. It has been associated with increased frequency of accidents and falls and therefore may be associated with increased mortality. Use of agents containing antihistamines are not recommended in the older adult because of the increased paradoxical effects including increased agitation.

The older adult may worry excessively about insomnia and the effect decreased sleep may be having on their overall health. Calm reassurance and treatment for anxiety including cognitive behavioral therapy may offer some relief (see Chapter 26).

Obstructive Sleep Apnea in the Older Adult

OSA occurs with increased frequency in the older adult compared to younger sleepers, but it is often much less symptomatic. For example, complaints of excessive daytime sleepiness are usually less severe in the older adult with untreated OSA. It is not clear whether this is due to decreased prevalence of the symptom, whether it is under-reported, or whether fewer demands of life make daytime sleepiness less noticeable. Age-dependent changes in respiratory drive, respiratory muscle strength, upper airway muscle tone, and airway size contribute to the increased risk of OSA in the older adult. Though the prevalence of OSA increases with age to a point, it appears that after the age of approximately 65, the prevalence of OSA remains relatively constant. Increased body weight, snoring, and witnessed apneic events are less consistent indicators for OSA in the older adult. In addition, the risk factors for OSA do not appear to have as strong a contribution as they do in a younger individual with OSA.

Sleep in the Institutionalized Older Adult

Sleep disruption is a significant problem for the institutionalized older adult (Figure 24-13). It is usually marked by disturbances in the sleep–wake cycle and frequent awakenings disrupting nighttime sleep. Napping often occurs during the day, sometimes because of lack of stimulation. Some residents of long-term care facilities develop a polyphasic sleep pattern in which multiple, relatively brief sleep

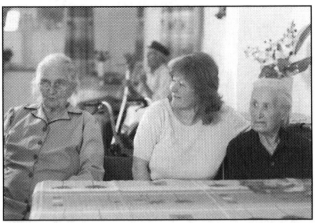

Figure 24-13. Institutionalization presents a number of challenges to the older sleeper. Nighttime sleep is frequently disrupted, and lack of daytime stimulation may lead to excessive napping. (From Fotolia.com)

episodes replace a single nocturnal sleep period. Though the shift from nocturnal sleep to a polyphasic sleep pattern can be related to comorbid conditions, many long-term care facilities are not conducive to nighttime sleep. Residents may be relatively inactive and understimulated. They tend to be allowed to nap frequently and often have limited light exposure. Excessive environmental noise, artificial light exposure, and interventions for care can disrupt sleep. Timing of medications according to staff preference rather than optimal patient efficacy may also contribute to chronic sleep disruptions in the institutionalized older adult.

SLEEP IN WOMEN

Women are more likely to have changes in sleep across their life span because of changes in the reproductive cycle. Cyclic changes in estrogen and progesterone during the menstrual cycle; during gestation, labor, delivery, and lactation; and during the perimenopausal and postmenopausal period can affect the quality and quantity of sleep in women. In general, women have more deep sleep, a slower age-related decline in slow-wave sleep, and twice as many sleep spindles compared to men of the same age.[37] However, women report more problems with insomnia than men. Forty-six percent of women complain of disrupted or nonrestorative sleep almost every night, according to a survey conducted by the National Sleep Foundation.[38] Factors that alter sleep in women also put women at increased risk of developing sleep disorders.

Sleep During the Menstrual Cycle

The menstrual cycle typically lasts 28 to 30 days and is divided into the follicular phase and the luteal phase. The follicular phase is dominated by the hormone estrogen and begins on the first day of menses. Rising estrogen and progesterone levels cause a surge of luteinizing hormone, which peaks and stimulates ovulation. Estrogen and progesterone levels begin to fall and lead to the onset of menses. Each phase lasts approximately 14 to 15 days. The follicular phase is associated with a lower mean body temperature compared to the luteal phase.

Many women report poorer quality of sleep immediately prior to and during the first days of menstruation, with the worst sleep occurring in the premenstrual period even though the duration of sleep is usually longer (Figure 24-14). The follicular phase is characterized by decreased sleep efficiency. Compared to the follicular phase, the luteal phase is characterized by increased NREM sleep, increased sleep spindles, and decreased REM sleep. During menstruation women often have increased sleep latency.

Oral contraceptives can change sleep architectures. They have been shown to increase NREM stage 2 sleep, decrease slow-wave sleep, and decrease REM sleep latency. Oral contraceptives have also been shown to increase mean levels of melatonin and mean body temperature during sleep. They are not associated with changes in daytime alertness or cognitive function. Use of oral contraceptives may resolve excessive daytime sleepiness that is associated with the premenstrual period suggesting that a hormonal imbalance may contribute to premenstrual hypersomnia.

Disorders of the menstrual cycle are associated with sleep disorders. For example, dysmenorrhea, which is defined as painful uterine cramps that occur during menstruation, can cause poor sleep quality, decrease sleep efficiency, decrease REM sleep, and increase daytime fatigue. Pain caused by endometriosis, sometimes a component of dysmenorrhea, can also lead to significant sleep disruption.

Premenstrual syndrome (PMS), which may be characterized by abdominal bloating, increased irritability, breast tenderness, and excessive daytime sleepiness, may also lead to poor-quality sleep. Poor-quality sleep may include insomnia, increased frequency of awakenings, unpleasant dreams, and excessive daytime sleepiness. Premenstrual dysphoric disorder (PMDD) shows increased severity of symptoms seen in PMS. Polysomnography also shows decreased sleep efficiency, increased NREM stage 2 sleep, and decreased REM sleep. Nocturnal levels of melatonin are decreased, and there is a later onset of nocturnal melatonin secretion during the luteal phase in women with PMDD.

Sleep During Pregnancy and the Postpartum Period

Sleep problems are a consistent complaint during pregnancy. In fact, 30% of women report rarely getting a decent night's sleep while pregnant, and the majority report significant sleep disruptions at least a few times per week during pregnancy[38] (Figure 24-15). Sleep disturbances include

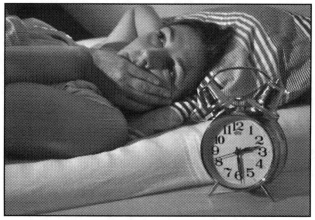

Figure 24-14. Many women report reduced sleep quality during menstruation. (From Fotolia.com)

snoring, sleep apnea, and/or restless leg/legs syndrome (RLS).

Sleep disruption gets worse as the pregnancy progresses, and especially during the third trimester, there is decreased total sleep time, increased insomnia, and increased nighttime awakenings.

Pregnant women often report more difficulty falling asleep than staying asleep, especially as pregnancy progresses. Sleep is commonly disrupted by physical discomfort, frequency of urination, back pain, leg cramps, and fetal movements. Women with severe sleep disruption during pregnancy have been found to have longer labors and are more likely to have a cesarean section.[39]

Snoring increases during pregnancy and symptoms of sleep apnea increase significantly from the first trimester to delivery. Snoring is associated with increased prevalence of hypertension and pre-eclampsia during pregnancy and has been associated with decreased growth in the fetus.

Sleep apnea increases particularly during the third trimester because of reduced functional respiratory residual capacity because of growth of the fetus and changes in the shape of the diaphragm and thorax. Ten percent of pregnant women are at risk for developing sleep apnea during pregnancy, and the risk increases with women who are overweight and have metabolic syndrome.[40] Pregnant women with sleep apnea are at increased risk of pre-term and low-birth weight infants and have a higher rate of pre-eclampsia and cesarean sections.[41]

Twenty to 25% of pregnant women experience RLS, especially during the second and third trimesters. Symptoms generally stop shortly after delivery, but this has been associated with recurrence of symptoms later in life.[42]

During the postpartum period, the majority of women, 84% according to one study, report insomnia at least a few nights per week following delivery.[39] The study also reported that 19% of postpartum women experience postpartum depression. After delivery, symptoms of sleep apnea generally improve significantly.

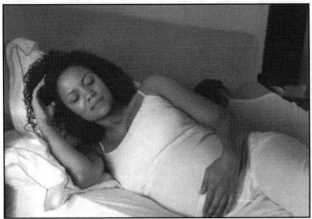

Figure 24-15. Pregnant women frequently report difficulty falling asleep and difficulty staying asleep. (From Fotolia.com)

Sleep and Menopause

Many postmenopausal women experience significant sleep complaints. The decline in estrogen and progesterone production, which brings about menopause, also increases the risk of developing sleep apnea. In fact, the severity of sleep apnea in postmenopausal women is equal to that found in men.[37] Other symptoms of menopause can cause sleep disruption. For example, hot flashes display circadian variation with a peak frequency occurring in the late evening, which appears to be related to changes in the central thermoregulatory response, although the precise mechanism is not clear. The majority of women who report severe hot flashes also suffer from chronic insomnia.[43]

Sleep Apnea in Women

Severe sleep apnea in women, with the exception of that which occurs during pregnancy, is found in 2% of middle-aged women compared to 4% in men of the same age.[44] Some of the gender difference found in sleep apnea occur because of increased fat distribution in the upper body of middle aged men compared to middle aged women. Progesterone also appears to allow increased ventilation and upper airway muscle activity.[45]

Women and Restless Leg/Legs Syndrome

RLS is a sensorimotor disorder characterized by an urge to move the legs and an uncomfortable sensation in the legs. Symptoms are usually increased at rest and aggravated in the evening and at night. Symptoms are only temporarily relieved by movement, walking, or stretching. RLS is frequently undiagnosed. Prevalence increases with age and is more common in women. Women who experience RLS

during pregnancy are more likely to experience a return of symptoms later in life. One study reported that women with children diagnosed with ADHD had an increased risk of RLS.[46] Women with RLS who also have hypertension and increased resting heart rate have an increased risk of cardiovascular disease than those without RLS.[47]

SUMMARY

Sleep disorders manifest themselves differently in various age and gender groups. As sleep architecture changes with age, different problems arise. Infants are polycyclic sleepers; they have multiple sleep and wake periods in a 24-hour day. It is very important to lay a foundation of good sleep habits in infancy and early childhood. These habits can translate into a lifetime of good sleep habits. Conversely, children who are not taught to self-soothe or who habitually do not get enough sleep may be developing sleep habits that are problematic as they grow into adolescents and adulthood. Children who are chronically sleep deprived are more likely to develop academic problems and have an increased prevalence of ADHD.

Teenagers are notorious for being chronically sleep deprived. Social, academic, athletic, and family life pressures compete for the teenager's time and sleep is often the victim. Teenagers also have a natural tendency to experience a shift in the circadian clock to mimic a delayed phase sleep disorder, which can add to sleep deprivation. School schedules and athletic schedules often do not take this into consideration and thus compound the problem. Puberty places one of the largest energy demands on the body that an individual will experience in a lifetime; therefore, the sleep requirements are actually slightly higher during this time. Poor quality and decreased quantity sleep can create neurocognitive deficits and add to an already chaotic emotional time for the teenager.

Older adults have the same sleep requirements that they did when they were younger, but the systems that generate and maintain sleep may begin to degenerate and lead to increased sleep fragmentation as these individuals age. Older adults often make up for sleep fragmentation at night with daytime naps. Advance phase sleep disorder and insomnia are often increasing problems for the aging population.

Sleep in women can become complicated because of the hormonal changes that occur cyclically throughout the adult life of most women. Changes in sleep are associated with the menstrual cycle, pregnancy, and menopause.

Clearly, specific populations have particular sleep needs and suffer from particular sleep disorders. This should be an important consideration in evaluating sleep and sleep disorders in each of these populations.

REFERENCES

1. BehaveNet. Trace alternant. Available at: http://behavenet.com/trace-alternant. Accessed August 4, 2012.

2. Weissbluth M. *Healthy Sleep Habits, Happy Child.* New York, NY: Random House Publishing Corp; 2003.

3. Peirano PD, Algarin CR. Sleep in brain development. *Biol Res.* 2007;40:471–478.

4. Penn AA, Shatz CJ. Brain waves and brain wiring: the role of endogenous and sensory-driven neural activity in development. *Pediatr Res.* 1999;45:447–458.

5. Katz LC, Shatz CJ. Symaptic activity and the construction of cortical circuits. *Science.* 1996;274:1133–1138.

6. Graven SN, Browne JV. Sleep and brain development: the critical role of sleep in fetal and early neonatal brain development. *Newborn Infant Nurs Rev.* 2008;8(4):173–179.

7. Marcus CL, Carrol JL, Koemer CB et al. Determinants of growth in children with the obstructive sleep apnea syndrome. *J Pediatr.* 1994;125:556–562.

8. Chan J, Edman JC, Koltai PJ. Obstructive sleep apnea in children. *Am Fam Physician.* 2004;69:1147–1154.

9. Lipton AJ, Gozal D. Treatment of obstructive sleep apnea in children: do we really know how? *Sleep Med Rev.* 2003;7:61–80.

10. Guilleminault C, Winkle R, Korbkin R, Simmons B. Children and nocturnal snoring: evaluation of the effects of sleep related respiratory resistive load and daytime functioning. *Eur J Pediatr.* 1982;139(3):165–171.

11. Gozal D. Sleep-disordered breathing and school performance in children. *Pediatrics.* 1998;102:616–620.

12. Owens J, Opipari L, Nobile C, Spirito A. Sleep and daytime behavior in children with obstructive sleep apnea and behavioral sleep disorders. *Pediatrics.* 1998;102:1178–1184.

13. Marcus CL, Omlin KJ, Basinki DJ et al. Normal polysomnographic values for children and adolescents. *Am Rev Respir Dis.* 1992;146:1135-1139.

14. Arens R, Sin S, McDonough JM, et al. Changes in upper airway size during tidal breathing in children with obstructive sleep apnea syndrome. *Am J Respir Crit Care Med.* 2005;171(11):1298–1304.

15. Arens R, McDonough JM, Costarino AT, et al. Magnetic resonance imaging of the upper airway structure of children with obstructive sleep apnea syndrome. *Am J Respir Crit Care Med.* 2011;183(6):782–787.

16. Goodwin JL, Babar SL, Kaemingk KL, et al. Symptoms related to sleep disordered breathing in white and Hispanic children: the Tucson Children's Assessment of Sleep Apnea study. *Chest.* 2003;124:196–203.

17. Chervin RD, Ruzicka D, Archbold KH, Dillon JE. Snoring predicts hyperactivity four years later. *Sleep.* 2005;28:885–890.

18. Gozal D. Obstructive sleep apnea in children: implications in the developing nervous system. *Semin Pediatr Neurol.* 2008;15:100–106.

19. Budhiraja R, Quan SF. Outcomes from the Tucson Children's Assessment of Sleep Apnea study. *Sleep Med Clin.* 2009;4:9–18.

20. Amin R, Somers VK, McConnell K, et al. Activity adjusted 24-hour ambulatory blood pressure and cardiac remodeling in children with sleep disordered breathing. *Hypertension.* 2008;51:84–91.

21. Bixler EO, Vgontzas AN, Lin HM, et al. Blood pressure associated with sleep-disordered breathing in a population sample of children. *Hypertension.* 2008;52:841–846.

22. Redline S, Storfer-Isser A, Rosen CL, et al. Association between metabolic syndrome and sleep disordered breathing in adolescents. *Am J Respir Crit Care Med.* 2007;176:401–408.

23. Tauman R, O'Brien LM, Gozal D. Hypoxemia and obesity modulate plasma C reactive protein and interleukin-6 levels in sleep disordered breathing. *Sleep.* 2007;11:77–84.

24. Carpenter S. Sleep deprivation may be undermining teen health. *Monitor.* 2001;32:42–45.

25. Better sleep is associated with increased academic success. *Science News.* Available at: http://www.sciencedaily.com/releases/2009/06/090610091232.htm. Accessed August 3, 2012.

26. Adolescents who sleep better score higher in math and physical education. *Science News.* Available at: http://www.sciencedaily.com/releases/2011/10/111020025758.htm. Accessed August 3, 2012.

27. Being a night owl in high school is linked with lower college GPA. *Science News.* Available at: http://www.sciencedaily.com/releases/2009/06/090609072813.htm. Accessed August 3, 2012.

28. Fenn KM, Nusaum HC, Margoliash D. Consolidation during sleep of perceptual learning of spoken language. *Nature.* 2003;425:614–616.

29. Hardman H. Sleep strengthens memories and makes them resistant to interfering information. Available at: http://news.bio-medicine.org/biology-news-3/Sleep-strengthens-memories-and-makes-them-resistant-to-interfering-information-6011-1/. Accessed August 3, 2012.

30. Memorizing in your sleep. *Science News.* Available at: http://www.sciencedaily.com/releases/1999/10/991026074517.htm. Accessed August 2, 2012.

31. Wolfson AR, Carskadon MA. Sleep schedules and daytime functioning in adolescents. *Child Dev.* 1998;69:875–887.

32. National Sleep Foundation. School start time and sleep. Available at: http://www.sleepfoundation.org/article/sleep-topics/school-start-time-and-sleep. Accessed August 2, 2012.

33. Carskadon MA, Wolfson AR, Acebo C, Tzischinshy O, Seifer R. Adolescent sleep patterns, circadian timing and sleepiness at a transition to early school days. *Sleep.* 1998;21:871–881.

34. Crowley SJ, Acebo C, Fallone G, Carskadon MA. Estimating dim light melatonin onset (DLMO) phase in adolescents using summer or school-year sleep/wake schedules. *Sleep.* 2006;29:1632–1641.

35. Carskadon MA. Factors influencing sleep patterns of adolescents. In: Carskadon MA, ed. *Adolescent Sleep Patterns: Biological, Social, and Psychological Influences.* Cambridge, UK: Cambridge University Press; 2002:4–26.

36. Dahl RE. Beyond raging hormones: the tinderbox in the teenage brain. *Cerebrum.* 2003;5(3):7–22.

37. Bixler EO, Papaliaga MN, Vgontzas AN, et al. Women sleep objectively better than men and the sleep of young women is more resilient to external stressors: effects of age and menopause. *J Sleep Res.* 2009;18:221–228.

38. National Sleep Foundation. Sleep in America poll. Available at: http://www.sleepfoundation.org/sites/default/files/nsaw/NSF%20Sleep%20in%20%20America%20Poll%20-%20Summary%20of%20Findings%20.pdf. Accessed August 5, 2012.

39. Gay CL, Lee KA, Lee SY. Sleep patterns and fatigue in new mothers and fathers. *Biol Res Nurs.* 2004;5:311–318.

40. Pien GW, Fife D, Pack AI, Nkwuo JE, Schwab RJ. Changes in symptoms of sleep-disordered breathing during pregnancy. *Sleep.* 2005;28:1299–1305.

41. Bourjeily G, Ankner G, Mohsenin V. Sleep-disordered breathing in pregnancy. *Clin Chest Med.* 2011;32:175–189.

42. Suzuki K, Ohida T, Sone T, et al. The prevalence of restless legs syndrome among pregnant women in Japan and the relationship between restless legs syndrome and sleep problems. *Sleep.* 2003;26:673–677.

43. Ohayon MM. Severe hot flashes are associated with chronic insomnia. *Arch Intern Med.* 2006;166:1262–1268.

44. Young T, Palta M, Dempsey J, Skatrud J, Weber S, Badr S. The occurrence of sleep-disordered breathing among middle-aged adults. *N Engl J Med.* 1993;328:1230–1235.

45. Kapsimalis F, Kryger MH. Gender and obstructive sleep apnea syndrome, part 2: mechanisms. *Sleep.* 2002;25:497–504.

46. Gao X, Lyall K, Palacios N, Walters AS, Ascherio A. RLS in middle aged women and attention deficit/hyperactivity disorder in their offspring. *Sleep Med.* 2011;12:89–91.

47. Pennestri MH, Montplaisir J, Colombo R, et al. Nocturnal blood pressure changes in patients with restless legs syndrome. *Neurology.* 2007;68:1213–1218.

25

Temporomandibular Joint Internal Derangement and Oropharyngeal Form and Function

Duane C. Keller, DMD, FAGD, Dip. IBO and Julie M. Hereford, PT, DPT

In any discussion of sleep-related breathing disorders (SRBDs), attention must be given to the function of the temporomandibular joint (TMJ) and its association with the structure of the upper airway. Dysfunction of the TMJ may contribute to the development and complication of SRBD because of the changes it causes in the structure and function of the oropharynx or upper airway.

It is widely accepted that oral devices can be used for amelioration of mild-to-moderate obstructive sleep apnea, perhaps the most common subgroup of SRBD. This is accomplished primarily by advancing the mandible and increasing the vertical dimension, thereby increasing the volume of the upper airway. Though many dentists use these devices, the method of determining bite position is often somewhat arbitrary and may or may not be the best desired functional position.

The device may succeed at improving airway function at night, but if it is not fitted properly with regard to the TMJ, the primary and secondary muscles of mastication, and the alignment of the head and neck, it may result in temporomandibular dysfunction (TMD) or compromises to the associated structures. TMD may involve painful contraction of the muscles of mastication or may be caused by arthritic changes in the TMJ or by an internal joint derangement including dislocation of the articular disc. Improper positioning of the joint by an oral device can aggravate preexisting joint derangement or muscle dysfunction or it may actually cause a new joint problem.

This chapter is intended to be an overview of treatment considerations for TMD, particularly as it relates to mandibular advancement for improving SRBD in regard to abnormal oropharyngeal form and function. It is not intended to be a comprehensive study of TMD; rather, it will focus on the most commonly occurring TMD and its relationship to disordered sleep. It should be noted that these authors strongly recommend a collaborative effort by dental and rehabilitative professionals to recognize and treat TMD and upper airway problems. As this chapter will discuss, it is difficult to achieve good, long-lasting treatment outcomes without addressing these problems from a multidisciplinary perspective.

Healthcare professionals are called upon to treat the cause of disease, not merely the effects of that disease, which are generally a host response. In order to do so in an effective manner, one must understand both the anatomy (form) and the physiology (function) of the structures involved. Form and function are said to be joined as 2 halves of an anatomic–physiologic association. As such, form and function affect one another. The lack of proper form is likely to cause a compensatory dysfunction, and a compromise of function may lead to an alteration of form, which, in turn, further changes function. This chapter will facilitate a better understanding of the problems with TMJ as it relates to oropharyngeal function and therefore as it relates to sleep-related breathing disorders.

The structures of the TMJ and the oropharynx are related in their structural, functional, and postural relationships. The oropharynx reaches from the uvula to the hyoid bone. It opens anteriorly through the isthmus faucium into the mouth. Residing in its lateral walls, between the 2 palatine arches, are the palatine tonsils. It is contiguous above with the nasopharynx and below with the laryngopharynx.

Hereford JM. *Sleep and Rehabilitation:
A Guide for Health Professionals* (pp 295-305).
© 2014 Taylor & Francis Group.

Oral structures and nasal function can affect pharyngeal relationships. For example, nasal obstruction can increase air resistance and flow velocity, which affects the pressure differential between the atmospheric and intrathoracic environment.[1-3] Obstruction may occur when inspiratory muscles pull on compliant soft tissue in the upper airway, sucking it closed. The nose accounts for half of the total respiratory system resistance.[4] The nose acts as a variable resistor to the upper airway that is prone to collapse. Flow limitation in the nasopharynx increases the likelihood of downstream pharyngeal collapse.[5] The structure of the nose is such that it can detain inspired air in the turbinate thus allowing for its warming and humidifying. Nasal resistance can be affected by temperature and humidity of the air supply, posture, nasal vasoconstriction, and mucosal changes.[3] Nasal mucosa responds to internal and external stimuli that lead to obstruction and irritation, which may therefore modulate air resistance. Significant acute or chronic nasal obstruction may lead to mouth breathing, which becomes a factor in maxillary and mandibular form and function. This may therefore be a contributing factor in SRBD and TMD.[6]

Oral structures may also affect the optimal maxillary–mandibular functional relationship and thus play a role in SRBD and TMD. For example, tongue volume and function play a substantial role in SRBD and may be implicated in the development of TMD. If the tongue volume is greater than normal, a condition that may be screened for by observing lateral scalloping, the tongue may have an increased tendency to fall into the airway during relative muscle relaxation that is associated with sleep. Additionally, abnormal tongue posture or activity may contribute to obstruction of the upper airway during sleep.[7]

The position of the tongue also plays an important role in function. Though it is common for newborns to have a lowered tongue posture,[8] the position of the adult tongue is elevated to conform to the roof of the mouth.[9] The function of the tongue against the palate is one of the factors that contributes to normal arch development. Normal maxillary arch development is an important determinant of nasal development. Restrictions of tongue position have resulted in abnormally deficient maxillary development, which has an effect on nasal development as well. Decreased mouth opening and limitation in jaw protrusion are independent predictors of difficult airway in patients.[10]

When evaluating the structures of the naso-oropharynx, it is important to consider the form and function of the TMJ in order to better determine the structural, postural, and functional relationships. It is also essential to understand how dysfunction of the TMJ can adversely affect form.

An evaluation of symmetry is one means used to compare form and function. Under ideal conditions, one side of the face of an individual should be a mirror image of the opposite side, and the right side should mirror function of

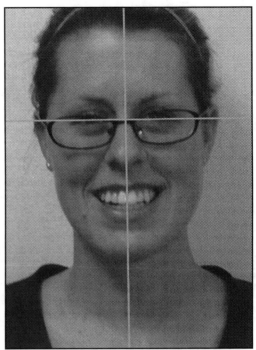

Figure 25-1. Typical facial asymmetry seen in the common compensatory pattern. Note asymmetry in left versus right sides of the face and horizontal asymmetry referenced from the true horizontal line. (Reprinted with permission from H. Vanderschaff.)

the left. Significant deviation from this symmetry can lead to abnormalities in form and function.[11]

Facial asymmetry may be an external indication of dental lesions and changes in the temporomandibular articulation and, according to Cathie, are capable of producing variable local and/or distant disturbances.[12] Myofascial restrictions of the head and neck that produce facial asymmetry can be reflected in the body in so-called descending lesions and, conversely, myofascial asymmetries in the body can directly contribute to TMD, known as *ascending lesions.*[13-17]

Facial and upper quadrant asymmetry can be documented by using a standard reference such as a true horizontal or true vertical reference that is superimposed over photographs and radiographs.[8] Photographs can be taken using a grid for easier analysis. It is also preferable to take the photograph with the shoulders and upper body visible in order to document other asymmetry of the upper quadrant.

Figure 25-1 demonstrates relative facial asymmetry in a patient with a dislocated right temporomandibular disc. Gelb described this dysfunction, which he reported was characteristically seen in individuals with a short right leg, who would develop a left-sided loss of vertical dimension in the jaw.[18] Travell and Simons noted in their seminal work *Myofascial Pain and Dysfunction* that observation of facial asymmetry is usually correlated with pelvic asymmetry and leg length discrepancy.[19]

Figure 25-1 shows characteristic facial changes, including increased right frontal bone prominence, right ear higher and closer to the head, right maxillary prominence, and right nostril enlarged. These changes are typically accompanied by the left side of the face appearing smaller, left orbit angle lower, left orbit appearing smaller, left ear lower and more flared from the skull, left mouth angle higher, and left mandible shifted left. The center line of the face does not correspond to the center line of the neck. The left cervical musculature is often tighter and more tender and the left shoulder is elevated in individuals with this typical compensatory pattern. Though other cranial torsions and facial asymmetries certainly occur, this pattern is the most commonly occurring compensatory pattern.

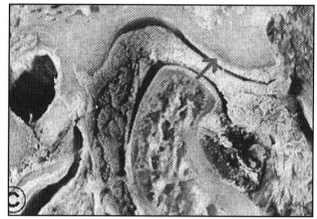

Figure 25-2. Cross section of a normal human temporomandibular joint. Note how the articular disc divides the joint into an upper and lower chamber. The red arrow indicates the proper functional joint and disc relationship. (Reprinted with permission from D. C. Keller.)

NORMAL TEMPOROMANDIBULAR FORM AND FUNCTION

Because normal form and function of the TMJ has a tremendous bearing on the functionality of the oropharyngeal region and thus the patency of the airway during sleep, it is essential to understand the structure and function of that joint. The joint is made up of the temporal fossa, which resides in the temporal bone of the skull, and the mandibular condyle. One of the unique characteristics of the TMJ is the fibrocartilage covering the anterior and superior aspect of the condyle, the fibrocartilaginous covering of the anterior fossa and the eminence of the glenoid fossa, and the interposed fibrocartilaginous articular disc. This disc divides the joint into 2 compartments. The lower joint compartment allows for rotational movement that is part of initial mouth opening. The upper compartment allows for translational movement that is seen as the jaw is opened wide.

The magnitude of mandibular movement is determined in part by the function of the components of the joint including the fossa/eminence, articular disc, and condyle. The movement of these interrelated structures is related to the structural relationships of the oropharyngeal structures, particularly the structural dimensions of the posterior pharynx.

Figure 25-2 shows a cross section of a normal TMJ. The mandibular condyle is seated against the relatively avascular central region of the articular disc, which, in turn, seats against the anterior slope of the eminence of the temporal fossa. The anterior and superior aspect of the mandibular condyle and the anterior slope of the eminence are covered with a dense layer of fibrocartilage.

The TMJ is a synovial joint whose capsule attaches to the articular eminence, the articular disc, and the neck of the mandibular condyle. The articular disc, an extension of the joint capsule, is a biconcave fibrocartilaginous tissue that attaches to the mandibular condyle medially and laterally. It divides the joint capsule into an upper and a lower chamber that allows for the unique movement of the joint. Anteriorly, the disc receives the attachment of the superior head of the lateral pterygoid muscle. Posteriorly, at the posterior bilaminar zone, some fibers continue as oto-mandibular ligaments that connect the middle ear with the TMJ, including the malleomandibular (Pinto's) ligament, which passes through the petrotympanic fissure to the middle ear. The remainder of the tissue comprises the posterior retrodiscal tissue. The retrodiscal tissue is comprised of adipose cells, elastic connective tissue, and the posterior synovial membrane. This tissue is highly vascular and is innervated by branches from the deep temporal, auriculotemporal, and masseteric nerves. It may therefore be a source of pain during disc dislocation as the mandibular condyle compresses the retrodiscal tissue against the posterior aspects of the temporal fossa. These tissues are relatively delicate and are not well suited to tolerate condylar compression and joint loading, especially with the presence of the posterior joint petrotympanic fissure.

The articular disc is uniquely shaped to afford temporomandibular function. The posterior aspect of the disc is slightly enlarged compared to the central region through hygroscopic properties of the intracellular matrix in a region known as the *bilaminar zone*. The development of the articular disc is dependent upon condylar forces being directed in an anterior and superior direction against the eminence of the glenoid fossa. This shape assists in joint function and increases the stability of the joint.

Because of the relative delicacy of the retrodiscal tissues and the placement of the articular disc, it is clear that this joint is designed to be loaded anteriorly and superiorly as is indicated in Figure 25-3. When loaded in an anterior and superior direction, the joint is able to withstand the considerable and repetitive compressive forces demanded

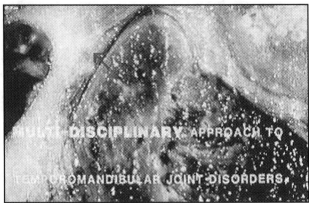

Figure 25-3. Sagittal section of an abnormal joint with a posterior and superior displaced joint with compression of the retrodiscal tissue. Note the arrow indicating changes in the retrodiscal region. (Reprinted with permission from D. C. Keller.)

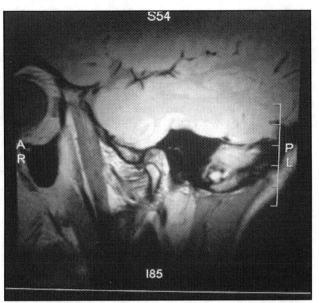

Figure 25-4. MRI of the temporomandibular joint. (Reprinted with permission from D. C. Keller.)

of it. Ward et al evaluated the loading capabilities of the TMJ and found that it has an adaptive capacity to loading in all directions except posteriorly.[20] The internal joint pressure was noted to become significantly elevated when the mandibular condyle compressive forces were directed in a posterior and superior direction (see Figure 25-3). Increased intracapsular pressure was also demonstrated to increase inflammatory chemokines and cytokines, especially interleukin 1β (IL-1β), an important mediator of the inflammatory response. The consequence of this is an increase in synovial fluid volume, increased joint instability, and, ultimately, the development of osteoarthritis.[21] Abnormal internal joint relationships adversely affect both joint mobility and muscle strength, and even surgical joint reconstruction does not always result in a return of muscle strength and joint mobility even with physical therapy modalities.[22]

If the mandible is dislocated in a posterior nonrecapturable position; that is, the disc cannot be repositioned into a normal relationship, any attempts to advance it in order to improve oropharyngeal airway volume will fail and may, in fact, increase symptoms of TMD. Unless the disc is recaptured, this dysfunction can become a permanent condition and will lead to significant joint destruction and debilitating symptoms.

Figure 25-4 shows a magnetic resonance image of an individual with a dislocated temporomandibular disc that is actually fused to the anterior slope of the temporal fossa. In this situation, the mandible cannot be advanced beyond this position and thus remains trapped in a posterior relationship. This disc dislocation and TMD will also cause a reduction in the volume of the posterior airway.

It is clear that abnormal joint form and function can result in significant dysfunction and may be experienced as jaw joint clicking, popping, or crepitus. It can cause facial pain and headaches. Some individuals with TMD may report tinnitus, dizzy spells, ear pain, or visual disturbances, among other symptoms. TMD is also a likely contributor to SRBD. Symptoms of TMD are often substantial and may create significant disability in the life of the sufferer.

The posterior bilaminar zone of the articular disc acts as a biomechanical lock to help maintain the disc in the proper relationship between the condyle and the fossa/eminence. A posterior movement of the mandible with either a superior or posterior–superior movement vector can compress the posterior bilaminar zone, resulting in a diminished thickness of the disc locking mechanism. A statistically significant difference in condylar position is seen in a symptomatic patient compared with an individual with reducible displaced discs.[23] Articular disc displacement increases as the condyle becomes more posteriorly displaced. When the mandibular condyle is in a posterior and superior position in the glenoid fossa, it is said to be in a pathologic position, because the joint cannot function normally in such an arrangement in which the joint components are in a distracted relationship.[24]

EVALUATING THE PATIENT WITH TEMPOROMANDIBULAR DYSFUNCTION

Evaluation of a patient suspected of having TMD begins with observation. As noted previously, facial asymmetry may offer the first clues of the disorder. These asymmetries should be documented with a photograph of the head, neck, and upper shoulders. A vertical and horizontal reference line can help to identify asymmetry as seen in Figure 25-1.

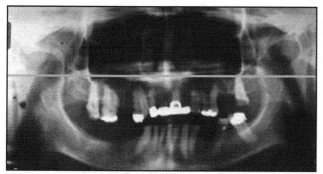

Figure 25-5. True horizontal superimposed on a standard panoramic film. Note the difference in the height of the mandibular condyles measured from the true horizontal. (Reprinted with permission from D. C. Keller.)

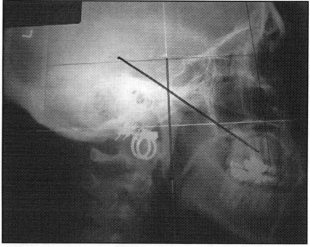

Figure 25-6. Radiograph of temporomandibular joint using horizontal and vertical reference lines to analyze structural changes. Note the tangential line indicating the slope of the temporomandibular fossa/eminence. (Reprinted with permission from D. C. Keller.)

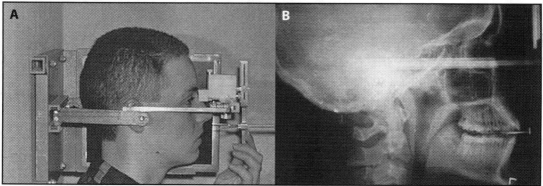

Figure 25-7. (A) Patient positioning for temporomandibular joint radiograph (B) and the resultant film. (Reprinted with permission from D. C. Keller.)

This method of documenting asymmetry can also be utilized to analyze a standard panoramic radiograph by superimposing a true horizontal line over the film. This enables a quick but comprehensive view of left and right symmetry, as seen in Figure 25-5. In this example, the maxilla and mandible are canted down on the right and up on the left. The difference in height of the left and right mandibular condyles can be measured to the true horizontal. Horizontal differences can be used to determine the scope and magnitude of the asymmetry.

The same horizontal and vertical reference lines can be superimposed on any radiograph and comparisons between different radiographs can be superimposed from one film to another using the standard reference planes. This can allow for documentation of structural changes rendered by the treatment plan (Figure 25-6).

Figure 25-7 shows the tangent of the eminence of one fossa/eminence taken from a joint radiograph superimposed on a cephalometric film to evaluate form and function and symmetry. This method can be used before treatment to help document the magnitude of the treatment that will be

necessary to restore symmetry. It may also be utilized after the completion of treatment to document treatment success and the status of the form which is linked to patient function.

Once the patient has been evaluated and appropriate photographs and radiographs have been obtained and analyzed, models can be mounted to a true horizontal to assist in the symmetrical analysis. In this manner, it is possible to evaluate and compare the anatomic relationships of the patient using photographs, radiographs, and mounted models using one common horizontal and vertical reference.

Figure 25-8 depicts models that were mounted to a true horizontal and vertical reference. The model on the left was taken at the patient's habitual bite. The model on the right was mounted with a diagnostic orthotic at the best functional maxillary/mandibular relationship as determined by a combination of physical medicine modalities and use of an intraoral orthotic. With this analysis, dental treatment can be designed that will facilitate better form and thus create a better functional relationship for this patient. The overall goal is to restore the dental occlusion to best functional

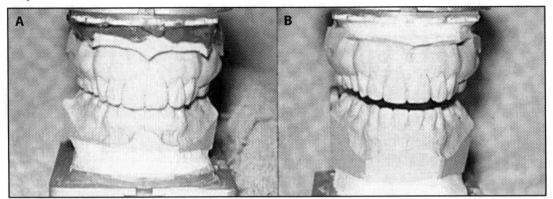

Figure 25-8. Mounted dental models. (A) This model captures the habitual bite of the patient. (B) This model depicts the best functional occlusal position for proper temporomandibular function. (Reprinted with permission from D. C. Keller.)

position of the maxillary–mandibular relationship and normalize the alignment and function of the upper quadrant. This treatment helps to restore joint function, normalize fascial restrictions, and improve muscular firing patterns. In this treatment model, orthodontic treatment may be necessary to maintain the corrected functional relationship.

TEMPOROMANDIBULAR DYSFUNCTION AND SLEEP-RELATED BREATHING DISORDER RELATED TO ABNORMAL OROPHARYNGEAL FORM

TMD and internal joint derangement has been shown to be related to decreased oropharyngeal airway volume. TMJs that have a history of locking are predictors of decreased airway function correlated with increased age.[25] Mandibular condyle positioned in a posterior–superior position has been correlated with an increased incidence of internal joint derangement and with decreased oropharyngeal airway volume.

Figure 25-9 shows a patient who has bilaterally dislocated articular discs in her habitual bite position as seen in this photograph. This bite maintains a posterior and superior position of the condyle in the fossa, which compromises the joint position and function and corresponds to a decreased airway.

Treatments that advance the mandible and restore a normal joint relationship result in more normal joint function produce an immediate and long-lasting increase in oropharyngeal airway dimensions.[24] Mandibular advancement with an increase in the vertical dimension and a counterclockwise mandibular rotation increase the middle and lower oropharyngeal airway dimensions. This increase remains stable over the postsurgical period, and the upper oropharyngeal airway space was shown to increase in long-term follow-up studies.[26]

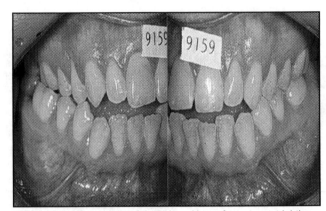

Figure 25-9. Photographs of the habitual bite of a patient with bilaterally dislocated temporomandibular joints. (Reprinted with permission from D. C. Keller.)

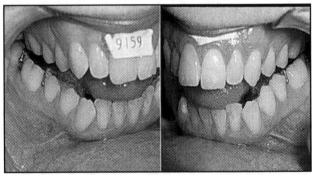

Figure 25-10. Photographs of the same patient in Figure 25-9 in the best functional position of the temporomandibular joint. Note the anterior open bite and the tongue thrust. Once the disc has been recaptured and the healing phase is completed, the dental structures will have to be restored in order to maintain the corrected bite position. This will reduce symptoms of TMD and will increase the volume of the upper airway. (Reprinted with permission from D. C. Keller.)

Joint recapture was possible using decompression techniques to move the mandible anterior and inferior and the disc repositioned into a recaptured joint position with an increased airway. Figure 25-10 shows the same patient with a mandibular advancement device that places her jaw joints in their best functional position.

If the mandible cannot be recaptured and then advanced due to internal joint derangement, the oropharyngeal airway dimension will be restricted. This situation will also lead to increased muscle activity and muscle dysfunction, leading to increased pain. If a mandibular advancement device is placed with the intent of improving mild-to-moderate obstructive sleep apnea, it may cause symptoms of TMD or may aggravate a preexisting condition.

Because of the potential consequences of internal joint damage, any guidance that directs the mandible in a posterior and superior direction may result in joint compression, restrict antero–posterior jaw movement, and predispose the TMJ to internal joint dysfunction and therefore should be avoided.[27]

Oral appliances are often used as diagnostic appliances to manage the position of the mandible in relationship to the maxilla and to establish an arbitrary diagnostic position in order to monitor patient response to the orthopedic appliance. Research has demonstrated that a mandibular repositioning device may increase the cross-sectional area of the soft palate.[28] This research has also demonstrated that a mandibular repositioning appliance is related to a reduction in apnea index. The study concluded that a mandibular repositioning appliance may be an effective treatment for obstructive sleep apnea and reduces the frequency of apneic events at least in mild-to-moderate disease.[25] Another study reported that subjects with a more posteriorly displaced mandible were found to have a statistically significant diminished airway volume. That is, a more distal mandibular position with respect to the cranial base decreases air volume.[29]

Though this study and others like it evaluate the efficacy of mandibular repositioning devices to improve airway function, they do not address the function of the TMJ, especially regarding internal joint derangement. Nor do these types of studies examine the impact internal joint derangement may have of oropharyngeal restrictions.

A posteriorly positioned mandible may lead to airway insufficiency, which is more symptomatic during sleep when general muscle tone is decreased. This situation may be further complicated by certain orthodontic corrections, particularly those that involve the removal of maxillary and mandibular bicuspids. It is this author's experience that removal of the bicuspids results in a posterior and superior movement of the mandibular condyle in the glenoid fossa. It is obvious that this potentiates a pathological force that can compress the posterior bilaminar zone, resulting in internal joint derangements as well as a diminished oropharyngeal airway. In addition, removal of maxillary bicuspids and closure of the maxillary dental spaces serves to decrease the magnitude of the maxillary arch dimensions.

In the patient pictured in Figure 25-11, treatment was initiated using splint therapy to find and hold the best functional position. Treatment of musculo-skeletal

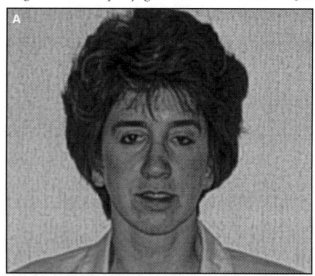

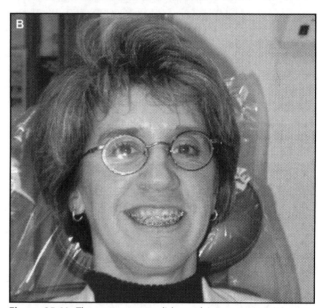

Figure 25-11. The pretreatment dislocated joint position (A) corresponds with a transverse decreased dimension of the maxilla and nasal airway. (B) The relationships at the recaptured joint position with the developed maxilla and nasal airway. (Reprinted with permission from D. C. Keller.)

components occurred in conjunction with serial splint adjustments. Once the optimal maxillary-mandibular relationship was achieved, the joint was allowed to heal. Phase 2 of treatment involved moving the teeth to support the optimal maxillary-mandibular relationship. The orthodontic treatments were initiated and completed without surgery at the recaptured joint relationship. The maxilla was developed with a combination of fixed and functional orthodontic and orthopedic appliances and resulted in a much more developed maxilla and a better functioning airway. Figure 25-11A shows the patient prior to any treatment. She suffered from debilitating headaches, jaw joint pain, and pain in the neck and upper back. Her jaw joint movement was also significantly limited and she reported

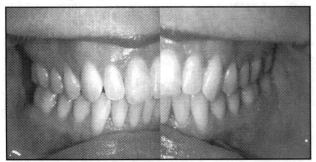

Figure 25-12. Photographs of the bite of the patient pictured in Figure 25-11B after completion of treatment. (Reprinted with permission from D. C. Keller.)

poor, nonrestorative sleep and snoring. Figure 25-11B shows the same patient after the completion of splint therapy and physical therapy to recapture her disc and correct her myofascial and skeletal restrictions and malalignment that were part of the precipitating or perpetuating factors in her TMD. In this figure, she is toward the end of orthodonture to correct her bite. Her symptoms have resolved completely, and her sleep is much improved and snoring is absent. Figure 25-12 shows the corrected bite position of the same patient.

Because the upper maxilla comprises the same structures that form the floor of the nasal passage, it follows that decreasing the dimensions of the maxilla will also decrease the dimension of the nasal passageway. Decreasing any airway will have an effect not only on air flow but also on the force required to move air through a restricted opening.

Physics applied to upper airway constriction can be understood by recalling the Venturi effect and Hagen-Poiseuille equation. The Venturi effect is an inverse association of gas or fluid pressure, velocity of flow, and restriction of passage of air flow that must pass through a constriction. The velocity of air flow would need to increase to push the same volume of air through a constriction. The increased pressure needed would require an increased muscular function that corresponds with the decreased structural dimension or a pressure differential that would require more effort to "shove" air through a constriction, or a decreased air flow potential.[30] The Hagen-Poiseuille equation, extrapolated to upper airway resistance to air flow, posits that small changes in the radius of the airway will cause a large change in airway resistance. Using this equation, for example, decreasing the radius of the airway by half would increase the resistance to that air flow by a factor of 16.[31]

The treatment described also served to improve the airway through mandibular advancement and the development of the maxilla and nasal passageway and therefore resulted in improved sleep. Treatment was performed to acquire a normal joint relationship from one that was dislocated. The recaptured joint resulted in an increased ability

to advance the mandible, which allows increased oropharyngeal airway volume. The development of the maxilla also increases the nasal passageway, resulting in decreased resistance to air flow. The final phase of treatment is completed with TMJ orthodontic correction so that the dental occlusion supports and maintains a functional joint position and a functional mandibular–maxillary relationship.

Another factor that helps to shape the airway and influences temporomandibular function is the posture of the head on the cervical spine and the effort required for normal respiration and respiration under stress.

The average adult breathes approximately every 4 to 6 seconds or between 12 to 18 times per minute, but a child will breathe slightly more often, around 20 to 22 times per minute.[32] Over the course of a day, this means a person will inspire and exhale around 26 000 times. In normal breathing, the diaphragm contracts causing an increase in the volume of the thoracic cavity, which reduces the intrathoracic pressure, allowing air to enter the lungs. During heavy breathing or if the airway becomes compromised, additional muscles are required to meet the increase in respiratory requirement. These muscles can include the intercostal musculature, the scalenes, pectorals, levator scapulae, and upper trapezius muscles. Respiration that requires increased musculature recruitment requires increased energy for these muscles to function. Constriction of the airway by TMD or malocclusion, for example, may result in increased muscle recruitment, increased muscle demand, increased airway resistance, decreased tidal volume, and greater residual volume. Overall, more energy will be required to move air through a constricted opening.

An individual with a posterior positioned mandible will have a slightly more forward head posture. Researchers have found an increase in the electromyographic activity of the masseter, temporal, and digastric muscles when comparing a "natural" head posture with a forward head posture. The more posterior the mandible was located corresponded with a more forward head posture.[33,34] Likewise, a forward head posture will increase the muscle demands of the posterior cervical region, neck, and upper back.

Ideal orthostatic head posture viewed in the sagittal plane has its center of gravity slightly anterior to the vertebral column. In order to maintain this posture, there must be a balanced tension between the anterior and posterior skeletal, musculature, and fascial structures. Any alteration in any of the structures anterior to the cervical spine will necessitate compensatory changes in the cervical spine and/or the posterior cervical structures.[35]

One of the most critical anterior structures that influences head posture is the dental occlusion. For example, an overbite or class 2 occlusion is often associated with forward head posture and increased cervical lordosis.[36–40] There is also some evidence that correcting total posture improves muscle firing patterns in the muscles of mastication in patients with malocclusion.[41,42] Wheaton also found that the resting position of the mandible was correlated with leg length discrepancy, noting that the mandible tends to deviate ipsilateral to the long leg and that muscle firing patterns adjust to support the asymmetry. This, in turn, generates other compensatory movement patterns locally and at regions distant to the jaw joint.[43]

Studies conducted by Gelb have shown that, over time, patients with a short leg developed a contralateral loss of vertical dimension in the jaw. Gelb also showed that subjects in these studies also developed characteristic ipsilateral facial changes that are consistent with the common compensatory pattern described earlier in this chapter.[44]

Rocabado proposed a postural model for ideal head posture based upon 3 parallel lines, including the bi-popular, vestibular, and transverse occlusal planes. He suggested that proper horizontal orientation of these planes allows the visual gaze and vestibular systems to remain level and functional.[45] Any deviation from horizontal or loss of the parallel relationship of one to another, and any of these relationships would result in compensatory adaptations of the cervical spine.[45,46]

Studies of the effect of malocclusion, head position, and scoliosis found a correlation among these factors. Huggare et al reported a correlation between cross-bite or lateral malocclusion and scoliosis. They found limited cranial tilt but significant side bending of the atlas with compensatory contralateral side bending of the axis and C_3.[47] They also found increased rotation of the orbit, maxilla, and mandible in the frontal plane in this population. The mandibular position is accompanied by loss of posterior vertical dimension on one side of the bite and loss of anterior vertical dimension on the opposite side.[48]

Royder suggested that the flexibility of the spine allows for the adjustment of the position of the head so that the eyes and the vestibular system can remain level and stable.[42] In a typical compensatory pattern, loss of left-sided vertical dimension of the mandible and a cephalometric tilting results in a compensatory scoliosis with cervical convexity to the right, thoracic convexity to the left, and lumbar convexity to the right. This causes a right sacral tilt and left-on-left forward sacral torsion. Muscular tightness and tenderness in this pattern is generally noted in the left cervicothoracic region and a dyssynchronous polyarticular muscle firing pattern (see Chapter 27). This compensatory pattern, if left untreated, will lead to myofascial strain, above and/or below the primary dysfunction, which can lead to movement patterns and dysfunction even at distant regions of the body. These dysfunctions can lead to neural facilitation and somatic dysfunction. Malocclusion and mandibular dysfunction can therefore result in localized pain or distant, seemingly unrelated symptoms and structural imbalances.[49] In fact, Zink suggested that TMJ pain and dysfunction are related to sacral dysfunction because of fascial influences on cranial and mandibular function

and, conversely, torsion of the sphenobasilar symphysis can produce a cranial torsion that can influence sacral position via fascial distortions.[50]

Forward head posture also causes an increased utilization of posterior cervical musculature, an increase in residual air volume, a decrease in tidal air flow, and compromise of swallowing. A comparison of patients with airway constriction compared to patients with normal airways demonstrated that the airway-constricted patients held their head and shoulders more forward, had a decreased chest wall expansion, experienced a decreased shoulder rotation capacity, and experienced decreased thoracic spine flexibility. The forward head posture and its associated decreased airway volume often are often related to increased headaches, cervical, thoracic, and shoulder pain.[51] Advancing the mandible will usually help to decrease this forward head posture.

Patients with a forward head posture were discovered to have increased activation amplitude from the cervicobrachial region when measured with normalized surface electromyographic (EMG) analysis. The muscles of the neck and shoulder region—levator scapula, upper trapezius, supraspinatus, posterior deltoid, masseter rhomboid major, cervical erector spinae, and sternocleidomastoid muscles—were more active with a forward head posture.[52]

Research has demonstrated that an orthotic used to reposition a recapturable internally deranged TMJ improves surface EMG activity of the masticatory, neck, and trunk musculature.[53] Studies of muscle activity on recapturable and nonrecapturable joints demonstrated decreased muscle activity if the joints were recaptured, but increased muscle activity in patients with nonrecapturable joints even to the point of muscle spasticity.[54]

Application of an orthotic to reposition the mandible anteriorly for the treatment of a recapturable TMJ has been shown to decrease EMG activity in masticatory musculature, decrease subjective reports of pain, and increase the vertical dimension of the oropharyngeal cavity, especially compared to the pretreatment maxillary–mandibular relationship.[55]

SUMMARY

This chapter discusses the relationship between mandibular position and TMJ dysfunction, particularly internal derangement in the form of disc dislocation. This situation has been shown to cause constriction of upper airway. It is also often related to forward head posture. All of this can lead to recruitment of primary and secondary muscles of mastication. Forward head posture associated with TMD can cause shoulder girdle pain and compromise of respiration with increased recruitment of accessory respiratory muscle function. This postural alteration can lead to increased posterior cervical and upper thoracic muscle activity. It can cause imbalance of the anterior and posterior cervical musculature, which leads to compensatory movement patterns and eventually may lead to structural compromise in the jaw, head, and neck and even at sites distant to the primary lesions via fascial plane torsions.

These postural changes have been shown to be related to TMD and dental malocclusion. Conversely, malocclusion may drive cranial distortions and compensatory vertebral malalignment. This leads one to the conclusion that one cannot successfully treat the anterior cervical components (TMJ) without also treating the posterior cervical components of the head and neck. In this way, the dental occlusion must be corrected to support the proper maxillary–mandibular relationship at the same time that abnormal postural and myofascial dysfunctions of the upper quadrant are addressed. This is best accomplished with a multidisciplinary treatment team that includes a dentist trained in evaluation and functional treatment of the TMJ and a physical therapist who understands the implications of the occlusion on the function of the craniomandibular unit and the entire upper quadrant. Biofeedback can also be a useful tool to help the patient relax and retrain masticatory and cervical musculature. Access to psychological services may also be useful to help manage the particular difficulties of this chronic pain disorder.

A sleep specialist is an important part of the treatment team to help evaluate disordered sleep, especially as it may impact the rehabilitation process. Polysomnography helps to define the severity of a sleep disorder. Mild and moderate disorders are particularly amenable to treatment with an oral device, but care must be taken to assure establishment and maintenance of a functional maxillary–mandibular relationship. Likewise, when dealing with severe obstructive sleep apnea, the position of the mandible may also need to be addressed even when using a continuous positive airway pressure device.

A TMJ that is not recaptured will result in sustained and sometimes spastic muscle activity both in the muscles of mastication and the musculature of the upper quadrant. This results in a mandible that is trapped in a posterior and superior position in the temporal fossa. Movement of the mandible in this direction reduces the dimensions of the posterior oropharyngeal airway. Constriction of the airway requires increased muscle function, which may contribute to forward head posture.

Treatment is designed to recapture the dislocated disc and normalize associated myofascial restriction and postural dysfunction. Once the disc is recaptured, the occlusion is corrected to support a functional relationship and rehabilitation of the upper quadrant assures maintenance of normal function. Treatment also improves the volume of the upper airway, therefore decreasing resistance to air flow. Improvement of the volume of the airway and reducing resistance to air flow will improve the quality of sleep, which, in turn, has been shown to improve quality of life. What is necessary for successful treatment of patients suffering from TMD that is contributing to airway constriction and sleep disturbance is to utilize the skills of a multidisciplinary team to analyze and balance form and function.

REFERENCES

1. Lavie P. Nasal obstructions, sleep and mental function. *Sleep.* 1983;6:244–246.
2. Papsidero MJ. The role of nasal obstruction in obstructive sleep apnea syndrome. *Ear Nose Throat J.* 1993;72:82–84.
3. Olsen KD, Kern EB. Nasal influences on snoring and obstructive sleep apnea. *Mayo Clin Proc.* 1990;65:1095–1105.
4. Proctor DF. The upper airways. Nasal physiology and defense of the lungs. *Am Rev Respir Dis.* 1977;115:97–129.
5. Shepard JW, Burger CD. Nasal and oral flow-volume loops in normal subjects and patients with obstructive sleep apnea. *Am Rev Respir Dis.* 1990;142:1288–1293.
6. Young T, Finn L, Kim H. Nasal obstruction as a risk factor for sleep-disordered breathing. *J Allergy Clin Immunol.* 1997;99:S757–S762.
7. Iida-Kondo C, Yoshino N, Kurabayashi T, Mataki S, Hasegawa M, Kurosaki N. Comparison of tongue volume/oral cavity volume ratio between obstructive sleep apnea syndrome patients and normal adults using magnetic resonance imaging. *J Med Dent Sci.* 2006;53:119–126.
8. Widström AM, Thingström-Paulsson J. The position of the tongue during rooting reflexes elicited in newborn infants before the first suckle. *Acta Paediatr.* 1993;82:281–283.
9. Benkert KK. The effectiveness of orofacial myofunctional therapy in improving dental occlusion. *Intl J Orofacial Myol.* 1997;23:35–46.
10. Asghar A, Shamim F, Aman AJ. Fiberoptic intubation in a paediatric patient with severe temporomandibular joint (TMJ) ankylosis. *J Coll Physicians Surg Pak.* 2012;22:783–785.
11. Keller DC. Three dimensional patient evaluation system. *J Gen Orthod.* 2000;11(4):19–28.
12. Cathie A. Fascia of the head and neck as it applies to dental lesions. A preliminary consideration. *J Am Osteopath Assoc.* 1952;51:260–261.
13. Royder J. Structural influences in temporomandibular join pain and dysfunction. *J Am Osteopath Assoc.* 1981;80:460–467.
14. Robinson, M. The influence of head position on temporomandibular joint dysfunction. *J Prosthet Dent.* 1966;1:169–172.
15. Lay E. Osteopathic management of temporomandibular joint dysfunction. In: Feely R, ed. *Clinical Cranial Osteopathy.* Sparta, NC: ID, The Cranial Academy; 1988:114–126.
16. Strachan F, Robinson M. Short leg linked to malocclusion. *Osteopath News.* April 1965:1–5.
17. Magoun H. *Osteopathy in the Cranial Field.* 3rd ed. Kirksville, MO: The Journal Printing Co; 1976.
18. Gelb H. Patient evaluation. In: Gelb H, ed. *Clinical Management of Head, Neck and TMJ Pain and Dysfunction.* St Louis, MO: Ishiyaku EuroAmerica; 1991:71–114.
19. Travell J, Simons D. *Myofascial Pain and Dysfunction: The Trigger Point Manual.* Vol 2. Baltimore, MD: Williams & Wilkins; 1992.
20. Ward D, Behrents R, Goldberg J. Temporomandibular synovial pressure responses to altered mandibular position. *Am J Orthod Dentofacial Orthop.* 1990;98:22–28.
21. Xie J, Naito M, Maeyama A. Intracapsular pressure and interleukin1ß cytokines in hips with acetabular dysplasia. *Acta Orthop.* 2010;81:189–192.

22. Hakkinen A, Gorg H, Kautiainen H, et al. Muscle strength and range of movement deficits 1 year after hip resurfacing surgery using posterior approach. *Disabil Rehabil.* 2010;32:483–491.

23. Kunita H, Ohtsuka A, Kobayashi H, Kurashina K. A study of the relationship between the position of the condylar head and displacement of the temporomandibular joint disk. *Dentomaxillofac Radiol.* 2001;20(3):162–165.

24. Ide Y, Nakazawa K. *Anatomical Atlas of the Temporomandibular Joint.* London, UK: Quintessence Publishing; 1991.

25. Yoshida H, Kashiwagi K, Sakata T, Tanaka M, Kawazoe T, Morita S. Prognostic factor of mandibular condylar movement exercise for patients with internal derangement of the temporomandibular joint on initial presentation: Preliminary Report. *J Craniomaxillofac Surg.* 2013;41(5):356–358.

26. Goncalves JR, Buschang PH, Concalves DG, Wolford LM. Postsurgical stability of oropharyngeal airway changes following counter-clockwise maxilla-mandibular advancement surgery. *J Oral Maxillofac Surg.* 2006;64:755–762.

27. Coleta KE, Wolford LM, Goncalves JR, et al. Maxillo-mandibular counter-clockwise rotation and mandibular advancement with TMJ Concepts total joint prostheses: part II—airway changes and stability. *Int J Oral Maxillofac Surg.* 2009;38:228–235.

28. Liu Y, Zeng X, Fu M, Huang X, Lowe AA. Effects of mandibular repositioner on obstructive sleep apnea. *Am J Orthod Dentofacial Orthop.* 2000;118:248–256.

29. El H, Palomo JM. Airway volume for different dentofacial skeletal patterns. *Am J Orthod Dentofacial Orthop.* 2011;139:511–521.

30. Konyukov Y, Takahashi T, Kuwayama N, et al. Estimation of triggering work of breathing. The depence of lung mechanics and bias flow during pressure support ventilation. *Chest.* 1994;105:1836–1841.

31. Hagen-Poiseuille law. Available at: http://web.archive.org/web/20080401045358/http://www.lib.mcg.edu/edu/eshuphysio/program/section4/4ch2/s4ch2_51.htm. Accessed April 2, 2013.

32. Ball WC. Interactive respiratory physiology. Available at: http://oac.med.jhmi.edu/res_phys/index.HTML. Accessed April 3, 2013.

33. Ohmure H, Miyawaki S, Nagata J et al. Influence of forward head posture on condylar position. *J Oral Rehabil.* 2008;35:795–800.

34. Olmos SR, Kritz-Silverstein D, Haligan W, Silverstein ST. The effect of condyle fossa relationship on head posture. *Cranio.* 2005;23:48–52.

35. Walther D. Applied kinesiology and the stomatognathic system. In: Gelb H. (ed). *New Concepts in Craniomandibular and Chronic Pain Management.* London: Mosby-Wolf; 1994:355–346.

36. Funakoshi M, Fujita N, Takehana S. et al. Relations between occlusal interference and jaw muscle activities in response to changes in head position. *J Dental Res.* 1976;55:684–690.

37. Levy P. Physiologic response to dental malocclusion and misplaced mandibular posture: the keys to temporomandibular joint and associated neuromuscular disorders. *Basal Facts.* 1981;4(4):103–122.

38. Milani RS, Periere DD, Lapeyre L, Pourreyron L. Relationship between dental occlusion and posture. *J Craniomandibular Pract.* 2000;19:127–133.

39. Fonder A. The dental distress syndrome. *Basal Facts.* 1984;6:17–29.

40. Manfredini D, Castroflorio T, Perinetti G, Guarda-Nardini L. Dental occlusion, body posture and temporomandibular disorders: where we are now and where we are heading for. *J Oral Rehabil.* 2012;39:463–471.

41. Robinson M. The influence of head position on temporomandibular joint dysfunction. *J Prosthet Dent.* 1966;1:169–172.

42. Royder J. Structural influences in temporomandibular join pain and dysfunction. *J Am Orthoped Assoc.* 1981;80:460–467.

43. Wheaton C. Mandibular rest position: relationship to occlusion, posture and muscle activity. In: Gelb H. (ed) *New Concepts in Craniomandibular and Chronic Pain Management.* London: Mosby-Wolf; 1994:163–175.

44. Gelb H. Patient evaluation. In: Gleb H. *Clinical Management of Head, Neck and TMJ Pain and Dysfunction.* St Louis, MO: Ishiyaku EuroAmerica; 1991:71–114.

45. Rocabado M, Johnston BE, Blakney MG. Physical therapy and dentistry: an overview. *J Craniomandibular Pract.* 1983;1:46–49.

46. MacConkey D. The relationship of posture and dental health. *Int J Orofacial Myol.* 1991;17(3):8–10.

47. Huggare J, Pirttiniemi P, Serlo W. Head posture and dentofacial morphology in subjects treated for scoliosis. *Proc Finn Dent Soc.* 1991;87:151–158.

48. Lieb M. Oral orthopedics. In: *Clinical Management of Head, Neck and TMJ Pain and Dysfunction.* Gelb H, ed. St Louis, MO: Ishiyaku EuroAmerica; 1991:31–70.

49. Greenman PE. *Principles of Manual Medicine.* 3rd ed. Philadelphia, PA: Lippincott Williams & Wilkins; 2003.

50. Zink GJ. Application of the osteopathic holistic approach to homeostasis. In: Cathie AG, (ed). *Museum of Osteopathic Medicine.* Kirksville, MO: AAO Year Book; 1973:37–48.

51. Lunardi AC, Marques da Silva CC, Rodriques Mendes FA, Marques AP, Stelmach R, Fernandes Carvalho CR. Musculoskeletal dysfunction and pain in adults with asthma. *J Asthma.* 2011;48:105–110.

52. McLean L. The effect of postural correction on muscle activation amplitudes recorded from the cervicobrachial region. *J Electromyogr Kinesiol.* 2004;15:527–535.

53. Tecco S, Tete S, D'Attilio M, Letizia P, Festa F. Surface electromyographic patterns of masticatory, neck and trunk muscles in temporomandibular joint dysfunction patients undergoing anterior repositioning splint therapy. *Eur J Orthod.* 2008;10:592–597.

54. Isberg A, Widmalm SE, Ivarsson R. Clinical, radiographic and electromyographic study of patients with internal derangement of the temporomandibular joint. *Am J Orthod.* 1985;88:453–460.

55. Hersek N, Uzun G, Cindas A, Kutsal YG. Effect of anterior repositioning splints on the electromyographic activities of masseter and anterior temporalis muscles. *Cranio.* 1988;16:11–16.

26

Insomnia and Nonpharmacological Management

Mark E. Murray, MS, BIAC, LPC and Julie M. Hereford, PT, DPT

Insomnia

Insomnia is one of the most common sleep disorders, affecting as many as 27% of the adult population, according to a Gallup poll conducted for the National Sleep Foundation[1] (Figure 26-1). Insomnia is defined as poor-quality and usually nonrestorative sleep that is characterized by extended time falling asleep (greater than 30 minutes); difficulty maintaining sleep, in which the sufferer awakens during the night and has difficulty falling back to sleep; or short sleep, in which the sufferer awakens in the early morning hours and is unable to return to sleep. Transient insomnia may last for 1 to 3 consecutive nights. This type of insomnia is extremely common in adults and can be a result of stressful events in a normal life. Insomnia may also be classified as short-term insomnia, which may last for up to a month. The far more problematic form of insomnia is the chronic variety, in which the insomnia may last for more than a month.

According to the American Academy of Sleep Medicine, the diagnostic criteria for insomnia include "(1) difficulty falling asleep, staying asleep or nonrestorative sleep; (2) this difficulty is present despite adequate opportunity and circumstance to sleep; (3) this impairment in sleep is associated with daytime impairment or distress; and (4) this sleep difficulty occurs at least 3 times per week and has been a problem for at least 1 month (p. S347)."[2] This definition is similar to that which appears as part of the *Diagnostic and Statistical Manual of Mental Disorders*, Fourth Edition, text

revision criteria for insomnia.[3] One third of the general population presents with at least one symptom of insomnia.[1]

A number of factors increase risk of and/or perpetuates the symptoms of insomnia. Risk factors may include gender, with women affected 1.5 times more than men. Depression often increases symptoms of insomnia; however, insomnia may also cause or worsen symptoms of depression, and the incidence of insomnia increases with age. Sleep-related breathing disorders are often found in individuals with insomnia because, paradoxically, there can be difficulty initiating or maintaining sleep as a consequence of sleep apnea or other sleep-related breathing disorders. Increased use of medication that may interfere with sleep onset or sleep maintenance tends to be more likely prescribed in an aging individual. Comorbidities of aging, which may include depression, can increase sleep fragmentation with reduced or absent slow-wave sleep and decreased rapid eye movement (REM) sleep. The presence of comorbid medical conditions may also contribute to insomnia in the older population.[2] Several studies have suggested that up to 40% of chronic insomnia may be related to psychiatric disorders.[4] Alzheimer's disease and other forms of dementia cause sleep fragmentation in early stages of the disease and may cause circadian disorders, with the sleep–wake cycle markedly disturbed as the disease progresses. Parkinson's disease is known to cause problems with initial insomnia and difficulties with sleep maintenance.

Among younger individuals, difficulty falling asleep is often associated with a phase delay syndrome and is a normal occurrence during puberty. This becomes an

Hereford JM. *Sleep and Rehabilitation:*
A Guide for Health Professionals (pp 307-317).
© 2014 Taylor & Francis Group.

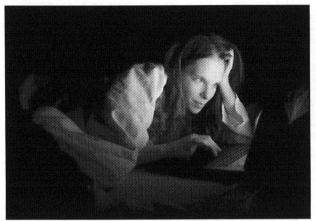

Figure 26-1. As many as 27% of adults in the United States suffer from insomnia. (From Fotolia.com)

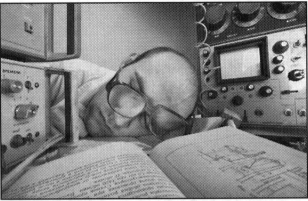

Figure 26-2. Excessive fatigue and daytime sleepiness from insomnia can negatively impact every aspect of a person's life and jeopardize physical and emotional health and the safety of the sufferer and those around the person. (From Fotolia.com)

interfering factor when academic, family life, or work obligations interfere with quantity of sleep. In older adults, phase advance syndrome results in reports of difficulty initiating sleep, difficulty maintaining sleep, and experiencing early morning awakenings.

The consequences of insomnia are similar to those occurring with other problems of nonrestorative sleep, including daytime fatigue, irritability, decreased memory, and poor concentration. Overall, there is a sense of a nonrestorative nature to sleep.

It is estimated that 75% to 90% of individuals who suffer from insomnia have an increased risk of comorbid medical conditions including hypoxemia and dyspnea, gastroesophageal reflux, pain, cardiovascular disease, and neurodegenerative disease. In fact, chronic illness is a significant risk factor for the development of insomnia.

The most common comorbidities associated with insomnia are psychiatric disorders. It is estimated that 40% of all individuals who suffer from insomnia also have a coexisting psychiatric condition.[5,6] Among these, depression is the most common, for which insomnia is one of the diagnostic criteria.[7]

It is often assumed that insomnia is a by-product of a psychiatric disorder, but it is possible that insomnia represents a significant risk for the development of a subsequent psychiatric disorder. A large-scale ($n = 14,915$) population-based study[8] conducted in Europe found that insomnia more often preceded a mood disorder than followed incident cases. This effect was even more pronounced for relapse of mood disorders, in which 56.2% of the subjects developed symptoms of insomnia preceding a relapse of a mood disorder. In contrast, in individuals who suffer from chronic insomnia with a comorbid anxiety disorder, the first episode of anxiety or a relapse of the disorder preceded insomnia in most incidences.

Several longitudinal studies have examined the evolution of psychiatric disorders among insomnia patients. These studies used follow-up periods ranging from 1 to 40 years, with the majority of follow-ups occurring in the 1- to 3-year period. In all of these studies, insomnia has been found to confer a substantial risk for the development of a depressive episode.[9,10] Though some studies also reported an increased risk of anxiety or drug abuse, neither of these were consistently found. Finally, longitudinal studies of subjects with affective disorders showed that depressed patients who experienced improvements in sleep also experienced a more rapid antidepressant response, whereas subjects in which insomnia persisted had a more rapid cycling into a depressive relapse.[11,12] Suggestions for further research include clinical trials to assess the impact of therapy for insomnia on the incidence of depression. Another study should look at the time to relapse in individuals who are in remission from depression but experience a recurrence of insomnia.

CONSEQUENCES OF INSOMNIA

Due to its chronicity, insomnia is associated with substantial impairments in an individual's quality of life (Figure 26-2). The primary complaint of individuals who suffer from insomnia is a decrease in quality of life because of excessive fatigue and daytime sleepiness. In several studies, insomniacs reported decreased quality of life on virtually all dimensions of the 36-item Short Form Health Survey of the Medical Outcomes Study (SF-36). The SF-36 is a valid reliable tool used to assess 8 domains, including (1) physical functioning; (2) role limitation due to physical health problems (role physical); (3) bodily pain; (4) general health perceptions; (5) vitality; (6) social functioning; (7) role limitations due to emotional health problems (role emotional); and (8) mental health.[13–15]

Individuals who suffer from severe chronic insomnia showed a numerically greater loss of function than patients with congestive heart failure. They also reported greater pain, emotional effects, and mental health effects. The chronic severe insomniac also reported more physical problems than those who suffer from depressive syndrome alone.[16]

Individuals who suffer from insomnia are more likely to have vehicular accidents and workplace accidents.[17] The incidence of auto accidents is 2.5 to 4.5 times greater than among normal sleepers. Insomniac workers have an industrial accident rate of 8%, compared to 1% for those reporting normal sleep. Work productivity also suffers in the insomniac population as evidenced by an increased rate of absenteeism, difficulty with concentration on the job, and difficulty performing work duties.[18,19]

Mean total health care expenditures have been reported to be as much as 60% higher in those suffering from insomnia compared to normal controls.[14] Approximately 10% of visits to the primary care provider report a major acute insomnia episode.[20] When further evaluated, these complaints were found to be associated with significantly greater functional impairment according to both the Brief Disability Questionnaire[21] and the Social Disability Schedule.[22] Individuals suffering from an acute episode of insomnia had more days of disability due to health problems and greater utilization of medical services. Of the patients with acute insomnia, only 28% received psychotropic medication—14% received benzodiazepines and 19% received an antidepressant.[23]

PATHOPHYSIOLOGY OF INSOMNIA

A leading theory of the pathophysiology of insomnia involves the concept that insomnia is related to a state of hyperarousal that is persistent throughout the day and spills over into nighttime when an individual is ready for sleep. One study selected groups of 10 individuals who were objectively defined as insomniacs paired with a control group of normal sleepers who were matched for age, sex, and weight. Subjects were evaluated on sleep, performance, mood, personality, and metabolic measures over a 36-hour sleep laboratory stay. Insomniacs were defined as those individuals who have increased wake time during the night, but who also had decreased stage 2 non-rapid eye movement (NREM) sleep and decreased REM sleep. As expected, the insomniac group reported increased confusion, tension, and depression and decreased vigor on the Profile of Mood States–Mood Scale[24] throughout the evaluation period compared to the normal sleepers. Insomniacs also had memory deficits on a short-term memory test and Memory and Search Test.[25] These performance and mood differences were determined not to be related to sleepiness because the insomniacs also had significantly increased sleep latency on the Multiple Sleep Latency Test[26] throughout the evaluation period. The insomniac group was shown to have a consistently elevated VO_{2max}, which is a measure

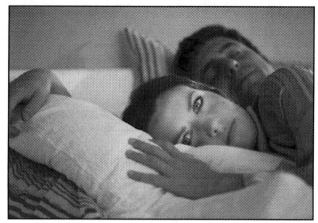

Figure 26-3. Insomniacs tend to have increased heart rate in all stages of sleep compared to normal sleepers. (From Fotolia.com)

of metabolic rate, when measured at intervals across the day and throughout one night of sleep compared to normal sleepers. The nocturnal increase in metabolic rate remained even after metabolic values from periods during the night containing wake time or arousals were eliminated from the data set. It was concluded that patients who report chronic insomnia may suffer from a more general disorder of hyperarousal, as measured in this study by the 24-hour increase in metabolic rate that may be responsible for both daytime symptoms and poor nighttime sleep.[27] Further study is needed to explore 24-hour insomnia treatment strategies that decrease hyperarousal.

Another factor that was evaluated in this study was heart rate variability. It was found that heart rate was increased in all stages of sleep in insomniacs compared to normal sleepers (Figure 26-3). Spectral analysis of heart rate variability reveals significantly increased low-frequency power and decreased high-frequency power in insomniacs compared to normal sleepers across all stages of sleep. Because increased low-frequency spectral power is an indicator of increased sympathetic nervous system activity, these data imply that chronic insomniacs may be at increased risk for developing diseases that are related to increase sympathetic nervous system tone such as coronary artery disease.[23]

The neuroendocrine system may also provide evidence of arousal as demonstrated by chronic activation of the stress response system. Several studies measuring 24-hour urinary excretion of free cortisol have found elevated levels in chronic insomniacs.[28,29]

Positron emission tomography has been used to assess cerebral glucose metabolism in insomnia patients. This is taken as an indirect measure of whole-brain metabolism.[30] Compared to normal sleepers, patients with insomnia exhibited greater cerebral glucose metabolism during wakefulness and during NREM sleep. Furthermore, insomnia patients demonstrated smaller reductions in relative metabolism from wakefulness to NREM sleep in wake-promoting

---

regions of the brain. These findings suggest that interacting neural networks including the general arousal system, the emotion-regulating system, and cognitive regions are involved in the inability to fall asleep.

A cognitive model of pathophysiology has also been suggested as a mechanism for insomnia. This model posits that worry and rumination about life stresses disrupt sleep, creating acute episodes of insomnia, especially for initiating sleep and returning to sleep upon waking after sleep onset.[31] Once the individual begins to experience sleep difficulties, worry and rumination shift from life events to worry about sleep itself and about the daytime consequences of not getting enough sleep. This can trigger emotional distress and increase autonomic arousal. Negatively toned cognitive activity is further fueled if a sleep-related threat is detected or a sleep deficit is perceived. This can escalate the worry and rumination and result in full-blown insomnia characterized by sleep deficit and interferences in neurocognitive function during the day.

There has been suggestion that insomnia may have a genetic link, but thus far, there has not been evidence of such a link. Rather, it appears that familial tendencies toward insomnia are due to learning of modeled behavior rather than genetic transmission. It is most likely that insomnia involves interplay among physiological, cognitive, and behavioral mechanisms, or the disorder may have multiple components in any given individual insomniac. These models will be reviewed.

The physiological model suggests that sleep and arousal are incompatible. In individuals with insomnia, there may be a state of hyperarousal that makes sleep problematic, including difficulties with initiation of sleep, frequent awakenings with difficulty returning to sleep, and/or early awakening with the inability of falling back to sleep. Therefore, treating the cause of the hyperarousal state should return the individual to a normal sleep pattern.

The cognitive model proposes that individuals who suffer from chronic insomnia are more likely to be individuals who tend to worry and ruminate. These individuals are more likely to reach a state of hyperarousal from daily events and are thus more likely to suffer from acute insomnia. These individuals are more likely to become inordinately worried and concerned over the possible consequences of the insomnia itself, thereby creating a chronic insomnia problem. Effectively addressing the preceding anxiety and rumination through cognitive behavioral techniques may be effective in treatment of this type of insomnia.

The behavioral model suggests that chronic insomnia is a consequence of behaviors that produce insomnia in the first place. That is, poor sleep hygiene habits will produce insomnia when normal sleep cues are ignored and perpetuation of these negative habits can produce a chronic insomnia with all of the relevant consequences. If one adequately addresses the behavioral issues, the insomnia is more likely to resolve.

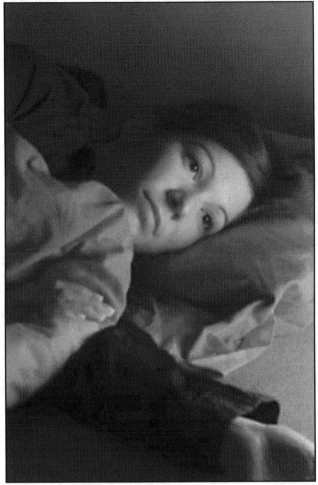

Figure 26-4. Insomnia patients often benefit from specific psychological counseling methodology of cognitive behavioral therapy for insomnia. (From Fotolia.com)

COGNITIVE BEHAVIORAL THERAPY FOR INSOMNIA

Cognitive behavioral therapy for insomnia (CBT-I) is defined as a structured program that helps to identify and replace thoughts and behaviors that can cause or increase insomnia with habits that promote normal sleep (Figure 26-4). The cognitive behavioral theory conceptualizes how acute insomnia can develop into chronic forms of the disorder and how to identify factors that can be targeted for effective treatment.

CBT-I is based upon 3 factors identified by Spielman et al, including predisposing factors, precipitating factors, and perpetuating factors.[32] Predisposing factors are those individual traits that set the stage for insomnia. Some psychological or biological characteristics increase vulnerability or predisposition to sleep difficulties. These may include female gender, older age, underlying anxiety, and hyperarousal. These factors are not a direct cause of insomnia, but they tend to increase the risk that an individual will develop sleep difficulties. These factors can fit across the entire biopsychosocial spectrum. Biological factors may be hyperarousal, hyperactivity, or a weak sleep-generating system. Psychological factors include excess worry or rumination. Social factors include work or social obligations or desires that interfere with a regular sleep–wake cycle.

Precipitating factors are described as stressors that push the limits of the individual sleeper (Table 26-1). These factors interact with the sleeper's predisposition for insomnia to produce transient sleep initiation and/or sleep maintenance problems. These factors also cross biopsychological borders. Biological precipitating factors may be such things as medical illness or injury that can have a direct or indirect causal relationship with insomnia. Psychological factors may include an acute stress reaction. Social factors may include a social environment that can disrupt preferred sleep patterns such as caring for an infant or for a sick family member.

Perpetuating factors for insomnia are those maladaptive strategies that the individual with transient insomnia adopts in an effort to get more sleep. These may include such things as spending too much time in bed in order to increase the likelihood of sleep. Instead of allowing the person to increase sleep periods, these maladaptive strategies often lead to a mismatch between sleep opportunity and sleep ability. The greater the mismatch, the more likely one will stay awake during a given sleep period. Another common perpetuating factor is non–sleep-related behaviors occurring in the bedroom. This is thought to produce stimulus dyscontrol, which may be defined as a decrease in the likelihood that the bed will elicit a singular response of sleep given that the stimulus has now been paired with a wide array of behaviors.

Conditioned arousal may be another perpetuating factor in insomnia. This concept suggests that using the bed for activities other than sleep sets the stage for a classical conditioning response. The pairing of sleep-related cues to wakefulness or arousal increases the likelihood that these cues will elicit arousal, regardless of any other intervening factors.

The nature of perpetuating factors makes it clear that behavioral management can offer the potential for effective treatment. If chronic insomnia is related to perpetuating factors, then eliminating those maladaptive behaviors will likely have a positive impact on insomnia.

The cognitive behavioral model considers behaviors that contribute to the mismatch between sleep opportunities and sleep ability. Stimulus control factors consider that non–sleep-related factors occur within the sleep environment, thus weakening the connections between sleep cues and sleep. Cognitive behavioral therapy works to identify and remove these behaviors and stimuli that perpetuate insomnia, thus relieving the symptoms. Classical conditioning is likely also a component of the perpetuating

Table 26-1.

Categories and Subtypes of Precipitating Factors in Insomnia

Activity	Precipitating Factor
Health	Pain
	Medical illness
	Hospitalization
	Menopause
Family	Separation
	Marital problems
	Family member illness
	Death of a significant person
	Sexual or physical abuse
	Birth of a child
	Caregiving
Work/school	Stress at work/school
	Rotating shift
	Employment change
	Retirement
Psychopathology	Major affective disorder
	Substance abuse

factors involved in insomnia. These factors elicit an arousal response in the absence of other factors that maintain insomnia.

Perlis suggests that the conditioned behavioral response may be the pathway to chronic insomnia.[33] That is, if aspects of stimulus control and sleep ability and associated maladaptive behaviors persist, insomnia becomes chronic. If the maladaptive behavior is modulated, then insomnia is likewise modulated. If, however, the maladaptive behaviors persist, the subsequent conditioned arousal may increase to a point that the originally connected behaviors are no longer a factor in the perpetuating of the insomnia. This becomes a self-perpetuating chronic insomnia that is much more difficult to treat with standard cognitive behavioral techniques.

CBT-I has been shown to be approximately 50% effective in reduction of symptoms of insomnia in the acute phase. This limited efficacy may be related to the sustaining affect that classical conditioning may have on insomnia. Over a longer period of up to 12 months, symptoms of insomnia continue to improve, which suggests that the conditioning component continues to abate over time. The repeated pairing of sleep-related cues with normal sleep extinguishes the conditioned arousal. Therefore, treating insomnia with cognitive and behavioral techniques must take the classical conditioning component into consideration.[32]

Table 26-2.

Psychological and Behavioral Interventions for Primary and Secondary Insomnia[a]

Treatment	Level of Evidence
Stimulus control therapy	Standard level of recommendation
Relaxation therapy	Meets standard level of recommendation
Sleep restriction therapy	Meets guideline level of recommendation
CBT-I with or without relaxation	Meets standard level of recommendation
Multi-component therapy without CBT-I	Meets guideline level of recommendation
Paradoxical intention	Meets guideline level of recommendation
Biofeedback	Meets guideline level of recommendation
Sleep hygiene therapy	Insufficient evidence (no recommendation level)
Imagery training	Insufficient evidence (no recommendation level)
Cognitive therapy alone	Insufficient evidence (no recommendation level)

[a]CBT-I indicates cognitive behavioral therapy for insomnia. (Adapted from Perlis ML, Junqqust C, Smith MT, Posner D. *Cognitive Behavioral Treatment of Insomnia: A Session-by-Session Guide.* New York, NY: Springer Science and Business Media; 2005.)

Though Perlis et al suggested classical conditioning as a fourth factor in the development of insomnia, particularly in its perpetuation, he also suggested that the improvement seen over time following CBT-I may be due to improved compliance with good maintenance strategies over time, decreased worry over time, or perhaps a neurohormonal or functional brain change following CBT-I that is yet to be described.[33]

PHARMACOLOGICAL TREATMENT FOR INSOMNIA

The most widely used treatment for insomnia is mild sedative medications and hypnotic pharmaceutical agents that are effective but only as short-term therapies, generally 3 to 6 months in duration. These agents have side effects, including sedation, which can interfere with next-day function. In addition, when these drug therapies are discontinued, insomnia often returns. Therefore, long-term use of medication for the treatment of insomnia is not generally recommended.

PSYCHOLOGICAL AND BEHAVIORAL TREATMENT FOR INSOMNIA

The Standards of Practice Committee of the American Academy of Sleep Medicine has updated recommendations of nonpharmacological treatment of insomnia.[34] The task force evaluated evidence for a variety of treatment modalities, including stimulus control therapy, relaxation therapy, CBT with or without relaxation, multi-component therapy without CBT, sleep hygiene therapy, and CBT alone, among others (Table 26-2). In general, the findings indicated that there is insufficient evidence to recommend one treatment over another or a single treatment modality vs combined treatments. There are, however, some treatment modalities that have better efficacy than others. Of particular interest is the classical sleep hygiene therapy, which continues to be widely recommended by primary care providers and sleep experts alike. There is insufficient evidence that these recommendations provide any benefit at all. It is possible that an individual who is already anxious about his or her sleep problems may ruminate excessively on these factors to his or her overall detriment.

INSOMNIA AND PAIN

Comorbid insomnia and depression can have a significant effect on pain sensitivity, tolerance, and perception. A survey study of pain clinics reported that 50% to 88% of patients who suffer from chronic pain also report impaired sleep.[35] Insomnia has been reported to correlate with higher pain intensity and greater levels of depression and anxiety.[36] However, higher pain levels are also reported in individuals who suffer from insomnia without depression. This is consistent with studies and patient reports of increased pain the day following a night of poor quality sleep.

Treatment for chronic insomnia requires a careful assessment of the individual, and it may be necessary to institute a multidisciplinary approach that addresses all of the psychophysiological components of the disorder in order to find the approach that is most affective and individualized to the patient.

Many studies have sought to investigate the relationship between sleep and pain, although the precise mechanisms subserving both remain unclear. There is evidence that neurotransmitters and neuropeptides involved in the onset and maintenance of sleep are involved in the modulation of pain, pain perception, and pain tolerance. For example, multiple studies have shown that there is a correlation between pain and serotonin levels, although the role of serotonin in pain tolerance and pain perception is open to continued study, and the precise mechanisms in pain and sleep are yet to be defined. In addition, an analogue of adenosine, which is a sleep promoter, has been administered both systemically and at the spinal cord level and has produced pain suppression in rodents.[37] Other studies correlating the neurochemistry that serves pain pathways and interactions with sleep pathways are ongoing.

Patients suffering from various types of chronic pain conditions may also be suffering from a sleep disorder. Failure to address one side of this equation may result in poor or inadequate control of the other. It has been shown that there is a circular relationship between sleep and pain; therefore, each must be considered in effective patient management. Even though there is a well-known interrelationship between sleep and pain, with the impact of one worsening the symptoms of the other, it is suggested that both pain and sleep disorders be evaluated separately in order to determine whether there is an independent cause of one that may be a contributing factor in the other. Some of the causes of sleep disturbance are more obvious like obstructive sleep apnea or insomnia, but a careful history and physical assessment can help to identify some of the more subtle contributors to the sleep and therefore pain problem.

NONPHARMACOLOGICAL TREATMENT FOR INSOMNIA

Sleep Hygiene Techniques

Sleep hygiene techniques are often recommended as a method of treatment for chronic or acute insomnia. However, there is no evidence that this treatment recommendation has any therapeutic value, particularly when it is the only form of intervention. This treatment involves patient education often merely in the form of a handout that recommends certain behaviors to try and to avoid to improve symptoms of insomnia. Some of the recommendations are useful especially when implemented in conjunction with other treatment modalities for insomnia.

Cognitive Behavioral Therapy for Insomnia

Cognitive behavioral therapy for insomnia is one nopharmacological treatment for insomnia that is designed to aid in changing maladaptive behaviors and dysfunctional beliefs and works to reduce physiological arousal. It has been shown to be one of the most efficacious treatments, particularly when used in combination with other modalities for the treatment of insomnia.[38,39] CBT-I is a structured program that works to help the insomniac to identify and replace thoughts and behaviors that cause or worsen sleep problems. These thoughts and behaviors are replaced with habits that promote sound sleep. Unlike sedative medication, when CBT-I is successful, it helps overcome the underlying psychophysiological causes of sleep problems, develop good sleep habits, and avoid behaviors that interfere with good sleep. CBT-I can contain multiple elements including sleep education, cognitive control and psychotherapy, sleep restriction, remaining passively awake, stimulus control therapy, sleep hygiene, relaxation training, biofeedback, and sleep diary.

Sleep education involves teaching the patient the basics of sleep. Increasing the understanding of the sleep cycle and learning how beliefs, behaviors, and outside factors can affect sleep can help in normalizing the insomnia experience, and decrease some cognitive arousal and anxiety related to sleep. Cognitive control and psychotherapy are aimed at identifying and eliminating thoughts and worries that interfere with sleep. It may also involve eliminating false or worrisome beliefs about sleep, such as that a single restless night causes illness. Sleep restriction involves limiting the time spent in bed to promote sleepiness when going to bed. The theory is that the sleepier a person is, the more likely he or she will be to fall asleep and stay asleep. Remaining passively awake involves avoiding any effort to fall asleep. Paradoxically, worrying about not being able to fall asleep can promote wakefulness. Letting go of worry can help the sleeper to relax and make it easier to fall asleep. Stimulus control therapy is a method of treatment that helps remove factors that condition the mind to resist sleep. For example, the patient may be coached to avoid the bed for any activities other than sex and sleep. Relaxation training is a specific method that teaches the patient ways to calm the mind and body. It may take different forms, including meditation, hypnosis, and progressive muscle relaxation. Biofeedback involves the use of sensitive instruments that can measure biological signs such as heart rate and muscle tension that can be used as indicators of increased stress and autonomic tone. This technique can be used to assist with relaxation training, and simple small portable units can be used in the home setting. The sleep diary also may be part of a treatment plan. This is a record kept by the patient that details sleep habits over a period of 1 or 2 weeks. The patient generally records when he goes

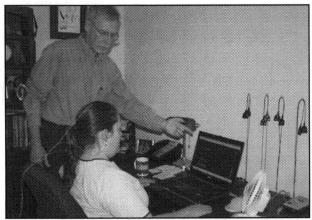

Figure 26-5. Neurofeedback uses operant conditioning of electroencephalogram (EEG) brainwaves by allowing the patient to see actual EEG results. Neurofeedback has developed video game interfaces in which the desired brainwave activity is rewarded through improved game performance. (Reprinted with permission from M. Murray and V. Mebruer.)

to bed, when he gets up, how much time he spends in bed unable to sleep, total sleep time, and other details about the sleep pattern.

One or more of these techniques may be used as part of CBT-I. CBT-I has been shown to be an effective treatment modality in approximately 50% of individuals and is generally more effective if it is used in conjunction with another form of treatment such as neurofeedback. In fact, the combination of neurofeedback and CBT-I has been shown to be one of the more effective methods of treatment for psychophysiological insomnia.[40-45] It also confers long-term relief, unlike pharmaceutical therapies and many other treatment modalities.

USE OF NEUROFEEDBACK FOR INSOMNIA

Several recent studies have suggested that an impairment of information processing due to the presence of cortical hyperarousal might interfere with normal sleep onset and/or consolidation. Because these findings suggest that a treatment modality that focuses on central nervous system arousal may be able to influence information processing and thus improve symptoms of acute and chronic insomnia, neurofeedback may prove to be a valuable tool in treating insomnia.

Neurofeedback is an operant conditioning technique used to shape brain activity toward more functional patterns through electroencephalography (EEG). The EEG allows a clinician to monitor brainwave activity in real time and reward or reinforce desired results using visual and auditory feedback, generally in the form of video games (Figure 26-5). When desirable activity is produced,

the subject advances in the game; dysfunctional patterns result in slower responses in the game and a reduced score. Over time, the brain becomes established in the functional range.

Neurofeedback is distinguished from biofeedback, which monitors various biological factors as they relate to relaxation or another defined behavior. Neurofeedback, however, modulates central nervous system function by monitoring real-time brainwave activity. Sensors are placed on the scalp to measure EEG activity that is detected by computer software and is then amplified and recorded. The therapist views the EEG activity while the patient sees and hears the video game format, which registers success or failure based on the EEG activity. The feedback to the patient is nearly instantaneous and allows the patient to experience immediate changes in brainwave patterns with behavioral, cognitive, or emotional input. With guidance from the practitioner, neurofeedback can help the patient create positive changes in brainwave patterns that allow permanent physical, emotional, and cognitive improvements.

In a typical neurofeedback setup, the patient may appear to just be watching a computer screen passively. However, because the game performance is linked directly to the brain activity, the patient is very engaged in essentially playing the game with his mind. For example, in a standard video road race game, the patient chooses a car and the race begins. There is no handheld controller, simply the electrodes on the patient's scalp reading brain activity. If desired EEG readings are detected, the car speeds ahead; if activity is out of desired range, other cars pass the patient's car and the car may even stop. It is not important that the patient understands how he is improving his score because neurofeedback works directly with the brain and essentially bypasses the conscious efforts of the patient. In fact, the patient generally performs worse if he is too actively trying to figure out how to improve his performance. Overthinking is often a symptom of the high beta activity associated with insomnia. The EEG detects this activity and game performance suffers. When the patient relaxes and beta activity decreases, the patient's game performance immediately improves.

It is helpful to think of neurofeedback as exercise for the mind. To achieve results, the patient must commit to a consistent regimen. Much like any physical exercise, it must be frequent enough to maintain and improve performance, but not so much to cause overfatigue. A course of neurofeedback treatment generally starts with twice-weekly sessions of around 30 minutes to 1 hour. In these first several sessions, the clinician is coaxing the brain toward the desired range. As the patient moves into that range over a course of weeks, sessions are spaced out to weekly, biweekly, etc. Unlike exercise, neurofeedback results become permanent. An occasional refresher may be desirable, and stressful circumstances may result in relapse, but subsequent treatment regimens can generally be much shorter. Once the brain has learned the more functional patterns and experienced the positive results, the functional patterns become their own reward, and treatment repetition is not necessary.

Recent studies have suggested that an impairment of information processing due to the presence of cortical hyperarousal might interfere with normal sleep onset and/or consolidation.[46–48] These findings suggest that a treatment modality that focuses on central nervous system arousal may be able to influence information processing and thus improve symptoms of acute and chronic insomnia.

One of the most dominant theoretical frameworks for the explanation of insomnia suggests that the presence of physiological or cognitive hyperarousal interferes with normal sleep-onset and sleep-maintenance processes.[31,32,49] In individuals with insomnia, cognitive arousal occurs close to bedtime, at sleep onset, or during periods of wakefulness after sleep onset.[50] Psychophysiological insomnia is the most common subtype of insomnia, representing 12% to 15% of all referrals to a sleep specialist. Diagnostic guidelines describe psychophysiological insomnia as an intrinsic sleep disorder involving both hyperarousal and learned sleep-preventing associations. Though evidence for the first component is reasonably compelling, evidence for learned or conditioned sleep effects is markedly lacking. Indeed, to date, no study has attempted to directly capture the conditioned arousal affect that is assumed to characterize this disorder. A study conducted by Robertson et al suggested that an impairment of information processing due to the presence of cortical hyperarousal might interfere with normal sleep onset and/or with normal sleep consolidation.[50] The reflection of hyperarousal during the day may manifest as cognitive arousal that occurs close to bedtime, at sleep onset, or during periods of wakefulness from sleep. As such, a treatment modality that focuses on central nervous system arousal, and thus influences information processing, may have significant therapeutic efficacy.

A study explored variations in subjective arousal over time in 15 subjects suffering from sleep-onset insomnia and 15 normal sleepers. Self-report measures of cognitive arousal, somatic arousal, and sleepiness were taken at 3 different intervals, including 3 hours before bedtime, 1 hour before bedtime, and at lights out across 4, 24-hour cycles. Fluctuations in mean arousal and sleepiness values and in day-to-day variation were then examined. Study participants who suffered from psychophysiological insomnia were significantly more cognitively aroused in the bedroom environment and significantly less sleepy compared to normal sleeping controls.[47]

Another component of arousal has been suggested by Perlis et al as part of a new perspective on insomnia called the *neurocognitive model*.[51] This theoretical framework is an extension of the behavioral model with the addition of a third arousal component. This third component is cortical arousal, which is reflected by increased levels of high-frequency EEG activity, primarily beta and gamma power. This elevated high-power EEG activity appears to occur in patients with insomnia and displays itself as higher levels of relative beta activity in the sleep-onset period and higher beta and gamma activity during NREM and REM sleep. Standard sleep staging as occurs in typical polysomnography does not perform a microanalysis of the sleep EEG, particularly high-frequency activity. This sort of analysis may reveal evidence of cortical activity characteristic of the insomniac because there is a strong correlation between stress, cognition, and cortical arousal. DeValck et al showed that the induced cognitive arousal is reflected by high beta power.[52] These subjects also showed increased sleep latency.

Animal research produced by Sterman et al showed that slow-wave EEG rhythm recorded from the sensorimotor cortex of the waking animal was correlated behaviorally with suppression of movement.[53] Facilitation of this rhythm through conditioning selectively enhanced the sleep spindle burst recorded during NREM stage 2 sleep. The training also produced longer periods of undisturbed sleep. The specific neural mechanisms manipulated during wakefulness appeared to function in sleep, and it was suggested that these mechanisms were also involved in regulation of phasic motor behavior.[53]

Hauri et al extended Sterman's work to a human insomniac population. They found significant improvement in subjects treated with neurofeedback.[54,55] Despite experimental evidence of the efficacy of the treatment presented several decades ago, the treatment was not considered very practical because of the size and complexity of equipment and the technical difficulties involved in processing of data. Recent technological advances and decreased cost of equipment has made neurofeedback instruments much more available in a clinical setting. These tools can now measure real-time *z* scores and allow for rapid computer analysis of EEG and instantaneous feedback of rewards and inhibits, making it a much more viable treatment option.

A recent study conducted by Cortoos et al demonstrated that sensorimotor rhythm (SMR) neurofeedback was superior to relaxation biofeedback in improving sleep behavior.[48] Hammer et al reported in a recent pilot study that either of 2 distinct neurofeedback protocols showed significant improvement in sleep behavior and in daytime functioning.[47] They demonstrated that treatment outcomes utilizing the simpler SMR protocol was just as efficacious as the more complex individualized protocol based on a full cap quantitative EEG.

Although there is insufficient research on neurofeedback at this time to meet the requirements of a standard recommendation, the available research strongly supports its use. It is one of the newest and most innovative treatments available for the treatment of psychophysiological insomnia.

SUMMARY

The most widely used treatments for insomnia are mild sedatives and hypnotic medications that are effective but are not recommended for long-term use. Though very effective for acute insomnia, particularly that due to acute stress, grief, or loss, these types of pharmaceutical agents have side effects including lingering next-day sedating effects. They are generally not recommended for use longer than 3 to 6 months. They also only treat the symptom of insomnia, rather than solving any underlying issues. Usually when these medications are discontinued, symptoms of insomnia often return. Nonpharmacological therapies for insomnia are generally focused on the cognitive behavioral model aimed at changing maladaptive behaviors and dysfunctional beliefs and reducing physiological arousal. The efficacy of CBT alone for the treatment of insomnia is variable, but adding neurofeedback to the treatment has been shown to be remarkably effective. With recent technological advances, neurofeedback has become a much more viable treatment option.

REFERENCES

1. Ascoli-Isreal S, Roth T. Characteristics of insomnia in the United States: results of the 1991 National Sleep Foundation Survey. *Sleep.* 1999;22(suppl 2):S347–S353.
2. Roth T. Insomnia: definitions, prevalence, etiology and consequences. *J Clin Sleep Med.* 2007;3(5 suppl):S7–S10.
3. American Psychiatric Association. *Diagnostic and Statistical Manual of Mental Disorders.* (4th ed, text rev.) Washington, DC: American Psychiatric Association; 1994.
4. Sateia M, Hauri P. *The International Classification of Sleep Disorders.* 2nd ed. Westbrook, IL: American Academy of Sleep Medicine; 2005.
5. McCall WV. A psychiatric perspective on insomnia. *J Clin Psychiatry.* 2001;62(suppl 10):27–32.
6. Ford DE, Kamerow DB. Epidemiologic study of sleep disturbances and psychiatric disorders. An opportunity for prevention? *JAMA.* 1989;262:1479–1484.
7. Ancoli-Israel S. The impact and prevalence of chronic insomnia and other sleep disturbances associated with chronic illness. *Am J Manag Care.* 2006;12:S221–S229.
8. Ohayon MM, Roth T. Place of chronic insomnia in the course of depressive and anxiety disorders. *J Psychiatr Res.* 2003;37:9–15.
9. Breslau N, Roth T, Rosenthal L, Andreski P. Sleep disturbance and psychiatric disorders: a longitudinal epidemiological study of young adults. *Biol Psychiatry.* 1996;39:411–418.
10. Chang PP, Ford DE, Mead LA, Cooper-Patrick L, Klag MJ. Insomnia in young men and subsequent depression. The Johns Hopkins Precursors Study. *Am J Epidemiol.* 1997;146:105–114.
11. Perlis ML, Giles DE, Buysse DJ, Tu X, Kupfer DJ. Self-reported sleep disturbance as a prodromal symptom in recurrent depression. *J Affect Disord.* 1997;42:209–212.
12. Fava GA, Grandi S, Canestrari R, Molnar G. Prodromal symptoms in primary major depressive disorder. *J Affect Disord.* 1990;19:149–152.
13. McHorney CA, Ware JE Jr, Raczek AE. The MOS 36-Item Short Form Health Survey (SF-36): II. Psychometric and clinical tests of validity in measuring physical and mental health constructs. *Med Care.* 1993;31:247–263.
14. McHorney CA, Ware JE Jr, Rogers W, Raczek AE, Lu JF. The validity and relative precision of MOS short- and long-form health status scales and Dartmouth COOP charts. Results from the Medical Outcomes Study. *Med Care.* 1992;30:MS253–MS265.
15. McHorney CA, Ware JE Jr, Lu JF, Sherbourne CD. The MOS 36-item Short-Form Health Survey (SF-36): III. Tests of data quality, scaling assumptions, and reliability across diverse patient groups. *Med Care.* 1994;32:40–66.
16. Katz DA, McHorney CA. The relationship between insomnia and health-related quality of life in patients with chronic illness. *J Fam Pract.* 2002;51:229–235.
17. Balter MB, Uhlenhuth EH. New epidemiologic findings about insomnia and its treatment. *J Clin Psychiatry.* 1992;53(suppl):34–39.
18. Leger D, Guilleminault C, Bader G, Levy E, Paillard M. Medical and socio-professional impact of insomnia. *Sleep.* 2002;25:625–629.
19. Kuppermann M, Lubeck DP, Mazonson PD, et al. Sleep problems and their correlates in a working population. *J Gen Intern Med.* 1995;10:25–32.
20. Sleep in America Polls. National Sleep Foundation. Available at: http://www.sleepfoundation.org/. Accessed May 7, 2012.
21. Von Korff M, Ustun TB, Ormel J, Kaplan I, Simon GE. Self-report disability in an international primary care study of psychological illness. *J Clin Epidemiol.* 1996;49(3):297–303.
22. Wiersma D, DeJong A, Omel J. The Groningen social disabilities schedule: development, relationship with ICIDH and psychometric properties. *Int J Rehabil Res.* 1988;11(3):213–224.
23. Simon GE, VonKorff M. Prevalence, burden, and treatment of insomnia in primary care. *Am J Psychiatry.* 1997;154:1417–1423.
24. Pollock V, Cho D, Reker D, Volavka J. Profile of mood states: the factors and their physiological correlates. *J Nervous Mental Dis.* 1979;167(10):612–614.
25. Sternberg S. Memory-scanning: mental processes revealed by reaction-time experiments. *American Scientist.* 1969;57:421–457.
26. Littner MR, Kushida C, Wise M, et al. Practice parameters for clinical use of the multiple sleep latency test and the maintenance of wakefulness test. *Sleep.* 2005;28(1):113–121.
27. Bonnet MH, Arand DL. 24-hour metabolic rate in insomniacs and matched normal sleepers. *Sleep.* 1995;18:581–588.
28. Vgontzas AN, Bixler EO, Lin HM, et al. Chronic insomnia is associated with nyctohemeral activation of the hypothalamic-pituitary-adrenal axis: clinical implications. *J Clin Endocrinol Metab.* 2001;86:3787–3794.
29. Vgontzas AN, Tsigos C, Bixler EO, et al. Chronic insomnia and activity of the stress system: a preliminary study. *J Psychosom Res.* 1998;45:21–31.
30. Nofzinger EA, Buysse DJ, Germain A, et al. Functional neuroimaging evidence for hyperarousal in insomnia. *Am J Psychiatry.* 2004;161:2126–2128.
31. Harvey AG. A cognitive model of insomnia. *Behav Res Ther.* 2002;40:869–893.
32. Spielman AJ, Caruso LS, Glovinsky PB. A behavioral perspective on insomnia treatment. *Psychiatr Clin North Am.* 1987;10:541–553.
33. Perlis ML, Junqqust C, Smith MT, Posner D. *Cognitive Behavioral Treatment of Insomnia: A Session-by-Session Guide.* New York, NY: Springer Science and Business Media; 2005.
34. Morgenthaler T, Kramer M, Alessi C, et al. Practice parameters for the psychological and behavioral treatment of insomnia: an update. An American Academy of Sleep Medicine report. Standards of Practice Committee of the American Academy of Sleep Medicine. *Sleep.* 2006;29:1415–1419.
35. Pilowsky I, Crettenden I, Townley M. Sleep disturbance in pain clinic patients. *Pain.* 1985;23:27–33.

36. Menefee L, Frank E, Doghramji K, et al. Self-reported sleep quality and quality of life for individuals with chronic pain conditions. *Clin J Pain.* 2000;16:290–297.

37. Sawynok J. Adenosine receptor activation and nociception. *Eur J Pharmacol.* 1998;347:1–11.

38. McCrae CS, Taylor DJ, Smith MT, Perlis ML. The future of behavioral sleep medicine: a report on the presentations given at Ponte Vedra Behavioral Sleep Medicine Consensus Conference. *Behav Sleep Med.* 2010;8(2):74–89.

39. National Institutes of Health. State of the science conference statement on manifestations and management of chronic insomnia disorder in adults. *NIH Consens State Sci Statements.* 2005;22(2):1–30.

40. Hammer BU, Colbert AP, Brown KA, Ilioi EC. Neurofeedback for insomnia: a pilot study of Z-score SMR and individualized protocols. *Appl Psycholphysiol Biofeedback.* 2008;33(4):51-64.

41. McCrae CS, Taylor DJ, Smith MT, Perlis ML. The future of behavioral sleep medicine. *Behav Sleep Med.* 2010;8(2):74–89.

42. Sterman MB, Egner T. Foundation and practice of neurofeedback for the treatment of epilepsy. *Appl Psychophysiol Biofeedback.* 2006;31(1):21–35.

43. Hauri PJ. Treating psychophysiologic insomnia disorder with biofeedback. *Arch Gen Psychiatry.* 1981;38(7):752–758.

44. Hauri PJ. EEG Biofeedback in the treatment of insomnia: A historical perspective. *Appl Psychophysiol BFB.* 2008;33(4):246-247.

45. Hauri PJ, Percy, L, Hellekson C, Hartmann E, Russ D. The treatment of psychophysiologic insomnia disorder with biofeedback: A replication study. *BFB Self-Reg.* 1982;7(2):223–235.

46. Cortoos A, DeValck E, Arns M, et al. An exploratory study on the effects of tele-neurofeedback and tele-biofeedback on objective and subjective sleep in patients with primary insomnia. *Appl Psychophysiol Biofeedback.* 2010;35:125–134.

47. Hammer BU, Colbert AP, Brown KA, Ilioi EC. Neurofeedback for insomnia: a pilot study of Z-score SMR and individualized protocols. *Appl Psycholphysiol Biofeedback.* 2011;36:251–264.

48. Bastien CH, St-Jean G, Morin CM, Turcotte I, Carrier J. Chronic psychophysiological insomnia: hyperarousal and/or inhibition deficits? *Sleep.* 2008;31:887–898.

49. Spielman AJ, Glovinsky PB. The diagnostic interview and differential diagnosis for complaints of insomnia. In: Pressman MR, Orr WC, eds. *Understanding Sleep: The Evaluation and Treatment of Sleep Disorders.* Washington, DC: American Psychological Association; 1997:125–160.

50. Robertson JA, Broomfield NM, Espie CA. Prospective comparison of subjective arousal during the presleep period in primary sleep-onset insomnia and normal sleepers. *J Sleep Res.* 2007;16:230–238.

51. Perlis ML, Giles DE, Mendelson WB, Bootzin RR, Wyatt JK. Psychophysiological insomnia: the behavioral model and a neurocognitive perspective. *J Sleep Res.* 2003;6(3):179-188.

52. DeValck E, Cluydts R, Pirrera S. Effect of cognitive arousal on sleep latency, somatic and cortical arousal following partial sleep deprivation. *J Sleep Res.* 2004;13:295-304.

53. Sterman MB, Howe RC, Macdonald LR. Facilitation of spindle-burst sleep by conditioning of electroencephalographic activity while awake. *Science.* 1970;167:1146-1148.

54. Hauri P. Treating psychophysiologic insomnia disorder with biofeedback. *Arch Gen Psychiatry.* 1981;38:752–758.

55. Hauri PJ, Percy L, Hellekson C, Hartmann E, Russ D. The treatment of psychophysiologic insomnia disorder with biofeedback: a replication study. *Biofeedback Self Regulat.* 1982;7:223–235.

27

The Influence of Mechanical Respiratory Dysfunction on Sleep Disturbance

Julie M. Hereford, PT, DPT

Obstructive sleep apnea is one of the most frequently diagnosed sleep disorders. The consequences of disordered sleep can be profound. It can impact multiple systems and has a deleterious effect on an individual's general health. It can interfere with neurocognitive function and can decrease overall quality of life.

Of particular concern to the rehabilitation professional are the effects that disordered sleep can have on pain, tissue regeneration and healing, motor learning and memory encoding, and athletic or exercise performance. Disordered sleep can cause increased pain sensitivity, which can disrupt sleep further, setting up a cycle of increased pain and poor-quality sleep. Disordered sleep can interfere in a patient's ability to recover from an injury or a surgical repair, particularly if sleep fragmentation disrupts non-rapid eye movement (NREM) stages 3 and 4 sleep, the sleep stages in which hormones responsible for tissue and nerve regeneration are secreted. Disordered sleep can interfere with motor learning and memory, which may impact a patient's ability to fully benefit from a rehabilitation program. Disordered sleep has been shown to decrease athletic performance. Although there are no studies available in the current body of literature, it can be extrapolated that therapeutic exercise, which is designed to correct faulty movement patterns and involves learning precise movements, may also suffer as a result of disordered sleep.

Significant data are available that show that sleep can improve performance on specific, relatively simple tasks, but this research has not been extended to the performance of therapeutic exercise, which generally involves more complex movement patterns. Sleep extension has been shown to improve athletic performance in many areas including speed, power, precision of movement, and endurance. One can reasonably speculate then that because sleep improves specific, simple tasks, and sleep extension significantly improves complex athletic performance, sleep will enhance therapeutic exercise designed to correct faulty movement patterns and restore movement after musculoskeletal injury or surgical repair. One may further speculate that because improvements in athletic performance involve improved neuromuscular control, sleep may be an important component of neurological rehabilitation.

Because sleep deprivation is known to interfere with performance, it will interfere with patient outcomes, and, therefore, it is important that rehabilitation professionals recognize manifestations and consequences of disordered sleep. Not only can disordered sleep interfere with rehabilitation goals directly, but it may also exacerbate comorbid conditions, which can complicate treatment and outcomes. Chapter 28 offers some guidelines for decision making regarding referral for evaluation of a suspected sleep disorder.

Because sleep-related breathing disorders are a significant component of most sleep problems, consideration should be given to the mechanics of respiration. If these mechanics are faulty or dysfunctional, they could contribute to increased resistance to respiration. Sleep has an inherent increased resistance to respiration because of decreased

Hereford JM. *Sleep and Rehabilitation: A Guide for Health Professionals* (pp 319-339).
© 2014 Taylor & Francis Group.

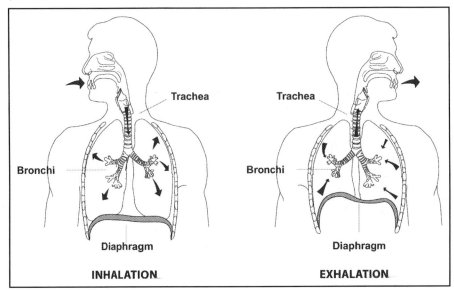

Figure 27-1. Normal inhalation and exhalation.

muscle tone during NREM sleep and atonia during rapid eye movement (REM) sleep and the increased tendency of the upper airway to collapse. If faulty mechanics of respiration contribute to the sleep-related respiratory changes, the resistance is compounded. Mechanical dysfunction will increase the workload required by the respiratory apparatus to effectively ventilate the individual. It is reasonable, therefore, to conclude that dysfunctional mechanical aspects of respiration contribute to sleep-related breathing disorders.

Manual therapy and therapeutic exercise, positional training, and neuromuscular re-education can be applied to improve the mechanical dysfunction within the respiratory system. Dysfunction may include stiffness in the thoracic spine and/or rib cage, chronic forward head posture, bias toward use of accessory respiratory musculature, dysfunction of the diaphragm including uncoordinated movement, weakness, and loss of the zone of apposition (ZOA).

This chapter will review the mechanics of respiration and discuss common mechanisms that underlie dysfunction within that system and how they impact sleep. It will also present recommendations for treatment.

Normal Breathing

The function of breathing is to allow for the exchange of gases involving the acquisition of oxygen (O_2) and the elimination of carbon dioxide (CO_2). Efficient exchange of these gases enhances cellular function and facilitates normal performance of the brain, organs, and tissues of the body. Normal breathing permits normal speech. It is also intimately involved in human nonverbal expression; for example, sighing or gasping in surprise. It assists in fluid movement, such as dilation and pulsation of lymphatics and for blood circulation. It helps maintain spinal mobility through regular mobilizing of the thoracic cage. It enhances

digestive function by rhythmic positive and negative pressure fluctuations when diaphragmatic function is normal.

Certain pathological states can affect the patency of the airway. Obstruction may be momentary or situational, such as restriction of the abdomen or chest as may occur with compression in a body hold or wearing a tight garment, or may occur in an individual with excess abdominal obesity who is lying prone. Changes in airway patency may increase resistance to air flow and necessitate a switch from quiet breathing using the diaphragm to a more labored breathing involving activity of the intercostal musculature or the anterior neck musculature. Increased resistance of the airway may necessitate a change to mouth breathing. Obstruction may occur in the presence of redundant or lax mucosal folds in the upper airway that cause obstruction during sleep.

Obstruction of the airway may be chronic as occurs with a deviated septum, exuberant distorted nasal conchae, enlarged adenoids, or hay fever. Space-occupying lesions may distort and constrict the upper airway and increase resistance. Chronic inadequately treated asthma may cause spasm of the bronchioles and produce an expiratory wheeze and breathlessness. Lung disease and heart disease can cause congestion in the airway and result in the need for accessory effort in order to adequately ventilate the individual.

Structural Features of Breathing

In normal, quiet, and unrestricted breathing, the diaphragm offers enough effort to allow an individual to breathe in a seemingly effortless fashion. On inhalation, the diaphragm contracts from the central tendon and the dome flattens. This increases the volume in the thoracic cavity and causes a negative pressure gradient causing air to rush in (Figure 27-1). If the abdomen is relaxed during quiet breathing, diaphragmatic contraction may cause the abdomen to bulge outward. Air enters the nasal cavity or mouth and passes via the trachea to the bronchi. Normal nasal function in respiration filters and warms the air as it passes through the nasal cavity to the pharynx and toward the trachea. The function of warming and filtering the air is lost if there is obstruction of the nasal portion of the airway or with chronic mouth breathers.

Air enters the trachea and moves to the bronchi. The structure of the trachea and bronchi includes supporting rings that are made up of varying proportions of cartilage for rigidity and elastic muscles to allow expansion. The trachea is wider superiorly and contains a larger proportion of cartilage. It narrows inferiorly and separates into the bronchi, which are almost entirely elastic. The bronchi separate to form four lobar bronchi and subsequently subdivide into ever narrower bronchi until, at the 11th subdivision, the airway is called a *bronchiole*.

Bronchioles terminate in alveoli, which are the functional units of the lung where gas exchange takes place. The alveoli have fine membranous capillaries that allow for this gas exchange to occur.

Quiet inhalation function should be effortless if all of the mechanical characteristics of the upper airway are optimal and the airway is patent. Altered compliance, which is the characteristic of the expansibility potential of the lungs and thoracic cage, and tissue resistance, which includes how elastic, fibrotic, and mobile the structures are, compounded with airway resistance, increase the amount of effort that is required to inhale.

Exhalation in quiet breathing is a relatively passive event. When the diaphragm relaxes from the central tendon, the dome regains its shape and the pressure gradient in the thoracic cavity is normalized. The elasticity of the lungs is a component of exhalation.

Quiet, relaxed breathing requires little energy. However, when the need arises for increased ventilation, as may occur during increased activity such as exercise, the abdominal musculature may act to resist expansion. This increased abdominal pressure tilts the diaphragm and rib cage upward and increases the volume of the thoracic cavity and allows for increased capacity into the lungs. Expiration usually follows simple relaxation of the diaphragm and abdominal musculature, but it can be increased by downward action of the abdominal muscles on the rib cage. Forced expiration increases pressure in the walls of the airway and may cause narrowing and wheezing. Intercostal musculature contract to change the stiffness and shape of the rib cage and contribute to forced inspiration and expiration. Scalene and sternocleidomastoid (SCM) musculature can also assist with respiration by pulling the sternum and first 2 ribs superiorly in an effort to change the shape and volume of the thorax.

For the lungs to expand and contract, the thoracic cavity must lengthen and shorten with the rise and fall of the diaphragm (Figure 27-2). In order for the diaphragm to be able to function normally, the ribs must be able to elevate and depress and rotate to produce an increase and decrease in the anteroposterior and lateral diameter of the rib cage. Any restriction by the thoracic facet joints or the costovertebral, costotransverse, or costochondral joints or dysfunction in the soft tissue will retard the efficiency of the pumping process of the diaphragm and will therefore restrict respiratory capacity.

Total lung capacity is defined as the amount of air the lung can contain at the height of maximum inspiratory effort. All other lung volumes are natural subdivisions of the total lung capacity. The average total lung capacity of an adult male is 6 L of air, but only a small amount of the total capacity is utilized during normal breathing. Tidal volume is defined as the volume of air that is inhaled or exhaled during normal resting breathing. Residual volume is defined as the volume of air remaining in the lungs after a maximal exhalation. Vital capacity is defined as the total lung capacity minus the residual volume. It is measured as the maximum amount of air a person can expel from their lungs after a maximum inhalation. This value can be measured with a regular spirometer. A normal adult has a vital capacity of 3 to 5 L of air, but variations in the vital capacity can depend on age, sex, height, weight, and ethnicity. For example, tall people, nonsmokers, and people who live at higher altitudes have larger lung volumes. Lung volume also changes in response to pregnancy because of compression of the diaphragm by the expanding uterus.

The average human infant breathes at 30 to 60 breaths per minute at birth. This respiratory rate decreases to an average of 10 to 14 breaths per minute in the adult.

Neural Regulation of Breathing

Respiratory centers are located in the most primitive part of the brain, the brain stem. Respiratory centers unconsciously influence and adjust alveolar ventilation to maintain arterial blood O_2 and CO_2 values at a relatively constant level in order to sustain life under varying conditions and requirements. Though breathing is normally controlled unconsciously, it can also be controlled consciously as may be seen during meditation, relaxation training, or yoga. During certain activities, including vocal training or swimming, an individual can learn to control breathing consciously in initial training, but as training progresses, breathing control becomes subconscious. Speech also requires a balance of inspiration and expiration that is normally unconscious but can be modified consciously as the need or situation arises.

Unconscious control of breathing is accomplished by brain stem centers in the medulla and pons that respond primarily to CO_2 and O_2 levels in the blood (Figure 27-3).

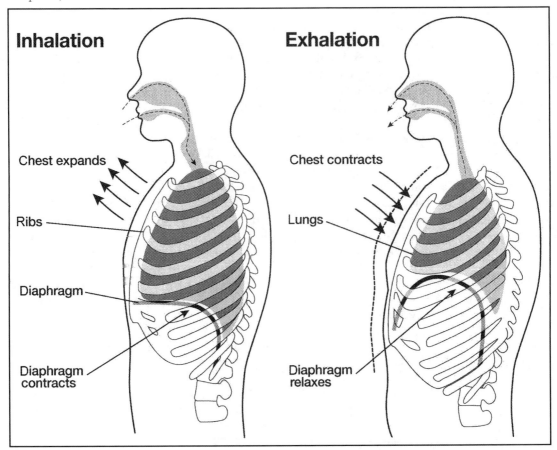

Figure 27-2. Chest movement and diaphragm movement during inhalation and exhalation.

The respiratory pattern is divided into inspiratory and expiratory phases. Inspiratory musculature, including the diaphragm and the dilator musculature of the upper airway, responds to a ramped increase in motor discharge that declines before the end of inspiration. The motor stimuli are silent during quiet expiration.

The dorsal respiratory nuclei in the medulla control motor activity and timing of inspiratory musculature. The ventral respiratory group increases the force of inspiration and control voluntary forced exhalation.

Pontine nuclei include the pneumotaxic center, which coordinates the transition between inhalation and exhalation and inhibits inspiration, which may act to fine-tune the respiratory rate. The apneustic center stimulates inspiration especially during long deep breaths. Further integration of respiration occurs in the anterior horn of the spinal cord subserving the musculature of respiration.

Respiratory rate is rigidly controlled by blood gas levels. Blood pH levels are sensed by chemoreceptors in the medulla, and O_2 and CO_2 levels are sensed by the carotid and aortic bodies. Afferent neurons from the carotid bodies ascend via the glossopharyngeal nerve and from the aortic bodies via the vagus nerve.

CO_2 levels rise when metabolic use of O_2 increases beyond the capacity of the lungs to expel CO_2. CO_2 is stored as bicarbonate (HCO_3^-) and H^+, which, when CO_2 builds up, decreases the pH of the blood. This is sensed by peripheral and central chemoreceptors, which stimulate respiratory centers to adjust the rate of respiration in order to blow off excess CO_2 and normalize metabolic balance. Mechanoreceptors in the airway and lung parenchyma are responsible for respiratory reflexes including coughing, sneezing, closure of the glottis, and hiccups. Nasothoracic reflexes trigger respiratory nuclei via the trigeminal nerve to increase the force of inspiration by increasing diaphragmatic and adding intercostal effort. Spinal cord reflexes activate accessory respiratory musculature to compensate for increased respiratory rate and volume demands.

Respiratory function can be influenced by emotional state via the limbic system or by temperature via the hypothalamus. Respiration can switch to voluntary control by centers in the cerebral cortex that take control of respiratory centers in the brain stem, although chemoreceptors can override conscious control when the demand presents itself.

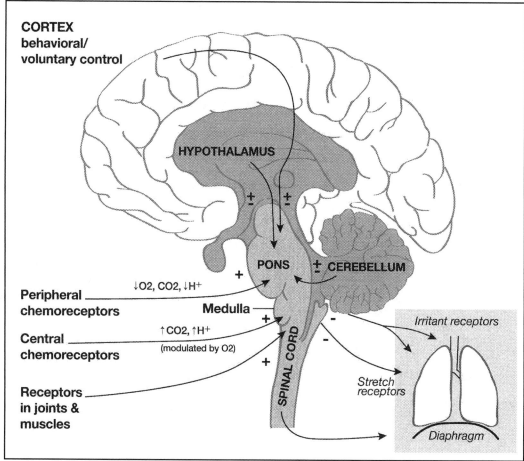

Figure 27-3. Neural pathways of respiration.

THE ANATOMY OF THE MECHANICS OF RESPIRATION

The anatomy of the mechanical respiratory system is usually considered to extend from the nose to the abdomen. Clinical experience suggests that structures that support and are involved in respiration likely begin in the cranium and extend as far as the feet. This is seen in the dysfunctional patient and can be best described by the common compensatory pattern (CCP) a pattern of structural asymmetry that promotes a dyssynchronous movement pattern has been noted by many osteopathic and rehabilitation clinicians (Figure 27-4).

The CCP was described by Zink[1] and Pope.[2] It theorizes that there is a predisposition of the neuro-myo-facioskeletal unit that leads to fascial bias, muscle imbalance, postural asymmetry, functional deficits, and common systemic complaints.[1] A number of mechanisms have been proposed to explain the origin of the CCP. One theory suggests a developmental fascial bias in which the position of the fetus in the uterine habitus begins the asymmetry that is carried forth through life. A second theory suggests

that the pattern begins from birth trauma that is never resolved. A third theory explains the origin of the CCP as a function of asymmetric leg growth in childhood that causes leg length discrepancy and leads to the most commonly found postural asymmetry.[3] Hruska suggested a fourth model for this compensatory pattern.[4] He suggests that the inherent asymmetry of the abdominal organs combined with the asymmetry of the diaphragm generates sagittal and transverse movement biases. This potential for asymmetrical patterned movement is habituated by muscle imbalance that facilitates joint position dysfunction. The movement patterns that are generated along polyarticular chains become established by habitual postures and biases in activities of daily living.[4]

Study of these theories suggests it is likely that the origin of asymmetrical dyssynchronous movement patterns is a complex interaction of a number of factors. Regardless, habitual postures and movement patterns contribute to the CCP.

The biases of the fascial planes that describe the CCP begin at the feet and are expressed through fascial planes up the appendicular and axial skeleton to the head. These biases are expressed as abnormal foot mechanics with the

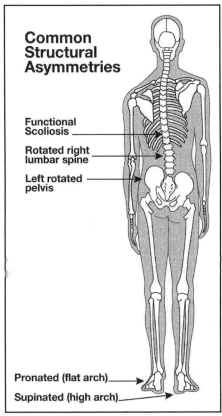

Common Structural Asymmetries

Functional Scoliosis

Rotated right lumbar spine

Left rotated pelvis

Pronated (flat arch)

Supinated (high arch)

Figure 27-4. Common structural asymmetries.

left foot relatively pronated and the right foot relatively supinated. Foot positional asymmetry causes a clinically short right leg, which produces asymmetrical tibial and femoral torsion. This causes a superior pube on the left, a posterior ilium on the left, and an anterior ilium on the right, and a left-on-left forward sacral torsion. L_5 is side bent left and rotated right. Right pelvic rotation causes the lower thoracic outlet to be rotated to the left and the upper thoracic outlet to be rotated to the right. Thoracic asymmetry produces rotation of the craniocervical junction to the left.

Compensatory patterns may be relatively adaptive, in which there is minimal abnormal loading that is transferred to adjacent areas. Individuals with a fully adaptive pattern generally do not have pain complaints. Sometimes, however, these adaptive patterns alternate directions at transition zones (Figure 27-5). These individuals generally do well and have fewer pain complaints as long as the compensation remains balanced, but when problems arise, they tend to be at the transition zones. These also may be sites of increased degenerative changes because of the compensatory pattern. Finally, there is the poorly compensated or uncompensated pattern in which the adaptive pattern is not balanced. This may be due to trauma to or exhaustion of the tissues' ability to compensate resulting in imbalance and usually pain and dysfunction, which may be seen as the CCP.

The CCP is marked by common muscular adaptations that produce tight, hypertonic postural musculature that is not effectively opposed by weak, overstretched, hypotonic dynamic musculature. Imbalances between paired antagonist muscle groups lead to compensatory side bending and rotational patterns. This describes a pattern of movement that is driven by asymmetrical alignment of the axial and appendicular skeleton. Muscles, tendons, fascia, ligaments, and joint capsules compensate to accommodate for the alignment and reorient the body segments from head to foot. The combined effect produces a malalignment syndrome. Treatment is aimed at inhibiting the hypertonic postural musculature, facilitating the hypotonic dynamic musculature and normalizing motor control.

In the context of this book, it is important to consider how the CCP affects diaphragmatic function. If the CCP decreases the strength or coordination of the diaphragm necessitating increased use of intercostal musculature and accessory respiratory musculature, particularly the left scalenes and right SCM, it may decrease vital capacity and alter ventilation. This change in pattern may be accommodated during wakefulness, but with the tonal changes that occur during sleep, this situation may increase resistance to respiration and complicate sleep-related breathing disorders. Manual therapy, therapeutic exercise, and neuromuscular reeducation can be implemented to correct the dysfunction in the diaphragm and improve the mechanics of respiration. Normalized respiratory function during wakefulness allows for improved respiratory function during sleep, even when breathing becomes unstable during REM sleep.

To understand this concept, understanding the anatomy of the mechanics of respiration is necessary. This chapter is not intended to be a definitive work on evaluation and treatment of the thoracic cage and diaphragm. Instead, the basic anatomy will be reviewed and the contribution of mechanical dysfunction within the respiratory apparatus will be discussed. The diaphragm will be discussed in more depth as some of the particular aspects of its anatomy impact somatic function and diaphragmatic action and therefore may give rise to respiratory dysfunction. In addition, some of the concepts of diaphragmatic dysfunction may be unfamiliar, so they will be discussed in greater detail.

The structure and function of the craniomandibular unit and its effect on the upper airway are discussed in greater detail in Chapter 25.

Postural influences in the function of the respiratory apparatus will be discussed in overview such that the reader may become familiar with habitual and adaptive movement patterns that may be addressed in order to improve the quality of sleep. For example, the position of the cervical spine in relation to the thorax is altered by habitual forward head position and influences the longitudinal architecture of the airway. Another example of postural influences on respiratory mechanics can be seen in slumped posture. For example, if the position of the diaphragm is altered

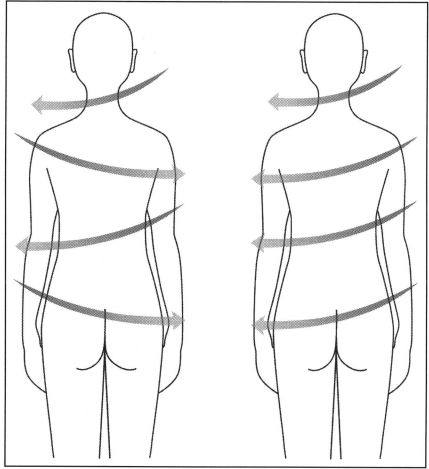

Figure 27-5. Alternating compensated and uncompensated patterns.

relative to its normal position because of slumped posture, the functional efficiency of breathing mechanisms may be compromised.

Thoracic Spine and Ribs

The rib cage is composed of the bony and cartilaginous structures that surround the thoracic cavity and support the shoulder girdle. A typical rib cage consists of 12 paired ribs, the sternum, costal cartilages, and 12 thoracic vertebrae. The rib cage is a component of the respiratory system that encloses the thoracic cavity and contains the lungs, the heart, and the mediastinal nerves and vessels.

The degree of movement in all directions allowed by the relatively rigid structure of the thorax is less than that which is available in the cervical or lumbar spines. This limitation acts to protect vital organs housed within the thoracic cavity. In most individuals, the thoracic spine has a kyphotic profile because of the slight decrease in height in the intervertebral disc from posterior to anterior. This change in dimension varies in degree from individual to individual. The thoracic spinous processes are especially prominent and therefore are easily palpated. Transverse

processes for T_1 to T_{10} carry the costotransverse joints for articulation with the ribs. The intervertebral facet joints are oriented in the frontal plane. The bodies of the thoracic segments are intermediate in size, and the size increases as the load-bearing need increases. That is, they are much smaller in the upper segments and get progressively larger in the lower segments. They are distinguished from vertebral segments in other regions by the presence of demifacets on the sides of the bodies that receive the articulation of the heads of the ribs, called the costovertebral joints, and facets on the transverse processes of the first 10 ribs that receive the articulation of the tubercles of the ribs and are called the costotransverse joints.

Rib Anatomy

All ribs are attached in the back to the thoracic vertebrae. The upper 7 true ribs are attached to the sternum via a costal cartilage. The eighth, ninth, and tenth ribs are known as the *false ribs*. They do not connect directly with the sternum but rather attach via the costal cartilages of the ribs above. The 11th and 12th ribs are known as the *floating ribs* because they only attach posteriorly and do not have an anterior attachment at all. The elasticity of the ribs and

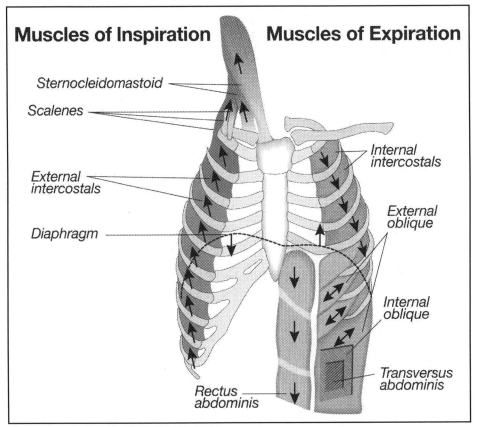

Figure 27-6. Muscles of inspiration and expiration.

costal cartilages allow movement during inhalation and exhalation.

The spaces between the ribs are known as the *intercostal spaces* and contain intercostal musculature and a neuro-vascular bundle that resides in a groove on the internal surface of the lower border of the each rib. Abnormalities of rib cage development may include pectus excavatum, also called *sunken chest*, and pectus carinatum, also called *pigeon chest*. In males, the rib cage expands as an effect of the testosterone surge that characterizes puberty. This contributes to the generally broader shoulders and expanded chest that allow adult males to inhale more to supply adequate oxygen to their increased muscle mass.

The rib cage is the structure from which musculature acts in order to accomplish respiration. Inhalation is accomplished when the diaphragm contracts and flattens, moving the floor of the thorax inferiorly, and the intercostal muscles lift the rib cage up and outward. Exhalation is generally a passive event, except in cases of forced exhalation.

Muscles of Respiration

Various muscles of respiration aid in both inspiration and expiration, which require changes in the pressure within the thoracic cavity (Figure 27-6). The primary muscles of inspiration are the diaphragm, the upper and more lateral external intercostals, and the parasternal portion of the internal intercostal muscles. Both the external intercostal muscles and the parasternal portion of the internal intercostal muscles elevate the ribs. This increases the width of the thoracic cavity, while the diaphragm contracts to increase the vertical dimensions of the thoracic cavity. The external intercostal muscles also aid in the elevation of the lower ribs. The levatores costarum are primary muscles of respiration that probably serve mostly a proprioceptive role.

The accessory muscles of inspiration include the scalenes, SCM, levator scapulae, and upper fibers of the trapezius, the iliocostalis thoracis, subclavius, and omohyoid. The serratus anterior and latissimus dorsi are accessory muscles of respiration with the upper extremities elevated. Accessory muscles of expiration include the interosseous internal intercostals, abdominal muscles, transversus thoracis, subcostalis, iliocostalis lumborum, quadratus lumborum, serratus posterior inferior, and latissimus dorsi. The accessory respiratory muscles are typically only used when the body needs to process energy quickly; for example, during heavy exercise, during the stress response, or during an asthma attack. When accessory muscles of respiration are habitually utilized and become part of the primary muscle recruitment pattern of respiration, dysfunction will follow. For example, decreased excursion of the diaphragm because of improper position will require the upper accessory musculature to increase activity for normal quiet respiration and the lower musculature to be added to the respiratory effort during times of increased respiratory demand as occurs with increased physical activity. If the SCM and scalenes are needed to expand the upper rib cage and the quadratus and psoas are needed to stabilize the lower rib cage, these muscles may become hypertonic and tight. The impact on the normal respiratory pattern can be significant. Accessory respiratory musculature is optimally designed to assist in increasing the expansion capacity of the thoracic cage in order to increase lung capacity at times of increased metabolic demand.

The diaphragm is crucial for breathing and respiration. During inhalation, the diaphragm contracts, thus enlarging the thoracic cavity. This reduces intrathoracic pressure; in other words, it enlarges the cavity and creates suction that draws air into the lungs. When the diaphragm relaxes, air is exhaled by elastic recoil of the lungs and the tissues lining the thoracic cavity in conjunction with the abdominal muscles, which act as an antagonist paired with diaphragmatic contraction. Humans have more control over the abdominal musculature and intercostals than over the diaphragm, which has fewer proprioceptive receptors. By training, proper posture, and balance in the rest of the body, the diaphragm naturally strengthens and works in concert with surrounding structures rather than in isolation. The diaphragm is also involved in non-respiratory function, helping to expel vomit, feces, and urine from the body by increasing intra-abdominal pressure and preventing acid reflux by exerting pressure on the esophagus as it passes through the esophageal hiatus.

Quiet expiration is accomplished by the elastic recoil of lungs, the diaphragm, pleura, and costal cartilages. At certain times, forced expiration is needed. Forced expiration is accomplished by the interosseous portion of the internal intercostals, abdominal muscles, transverse thoracis, subcostales, iliocostalis lumborum, quadratus lumborum, serratus posterior inferior, and latissimus dorsi.

The intercostal musculature comprise several groups of muscles that run between the ribs and help form and move the chest wall. There are 3 principal layers of intercostals. The external intercostal muscles assist with quiet inspiration and act as accessory muscles during forced inhalation. They are 11 paired muscles that originate starting on the first rib and inserting on the next lower rib. Each external intercostal arises from the lower border of the rib above and inserts into the upper border of the rib below. They extend from the tubercles of the ribs behind the cartilages of the ribs in front where they end in thin membranes, known as the *anterior intercostal membrane*, which continues forward to the sternum. They are thicker than the internal intercostals, and their fibers are directed obliquely downward and laterally on the back of the thorax and downward, forward, and medially in front. The external intercostals are responsible for the elevation of the ribs and expanding the transverse dimensions of the thoracic cavity.

Quiet expiration is a relatively passive process. The internal intercostal muscles aid in forced expiration. They are 11 pairs of muscles that originate anteriorly at the sternum in the interspaces between the cartilages of the true ribs and at the anterior extremities of the cartilages of the false ribs. They originate on the inner surface of the upper border of the rib below, as well as from the corresponding costal cartilage and insert into the lower border of the rib above. They extend backward as far as the angles of the ribs where they are continued to the vertebral column by a thin aponeurosis known as the posterior intercostal membrane. Fibers are directed obliquely by passing in the direction opposite to those of the external intercostals. The internal intercostals are responsible for the depression of the ribs and decrease the transverse dimension of the thoracic cavity.

The innermost intercostal muscles are the deep layers of the intercostal muscles, which are separated by the intercostal neurovascular bundle that corresponds to each rib. The subcostal muscles, which elevate the ribs arise from the ribs posteriorly and insert into the second or third rib below. The transversus thoracis, which acts in forced expiration, arises from the posterior surface of the xiphoid process and body of the sternum and is inserted posteriorly into several costal cartilages.

The transversus thoracis lies anteriorly on the internal surface of the internal thoracic cage. It resides in the same plane as the subcostales musculature. It arises on either side from the lower third of the posterior surface of the body of the sternum, from the posterior surface of the xiphoid process, and from the sternal ends of the costal cartilages of the lower 3 or 4 true ribs. Fibers diverge upward and laterally to insert by slips into the lower borders and inner surfaces of the costal cartilages on the second, third, fourth, fifth, and sixth ribs. The lowest fibers are oriented horizontally and are continuous with fibers of the transverse abdominus. The intermediate fibers are oriented obliquely, and the highest fibers are oriented nearly vertically. This muscle has variation from side to side and individual to individual. The transversus thoracis contracts during exertional expiration by decreasing the transverse diameter of the thoracic cage.

The subcostales consists of muscular and aponeurotic slips that are usually well developed only in the lower part of the thorax. Muscular slips originate from the internal surface of one rib and insert into the internal surface of the second or third rib above, near the rib angle. Fibers run obliquely in the same direction as the internal intercostals.

Expansion of the Rib Cage

Expansion of the rib cage normally occurs in 3 planes: vertical, anteroposterior, and transverse (Figure 27-7). Vertical expansion is accomplished by a coordinated effort of the diaphragm flattening and applying downward pressure against the abdominal visceral. This pressure is opposed by the abdominal musculature. The vertical

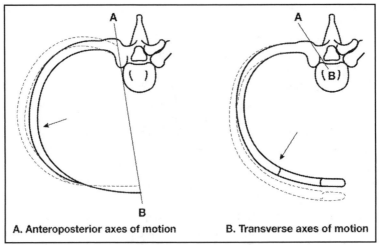

A. Anteroposterior axes of motion

B. Transverse axes of motion

Figure 27-7. Motion of the costovertebral and costotransverse joints with associated rib movement.

dimension can be further expanded by the diaphragm moving downward rather than simply flattening. The rib cage expands in an anteroposterior dimension by a movement known as a pump-handle movement of the ribs. This pump-handle movement occurs as the ribs attach posteriorly to the vertebrae at the costovertebral joints then slope downward to attach to the costal cartilages anteriorly, which, in turn, attach to the sternum. The external intercostal muscles contract and lift the ribs, pushing them into the sternum, which then moves up and out, thereby increasing the anteroposterior dimension of the rib cage. The rib cage can increase its transverse dimension, primarily the lower ribs. When the diaphragm contracts, and with the central tendon of the diaphragm acting as a fixed point, the ribs move up and out in a bucket-handle movement pattern, gliding at the costovertebral joints. This increases the lower transverse diameter of the rib cage as the lungs expand. During normal respiration, the adult rib cage expands approximately 3 to 5 cm during inspiration.[5]

Respiration may be assisted by accessory respiratory musculature, which is any musculature that attaches onto the ribs such as the SCM, pectoral muscles, and scalene muscles or acts to change the shape of the thorax such as the psoas or latissimus dorsi musculature, which aids in forced expiration.

In most circumstances during quiet breathing in a healthy individual, inspiration is almost unnoticeable event, and expiration is completely passive, carried out by the elastic recoil of the thoracic cage and lungs and relaxation of the diaphragm. However, during exercise or other forms of physiological stress, the body is required to force expiration in order to assist in greater expansion and to speed the rate of respiration when metabolic needs demand it. In these situations, accessory respiratory musculature is recruited to accomplish this. For example, the SCMs pull the sternum upward and the pectoralis major and minor pull the upper anterior ribs outward, increasing the anteroposterior diameter of the thoracic cage. The scalene

musculature pulls the upper two ribs superiorly and is often opposed by the iliopsoas musculature inferiorly. The action of these muscles increases the vertical dimension of the rib cage. The anterior abdominal wall, excluding the transversus abdominus, helps depress the lower ribs and the latissimus dorsi can also aid in deep, forced expiration.

The thoracic cavity can expand during so-called belly breathing, in which the lower ribs stabilize and the diaphragm contracts, moving the central tendon down, compressing the abdominal cavity, and allowing the thoracic cavity to expand downward.

The Respiratory Diaphragm

Because of the central function of the diaphragm in breathing and the role that dysfunction of diaphragmatic breathing can play in sleep-related breathing disorders, it is important to understand the functional anatomy of the diaphragm (Figure 27-8).

The respiratory diaphragm is a dome-shaped musculofibrous septum that separates the thoracic cavity from the abdominal cavity. At its peripheral dimension, the diaphragm consists of muscular fibers that take origin from the circumference of the inferior thoracic aperture and converge to be inserted into a central tendon. The muscular fibers are grouped according to their origins and are generally considered in 3 parts. The sternal part takes origin from 2 fleshy slips from the internal surface of the xiphoid process. The costal portion takes origin from the internal surfaces of the cartilages and adjacent part of the lower 6 ribs on either side. The costal fibers of the diaphragm interdigitate with fibers of the transversus abdominus muscle. The lumbar portion of the diaphragm arises from aponeurotic arches, known as *lumbocostal arches*, and from 2 pillars of muscle known as the *crura*. The crura begin as tendons and blend with the anterior longitudinal ligament of the vertebral column. The right crus is larger and longer

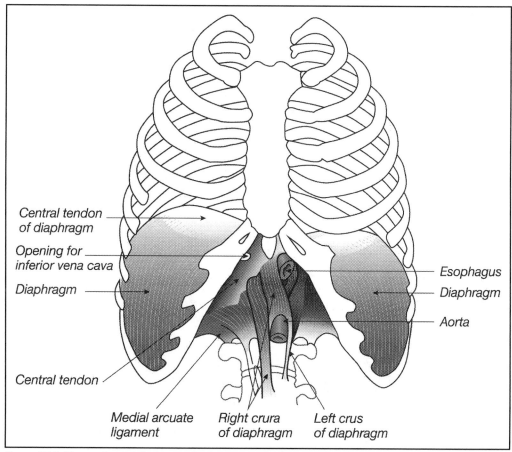

Central tendon
of diaphragm

Opening for
inferior vena cava

Diaphragm

Central tendon

Esophagus

Diaphragm

Aorta

Medial arcuate
ligament

Right crura
of diaphragm

Left crus
of diaphragm

Figure 27-8. The respiratory diaphragm. Note variation of right and left leaflets, especially in relationship to the position of internal organs. For example, the right leaflet is held in apposition by the liver. Asymmetry of the crura, especially the origin off the lumbar spine, facilitates lumbar rotation.

than the left, arising from the anterior surface of the body and intervertebral fibrocartilages of the upper three lumbar vertebrae. The left crus arises from the intervertebral fibrocartilages of only the upper 2 lumbar vertebrae. The medial tendinous margins of the crura pass anteriorly and medially and meet in the midline to form a relatively poorly defined arch, which crosses anterior to the aorta.

The posterior attachment of the diaphragm is marked by several specialized areas that form openings through which vital structures pass. The medial lumbocostal arch, also known as the *medial arcuate ligament,* is a tendinous portion of the fascia that arches over the psoas major muscle as it passes under the diaphragm. It is not uncommon to find tendinous slips from either muscle interdigitate with the other. The medial arcuate ligament is an arch that is attached to the side of the body of the first or second lumbar vertebra and laterally to the front of the transverse process of the first and sometimes the second lumbar vertebra. It lies between the lateral arcuate ligament and the midline median arcuate ligament. The sympathetic chain enters the abdomen by passing deep to this ligament.

The lateral lumbocostal arch, also known as the *lateral arcuate ligament,* arches across the upper part of the quadratus lumborum. It is traversed by the subcostal neurovascular bundle. It runs from the front of the transverse process of the first lumbar vertebra and proceeds laterally to the tip and lower margin of the 12th rib.

The median arcuate ligament is made up of the convergence of the right and left diaphragmatic crura in the midline. The area behind the arch is known as the aortic hiatus. The aorta, the azygos vein, and thoracic duct pass through the aortic hiatus. The celiac artery and celiac ganglia also pass through the hiatus.

All of the fibers of origin of the diaphragm converge from various directions and insert into a common central tendon, which is a thin but strong aponeurosis that is situated near the center of the vault formed by the diaphragm but is closer to the front than to the back of the thorax. This makes the posterior fibers somewhat longer than the anterior muscle fibers. Fibers attaching to the xiphoid process are very short and occasionally aponeurotic. Fibers from the medial and lateral arcuate ligaments and fibers from the ribs and their cartilages are longer and curved markedly as they ascend and converge into the central tendon. Fibers from the right and left crura diverge as they ascend with the most lateral fibers projecting superior and lateral

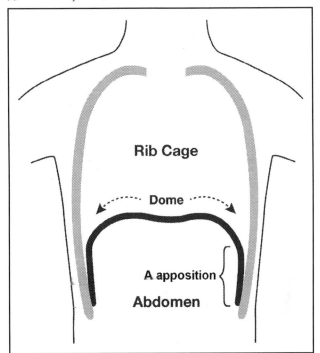

Figure 27-9. Zone of apposition of the respiratory diaphragm. When the diaphragm is properly positioned in apposition to the internal chest wall, the abdominal musculature can oppose its function.

into the central tendon. The medial fibers of the right crus ascend on the left side of the esophageal hiatus and occasionally a fasciculus of the left crus crosses the aorta and runs obliquely through the fibers of the right crus toward the opening for the vena cava. The central tendon sits immediately below the pericardium and is partially blended with it. There is an opening at about the level of T_8 through which the vena cava passes. The central tendon is shaped somewhat like a trefoil leaf, consisting of 3 leaflets that are separated from one another by slight indentations. The right leaflet is the largest, the middle leaflet is directed toward the xiphoid process, and the left leaflet is the smallest. The tendon is composed of several planes of fibers that intersect with one another at various angles and unite into bundles of fibers that are either straight or curved in an arrangement that gives it additional strength.

During respiration, the diaphragm contracts, which causes the central tendon to be drawn inferiorly, partially flattening the dome. This enlarges the thoracic cavity and decreases the intrathoracic pressure, which causes air to rush into the lungs. Diaphragmatic contraction also enhances venous return to the heart. During inspiration, the central tendon retains its shape due to its tendinous nature. This prevents constriction of the inferior vena cava or the aorta; however, the esophagus is surrounded by muscle at the esophageal hiatus and can become constricted.

There are multiple openings in the diaphragm that have been mentioned previously, but should be discussed in further detail. The anatomy of the diaphragm and the manner in which structures pass through anatomical openings in the diaphragm is important in understanding how diaphragmatic dysfunction may play a part in certain symptoms. Careful consideration of the anatomy of the diaphragm and related structures will also help the clinician to understand certain aspects of its rehabilitation.

The caval opening is a hiatus in the diaphragm through which the inferior vena cava and some branches of the right phrenic nerve pass. The walls of the vena cava are adherent of the margins of the opening. It is located at the level of the eighth thoracic vertebra and passes through the central tendon of the diaphragm at the junction of the right and middle leaflets. Since it is situated in the tendinous part of the diaphragm, the vena cava is stretched open during each inspiratory contraction. Because intrathoracic pressure decreases upon inspiration, blood in the vena cava is pushed upward toward the right atrium. When the caval opening increases in size, it allows more blood to return to the heart, thus maximizing the efficacy of the lowered thoracic pressure returning blood to the heart.

The esophageal hiatus is an opening in the diaphragm through which the esophagus passes. It is located in the right crus of the diaphragm at approximately the 10th thoracic vertebra. It is situated in the muscular part of the diaphragm and is superior, anterior, and slightly to the left of the aortic hiatus. It transmits the esophagus, the vagus nerves, and some small esophageal arteries. The right crus of the diaphragm loops around, forming a sling around the esophagus. Upon inspiration, this sling constricts the diaphragm, forming an anatomical sphincter that prevents stomach contents from refluxing up the esophagus when intra-abdominal pressure increases during inspiration.

The aortic hiatus is the lowest and most posterior of the large apertures in the diaphragm. It is an opening between the muscle and the body of the first lumbar vertebra. Occasionally, some tendinous fibers from the medial aspects of the lower ends of the crura pass between the aorta and the vertebra, forming a fibrous ring. The hiatus is situated slightly to the left of the midline. It carries the aorta, the azygos vein, and the thoracic duct.

Zone of Apposition

A number of researchers have considered the dual role of the diaphragm in postural stability and respiration.[4,6-9] The maintenance of optimal balance of the respiratory function of the diaphragm and the postural musculature can create a challenge, particularly in the individual who has postural alignment issues and faulty muscle firing patterns. Achieving and maintaining an optimal ZOA of the diaphragm is key to this balance (Figure 27-9). An important concept in the discussion of dysfunction of the diaphragm is the structure and function of the ZOA. *Apposition* is defined as placing something side by side or next to another. It may also be described as the growth of

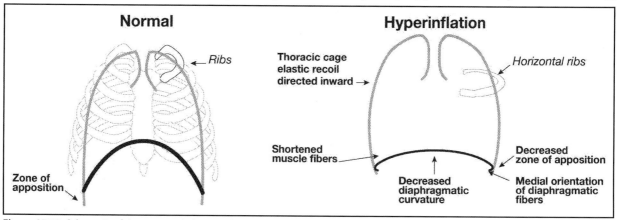

Figure 27-10. Schematic of the structural changes that occur when the lungs are hyperinflated, as occurs in mechanical dysfunction of the diaphragm and increased activity of accessory respiratory musculature.

successive layers of a cell wall. This term is to be distinguished from *opposition*, which is defined as the placement of something opposite to or in contrast to another. These terms will be important to distinguish when discussing the mechanics of the diaphragm and the abdominal wall.

If the diaphragm is considered as the top of a domed cylinder, the cylindrical aspect of the diaphragm lays against the inner aspect of the rib cage and lower mediastinal wall. This area where the diaphragm lays against the internal wall of the rib cage is the ZOA. The ZOA is controlled by the abdominal muscles and affects diaphragmatic tension.[4] The efficiency of the diaphragm is largely dependent upon its position and anatomical relationship with the lower rib cage. A suboptimal ZOA may cause inefficient respiration because of decreased transdiaphragmatic pressure. That is, the smaller the ZOA, the smaller mechanical action the diaphragm can exert on the rib cage. Suboptimal ZOA will also lead to decreased activation of the abdominal wall which should act in opposition to the diaphragm. Dyssynchronous muscle firing pattern may lead to decreased spinal stabilization. Selective weakness in the transversus abdominus results in decreased tension on the thoracolumbar fascia. Decreased tension on the thoracolumbar fascia changes the length-tension ratio of the multifidi musculature, reducing their ability to provide segmental stability of the spine. Therefore, suboptimal ZOA, particularly of the left crus of the diaphragm can lead to decreased spinal stabilization.

The ZOA and the dome shape of the diaphragm are maintained during inspiration by the resting tension of the abdominal muscles supporting the abdominal viscera against the undersurface of the diaphragm. The ZOA comprises a variable area depending upon structural changes and respiratory environment. In an adult, standing and breathing quietly, the ZOA represents about 30% of the total surface of the internal rib cage.[10] The crural portion of the diaphragm contracts and descends during inspiration. Normally, the dome of the diaphragm maintains its size and shape because of the stiffness of the central tendon.

However, the ZOA decreases by approximately 15 mm during quiet inspiration, it may be reduced to near zero during maximal inspiration. The resting tension of the abdominal musculature opposes the inspiratory action of the diaphragm by facilitating an increasing of the abdominal pressure rather than outwardly protruding of the abdomen during diaphragmatic contraction. The diaphragm and the abdominal musculature are always mechanically coupled throughout the ZOA.

If the diaphragm does not function with optimal ZOA and is appropriately opposed by the abdominal musculature, the diaphragm will lose its characteristic dome and will distort the shape of the lower rib cage. While this can occur on either side, this is most likely to occur on the left side because there are no other structures that help to maintain its shape and apposition as occurs on the right side of the diaphragm. This distortion causes a change of muscle pull because of the change of orientation of muscle fibers due to the change in shape of the diaphragm. The change in muscle action distorts the lower rib cage, in particular, causing external rotation of the lower ribs resulting in a rib flare (Figure 27-10). The change in shape of the lower rib cage then causes a change in the length–tension ratio of the abdominal musculature, particularly on the left anterior abdominal wall. This weakness reduces abdominal musculature opposition to diaphragmatic action during inspiration.

The functional relationship between the diaphragm and the abdominal musculature is further illustrated by observing that in the presence of increased demand for spinal stability, the diaphragm contracts concentrically and specific abdominal musculature contracts eccentrically during inspiration.

When the mechanics of the diaphragm and opposing abdominal musculature break down, a faulty breathing pattern is established and spinal stabilization becomes inefficient. This may lead to increased use of accessory respiratory musculature, particularly in the right upper quadrant. This cascade of events, which begins with the loss of a ZOA of the diaphragm, usually on the left, may lead to other clinical conditions including lower back pain, pelvic floor dysfunction, and neck and shoulder pain. It may contribute to forward head posture. All of this causes suboptimal respiration.

In the context of this book, dysfunction of the mechanics of respiration that leads to suboptimal function of the diaphragm is likely to lead to depressed respiration during sleep. It is reasonable to consider that mechanical respiratory dysfunction during wakefulness will be compounded during sleep, when respiration is typically depressed and becomes unstable, especially during REM sleep. Because of this, it is important to understand the signs and symptoms of faulty respiratory function, particularly that which is mechanically driven. Position and function of the diaphragm becomes paramount in optimizing respiration during sleep. This can be accomplished in a variety of ways. Specific techniques for restoring the ZOA and maintaining optimal diaphragmatic position, strength, and endurance are beyond the scope of this book. The clinician is directed to other resources such as Chaitow's *Multidisciplinary Approaches to Breathing Pattern Disorders*[5] and Hruska's "Postural Respiration."[4] A general discussion on restoration of the ZOA is merited.

THORACIC FORM AND FUNCTION

The body continually contends with the influence of gravity while sitting and standing. In fact, the Nobel laureate Sperry suggested that 90% of the brain's energy is spent in activities that are geared toward dealing with the effects of gravity.[11] The adoption of an upright posture, however, suggests the existence of some reflexive mechanisms to maintain tone in order for purposeful activity to take place. Distortions of the body as may occur with faulty posture may alter the function of the musculature. For example, the gravitational pull of upright posture relaxes the lower abdomen and diaphragm, which puts it at a functional disadvantage. Postural alignment, therefore, is an important component of normal diaphragmatic function. Postural habits that deform the thorax and cause the diaphragm to function in a suboptimal fashion need to be corrected.

Positional correction of the diaphragm is a bit more complex than other skeletal muscle rehabilitation. Because the diaphragm has relatively few proprioceptors, it is likely that it is not guided by stretch reflex; instead, it appears to be controlled by a reflexive mechanism. The close functional relationship of the intercostal muscles and diaphragm, as well as the intimate anatomical relationship between the diaphragm and the lower part of the rib cage, supports the idea of a reflexive mechanism between the two muscles. Autogenetic facilitation, which is the process of inhibiting the muscle that generated a stimulus while providing an excitatory impulse to the antagonist muscle,

has been demonstrated for the external intercostal muscle. This is part of an intercostal-to-phrenic reflex that ties the function of the diaphragm to the external intercostal musculature, although the precise mechanism remains unclear.[12,13] It has been suggested that phrenic motorneurons are controlled by reflexes elicited by afferent stimulation of the lower intercostal nerves and dorsal rami of the lower thoracic spinal nerves. The intercostal-to-phrenic reflex can also be facilitated under conditions of gravity with proper lower thoracic alignment and postural support. It is further postulated that increased phrenic motorneuron activity has an excitatory effect on the diaphragm during mechanical stimuli to the lower rib cage. Afferent stimulation in the mid-thoracic region has been shown to inhibit phrenic motorneuron activity. This is the neurological basis for manual techniques designed to optimize the ZOA of the diaphragm and thus improve respiratory function.

RESTORATION OF THE ZONE OF APPOSITION

The ZOA may become suboptimal unilaterally, almost always on the left because of the capacity for the shape and pressure of the liver on the right help the right side of the diaphragm to maintain its ZOA. Assuming the loss of the ZOA on the left side of the diaphragm, the abdominal muscles, particularly the left internal oblique and the transversus abdominus, are primarily responsible for opposition to the left leaflet of the diaphragm. This assists with maintaining the ZOA on the left side of the diaphragm during inspiration. It induces expansion in the opposite apical chest wall and upper rib cage especially during trunk rotation or during gait. Loss of control of the internal abdominal oblique either on the left or bilaterally may cause suboptimal apposition of the diaphragm and, therefore, suboptimal respiration. This would trigger firing of accessory respiratory musculature on the opposite upper rib cage and may cause hyperinflation in the apical chest. Changes in diaphragmatic dimensions may be produced by chronic hyperinflation and result in chronic increased tone corresponding in the accessory respiratory musculature.[4]

Reducing the physical and physiological symptoms associated with hyperinflation, paradoxical and accessory respiratory muscle overuse requires repositioning and retraining of the diaphragm to establish and maintain a normal ZOA. Manual techniques and exercise can improve rib cage and diaphragm position in which the left side of the diaphragm regains its proper mechanical advantage to efficiently contract through the central tendon. The dome of the diaphragm can rest at expiration, since tangential force is no longer required for postural stabilization.[4]

The proper position of the diaphragm is reached when expansion of the abdominal wall is no longer required during maximal opposition in inspiration. Simultaneous belly expansion and chest wall expansion is desirable upon inhalation through the nose without use of the accessory respiratory muscles of the neck. Contralateral apical flexibility and chest wall mobility are needed during same-side diaphragm apposition contraction for diaphragmatic breathing to occur effortlessly with assistance from external barometric pressure, chest wall recoil, pleural elasticity, and negative internal mediastinal pressure.[4]

An active ZOA occurs when an individual can perform a standing forward bend test, touching fingers to toes, and is able to inhale with anterior mediastinal compression and posterior mediastinal expansion.[4] These concepts and techniques for reestablishing and maintaining an optimal ZOA have been described by Ron Hruska, PT, of the Postural Restoration Institute.[14]

FORWARD HEAD POSTURE

Other postural compromises can have a significant impact upon the respiratory capacity of an individual. For example, forward head posture is a common clinical and societal finding (Figure 27-11). It is linked to negative metabolic state, including reduced blood and lymphatic flow, fatigue, and neck pain. Forward head posture presents with a head that has migrated anteriorly on the neck. Kapandji stated that for every inch the head migrates anterior to its optimal alignment, the gravitational pull on the musculature increases by 10 pounds.[15] For example, assuming that a patient's head weighs 15 pounds and is displaced 2 inches anteriorly of its optimal position, the restraining force that must be sustained by the axial musculature in the upper quadrant is 35 pounds. This is not an uncommon finding in probably the majority of patients seen in a clinical setting, regardless of their presenting complaint. Symptoms can occur if the posture is maintained for as little as 10 minutes.[16] With chronic forward head posture, excessive gravitational pull has been linked to ligamentous laxity. Because the ligaments are responsible for protecting the intervertebral discs and facet joints, disruption of their integrity predisposes the neck to injury. Once the tissue is strained, it is difficult for it to return to its original length.

Cailliet suggested that forward head posture can add up to 30 pounds of abnormal forces to the intervertebral disc, uncovertebral joints, and facet joints.[17] This abnormal and asymmetrical pull can result in multiple levels of spinal malalignment. Cailliet also reported that forward head posture can result in 30% reduction of pulmonary vital capacity. The change in respiratory function produced by forward head posture is primarily due to changes in cervical alignment. It interferes with the action of the infrahyoid musculature, which works with the scalenes to lift the first rib during normal inspiration.[17]

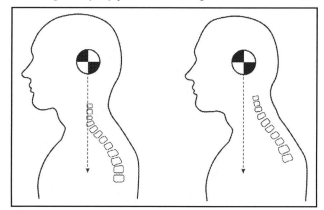

Figure 27-11. Anatomy of forward head posture.

An important function of the position of the head on the neck is to maintain horizontal gaze, and movement is necessary in order to engage the vestibule-ocular reflex and pursue objects in the visual field. Head-on-neck position is also important to the function of the vestibular apparatus that helps to maintain balance. This is the primary postural consideration.

Abnormal upper cervical position as seen in forward head posture causes muscular imbalance in which the suboccipital musculature is hypertonic and the antagonists, the short flexors, longus capitis, and longus colli, become overstretched and weak. This causes the synergists, the SCMs, to activate. The normal muscle firing pattern for cervical flexion is as follows: first, the intrinsic flexors and then the longus capitis and longus colli. Once segmental upper cervical flexion has been established, the SCMs and scalene muscles fire to enhance cervical flexion. If the SCMs fire first, the occiput is extended over the atlas because of the attachment of the SCM on the mastoid process. This can cause compression of the dorsal root ganglia and the vascular structures in the suboccipital triangle, as well as increased compressive load on the posterior aspect of the occipito-atlantal joints. Increased pain can increase the muscle tone and set up a cycle of pain and muscle spasm. It will also habituate the postural malalignment.

When this pattern is established, it causes other cervical extensors such as the semispinalis, splenius, and longissimus to become tight and shortened. Their action overpowers the overstretched and weakened longus colli that can lead to overstretching of the anterior longitudinal ligament, which, in turn, causes increased lordosis in the mid-cervical region. This leads to increased cervical facet dysfunction and spurring at the uncovertebral joints primarily at C_{4-5} and C_{5-6} and can cause neck pain and cervical radiculopathy.

Forward head posture can cause abnormal mandibular position (Figure 27-12). For example, changes in the normal cervical lordosis can cause a change in position of the hyoid bone, causing hypertonic suprahyoid and digastric musculature. This can cause a repositioning of the mandible

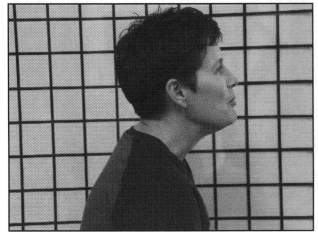

Figure 27-12. Forward head posture. It is a good idea to photograph the patient in front of a postural grid. Note increased tone in anterior cervical musculature and posterior cranial rotation with increased extension of upper cervical segments and compensatory increase in thoracic kyphosis. There is also a change in craniomandibular position. (Reprinted with permission from L. Brinkman.)

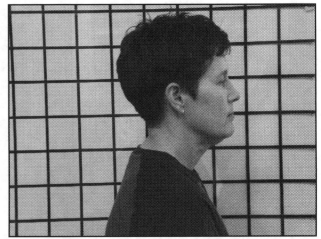

Figure 27-13. Improvement of forward head posture. Note the decreased tone in the anterior cervical musculature and the improved position of the occiput on the cervical spine. (Reprinted with permission from L. Brinkman.)

posteriorly as the head moves anteriorly. To keep the mouth from hanging open, bilateral temporalis and masseter musculature co-contract. This muscular effort compresses the mandibular condyles into the fossa and can compress the intra-articular disc and may contribute to disc displacement and temporomandibular pain. Unilateral muscle spasm and disc displacement is reflected in occipito-atlantal alignment and vice versa.

The forces that generate and perpetuate forward head posture also distort the position and increase the flexure of the airway, which increases resistance to air flow. If the airway is already compromised by changes in anatomical size or shape, forward head posture will add to airway restriction. Changes in airway patency caused by postural dysfunction will compromise respiratory efficiency.[18] Because the airway has an increased tendency toward collapse during sleep due to the decrease in muscle tone that is part of NREM sleep and muscle atonia that is part of REM sleep, any problems in the airway size or shape caused by postural habits will increase the risk of sleep-related breathing disorders. In addition, an individual who has problems with the size or shape of the airway may position his head on the neck in such a manner that will help to increase airway patency. These postures may help to maintain the airway during sleep but may result in increased compression of upper cervical structures and increased pain and, in particular, contribute to morning headaches. Improvement of muscle firing patterns and normalizing cervical segmental mobility to reduce forward head posture may improve airway patency during wakefulness and during sleep (Figure 27-13).

NORMALIZING MOBILITY IN THE THORACIC CAGE

Segmental mobility within the thoracic cage is an important factor to consider when rehabilitating the mechanics of respiration. In a normal, healthy thoracic cage, there are many moving parts, although there is inherent stiffness because of the structure of these parts. For example, the existence of the rib cage with the sternum increases the stiffness of the thoracic spine by about 2.5 times, more so when the spine is in extension and less so when the spine is in flexion. Compressive loading capacity of the thoracic spine increases significantly by 3 to 4 times with the addition of the rib cage.[19]

Biomechanics of Thoracic Motion

Flexion of the thoracic spine occurs in the sagittal plane during forward bending of the trunk and during exhalation. Flexion of a functional unit of the thorax includes translation anteriorly and slight distraction of the segments. The orientation of the thoracic articular facets supports motion of the superior vertebra gliding upward and slightly forward on the inferior segment.[20] During flexion, the superior segment of the thoracic spine translates anteriorly, thus moving the superior demifacet of the costovertebral joint forward. This causes the attached rib to rotate anteriorly because the demifacet pushes downward on the head of the rib. Because of the configuration of the concave demifacet on the convex rib head in the mid thoracic segments, during flexion in the mid thorax, anterior rotation of the rib at the costovertebral joint is accompanied by a superior glide at the costotransverse joints. In the lower thoracic segments, the amount of rotation diminishes especially in the 11th and 12th ribs because they have no corresponding costotransverse joints.[21]

Extension of the thorax occurs during backward bending, during forward flexion of the arms, and during deep inspiration. Thoracic extension occurs in the sagittal plane and includes a posterior translation and slight distraction as the inferior facets of the superior segment glide posterior and inferiorly. This motion causes compression of the superior facet onto the inferior segment. Thoracic extension facilitates posterior rotation of the corresponding rib at the costovertebral joint and an inferior glide at the costotransverse joint.

Side bending of the thorax occurs in the frontal plane. During side bending of the trunk, the vertebra side bend in one direction and rotate in the opposite direction. The vertebra translate toward the side of side bending. The ribs on the ipsilateral side of the side bending approximate before intervertebral facet joint motion has reached its limit; therefore, the rib stops the motion. Because of this movement limitation, the rib facet on the transverse process moves superiorly, which causes the rib to rotate anteriorly (also known as internal rotation of the rib). This motion is a function of the concave surface of the facet on the transverse process and the concave surface of the rib tubercle. The anterior or internal rotation of the rib head causes the superior vertebra to move forward at the costovertebral joint.[19,20] On the contralateral side, the ribs distract but are limited in this motion by the intercostal muscles. The ribs on the contralateral side of the side bend move inferiorly at the costotransverse joint as the transverse process moves superiorly. This results in posterior (or external) rotation of the head of the rib as the superior vertebra moves backward. In summary, during side bending of the thorax, the ribs on the ipsilateral side of the side bend will rotate anteriorly or internally, and the ribs contralateral to the side bend will rotate posteriorly or externally.

Rotation of the thorax couples rotation with ipsilateral side bending. The translation will pull the ipsilateral rib and push the contralateral rib. Therefore, the superior segment rotates in one direction and translates in the opposite direction, which results in posterior or external rotation of the ipsilateral rib and anterior or internal rotation of the contralateral rib.

Normal rib cage motion during respiration has been discussed earlier, but in light of the discussion of the mechanics of the rib cage, it bears repeating. Movement of the upper ribs during respiration involves rotation occurring at the costovertebral and translation occurring at the costotransverse joints. The axis of motion of the upper ribs falls between the costovertebral and costotransverse joints. That motion allows for lifting of the anterior aspect of the rib as it attaches via the chondral cartilages to the sternum. This is known as the so-called pump-handle movement that characterizes upper rib motion. The axis of rotation for the lower ribs, excluding the 11th and 12th ribs, is more

in the sagittal plane; therefore, motion of the lower ribs is more oblique and occurs more in the frontal plane and thus is designated as a bucket-handle motion. Overall, the ribs move upward and outward in order to increase the volume of the thorax during inspiration.

Dysfunction in the Thoracic Cage

Discussion of the segmental mechanics of the thoracic cage demonstrates that mobility of the thoracic spine and rib cage are essential for normal efficient respiratory function. If a single segment is restricted, immobile, or stiff because of its close attachment to and functional linkage to the rest of the thoracic cage, that movement impairment will be translated to other segments as they attempt to compensate for the alteration in mechanics. In addition, generalized restriction in thoracic segments that may occur with deconditioning, postural habits, or systemic illness can decrease respiratory efficiency during daytime wakefulness and may contribute to sleep-related breathing disorders. Research is scant in this area, but clinical data have shown that improvement in the mechanics of respiration can improve respiratory efficiency during daytime wakefulness. It is reasonable to speculate that this will translate to improved respiratory patterns during sleep.

Improving the mechanics of the thoracic cage includes increasing the segmental mobility of the thoracic spine and rib cage. It is important to remember that each functional unit of the thorax includes 2 adjacent vertebra and 4 ribs that attach posteriorly at a demifacet on the inferior border of the vertebra above and on the superior border of the demifacet below. Some segmental variations do exist. Most ribs also attach at a costotransverse joint on each side. The ribs attach anteriorly to the sternum (true ribs) or via costal cartilages to the ribs above (false ribs). It is important to keep all of these articular structures in mind when mobilizing the thoracic cage. Consideration should also be given to the myofascial structures that support the thoracic cage. Though it is outside the scope of this book to provide detailed instruction in myofascial and soft tissue therapy, the clinician should review these structures, particularly as they relate to respiratory dysfunction. It should be noted that Janda's upper-crossed syndrome and lower-crossed syndrome[22] are excellent descriptions of the manner in which upper and lower quadrant problems contribute to and are influenced by respiratory function and dysfunction.

THE STRUCTURE OF DYSFUNCTION

Prolonged modifications of function such as uncoordinated or dysfunctional respiratory patterns displayed during hyperventilation or in a state of chronic hyperinflation induce structural changes. For example, the increased activity of the accessory respiratory muscles that occurs in an attempt to increase ventilation causes hypertrophy and shortening of these muscles. There may also be structural changes in the cervical facet joints from chronic forward head posture or changes in the thoracic articulations. These changes can develop into a self-perpetuating cycle of functional change creating structural modification leading to reinforced dysfunctional tendencies. These changes occur from whichever direction the dysfunction begins. For example, structural adaptations can prevent normal breathing function, and abnormal breathing function ensures continued structural adaptation stresses leading to decompensation. Restoration of normal function requires restoration of adequate mobility of the structural component. This requires that function, or how an individual breathes, should be normalized through re-education and training. Functional changes in respiration may be pathological, or they may be habitual and functional. Either way, the impact of altered respiratory physiology caused by hyperventilation of the apical lung as is part of the pattern involved in loss of ZOA of the left side of the diaphragm can be profound. This could lead to significant health problems ranging from anxiety and panic attacks to fatigue and chronic pain. One of the most significant problems of waking respiratory dysfunction is its contribution to sleep-related breathing disorders. The likelihood of sleep-related hypoventilation is significantly higher in individuals who experience decreased efficiency of respiration during wakefulness. Changes in respiration may be due to biomechanical factors such as postsurgical factors or postural factors; biochemical contributors such as allergic or infectious factors; or psychological factors including chronic emotional states like anxiety or anger.

The rehabilitation professional is in an advantageous position to evaluate the mechanical respiratory function of the patient and to correlate this with signs and symptoms of disordered sleep. The rehabilitation professional is also able to apply a number of treatment techniques aimed at improving waking respiratory function. Possible contributors to dysfunction in the mechanics of respiration may include forward head posture, suboptimal ZOA of the diaphragm, abnormal hyoid position, or restrictions in the thoracic cage.

The goals of such treatment should include improving forward head posture and restoring normal balance in the cervical flexors and extensors, restoring and maintaining a normal ZOA, and reducing abnormal accessory respiratory musculature activity. Mechanics of respiration should be addressed by normalizing segmental mobility in the thoracic cage. Correction of hyoid position may include evaluation and treatment of the craniomandibular complex.

Treatment strategies should be aimed toward reducing the abnormal loads impacting the body by taking away as many of the undesirable adaptive factors as possible. Treatment should consist of strategies that enhance and improve normal neuromusculoskeletal control. Along the way, symptoms should be treated while making sure that nothing is being done to add further to the burden the system.

EVALUATION OF THE MECHANICS OF RESPIRATION

Evaluation of the mechanics of respiration and its correlation to sleep-related breathing disorders should become a standard part of patient evaluation in the rehabilitation setting. This can certainly be undertaken by therapists from different clinical disciplines, including physical therapy, occupational therapy, speech and language pathology, and respiratory therapy. The advantage that rehabilitation clinicians have is the amount of time that is spent with the patient over a period of weeks or months. Normally, a physician or dentist sees a patient for an office visit once or twice a year unless the patient has on ongoing medical or dental condition that requires closer monitoring. Even then, the amount of contact time that a rehabilitation professional has with a patient is significantly greater; therefore, the burden of recognizing the manifestations and consequences of disordered sleep should naturally be part of the clinical knowledge of rehabilitation providers. This section will provide some recommendations for screening of a patient suspected of having dysfunction in the mechanics of respiration, especially as they may relate to sleep-related breathing disorders.

Clinical Observation of Respiration

First, caution should be exercised to ensure that the patient does not have serious respiratory or other systemic disease before undertaking efforts to treat them for mechanical dysfunction. A discussion of respiratory pathology is outside the scope of this book, but it is recommended that clinicians familiarize themselves with signs of serious disease and send any patient suspected of having undiagnosed pulmonary disease for medical evaluation. The presence of diagnosed pulmonary disease is not necessarily a contraindication for treatment of mechanical restrictions and dysfunction. In fact, it may allow the patient to maximize available pulmonary function.

Resting respiratory rate should be observed. The normal adult range is 10 to 14 breaths per minute. Respiratory rate that is significantly higher than 10 to 14 may be related to respiratory distress, systemic disease, or anxiety. Increased respiratory rate may be adopted to blow off accumulating CO_2 and in an attempt to increase O_2 saturation.

It should be noted whether the patient is a nose breather or a mouth breather. Nasal congestion can be a significant problem that increases respiratory effort during wakefulness and sleep because of the increased resistance to air flow. Chronic nasal congestion may be a symptom of upper respiratory infection, allergies, sinus disorders, or structural disorders in the nasal passages or sinuses and should be evaluated by a physician. Mouth breathing, especially when it is chronic or found in children, can create myriad

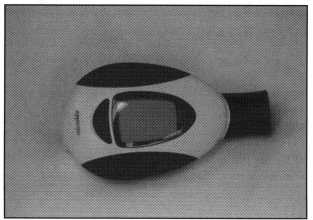

Figure 27-14. Peak expiratory flow spirometer. (Reprinted with permission from CORE Services, Inc.)

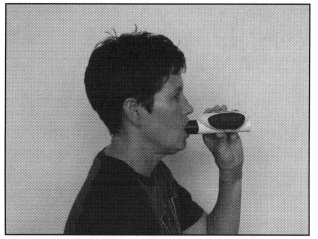

Figure 27-15. Patient blowing into a spirometer to determine peak expiratory flow rate. This test can be used to determine "lung power." It can also be used as a measure of clinical progress in a treatment program. (Reprinted with permission from L. Brinkman.)

problems in craniofacial and craniomandibular dysfunction (see Chapter 25).

The resting respiratory pattern should be noted. Is respiration effortless, or is there evidence of accessory muscle use or upper chest hyperinflation? Does the patient display frequent sighs or yawning, throat clearing, or air gulping? These may be signs of feeling air-starved. Does the patient appear to hold his or her breath for periods of time? Is there evidence of abdominal splinting? Does the respiratory pattern seem chaotic or erratic? Respiratory pattern should be observed with the patient lying prone with the face in a cutout. A normal deep inspiration pattern in this position appears to begin at the sacrum and progresses up the thorax to the neck. In an individual with mechanical respiratory dysfunction, particularly that involving segmental limitations in the thoracic cage, the thoracic spine will tend to rise as a block and the ribs will appear to move as a shield. Often there is very little movement above the lower third of the thoracic region. The respiratory pattern should be observed in sitting and in supine. Evidence of increased accessory respiratory muscle function, such as SCMs, upper trapezius, levator scapulae, and scalenes should be noted. These muscles may also be sites of trigger point activity. This may occur as a result of paradoxical breathing, also known as *upper-chest breathing*. In this respiratory pattern, as described by Travel and Simons, the diaphragm changes function to act as a muscle of exhalation and the chest musculature acts as during inspiration. This action does not allow for proper ventilation so the accessory respiratory musculature must overwork to increase tidal volume.[23]

The patient should be observed for postural tension or malalignment. Forward head posture should be measured and can be easily done with a simple grid that can measure the amount of forward displacement of the head on the axial skeleton. This can be measured and photographed and used as a gauge of progress. The face and jaw should be observed for increased tension, tremor, or twitches and

facial asymmetry. It is a good idea to obtain photos of the frontal and sagittal view of the face in order to better identify facial asymmetry. An additional facial view that is helpful in identifying facial asymmetry, particularly when treating a temporomandibular or cranial dysfunction that can be a part of upper airway dysfunction, is one taken while the patient lies supine and the photographer is positioned above the head.

The patient should also be observed for abnormalities of the chest wall, which may include pectus carinatum or pectus excavatum. Kyphosis, scoliosis, or kyphoscoliosis should be noted. Adaptive changes in the upper thoracic or shoulder or scapular musculature should be noted, including elevated or rounded shoulders or protracted scapulae.

Several breathing function tests can be performed in the standard clinical setting. These include the breath-holding test and peak expiratory flow rate. Although there are no standardized data regarding the amount of time an adult should be able to hold his or her breath, one source suggests that inability to hold the breath for 30 seconds is a sign of chronic hyperventilation on hyperinflation. Another test that is easy to perform in a normal clinical setting is peak expiratory flow rate (Figure 27-14). This is performed with an inexpensive instrument that measures maximum forced expiratory flow following a maximum effort inspiration (Figure 27-15). It measures the elasticity of the lungs and air flow resistance. In an individual who has dysfunction in the mechanical respiratory apparatus, this can quantify chronic air flow limitations or "lung power." It can also be used as a measure of clinical progress in a treatment program. Again, caution should be used in interpreting results. Values should be used as a general guide to treatment rather than as a diagnostic tool. In the event of significant loss of expiratory function, the patient

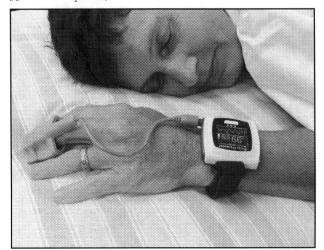

Figure 27-16. Pulse oximeter. (Reprinted with permission from L. Brinkman.)

should be referred to his or her primary care physician for further evaluation.

Pulse oximetry is a noninvasive method of accurately monitoring O_2 saturation that was developed in the 1940s. The device uses a pulsating red and infrared light that passes through the vascular bed usually in the fingertip or ear lobe (Figure 27-16). A microprocessor on the device measures the changing absorbance of the two different wavelengths as they pass through pulsating arterial blood. It has been shown to be reasonably accurate compared to obtaining actual arterial blood gasses above 75% O_2 saturation.[24] Normal resting oxygen saturation as measured by a pulse oximeter is 95% to 98%. Oxygen desaturation is considered to be a 4% drop in level. Caution should be exercised in using this device, since certain conditions can lead to an inaccurate reading, such as hypotension, anemia, hypervolemia, peripheral vascular disease, and some vasopressor medications. Stains on the fingers, such as nicotine stains and some nail polish, can also lead to inaccurate readings.[25] Monitoring O_2 saturation during breathing retraining can be used as a safety cross-check device if the patient has cardiovascular or pulmonary disease. It can offer reassurance to a patient who may have anxiety related to breathlessness that is associated with mechanical respiratory dysfunction. It is important to note hypoxemia, because it is evidence of decreased respiratory function, and decreased respiratory function in the daytime is associated with increased prevalence of sleep-related breathing disorders. Sleep-related breathing disorders that are associated with dysfunctional mechanics of respiration, particularly suboptimal diaphragmatic function, are characterized by increased frequency of arousals, increased wake time after sleep onset, and decreased REM sleep on polysomnography.

It is beyond the scope of this chapter to describe evaluation techniques for the thoracic cage, cervical spine,

and diaphragm. There are a number of very complete textbooks readily available that can guide the reader in this area, particularly manual therapy and osteopathic books. Regardless of the methodology, mobility and alignment of the thoracic spine and rib cage and the cervical spine should be evaluated. Deficits should be noted, and treatment plans should include breathing retraining as appropriate. This is particularly important if evidence of a mechanical respiratory dysfunction is present and the patient displays manifestations or consequences of disordered sleep.

How Can Dysfunctional Respiratory Mechanics Contribute to Sleep Dysfunction?

The likelihood of sleep-related hypoventilation is greater in individuals with daytime hypoxemia and hypercapnea. If an individual has stiffness in the thoracic cage that increases resistance to expansion that is necessary to inhale, the individual may have decreased vital capacity. Normal effort will not produce enough force to overcome the movement restriction, so accessory respiratory musculature will be recruited in order to have sufficient air exchange. Increased accessory muscle activity will cause these muscles to overwork and lead to compensatory changes, including forward head posture and discoordination of the respiratory apparatus. It may lead to or be caused by suboptimal ZOA of the diaphragm. Suboptimal diaphragmatic function, particularly on the left, will cause overstretching and weakness in the opposing abdominal musculature. It can lead to postural and fascial biases that occur as adaptive changes in other regions of the body, which may tend to habituate the compensatory movement pattern. The overall effect of this is suboptimal respiratory function and increased effort required for sufficient air exchange. The stereotypic postures of sleep also increase resistance in the upper airway. This combined increased resistance of the upper airway, discoordination of the diaphragm, and stiffness of the thoracic cage is likely to contribute to sleep-related breathing disorders. When overall tone is decreased during NREM sleep and when respiration becomes unstable during REM sleep, the added workload needed to overcome dysfunction in the mechanics of respiration may be a significant contributing factor to the development of apnea and hypopnea during sleep. Although there have not been any specific studies, it is reasonable to consider that effective treatment of the mechanics of respiration that improve daytime respiratory function will have a positive effect on sleep-related breathing disorders.

SUMMARY

From the previous description of the mechanics of the thoracic cage, postural habits, and the function of the diaphragm and other muscles of respiration, it is clear that the coordination of normal breathing involves a well-choreographed pattern of movement. Dysfunction in a single segment of this apparatus can lead to a cascade of compensatory movements that can end in disturbance of respiration. Diminished respiratory efficiency during wakefulness very likely will result in a sleep-related breathing disorder. This is an important area in which the rehabilitation professional can have a substantial impact on improving respiratory function. Improvements in respiratory function during daytime wakefulness are likely translated into improved effective ventilation during sleep. With that in mind, it is important to understand how to identify areas of restriction and dysfunction in the mechanics of the respiratory apparatus. All patients breathe and all patients sleep, and these 2 areas of function are often linked. Any patient who reports nonrestorative sleep, sleep disruption, or snoring should also be carefully observed for signs of dysfunction in respiratory mechanics. If patients show manifestations of disordered sleep or have consequences that may be related to disordered sleep, they should be observed for signs of dysfunction in respiratory mechanics. These dysfunctions can then be addressed in a patient's overall treatment.

REFERENCES

1. Zink JG, Lawson W. An osteopathic structural examination and functional interpretation of the soma. *Osteopathic Annals.* 1979;7:12-19.
2. Pope RE. The common compensatory pattern. Available at: http://erikdalton.com/article_pdfs/articleCCPThesis.pdf. Accessed August 6, 2012.
3. Somatics. Short right leg syndrome. Available at: hhttp://www.somatics.de/ShortRightLeg1.pdf. Accessed October 2, 2013.
4. Hruska R. *Postural Respiration.* [lecture notes]. Tulsa, OK: Postural Restoration Institute; 2007.
5. Chaitow L, Bradley D, Gilbert C. *Multidisciplinary Approaches to Breathing Pattern Disorders.* New York, NY: Churchill Livingstone; 2002.
6. Boyle KP, Olinick J, Lewis C. The value of blowing up a balloon. *N Am J Sports Phys Ther.* 2010;5(3):179-188.
7. Kolar P, Neuwirth J, Sanda J, et al. Analysis of diaphragm movement during tidal breathing and during its activation while breath holding using MRI synchronized with spirometry. *Physiol Res.* 2009;58:383-392.
8. Hodges PW, Jutler JE, McKenzie DK, Gandevia SC. Contraction of the human diaphragm during rapid postural adjustments. *J Physiol.* 1997;505:539-548.
9. Kolar P, Sulc J, Kyncl M, et al. Stabilizing function of the diaphragm: dynamic MRI and synchronized spirometric assessment. Available at: http://www.rehabps.com/REHABILITATION/Literature_Research_files/Stabil%20Function%20Diaphragm.pdf. Accessed August 6, 2012.
10. Mead J. Functional significance of the area of apposition of diaphragm to rib cage. *Am Rev Respir Dis.* 1979;119(suppl):31-32.
11. Sperry RW. Roger Sperry's Brain Research – Mind in the driver's seat – Science not in the traditional sense of reducing everything including the human psyche to quantum mechanics – A new philosophy and a new world view. Kannan A (ed). *Bull Theosophy Sci Study Grp-India.* 1988;26(3-4):27-28.
12. Von Euler C. The role of proprioceptive afferents in the control of respiratory muscles. *Acta Neurobiol Exp.* 1973;33:329-341.
13. Jammes Y, Speck DF. Respiratory control by diaphragmatic and respiratory muscle afferents. In: Dempsey JA, Pack AI, eds. *Regulation of Breathing.* 2nd ed. New York, NY: Marcel Dekker; 1995:543-582.
14. Hruska R. *Myokinematics.* [lecture notes]. St. Louis, MO: Postural Restoration Institute; 2008.
15. Kapandji IA. *The Physiology of the Joints: The Trunk and the Vertebral Column.* (Vol 3, 2nd Ed.) London, UK: Churchill Livingstone; 1974. pp 256.
16. Sato H, Ohashi J, Owanga K, et al. Endurance time and fatigue in static contractions. *J Hum Ergon.* 1984;3:147-154.
17. Cailliet R. *Pain: Mechanisms and Management.* Philadelphia, PA: FA Davis; 1993.
18. Lewit K. Relation of faulty respiration to posture. *J Am Osteopath Assoc.* 1980;79:525-529.
19. Andriacchi T, Schultx A, Belytschko T, et al. A model for studies of mechanical interactions between the human spine and rib cage. *J Biomech.* 1974;7:497-507.
20. Panjabi MM, Brand RA, White AA. Mechanical properties of the human thoracic spine. *J Bone Joint Surg.* 1976;58:642-652.
21. Lee D. Biomechanics of the thorax: a clinical model of in vivo function. *J Man Manip Ther.* 1993;1:13-21.
22. Janda V. Introduction to functional pathology of the motor system. Paper presented at: Seventh Commonwealth and International Conference on Sport. Glasgow, UK; 1982.
23. Travell J, Simons D. *Myofascial Pain and Dysfunction.* Vol 2. Baltimore, MD: Williams & Wilkins; 1992.
24. Durbin CG. Monitoring gas exchange. *Respir Care.* 1994;39:123-137.
25. Millikan GA. The oximeter: an instrument for measuring continuously oxygen-saturation of arterial blood in man. *Rev Sci Instrum.* 1942;13:434-444.

28

Practical Issues for the Rehabilitation Professional

Julie M. Hereford, PT, DPT

GENERAL REVIEW OF SLEEP AND REHABILITATION

Sleep occupies one third of human life. It has been shown to be vital to mental and physical health. The quality and quantity of sleep affect almost every physiological and psychological process. Changes in physiological or psychological processes can either interfere with sleep or enhance it. Disordered sleep has been shown to result in a variety of dysfunctions, including problems with neurocognitive function, and it may also contribute to the development of new illness or exacerbation of existing illness.

This text has given an overview of the basic science of sleep. It has described the biology of sleep, which consists of 2 distinct states—non-rapid eye movement (NREM) and rapid eye movement (REM) sleep. Each sleep state is composed of a constellation of neurological and physiological activity that usually occurs in a predictable pattern. NREM and REM sleep occur cyclically throughout the night, beginning with NREM sleep. As a general rule, a sleep cycle lasts approximately 90 to 110 minutes in an adult and is repeated at least 3 times in a normal night's sleep. As sleep progresses across the night, the amount of NREM sleep decreases and the amount of REM sleep increases. Also described in this book is a current understanding of how sleep is actively generated and maintained by the discharge and inhibition of specific neurons in distinct regions and nuclei of the brain (Table 28-1).

Particular physiological functions have been linked to the sleep–wake cycle (Table 28-2). For example, certain hormone secretions occur almost exclusively during specific sleep stages. Growth hormone is secreted during NREM stage 3 and 4 sleep, also known as slow-wave sleep or restorative sleep. Prolactin secretion peaks later during NREM stage 4 sleep. Gonadotropin secretion occurs predominantly during sleep in puberty. Secretion of thyroid-stimulating hormone peaks in the evening and is inhibited during sleep.

Theories regarding the possible functions of sleep were discussed in the basic science section of this book and were elaborated upon throughout the rest of the book, particularly as sleep relates to rehabilitative functions. Evidence does not support some of the early and perhaps commonly held theories regarding the function of sleep. For example, the energy conservation theory seems unlikely because though energy is conserved during sleep, it is about the same amount of energy that would be conserved by an animal that is resting quietly while remaining vigilant to predators. The restoration and recovery theory seems to have some merit, but protein synthesis actually increases rather than decrease during sleep, so it does not seem to be a comprehensive theory.

All mammals sleep and all mammals have NREM and REM sleep. Small mammals may sleep up to 20 hours a day and most large mammals sleep less, often less than 5 hours per day. Birds experience rapid cycling between NREM and REM sleep, which is thought to be an adaptive mechanism to allow them to fly long distances or perch while sleeping. Reptiles only exhibit NREM sleep, and amphibians and fish have rest–activity cycles but do not display electroencephalogram activity consistent with NREM and REM sleep.

Hereford JM. *Sleep and Rehabilitation:*
A Guide for Health Professionals (pp 341-351).

Table 28-1.

Electroencephalogram, Electrooculogram, and Electromyogram Activity During a Normal Sleep Cycle

	Non-rapid Eye Movement Sleep	Tonic Rapid Eye Movement Sleep	Phasic Rapid Eye Movement Sleep
EEG	N_1: low voltage, mixed frequency N_2: low voltage, 12- to 14-Hz spindles, K-complexes N_3: >50% delta waves (0.5–2 Hz) N_4: <50% delta	Low voltage, mixed frequency	Low voltage, mixed frequency
EOG	Slow rolling	Isolated REM	Clusters of REM
EMG	Moderate activity	Atonia in most skeletal muscles	Atonia plus myoclonic twitches

Table 28-2.

Changes in Physiological Activity During a Normal Sleep Cycle

	Non-rapid Eye Movement Versus Wake	Tonic Rapid Eye Movement Versus Non-rapid Eye Movement	Phasic Rapid Eye Movement Versus Tonic Rapid Eye Movement
Cerebral activity	Decrease	Increase	Further increase
Heart rate	Slows	Same	Increase, variable
Blood pressure	Decrease	Same	Increase, variable
Cerebral blood flow	Same	Increase	Further increase
Respiration	Decrease	Increase, variable	Further increase, variable
Airway resistance	Further increase	Increase, variable	Increase, variable

Sleep varies across the life span. Sleep can first be identified in fetal life at approximately 23 weeks of gestation. Over 80% of fetal sleep is spent in REM sleep. Newborn infants sleep approximately 16 to 18 hours per 24-hour period. Young children under the age of 5 generally sleep 10 to 12 hours per 24-hour period. Prepubescent children sleep 8 to 9 hours per day, but the remarkable energy demands of puberty require increased sleep during the mid-teen years. Unfortunately, the average teenager tends to stay up late because of the natural drift of the circadian clock, but the demands of the school day usually require teenagers to awaken early. Thus, many of today's teenagers are chronically sleep deprived. The consequences of chronic sleep deprivation in this age group can be substantial and can set up lifelong disordered sleep. Generally, this chronically sleep-deprived group does not perform as well in school or athletics as their well-rested counterparts. Adults require 7 to 9 hours of sleep and, contrary to popular belief, older adults require the same amount of sleep but generally have more difficulty attaining it because of the increased propensity toward sleep fragmentation as one ages. The decrease in nocturnal sleep often seen in older adults is sometimes replaced with daytime napping. The distribution of NREM sleep gradually declines as an individual ages, whereas the amount of REM sleep remains the same, consisting of approximately 20% to 25% of total sleep time from preteen years to old age.

Dreams occur in all stages of sleep and the majority of dreams are mundane, although some can be truly bizarre. The exact function of dreams is not clearly understood, but there is some evidence that dreams reflect the emotional state and personality of the dreamer. Contrary to commonly held beliefs, external stimuli during wakefulness are not readily incorporated into dreams.

Initiation and maintenance of sleep and wakefulness is regulated by particular regions and nuclei in the brain. Wakefulness depends principally upon the functioning of the reticular activating system in the brain stem. NREM is promoted by areas in the basal forebrain, whereas REM sleep depends upon the dorsolateral pontine tegmentum.

Wakefulness depends upon cortical noradrenaline as well as dopamine and acetylcholine from brain stem neurons. NREM sleep is maintained by gamma-aminobutyric acid (GABA) from neurons in the basal forebrain. REM sleep is initiated by acetylcholine that activates pontine neurons.

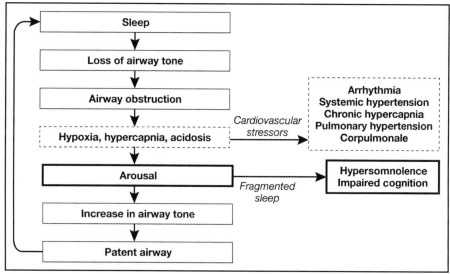

Figure 28-1. Consequences of sleep-related breathing disorder.

Circadian regulation of sleep and wakefulness is carried out by the suprachiasmatic nucleus. The timing of sleep, but not the quantity of sleep, is regulated by this circadian clock. In some free-running time experiments, the circadian clock was seen to drift toward a 25-hour day; however, that research has come under some question. The circadian clock regulates many physiological processes that interact with sleep, including temperature regulation. Gradual degeneration of the suprachiasmatic nucleus that may occur with normal aging is thought to play a role in the increased fragmentation of sleep that often occurs in older adults.

The manifestations and consequences of disordered sleep have been discussed (Figure 28-1). Because of the amount of patient contact, the rehabilitation professional is in a unique position to recognize these and educate the patient and refer them for appropriate evaluation. This text also has provided a review of common techniques for evaluation of sleep. Common abnormalities often encountered during polysomnography that help identify disordered sleep were reviewed. A number of primary sleep disorders were identified, including narcolepsy, characterized by irresistible sleep attacks during the day, and may also involve cataplexy, sleep paralysis, and hypnagogic hallucinations. Parasomnias, or abnormal movements that occur during sleep, including restless leg/legs syndrome, periodic limb movement syndrome, and REM sleep behavior disorder, were discussed.

Sleep-related breathing disorders were examined at length. The contribution of these disorders to excessive daytime sleepiness and decreased neurocognitive and physical performance during the day can be significant. This may translate directly to the rehabilitation setting, in which the manifestations or consequences of disordered sleep can interfere with a patient's ability to fully engage in, and gain maximum benefit from, a rehabilitation program. Mechanical dysfunction in the respiratory apparatus is not commonly considered in sleep medicine, but it is reasonable to consider its contribution to sleep-related breathing disorders. Increased resistance to air flow from a stiff thorax or increased utilization of accessory respiratory musculature may contribute to, or be a result of, a loss of the zone of apposition and of strength in the diaphragm. This reduces the efficiency of the respiratory apparatus while awake. Because sleep reduces overall muscle tone, dysfunctional breathing may be further compromised by the changes in respiratory function that are characteristic of sleep, especially REM sleep. Further, increased accessory respiratory muscle activity may foster the forward head posture known to change the architecture of the upper airway and may additionally contribute to increase resistance during sleep. This is an area that rehabilitation clinicians may impact directly by proper evaluation and application of manual techniques and therapeutic exercise to improve the mechanics of respiration.

Increased resistance in the upper airway is implicated in the occurrence of sleep-related breathing disorders. Part of this increased resistance may be related to the shape and function of the mouth and jaw (Figure 28-2). The Mallampati Scale is often used to qualify the degree of narrowing of the oropharynx. Narrowing may be caused by increased tongue volume, elevated tongue posture, and enlarged tonsilar or adenoid tissue. Consideration of the structure and function of the temporomandibular joint and dental component of the airway is also important. It is recommended that rehabilitation professionals develop a good working relationship with a dentist who specializes in treatment of temporomandibular joint dysfunction and understands its importance in the application of oral appliances designed to improve upper airway function during sleep. Failure to properly position the jaw joint or treat an underlying temporomandibular dysfunction may contribute to increased pain and loss of function.

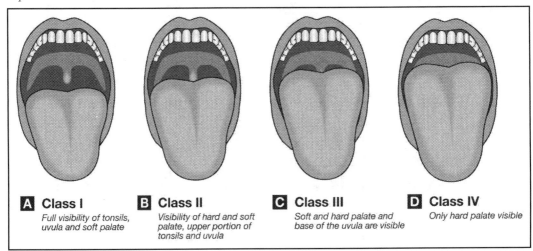

A **Class I**
Full visibility of tonsils, uvula and soft palate

B **Class II**
Visibility of hard and soft palate, upper portion of tonsils and uvula

C **Class III**
Soft and hard palate and base of the uvula are visible

D **Class IV**
Only hard palate visible

Figure 28-2. Mallampati Scale.

Sleep plays a significant role in episodic and procedural memory consolidation and in perceptual memory encoding. Multiple studies have shown that sleep enhances memory and learning and that it improves physical performance, particularly athletic performance. There is ample evidence offered in this book that sleep is important in normal brain growth and development. Sleep is involved in programming innate behavior and in processing emotions.

It is suggested that this evidence could be extrapolated to the practice of rehabilitation and therapeutic exercise to improve performance and patient outcomes. It is also suggested that sleep deprivation and sleep fragmentation, in the manner that occurs in sleep disorders, particularly sleep-related breathing disorders, may interfere with tissue healing and nerve regeneration. Sleep deprivation, like the one occurring with sleep fragmentation, has been shown to interfere with memory consolidation and to disrupt performance of physical activities including decreased precision, power, speed, and endurance. Conversely, sleep extension has been shown to improve performance in each of these areas. Therefore, it is reasonable to consider sleep as an essential component of any rehabilitation program. Clinicians should be able to identify the manifestations and consequences of disordered sleep in their patients.

The rehabilitation professional should understand when a patient should be referred for further evaluation of a potential sleep disorder. It is also important to have familiarity with treatments available to improve sleep, including CPAP, oral appliance therapy, neurofeedback, and medication. The clinician should also be able to educate the patient regarding sleep issues including techniques that may improve sleep such as good sleep hygiene (Table 28-3).

ASSESSMENT TOOLS

The remainder of this chapter offers some commonly used tools to assist the clinician in identifying a patient with a sleep disorder that is interfering in daytime function. All of these tools do not directly assess sleep. Some of the suggested tools are used to measure related factors, such as fatigue, oropharynx restrictions, and pain. These factors may be contributors to disordered sleep and may help the clinician to determine the interrelationships which help to inform the treatment plan. Included are a number of tools that have been validated and have been found reliable. The Stanford Sleepiness Scale may be used to identify excessive daytime sleepiness.[1] Information gathered with this tool can be gathered in a week-long recording chart that can be used in conjunction with the scoring method of the scale to help identify patterns of alertness. This information can help with activity planning and may be helpful in guiding the rehabilitation process. The Epworth Sleepiness Scale, which is readily available online, is often used to identify excessive daytime sleepiness.[2]

A visual analogue scale is a tool used to measure a characteristic or attitude that ranges across a continuum and cannot be easily measured. This allows for measurement of pain values that are experienced as continuous and that do not take a discrete jump in degree as a numeric or descriptive system might. The patient marks a point on the line that represents his or her current perception of his or her pain level. The visual analogue scale score is determined by measuring from the left end of a 100-mm line to the point indicated by the patient. This information may be combined with data collected regarding sleep to better inform treatment planning.[3]

Table 28-3.

Dos and Don'ts of Sleep Hygiene[a]

Do	Don't
Go to bed at the same time each day	Exercise just before bed
Get up at the same time each day	Engage in stimulating activity before bed
Get regular exercise—stretching and aerobic	Have caffeine in the evening
Get regular exposure to sunlight	Read or watch TV in bed
Keep bedroom temperature comfortable	Use alcohol to help go to sleep
Keep bedroom quiet during sleep	Go to bed too hungry or too full
Keep bedroom dark	Take another person's sleeping pills
Take medication as directed	Take over-the-counter sleeping pills
Use relaxation exercises	Take daytime naps
Keep feet and hands warm	Command yourself to sleep

[a]If you lie awake for more than 20 to 30 minutes, get up and go to a different room or different part of the bedroom, participate in a quiet activity such as non-stimulating reading or television, and return to bed when sleepy. Do this as many times during the night as needed.

The Epworth Sleepiness Scale

The Epworth Sleepiness Scale is a general measurement of an individual's perceived level of sleepiness. It is composed of a description of 8 situations and asks the respondent to use a number scale to describe the level of sleepiness in each situation. A quantitative measure of sleepiness is derived from the answers. A copy of the scale can be found at http://www.stanford.edu/~dement/epworth.html.

McGill Pain Questionnaire

The McGill Pain Questionnaire[4] is a pain rating scale consisting primarily of 3 major classes of word descriptions (sensory, affective, and evaluative) that are used by respondents to describe their subjective pain experience. It also contains an intensity scale and other items to determine additional aspects of the pain. The full McGill Pain Questionnaire and the short form are available online.[5,6]

Pain Disability Index

The Pain Disability Index (see Table 20-2) is an easy-to-administer, 7-item tool that is used to help patients measure the degree to which chronic pain is interfering with daily life.[7] This tool, combined with information gathered from sleep or fatigue measurement tools, can be used to quantify and qualify the interaction between sleep and pain. It may also be used to measure patient status over time.

Stanford Sleepiness Scale

The Stanford Sleepiness Scale (see Table 20-3) is a quick way to measure sleepiness and alertness. It is extremely easy to use and can be tracked at intervals over a week's time to determine optimal alertness. This may guide treatment planning.

Fatigue Severity Scale

Because sleepiness and fatigue are 2 different qualities that have different meanings in the clinical setting, it is important to distinguish between the two. The Fatigue Severity Scale (Table 28-4)[8] is a tool used to measure the impact that fatigue has on daily living. Often, for example, individuals with fibromyalgia may complain of fatigue, but not complain of or exhibit symptoms of excessive daytime sleepiness.

Mallampati Scale

The Mallampati grading system[9] to describe the size of the oropharynx is commonly used as a diagnostic and communication tool for those evaluating a patient's airway (see Figure 28-2). This examination asks the clinician to attempt to visualize 4 normally visualized structures: the soft palate, hard palate, uvula, and pharyngeal tonsils. Patients who present with an indistinctly visible posterior pharyngeal wall (class III and IV Mallampati) will have a higher predisposition toward a compromised airway and a tendency for obstructive sleep apnea.

Portable Recording Pulse Oximetry

Use of a recording pulse oximeter (Figure 28-3) is another tool that can help to identify the presence of a sleep disorder. This simple device, which indirectly measures the amount of oxygen in the blood, can be given to a patient to use over several nights. Data regarding the level of oxygen saturation during sleep are stored in the device and can be downloaded to a computer. This information may be used clinically to help identify a patient who requires further evaluation. If the patient exhibits multiple episodes of oxygen desaturation as measured by a portable recording pulse oximeter, the patient should be referred for more thorough sleep evaluation.

Table 28-4.

Fatigue Severity Scale[a]

The Fatigue Severity Scale is a method of evaluating the impact of fatigue on an individual. This is a short questionnaire that requires the individual to rate the level of fatigue. The Fatigue Severity Scale contains 9 statements that rate the severity of fatigue symptoms. Responses should rate symptoms based upon the level of fatigue over the past week. It is important to indicate a response to each question.

- 1 = strong disagreement
- 7 = strong agreement

During the past week, I have found that:	Disagree		→			Agree	
1. My motivation is lower when I am fatigued.	1	2	3	4	5	6	7
2. Exercise brings on my fatigue.	1	2	3	4	5	6	7
3. I am easily fatigued.	1	2	3	4	5	6	7
4. Fatigue interferes with my physical functioning.	1	2	3	4	5	6	7
5. Fatigue causes frequent problems for me.	1	2	3	4	5	6	7
6. My fatigue prevents sustained physical functioning.	1	2	3	4	5	6	7
7. Fatigue interferes with carrying out certain duties and responsibilities.	1	2	3	4	5	6	7
8. Fatigue is among my 3 most disabling symptoms	1	2	3	4	5	6	7
9. Fatigue interferes with my work, family, or social life.	1	2	3	4	5	6	7
Total Score:							

[a]Scoring: < 36 suggests that fatigue is not a primary symptom; > 36 suggests that fatigue is a significant factor and should be evaluated by a physician.

THERAPEUTIC EXERCISE TO IMPROVE MECHANICAL RESPIRATORY FUNCTION

Respiratory dysfunction that occurs during the day because of faulty postural alignment including forward head posture, muscular weakness, and/or asymmetry, paradoxical breathing pattern or hyperinflation will increase the resistance in the airway during sleep when compensatory mechanisms are less effective. This can be a contributing factor in sleep-related breathing disorder. Individuals who have decreased ventilation that results in hypoxemia and hypercapnea during the day have respiratory compromise during sleep. With proper evaluation and therapeutic intervention of the mechanics of respiration and postural control, rehabilitation clinicians may be able to improve respiratory function during both wakefulness and sleep.

If an individual is not able to easily and fully exhale at rest, inhalation will also be difficult because of imbalance between the diaphragm and the abdominal oblique muscles.[10] If the diaphragm is incapable of normal action because of improper positioning, it may cause the lower rib cage to flare. This causes a change in function of the abdominal oblique musculature because of stretch weakness. Therefore it is not able to provide proper opposition to the diaphragm and will contribute to the loss of apposition of the diaphragm against the inner thoracic cage. This, in turn, decreases the mechanical efficiency of the diaphragm and therefore decreases its ability to provide sufficient ventilation. Because of the loss of diaphragmatic action, accessory respiratory musculature must activate to provide proper ventilation. This musculature includes the scalenes, upper trapezius, levator scapulae, and sternocleidomastoid, among others.

When the upper trapezius are hyperactive during normal activities of daily living, the levator scapulae and sternocleidomastoid become agonists and the primary musculature of respiration, acting as upper cervical extenders, assisting in exhalation, because of postural alignment changes, and are activated during mandibular opening. They thus contribute to respiratory dysfunction and may be implicated in mechanical temporomandibular dysfunction.[11,12]

There are many exercise techniques that may be implemented to improve the mechanics of respiration. Figures 28-3 to 28-9 offer several examples of these. These exercises are part of a program designed to address faulty respiratory mechanics developed by Ron Hruska of the Postural Respiration Institute. Most of the examples given here are specifically used to promote improved diaphragmatic function by optimizing the zone of apposition. This allows the

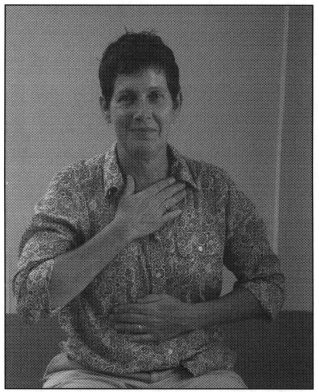

Figure 28-3. Breathing exercise. In normal respiration, the patient should feel expansion of the diaphragm before expansion of the upper chest during inspiration and the reverse pattern during expiration. In paradoxical breathing, the upper chest may expand prior to or simultaneously with diaphragmatic movement. (Reprinted with permission from L. Brinkman.)

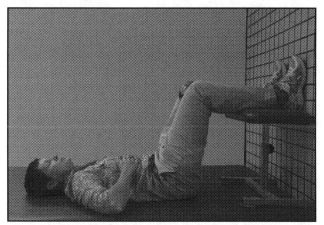

Figure 28-5. A 90/90 hip-lift exercise. Once the patient is able to establish and maintain a normal coordinated breathing pattern, he or she should begin to incorporate more complex movements while maintaining a normal diaphragmatic respiratory pattern. In this exercise, the patient is positioned in supine with legs elevated so that the hips and knees are at 90 degrees. A 4- to 6-inch ball is placed between the knees and the patient compresses the ball, thus engaging hip adductor musculature. This is done to inhibit hip adductors. Lower legs are pressed down onto the stool to engage the hamstrings and the patient is coached to perform a posterior pelvic tilt to inhibit the back extensors. Hands are placed on the lower rib cage to remind the patient to perform diaphragmatic respiration. Special attention should be paid to maintaining a relaxed state in the anterior cervical musculature. (Reprinted with permission from L. Brinkman.)

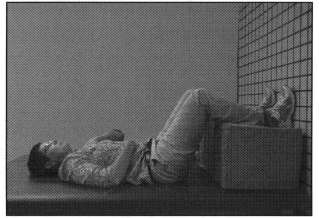

Figure 28-4. Breathing exercise. The patient is positioned in supine with legs supported by a bolster. This helps to inhibit hip flexor musculature from stabilizing the lower thoracic spine and thus assisting in a dysfunctional respiratory pattern. One hand is placed on the abdomen and the other hand on the upper chest. Normal respiratory pattern involves expansion of the diaphragm and abdomen prior to expansion of the upper chest during inspiration. During expiration, the chest should relax prior to the diaphragm and abdomen. The anterior cervical musculature should be quiet throughout this breathing exercise. (Reprinted with permission from L. Brinkman.)

diaphragm to act as a primary muscle of respiration rather than being utilized as a spinal stabilizer (see Chapter 27).

Bias of accessory respiratory musculature is a contributing factor in the development of forward head posture. Forward head posture, in turn, increases the bias toward use of accessory respiratory musculature and can contribute to dysfunction of the diaphragm, particularly on the left side. This then contributes to weakening of the abdominal oblique musculature, which is then less able to oppose the action of the diaphragm. In addition, this can lead to tightness in the latissimus dorsi and pectoralis major musculature.

In order to correct this complex mechanical dysfunction, correction of forward head posture, reestablishment of the zone of apposition of the diaphragm, stretching of the latissimus dorsi and pectoral musculature, and strengthening of the abdominal musculature must occur. Strengthening of the abdominal musculature must be accomplished without engaging the upper trapezius or anterior cervical musculature. Figures 28-4 through 28-9 are examples of therapeutic exercises that are helpful in reestablishing a coordinated diaphragmatic respiratory pattern without involving accessory respiratory musculature. The therapeutic exercises presented are not intended to be an exhaustive list but suggestions of activities that can work to improve normal respiratory pattern. Any treatment program designed to improve respiratory pattern should consider the importance of reestablishing the diaphragmatic zone of apposition, increasing strength of abdominal oblique musculature to oppose the diaphragm, and inhibiting cervical accessory respiratory musculature.

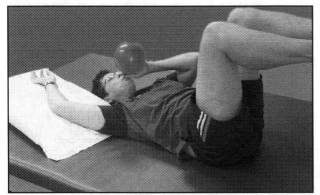

Figure 28-6. A 90/90 while blowing into a balloon. In this exercise, the patient uses a balloon to apply some resistance to diaphragmatic activity in order to strengthen it and to improve coordinated function. The patient is positioned in supine with feet on the wall so that the hips and knees are bent to 90 degrees. In this example, the right arm is positioned above the head and a balloon is held in the opposite hand. The patient performs a posterior pelvic tilt, keeping the low back flat during the entire exercise. The patient inhales through the nose and slowly blows out into the balloon. The patient pauses for 3 seconds with the tongue on the roof of the mouth to prevent air flow out of the balloon. Without pinching the neck of the balloon, the patient takes another breath in through the nose and then slowly blows out again, stabilizing the balloon with the hand. It is important that the patient does not strain the anterior neck or cheeks as he or she blows into the balloon. This technique is repeated for 4 breaths and then the balloon is removed and the patient relaxes completely. (Reprinted with permission from L. Brinkman.)

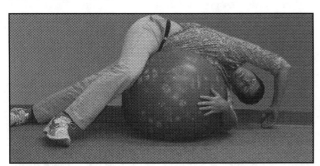

Figure 28-8. Side bending over a ball. This exercise allows approximation of the left lateral thoracoabdominal wall and compression of the left lower rib cage. Because the left leaflet of the diaphragm is the most likely to lose its zone of apposition, this activity assists in mechanical function of the left side of the diaphragm. It also stretches the right latissimus dorsi and lateral thoracoabdominal wall. (Reprinted with permission from L. Brinkman.)

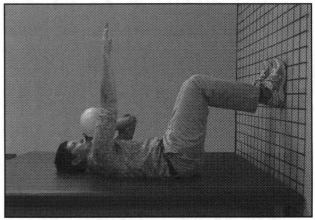

Figure 28-7. Breathing exercise while blowing up a balloon. This is an advancement of the previous exercise. The exercise is performed identically to the previous description, but instead of relaxing the right arm in an elevated position, the patient reaches toward the ceiling, thus engaging the serratus anterior. Special attention is given to the anterior cervical accessory respiratory musculature to maintain it in a relaxed state. (Reprinted with permission from L. Brinkman.)

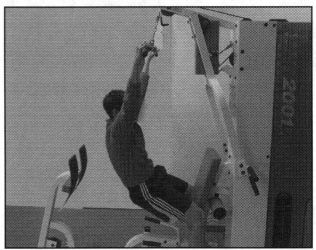

Figure 28-9. Latissimus dorsi and pectoralis major stretching while using diaphragmatic breathing and engaging the anterior abdominal wall. (Reprinted with permission from L. Brinkman.)

SUMMARY

This chapter offers a number of screening tools that may be utilized in clinical practice to identify patients who may be suffering from disordered sleep. Several tools are also suggested to assess the impact that pain and mood may have on the functional status of the patient. It is important to realize that pain, mood, and sleep interact and may each contribute to dysfunction. Table 28-5 presents a form which can be utilized to gather data regarding the sleep habits of a patient. This form prompts the clinician to ask particular questions regarding sleep quality and quantity. Scores for other tools that measure sleepiness, fatigue, pain, and mood can be reported here. It provides an area to gather important data from a previous sleep study. This screening tool may also be used to gather objective data regarding the structure and function of respiratory mechanics. The purpose of this tool is to provide one place to gather subjective and objective information about the sleep habits and sleep issues of a patient. These data can inform treatment decisions. It can help to identify a patient that may need referral for further testing and will allow for more efficient communication of a suspected sleep disorder to a sleep specialist. The rehabilitation professional is in a unique position to identify the manifestations and consequences

Table 28-5.

CORE Sleep Screening Tool

Patient Name: _____ **DOB:** _____ **Date:** _____

Special Questions

			Description
Sleep aids	Y	N	
Shift work	1	2	3
Snoring	Y	N	
Apneic event	Y	N	
PAP device	Y	N	
Oral appliance	Y	N	
Sleep study	Y	N	
Sleep diagnosis	Y	N	

Sleep Quantity

Lights out	
Lights on	
# of Awakenings	
Total sleep time	

Sleep Quality

Restorative	Y	N	
Nonrestorative	Y	N	
Other			

Observation of Respiratory Function — Comments

			Comments
Respiratory rate			
Respiratory rhythm	Effortless	Erratic	
Wheezing	Y	N	
Accessory m function	Y	N	
Mallampati score	Y	N	
Tongue scalloping	Y	N	
Nasal congestion	Y	N	Chronic/acute
Nose breather	Y	N	
Mouth breather	Y	N	

Posture and Symmetry — Comments

				Comments
Hyoid position	Normal	High	Low	
Forward head	Y	N		
Facial symmetry	Normal	Asymmetry:		
TMD	Deviation	R	L	
Orthodontics	Y	N	When:	
Postural tension	Y	N	Where:	
Kyphosis	Y	N		
Scoliosis	Y	N		
Kyphoscoliosis	Y	N		

(continued)

Table 28-5 (continued).

CORE Sleep Screening Tool

Patient Name: _____ **DOB:** _____ **Date:** _____

Respiratory Pattern

3-Minute nose breathing test	Able	Unable	
Rib cage			

	Inferior rib flare	L	R	
	Pectus excavatum	Pectus carinatum		

Hyperinflation: Y N		
Frequent yawning/throat clearing/air gulping	Y	N
Does patient hold breath		
Abdominal splinting		

Observation of Respiratory Pattern in Prone:

Does breath start from sacrum and progress up thorax to neck? Y N

Level of specific segmental limitation: _____

Segmental movement vs. moving as a block

Respiratory Tests

Breath holding test (30 s)	
Peak expiratory flow rate	
O2 saturation	

Sleep Study: Y N

Results of Sleep Study:

TST	Sleep Efficiency	Sleep Latency	REM Latency	N1	N2	N3	AHI	RDI

Diagnosis: _____

Referred to sleep study: Y N

PAP indicates positive airway pressure; TMD, temporomandibular joint disorder; TST, total sleep time; REM, rapid eye movement; N1, N2, N3, sleep stages; AHI, apnea hypopnea index; RDI, respiratory disturbance index.

Reprinted with permission from Hereford JM. CORE Sleep Screening Tool. Available at www.coreservices.org. Accessed August 24, 2012.

of disordered sleep. Part of this opportunity occurs because of the extended patient contact time that the rehabilitation professional has. It is therefore very important to also be able to recognize these signs and symptoms and further recognize the impact they may have on the overall health of the patient. In addition to the impact that disordered sleep may have on general health, it may have a negative impact on the rehabilitation process. This book has outlined the importance of sleep in processing of memory, particularly motor memory. The book has also shown that sleep disruption can increase pain sensitivity and interfere with tissue regeneration and repair.

Mechanics of respiration were reviewed, and suggestions were made for the rehabilitation of dysfunctional respiratory patterns. Improving respiratory function during wakefulness likely improves respiratory function during sleep. Management of sleep including identifying disordered sleep therefore becomes an important factor in any rehabilitation program.

REFERENCES

1. Hoddes E, Zarcone V, Smythe H, Phillips R, Dement WC. Quantification of sleepiness: a new approach. *Psychophysiol.* 1973;10(4):431–436.

2. Johns MW. A New Method for Measuring Daytime Sleepiness: The Epworth Sleepiness Scale. *Sleep.* 1991;14(6):540–545.

3. Wewers ME, Lowe NK. A critical review of visual analogue scales in the measurement of clinical phenomena. *Res Nurs Health.* 1990;13:227–236.

4. Melzack R. The McGill Pain Questionnaire: major properties and scoring methods. *Pain.* 1975;1:277–299.

5. McGill Pain Questionnaire. Available at: http://en.wikipedia.org/wiki/McGill_Pain_Questionnaire. Accessed July 10, 2013.

6. McGill Short Form Pain Questionnaire. Available at: http://www.ncbi.nlm.nih.gov/pubmed/3670870. Accessed October 2, 2013.

7. Tait RC, Pollard CA, Margolis RB, Duckro PN, Krause SJ. The pain disability index: psychometric and validity data. *Arch Phys Med Rehabil.* 1987;68(7):438–441.

8. Krupp LB, LaRocca NG, Muir-Nash J, Steinberg AD. The fatigue severity scale: application to patient with multiple sclerosis and systemic Lupus erythematosus. *JAMA Neurol.* 1989;46(10):1121–1123.

9. Nuckton TJ, Glidden DV, Browner WS, Claman DM. Physical examination: Mallampati score as an independent predictor of obstructive sleep apnea. *Sleep.* 2006;29:903–908.

10. Hruska RH. Influences of dysfunctional respiratory mechanics of orofacial pain. *Dent Clin North Am.* 1997;41:211–227.

11. Enivemeka CS, Bonet IM, Ingle J et al. Postural correction in persons with neck pain: Part 1. A survey of neck positions recommended by physical therapists. *J Orthop Sports Phys Ther.* 1986;8:235–239.

12. Enivemeka CS, Bonet IM, Ingle J, et al. Postural correction in persons with neck pain: Part II. Integrated electromyography of the upper trapezius in three simulated neck positions. *J Orthop Sports Phys Ther.* 1986;11:240–242.

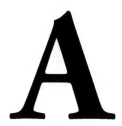

Sample Sleep Studies

SLEEP STUDY EXAMPLE ONE

Patient A is a 27-year-old female who was referred for evaluation and treatment of chronic daily headaches. During the initial evaluation, she noted multiple concussions from athletic injuries. She reported excessive daytime sleepiness and scored 13 on the Epworth Sleepiness Scale. She denied snoring. Because of her history of chronic headache and multiple mild traumatic brain injuries, she was sent for a sleep study. Although her findings were normal, it is reasonable to have baseline information on a patient with this history.

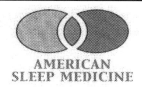

**AMERICAN
SLEEP MEDICINE**

*727 Craig Road # 101
St. Louis, MO 63141
(314) 994-9499*

Polysomnography Report

NARRATIVE REPORT

PATIENT'S NAME:
DOB: 1985
DATE OF RECORDING:
REQUESTING M.D.:
ATTENDING M.D.:

Study Performed: Nocturnal Polysomnography

HISTORY: This is a 27 year old female who presented for a sleep study to rule out obstructive sleep apnea. She has a history of asthma, traumatic brain injuries and concussions. Her Epworth Sleepiness Scale score is 15.

PROCEDURE: This is a nocturnal technician attended polysomnography using the American Sleep Medicine Protocol utilizing continuous digital recording. Recorded channels included: EEG (international 10-20 electrode placement), eye movement, chin EMG, nasal and oral airflow, ECG, respiratory effort, oximetry, body position, snoring sound, pulse rate and limb movement. All events are scored according to the current AASM criteria. Hypopneas (4a) have a 30% reduction in airflow and at least a 4% desaturation and are calculated within the AHI. Alternative Hypopneas (4b) have a 50% reduction in airflow and are accompanied by either a 3% desaturation or an arousal and is calculated within the RDI.

SUMMARY:
1. Sleep Architecture: Lights out occurred at 23:38:27. Lights on occurred at 05:50:28. Total recorded time was 536.3 minutes, with a total sleep time of 340.5 minutes and a sleep efficiency of 91.5 %. The patient's sleep latency was 18.5 minutes. Latency to REM was 127.5 minutes. There was 5.9% of Stage N1 sleep, 49.3% stage N2 sleep, 25.7% stage N3 sleep, and 19.1% REM sleep. Total number of arousals was 56. Arousal index was 9.9.

2. Respiratory Data: During the study the patient had 1 episodes of apneas and (4a) hypopneas (4% oxygen desaturations or greater) making the **Apnea/Hypopnea Index (AHI) 0.2** events per sleep hour. Mean length of the apnea/hypopnea was 22.4 seconds and the longest was 22.4 seconds. During **REM** sleep the **Apnea/Hypopnea Index was 0.0** events per sleep hour.

In addition to the above events, there were other hypopneas (4b) and "respiratory arousals" which did not strictly fulfill CMS criteria for desaturation, but were associated with arousals or sleep disruption. When these were considered, the total **Respiratory Disturbance Index (RDI)** was **0.7** events per sleep hour. Respiratory disturbance index during sleeping in the supine position was **0.0** events per sleep hour and the patient slept **191.5** minutes in the supine position. Respiratory disturbance index while sleeping on both sides was **0.4** events per sleep hour, and the patient slept for 149.0 minutes on both sides.

3. Oxygen Data: The patient spent 99.9 percent of sleep time with oxygen saturation above 90 percent, the patient spent 0.0 percent of sleep time with oxygen saturation below 88 percent and the lowest oxygen saturation was **95%**.

4. EKG Data: No arrhythmias were noted during the sleep study.

Figure A-1. Sleep study for patient A. (Reprinted with permission from American Sleep Medicine of St. Louis.)

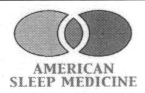

**AMERICAN
SLEEP MEDICINE**

*727 Craig Road # 101
St. Louis, MO 63141
(314) 994-9499*

Polysomnography Report

PATIENT'S NAME:
DOB: '1985
DATE OF RECORDING:

5. Other Data: No periodic leg movements were noted. The patient had a PLM index of 0.0 and a leg movement arousal index of 0.0.

6. Scorer's Comments: This study showed very mild and rare snores. She slept on her left side for the first half of the study and supine for the second half. There was 5.9% of Stage N1 sleep, 49.3% stage N2 sleep, 25.7% stage N3 sleep, and 19.1% REM sleep. The total number of arousals was 56 and her arousal index was 9.9.

CONCLUSION:

1. The study showed no evidence suggestive of underlying obstructive sleep apnea syndrome. This is based on an apnea hypopnea index of of **0.2** events per sleep hour as compared to a normal of 5 or less. The respiratory disturbance index is **0.7**.

2. The study showed normal sleep architecture with a slight delayed REM onset and decrease REM.

DIAGNOSIS:

1. Excessive Daytime Sleepiness (780.54) unspecified
2. Very Mild and Rare Snoring (786.09)

RECOMMENDATION:

1. The patient is scheduled for a follow-up appointment on 9/25/2012 to discuss the results of the study and treatment options.
2. If you would like to discuss this case feel free to call me
3. The patient was instructed not to drive or operate heavy machinery if having symptoms of sleepiness.

Diplomate, American Board of Sleep Medicine, ABSM
Diplomate, Pulmonary Critical Care and Sleep Medicine

Figure A-1 (continued). Sleep study for patient A. (Reprinted with permission from American Sleep Medicine of St. Louis.)

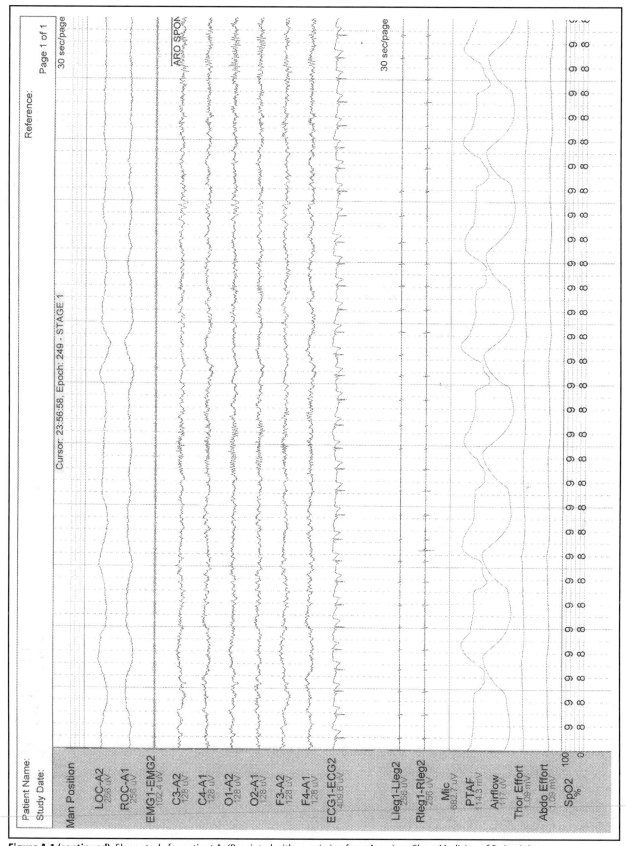

Figure A-1 (continued). Sleep study for patient A. (Reprinted with permission from American Sleep Medicine of St. Louis.)

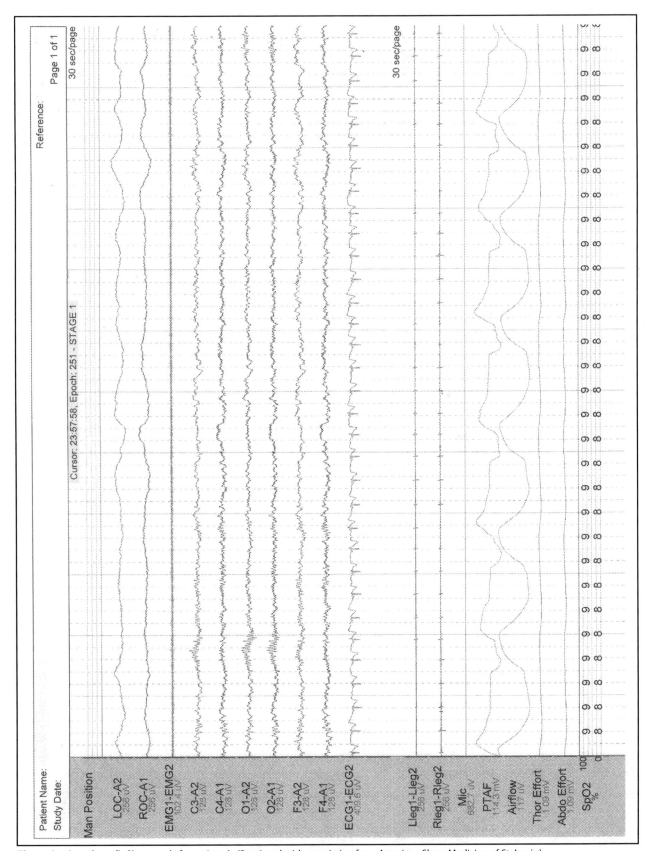

Figure A-1 (continued). Sleep study for patient A. (Reprinted with permission from American Sleep Medicine of St. Louis.)

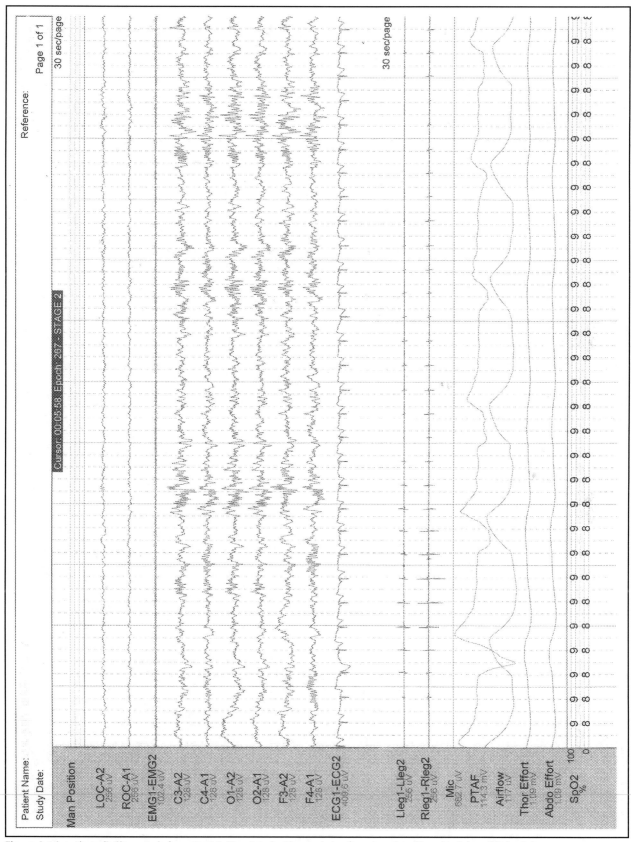

Figure A-1 (continued). Sleep study for patient A. (Reprinted with permission from American Sleep Medicine of St. Louis.)

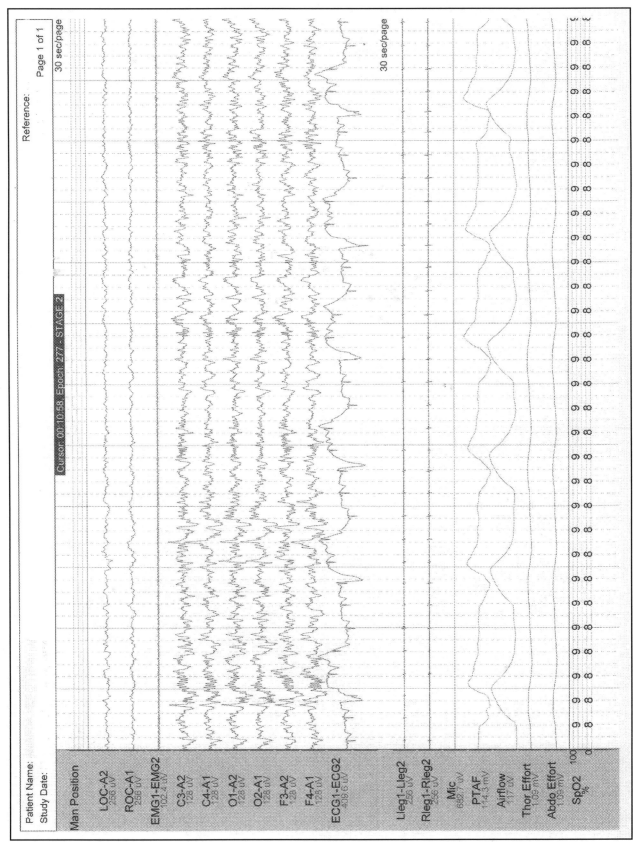

Figure A-1 (continued). Sleep study for patient A. (Reprinted with permission from American Sleep Medicine of St. Louis.)

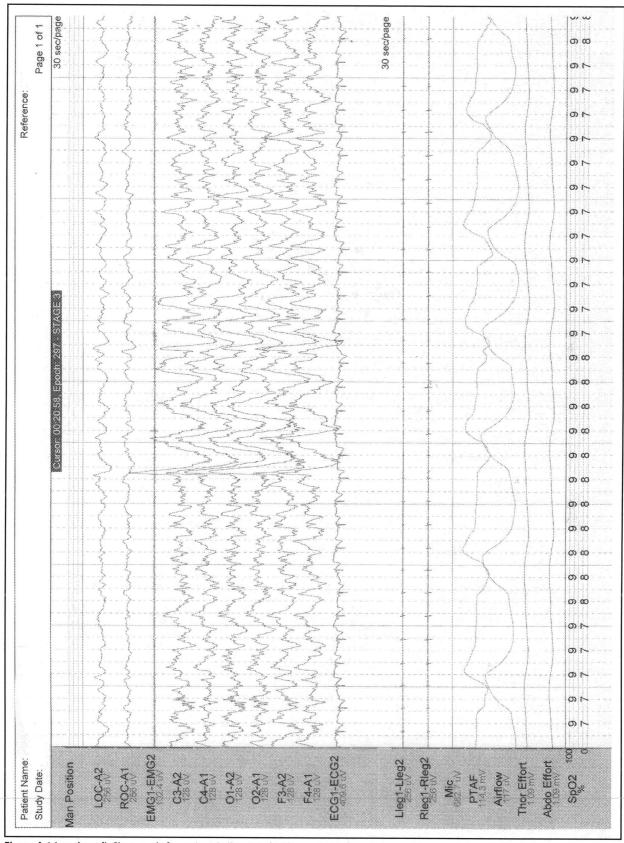

Figure A-1 (continued). Sleep study for patient A. (Reprinted with permission from American Sleep Medicine of St. Louis.)

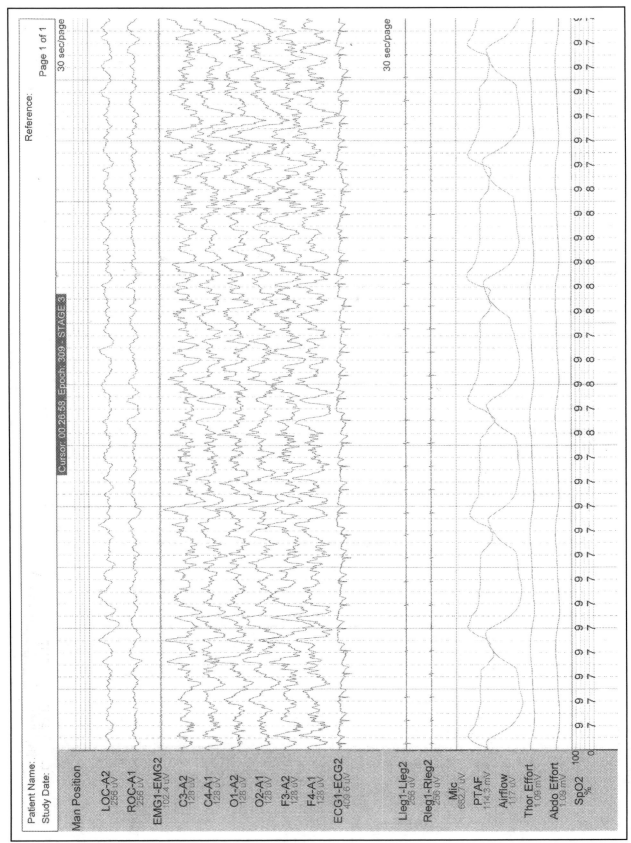

Figure A-1 (continued). Sleep study for patient A. (Reprinted with permission from American Sleep Medicine of St. Louis.)

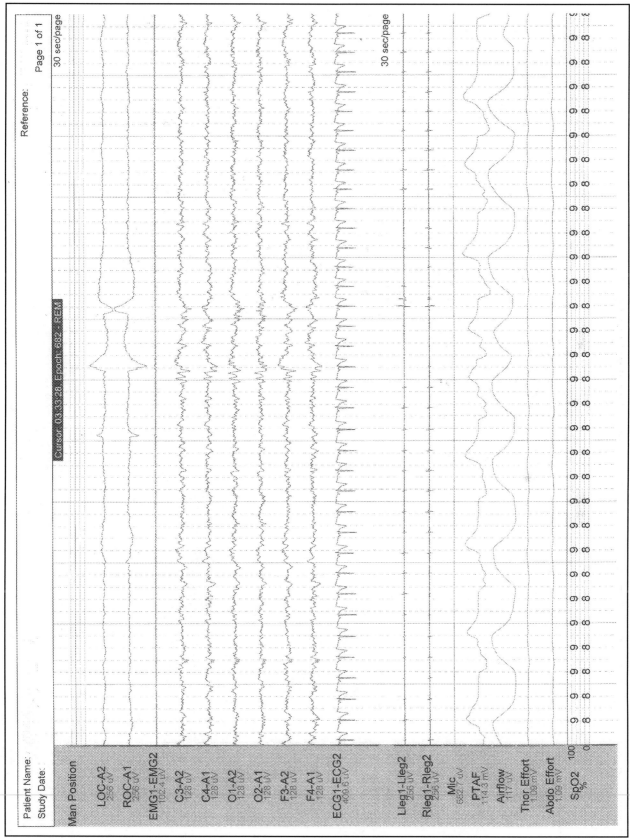

Figure A-1 (continued). Sleep study for patient A. (Reprinted with permission from American Sleep Medicine of St. Louis.)

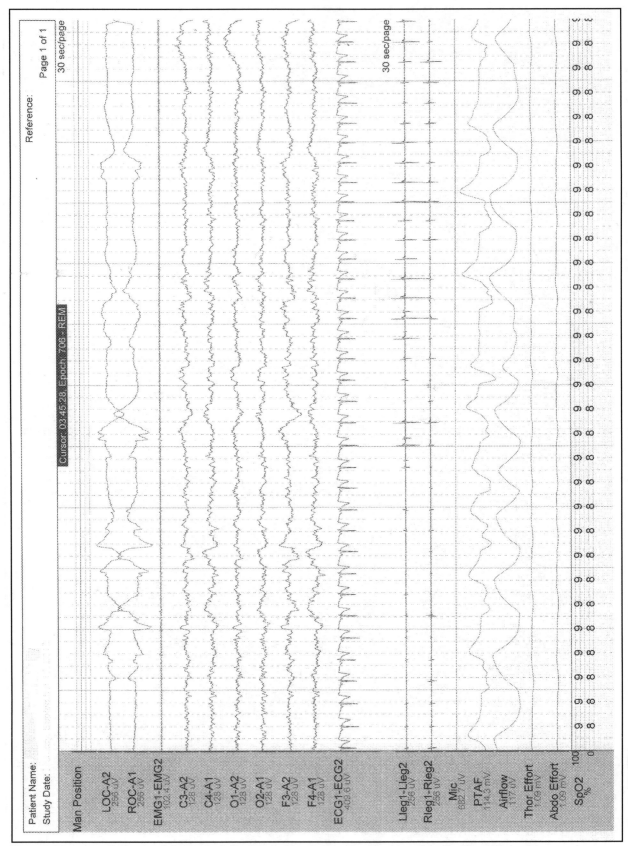

Figure A-1 (continued). Sleep study for patient A. (Reprinted with permission from American Sleep Medicine of St. Louis.)

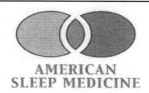

**AMERICAN
SLEEP MEDICINE**

*727 Craig Road # 101
St. Louis, MO 63141
(314) 994-9499*

Polysomnography Report

Summary

Study Information

Name:		Date of Study:	
Date of Birth:		Sex: Female	
Height: 5'6.5"	Wt: 139 lbs.		BMI: 22.1
Requesting Physician:		Diagnosis:	

Staging Summary Information

Recording Start Time:	21:52:58	Recording End Time:	06:49:13
Lights Out:	23:38:27	Lights On:	05:50:28
Total Recording Time (min) :	8:56.3	Total Sleep Time:	5:40.5
Sleep Efficiency (%):	91.5	Number of Awakenings:	12
Sleep Onset Latency (min):	18.5	Stage REM Latency (min):	127.5
(Lights Out to first epoch of 3 consecutive sleep epochs, stg. 1, 2, 3, 4, or one epoch of REM)		(Sleep onset to first REM epoch)	
Wake After Sleep Onset (min):	13.0		

Staging Table

Sleep Stage	Duration (min)	% Sleep Time	% Normal
Wake	13.0		
Stage N1 Sleep	20.0	5.9	10%
Stage N2 Sleep	168.0	49.3	50%
Stage N3 Sleep	87.5	25.7	15%
Stage REM	65.0	19.1	25%

SaO2 Summary

SaO2 Awake Average (%)	98
Lowest SaO2 (%)	95

Saturation Levels

Saturation Levels	Hours/Minutes
Time Equal to or Below 95%	0:00:2.0
Time Equal to or Below 90%	0:00:0.0
Time Equal to or Below 85%	0:00:0.0

Figure A-1 (continued). Sleep study for patient A. (Reprinted with permission from American Sleep Medicine of St. Louis.)

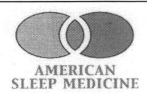

AMERICAN
SLEEP MEDICINE

727 Craig Road # 101
St. Louis, MO 63141
(314) 994-9499

Polysomnography Report

Name:	Date of Birth:	/1985	Date of Study:

Heart Rate Summary

Average Heart Rate	69
Slowest Heart Rate	44
Fastest Heart Rate	100
Number of Bradycardic Periods	0
Number of Tachycardic Periods	0

Arousal Summary

Number of	REM	Non-REM	Sleep
Respiratory Arousal	1	2	3
Limb Arousal	0	0	0
Spontaneous Arousal	13	40	53
Total			56
Per Hour			
Respiratory Arousal	0.9	0.4	0.5
Limb Arousal	0.0	0.0	0.0
Spontaneous Arousal	12.0	8.7	9.3
Total			9.9

Leg Movements Summary

	REM	NREM	Total
Number of Limb Movement Associated Arousals	0	0	0
PLM Episodes	0	0	0
Number of Limb Movements per Hour	0.0	0.0	0.0
PLM Index	0.0	0.0	0.0
Limb Movement Arousal Index	0.0	0.0	0.0

A PLM index of less than 5 is considered normal.
  Ref: THE INTERNATIONAL CLASSIFICATION OF SLEEP DISORDERS Diagnostic and Coding Manual,
                                      1990

Figure A-1 (continued). Sleep study for patient A. (Reprinted with permission from American Sleep Medicine of St. Louis.)

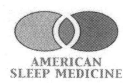

**AMERICAN
SLEEP MEDICINE**

*727 Craig Road # 101
St. Louis, MO 63141
(314) 994-9499*

Polysomnography Report

Name:	Date of Birth:	1985	Date of Study:

Respiratory Events Summary

Parameter	Obstructive	Mixed	Central	Total Apnea	Hypopnea	Alternative Hypopnea	RERA
Number	0	0	0	0	1	1	2
Index (per hour)	0.0	0.0	0.0	0.0	0.2	0.2	0.4
Average Duration (sec)	0.0	0.0	0.0	0.0	22.4	14.7	13.7
Longest Duration (sec)				-	22.4		14.0
Number in NREM	0	0	0	0	1	0.0	0
Number in REM	0	0	0	0	0	0.9	2

Respiratory Events – REM/NREM

Parameter	REM	Non-REM	Sleep
Apneas	0	0	0
Hypopneas (4%)	0	1	1
Apneas + Hypopneas	0	1	1
Alternative Hypopneas (3%)	1	0	1
RERA's (Respiratory limitation with arousal and 2% or less desaturation)	0	2	2
Duration in Apnea (min)	0.0	0.0	0.0
Duration in Hypopnea (min)	0.0	0.4	0.4
Duration in Apnea + Hypopnea (min)	0.0	0.4	0.4
AHI (/hr) Apnea/Hypopnea with 4 % oxygen desaturation or greater	0.0	0.2	0.2
RDI (/hr) AHI plus hypopneas with 3% oxygen desaturations and RERAs	0.9	0.7	0.7

Respiratory Events Index (/hr) by Position (sleep time)

Position	Obstructive	Mixed	Central	Hypopnea	Alternative Hypopnea	RERA
Index Supine	0.0	0.0	0.0	0.0	0.3	0.3
Index Non-Supine	0.0	0.0	0.0	0.4	0.0	0.4

Figure A-1 (continued). Sleep study for patient A. (Reprinted with permission from American Sleep Medicine of St. Louis.)

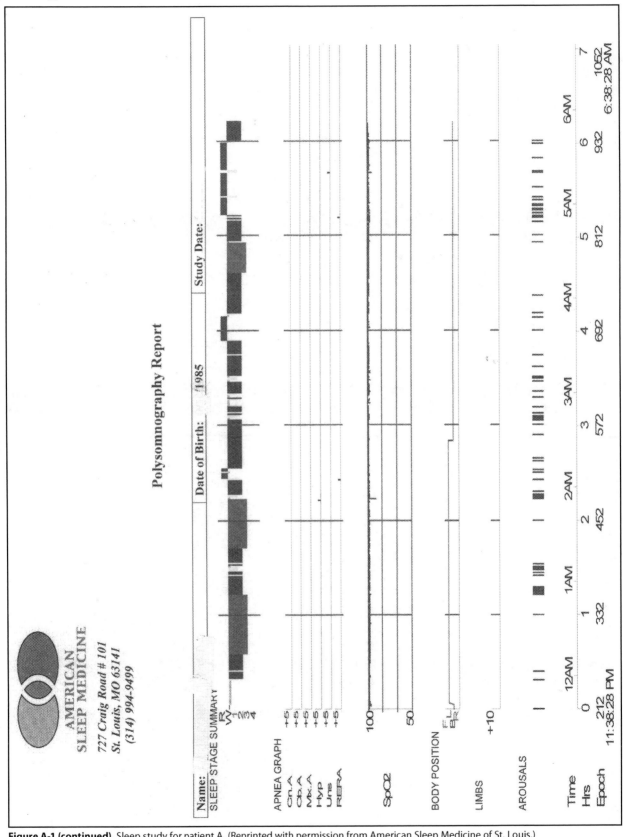

Figure A-1 (continued). Sleep study for patient A. (Reprinted with permission from American Sleep Medicine of St. Louis.)

SLEEP STUDY EXAMPLE TWO

Patient B is a 59-year-old male who suffered a work-related lumbosacral injury. On initial evaluation, he reported previous lumbar decompression surgery. He reported a history of a multivessel coronary artery bypass and hypertension, benign prostatic hypertrophy, and an ill-defined rheumatologic disorder. He reported that his wife complained of his loud snoring, such that she often sleeps in another room. He noted fatigue and had elevated scores on the Fatigue Severity Scale (FSS) and the Epworth Sleepiness Scale. He was noted to have hyperactivity of his upper respiratory musculature. Because of his underlying cardiovascular disease, pain, rheumatologic disease, snoring, and altered respiratory mechanics and scores on FSS and Epworth, he was referred for a sleep study. Patient B was found to have severe obstructive sleep apnea with an apnea/hypopnea index of 91. His study is what is known as a *split-night study*. Because of the severity of his apnea, the study was interrupted, and continuous positive airway pressure was immediately applied. His severity of disease considerably increased his risk of death from cardiovascular disease. It also had an impact on his rheumatologic disease and his pain problems. He had been on continuous positive airway pressure for 6 months at the time of writing this book and noted significant improvement in his energy level and control of some of his other symptoms.

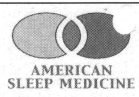

**AMERICAN
SLEEP MEDICINE**

*727 Craig Road # 101
St. Louis, MO 63141
(314) 994-9499*

Polysomnography Report 1

NARRATIVE REPORT

PATIENT'S NAME:
DOB:
DATE OF RECORDING:
REQUESTING M.D.:
ATTENDING M.D.:

Study Performed: Nocturnal Polysomnography, split night study, diagnostic/CPAP Titration

HISTORY: This is a 64 year old male who presented for a sleep study to rule out obstructive sleep apnea. He has a history of seasonal allergies, depression, anxiety, heart disease, arthritis, coronary artery bypass graft, and orthopedic surgery. His Epworth Sleepiness Scale score is 8.

PROCEDURE: This is a nocturnal technician attended polysomnography using the American Sleep Medicine Protocol utilizing continuous digital recording. Recorded channels included: EEG (international 10-20 electrode placement), eye movement, chin EMG, nasal and oral airflow, ECG, respiratory effort, oximetry, body position, snoring sound, pulse rate and limb movement. All events are scored according to the current AASM criteria. Hypopneas (4a) have a 30% reduction in airflow and at least a 4% desaturation and are calculated within the AHI. Alternative Hypopneas (4b) have a 50% reduction in airflow and are accompanied by either a 3% desaturation or an arousal and is calculated within the RDI. The initial portion of the study was undertaken to evaluate the severity of the suspected obstructive sleep apnea and the second portion for initiation of treatment with Nasal CPAP.

SUMMARY: PART I
1. **Sleep Architecture:** Lights out occurred at 23:15:12. Lights on occurred at 02:10:43. Total recording time was 609.8 minutes, with a total sleep time of 137.5 minutes and a sleep efficiency of 78.3 %. The patient's sleep latency was 30.0. Latency to REM was - minutes. There was 26.5% of Stage N1 sleep, 73.5% Stage N2 sleep, 0.0% Stage N3 sleep, and 0.0% REM sleep. Total number of arousals was 170. Arousal index was 74.2.

2. **Respiratory Data:** During the study the patient had 91 episodes of apneas and (4a) hypopneas (4% oxygen desaturations or greater) making the **Apnea/Hypopnea Index (AHI) 39.7** events per sleep hour. Mean length of the apnea/hypopnea was 18.8 seconds and the longest was 30.7 seconds. During **REM** sleep the **Apnea/Hypopnea Index was 0.0** events per sleep hour.

In addition to the above events, there were other hypopneas (4b) and "respiratory arousals" which did not strictly fulfill CMS criteria for desaturation, but were associated with arousals or sleep disruption. When these were considered, the total **Respiratory Disturbance Index (RDI)** was **71.6** events per sleep hour. Respiratory disturbance index during sleeping in the <u>supine position</u> was **0.0** events per sleep hour and the patient slept **0.0** minutes in the supine position. Respiratory disturbance index while sleeping <u>on both sides</u> was **39.7** events per sleep hour, and the patient slept for 137.5 minutes on both sides. Moderate snoring was noted.

Figure A-2. Split-night sleep study for patient B. (Reprinted with permission from American Sleep Medicine of St. Louis.)

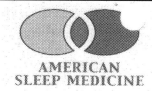

**AMERICAN
SLEEP MEDICINE**
*727 Craig Road # 101
St. Louis, MO 63141
(314) 994-9499*

Polysomnography Report 1

PATIENT'S NAME:
DOB: /1947
DATE OF RECORDING:

3. Oxygen Data: The patient spent 76.4 percent of sleep time with oxygen saturation above 90 percent, the patient spent 16.7 percent of sleep time with oxygen saturation below 88 percent and the lowest oxygen saturation was 83%.

4. EKG Data: No arrhythmias were noted during the sleep study.

5. Other Data: Periodic leg movements were noted. The patient had a PLM index of 1.7 and a leg movement with arousals index of 0.9. The patient spent 0% of sleep time in stage 3 and 0% in REM sleep which is abnormal. Sleep Efficiency was normal at 79%.

Figure A-2 (continued). Split-night sleep study for patient B. (Reprinted with permission from American Sleep Medicine of St. Louis.)

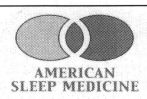

**AMERICAN
SLEEP MEDICINE**

*727 Craig Road # 101
St. Louis, MO 63141
(314) 994-9499*

Polysomnography Report 2

NARRATIVE REPORT

PATIENT'S NAME:
DOB: /1947
DATE OF RECORDING:
REQUESTING M.D.:
ATTENDING M.D.:

SUMMARY: PART II – CPAP

1. Sleep Architecture: The sleep architecture improved with nasal CPAP with periods of REM and Non REM sleep recorded. Total recording time was 609.8 minutes, with a total sleep time of 193.5 minutes and a sleep efficiency of 78.3 %. The patient's sleep latency was 32.5 minutes. Latency to REM was - minutes. There was 25.8% of stage N1 sleep, 74.2% stage N2 sleep, 0.0% stage N3 sleep, and 0.0% REM sleep. Total number of arousals was 136. Arousal index was 42.2 per hour.

2. Respiratory Data: Due to the frequency and severity of the above respiratory arousals, the patient was placed on CPAP at a pressure of 4 cm and titrated upwards sequentially for the eradication of apneas, hypopneas, and snoring. The best controlled events were achieved with CPAP at a setting of **11 cm H20**. The duration of sleep at the setting of **11 cm H20** was eleven minutes.

3. Oxygen Data: The patient spent 98.3 percent of sleep time with oxygen saturation above 90 percent, and the lowest oxygen saturation was **87%.**

4. EKG Data: No arrhythmias were noted during the study.

5. Other Data: Periodic leg movements were noted. The patient had a PLM index of 3.1 and leg movement with arousals index of 5.9.

Figure A-2 (continued). Split-night sleep study for patient B. (Reprinted with permission from American Sleep Medicine of St. Louis.)

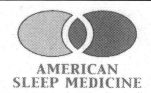

AMERICAN SLEEP MEDICINE

727 Craig Road # 101
St. Louis, MO 63141
(314) 994-9499

Polysomnography Report 2

PATIENT'S NAME:
DOB: /1947
DATE OF RECORDING:

CONCLUSION:

1. The first portion of this study showed **obstructive sleep apnea syndrome**. This is based on an apnea/hypopnea index of **39.7** events per sleep hour as compared to a normal of 5 or less.

2. The first portion of this study shows transient hypoxia, with the lowest saturation of **83 %.** The patient spent **16.7** percent of sleep time with oxygen saturation below 88 percent. The lowest oxygen desaturation on **11 cm H2O** was 89%.

3. This study showed improvement of the respiratory events and hypoxemia with positive airway pressure. At a pressure of **11 cm H20** the respiratory events decreased to 5.7 per hour. The patient did not achieve REM Sleep in the supine position during this pressure.

4. The patient had a sleep efficiency of 78.3% on CPAP, which is normal. He spent 0% of sleep time in stage 3 and REM sleep, which is abnormal.

DIAGNOSIS:

1. Severe Obstructive Sleep Apnea (327.23) reversed with CPAP
2. Sleep Related Hypoxia (799.02) reversed with CPAP
3. Snoring (786.09)

RECOMMENDATION:

1. Start CPAP at **11 cm H20** utilizing Respironics CPAP machine with a small Easy Life mask, headgear, chinstrap and heated humidifier.
2. The patient will be scheduled for a follow up appointment to check compliance and symptom relief.
3. Other measures which are known to benefit patients with obstructive sleep apnea syndrome include weight reduction and correction of upper airway abnormalities.
4. Avoidance of sedatives and alcohol should be discussed.
5. The patient will be instructed not to drive or operate heavy machinery if having symptoms of sleepiness.
6. If you would like to discuss this case feel free to call me

Figure A-2 (continued). Split-night sleep study for patient B. (Reprinted with permission from American Sleep Medicine of St. Louis.)

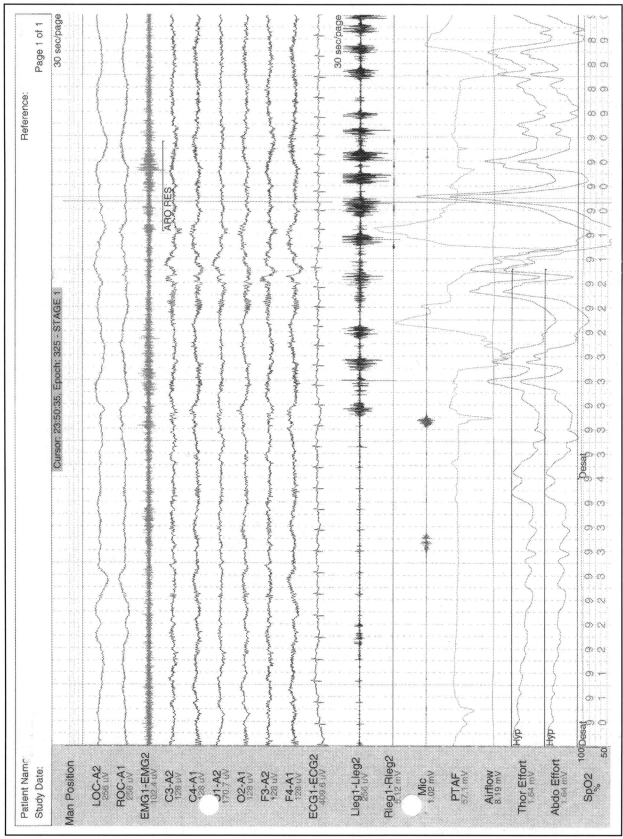

Figure A-2 (continued). Split-night sleep study for patient B. (Reprinted with permission from American Sleep Medicine of St. Louis.)

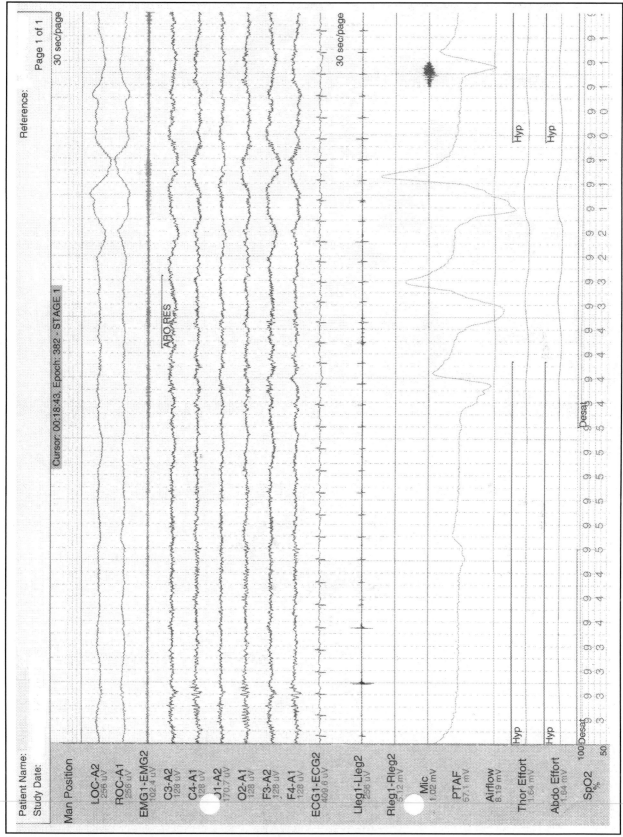

Figure A-2 (continued). Split-night sleep study for patient B. (Reprinted with permission from American Sleep Medicine of St. Louis.)

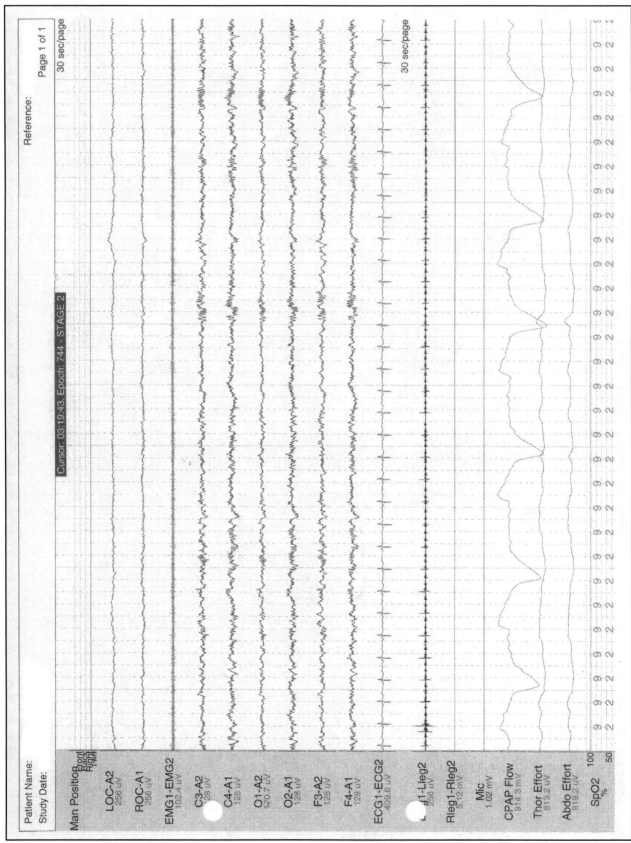

Figure A-2 (continued). Split-night sleep study for patient B. (Reprinted with permission from American Sleep Medicine of St. Louis.)

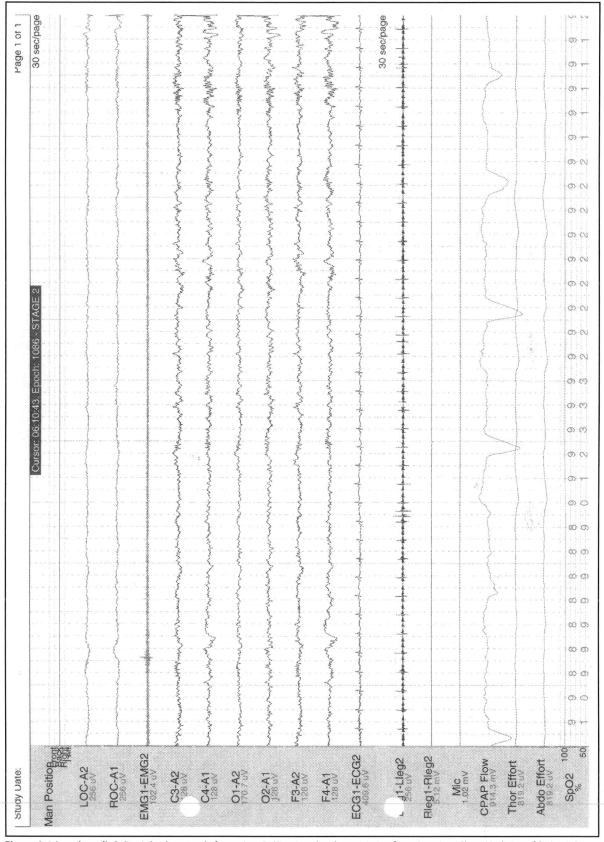

Figure A-2 (continued). Split-night sleep study for patient B. (Reprinted with permission from American Sleep Medicine of St. Louis.)

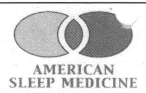

**AMERICAN
SLEEP MEDICINE**

*727 Craig Road # 101
St. Louis, MO 63141
(314) 994-9499*

Polysomnography Report 1

Summary
Part 1

Study Information

Name:		Date of Study:	
Date of Birth: 1947		Sex: Male	
Height: 5'12"	Wt: 189 lbs.		BMI: 25.6
Requesting Physician:		Diagnosis: Obstructive Sleep Apnea	

Staging Summary Information

Recording Start Time:	21:08:13	Recording End Time:	07:18:01
Lights Out:	23:15:12	Lights On:	02:10:43
Total Recording Time (min) :	10:9.8	Total Sleep Time:	2:17.5
Sleep Efficiency (%):	78.3	Number of Awakenings:	12
Sleep Onset Latency (min):	30.0	Stage REM Latency (min):	-
(Lights Out to first epoch of 3 consecutive			
sleep epochs, stg. 1, 2, 3, 4, or one epoch of REM)		(Sleep onset to first REM epoch)	
Wake After Sleep Onset (min):	7.0		

Staging Table

Sleep Stage	Duration (min)	% Sleep Time	% Normal
Wake	7.0		
Stage N1 Sleep	36.5	26.5	10%
Stage N2 Sleep	101.0	73.5	50%
Stage N3 Sleep	0.0	0.0	15%
Stage REM	0.0	0.0	25%

SaO2 Summary

SaO2 Awake Average (%)	92
Lowest SaO2 (%)	83

Saturation Levels

Saturation Levels	Hours/Minutes
Time Equal to or Below 95%	2:15:51.0
Time Equal to or Below 90%	0:31:9.0
Time Equal to or Below 85%	0:01:18.0

Figure A-2 (continued). Split-night sleep study for patient B. (Reprinted with permission from American Sleep Medicine of St. Louis.)

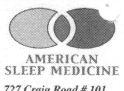

**AMERICAN
SLEEP MEDICINE**

727 Craig Road # 101
St. Louis, MO 63141
(314) 994-9499

Polysomnography Report 1

Name:		Date of Birth:	'1947	Date of Study:

Respiratory Events Summary

Parameter	Obstructive	Mixed	Central	Total Apnea	Hypopnea	Alternative Hypopnea	RERA
Number	26	0	0	26	65	50	23
Index (per hour)	11.3	0.0	0.0	11.3	28.4	21.8	10.0
Average Duration (sec)	15.9	0.0	0.0	15.9	20.0	19.0	17.0
Longest Duration (sec)				23.6	30.7		27.8
Number in NREM	26	0	0	26	65	21.8	0
Number in REM	0	0	0	0	0	0.0	23

Respiratory Events – REM/NREM

Parameter	REM	Non-REM	Sleep
Apneas	0	26	26
Hypopneas (4%)	0	65	65
Apneas + Hypopneas	0	91	91
Alternative Hypopneas (3%)	0	50	50
RERA's (Respiratory limitation with arousal and 2% or less desaturation)	0	23	23
Duration in Apnea (min)	0.0	6.9	6.9
Duration in Hypopnea (min)	0.0	21.6	21.6
Duration in Apnea + Hypopnea (min)	0.0	28.5	28.5
AHI (/hr) Apnea/Hypopnea with 4 % oxygen desaturation or greater	0.0	39.7	39.7
RDI (/hr) AHI plus hypopneas with 3% oxygen desaturations and RERAs	0.0	71.6	71.6

Respiratory Events Index (/hr) by Position (sleep time)

Position	Obstructive	Mixed	Central	Hypopnea	Alternative Hypopnea	RERA
Index Supine	0.0	0.0	0.0	0.0	0.0	0.0
Index Non-Supine	11.3	0.0	0.0	28.4	21.8	10.0

Figure A-2 (continued). Split-night sleep study for patient B. (Reprinted with permission from American Sleep Medicine of St. Louis.)

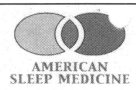

AMERICAN SLEEP MEDICINE

727 Craig Road # 101
St. Louis, MO 63141
(314) 994-9499

Polysomnography Report 1

Name:	Date of Birth:	1947	Date of Study:

Heart Rate Summary

Average Heart Rate	**72**
Slowest Heart Rate	65
Fastest Heart Rate	79
Number of Bradycardic Periods	0
Number of Tachycardic Periods	0

Arousal Summary

Number of	REM	Non-REM	Sleep
Respiratory Arousal	0	135	135
Limb Arousal	0	2	2
Spontaneous Arousal	0	33	33
Total			170
Per Hour			
Respiratory Arousal	-	58.9	58.9
Limb Arousal	-	0.9	0.9
Spontaneous Arousal	-	14.4	14.4
Total			74.2

Leg Movements Summary

	REM	NREM	Total
Number of Limb Movement Associated Arousals	0	2	2
PLM Episodes	0	1	1
Number of Limb Movements per Hour	0.0	3.5	3.5
PLM Index	0.0	1.7	1.7
Limb Movement Arousal Index	-	0.9	0.9

A PLM index of less than 5 is considered normal.
 Ref: THE INTERNATIONAL CLASSIFICATION OF SLEEP DISORDERS Diagnostic and Coding Manual, 1990

Figure A-2 (continued). Split-night sleep study for patient B. (Reprinted with permission from American Sleep Medicine of St. Louis.)

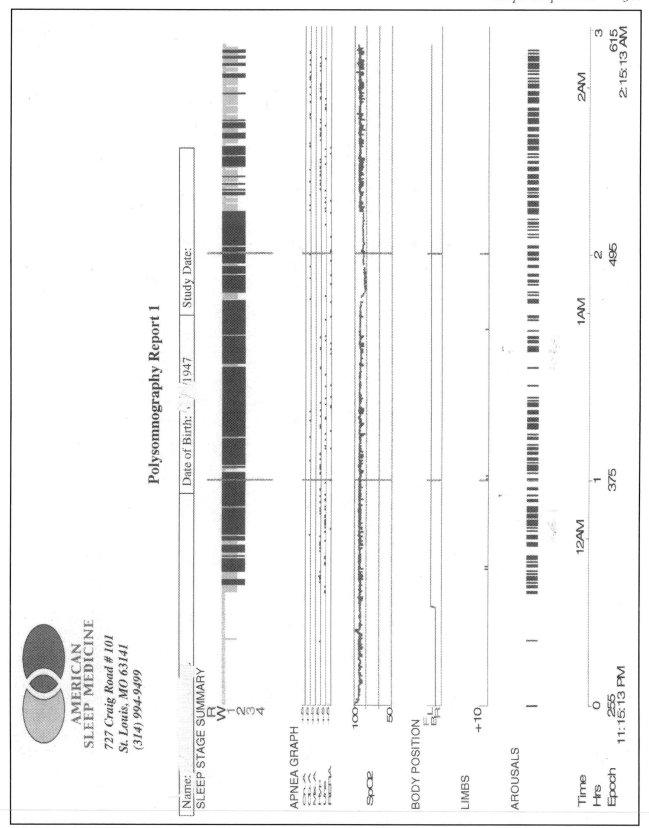

Figure A-2 (continued). Split-night sleep study for patient B. (Reprinted with permission from American Sleep Medicine of St. Louis.)

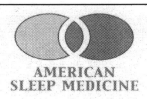

**AMERICAN
SLEEP MEDICINE**

*727 Craig Road # 101
St. Louis, MO 63141
(314) 994-9499*

Polysomnography Report 2

Summary
Part 2

Study Information

Name:		Date of Study:	
Date of Birth: 1947		Sex: Male	
Height: 5'12"	Wt: 189 lbs.		BMI: 25.6
Requesting Physician:		Diagnosis: Obstructive Sleep Apnea	

Staging Summary Information

Recording Start Time:	21:08:13	Recording End Time:	07:18:01
Lights Out:	02:15:42	Lights On:	06:22:43
Total Recording Time (min) :	10:9.8	Total Sleep Time:	3:13.5
Sleep Efficiency (%):	78.3	Number of Awakenings:	19
Sleep Onset Latency (min):	32.5	Stage REM Latency (min):	-
(Lights Out to first epoch of 3 consecutive sleep epochs, stg. 1, 2, 3, 4, or one epoch of REM)		(Sleep onset to first REM epoch)	
Wake After Sleep Onset (min):	19.5		

Staging Table

Sleep Stage	Duration (min)	% Sleep Time	% Normal
Wake	19.5		
Stage N1 Sleep	50.0	25.8	10%
Stage N2 Sleep	143.5	74.2	50%
Stage N3 Sleep	0.0	0.0	15%
Stage REM	0.0	0.0	25%

SaO2 Summary

SaO2 Awake Average (%)	93
Lowest SaO2 (%)	87

Saturation Levels

Saturation Levels	Minutes
Time Equal to or Below 95%	3:09:50.0
Time Equal to or Below 90%	0:03:10.0
Time Equal to or Below 85%	0:00:0.0

Figure A-2 (continued). Split-night sleep study for patient B. (Reprinted with permission from American Sleep Medicine of St. Louis.)

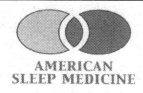

**AMERICAN
SLEEP MEDICINE**

*727 Craig Road # 101
St. Louis, MO 63141
(314) 994-9499*

Polysomnography Report 2

Name:				Date of Birth:	1947		Date of Study:	

Respiratory Events Summary

Parameter	Obstructive	Mixed	Central	Total Apnea	Hypopnea (4% or >)	Alternative Hypopnea	RERA
Number	5	0	0	5	28	21	5
Index (per hour)	1.6	0.0	0.0	1.6	8.7	6.5	1.6
Average Duration (sec)	14.6	0.0	0.0	14.6	20.6	19.0	18.7
Longest Duration (sec)				15.3	28.6		24.0
Number in NREM	5	0	0	5	28	6.5	0
Number in REM	0	0	0	0	0	0.0	5

Respiratory Events – REM/NREM

Parameter	REM	Non-REM	Sleep
Apneas	0	5	5
Hypopneas (4% or >)	0	28	28
Apneas + Hypopneas	0	33	33
Alternative Hypopneas (3%)	0	21	21
RERAs (Respiratory limitation with arousal and 2% or less desaturation)	0	5	5
Duration in Apnea (min)	0.0	1.2	1.2
Duration in Hypopnea (min)	0.0	9.6	9.6
Duration in Apnea + Hypopnea (min)	0.0	10.8	10.8
AHI (/hr) Apnea/Hypopnea with 4 % oxygen desaturation or greater	0.0	10.2	10.2
RDI (/hr) AHI plus hypopneas with 3% oxygen desaturations and RERAs	0.0	18.3	18.3

Respiratory Events Index (/hr) by Position (sleep time)

Position	Obstructive	Mixed	Central	Hypopnea	Alternative Hypopnea	RERA
Index Supine	12.0	0.0	0.0	43.2	19.2	4.8
Index Non-Supine	0.0	0.0	0.0	3.6	4.6	1.1

Figure A-2 (continued). Split-night sleep study for patient B. (Reprinted with permission from American Sleep Medicine of St. Louis.)

Polysomnography Report 2

AMERICAN SLEEP MEDICINE
727 Craig Road # 101
St. Louis, MO 63141
(314) 994-9499

Name: _____   Date of Birth: 1947   Date of Study: _____

CPAP/Bilevel/Oxygen Titration Table

CPAP/ Bilevel	Duration Report Time	Duration Sleep Time	Duration REM	Duration NREM	No. of Hypop.	No. of Central Apneas	No. of Obstr. Apneas	No. of Mixed Apneas	AHI	RERA	RDI
4/4/0	0:38:51.0	0:08:30.0	0:00:0.0	0:08:30.0	0	0	0	0	0.0	2	14.1
6/6/0	2:04:43.0	1:55:13.0	0:00:0.0	1:55:13.0	7	0	0	0	3.6	1	4.2
8/8/0	0:17:45.0	0:16:45.0	0:00:0.0	0:16:45.0	15	0	3	0	64.5	2	71.6
10/10/0	0:48:2.0	0:42:2.0	0:00:0.0	0:42:2.0	5	0	2	0	10.0	0	10.0
11/11/0	0:15:30.0	0:11:0.0	0:00:0.0	0:11:0.0	1	0	0	0	5.5	0	5.7

SLEEP TIME

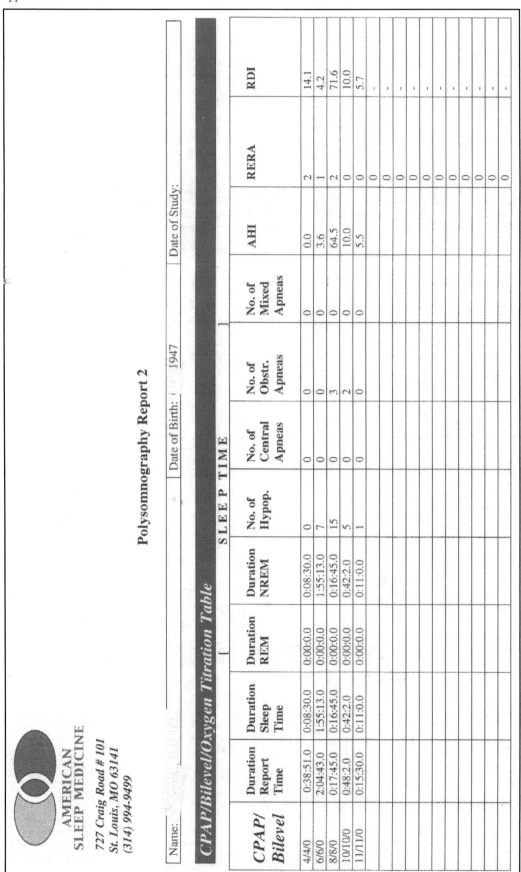

Figure A-2 (continued). Split-night sleep study for patient B. (Reprinted with permission from American Sleep Medicine of St. Louis.)

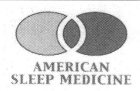

**AMERICAN
SLEEP MEDICINE**

727 Craig Road # 101
St. Louis, MO 63141
(314) 994-9499

Polysomnography Report 2

Name:	Date of Birth: 1947	Date of Study:

Heart Rate Summary

Average Heart Rate	**0**
Slowest Heart Rate	-
Fastest Heart Rate	-
Number of Bradycardic Periods	0
Number of Tachycardic Periods	0

Arousal Summary

Number of	REM	Non-REM	Sleep
Respiratory Arousal	0	46	46
Limb Arousal	0	19	19
Spontaneous Arousal	0	71	71
Total			136
Per Hour			
Respiratory Arousal	-	14.3	14.3
Limb Arousal	-	5.9	5.9
Spontaneous Arousal	-	22.0	22.0
Total			42.2

Leg Movements Summary

	REM	NREM	Total
Number of Limb Movement Associated Arousals	0	19	19
PLM Episodes	0	2	2
Number of Limb Movements per Hour	0.0	27.3	27.3
PLM Index	0.0	3.1	3.1
Limb Movement Arousal Index	-	5.9	5.9

A PLM index of less than 5 is considered normal.
   Ref: THE INTERNATIONAL CLASSIFICATION OF SLEEP DISORDERS Diagnostic and Coding Manual, 1990

Figure A-2 (continued). Split-night sleep study for patient B. (Reprinted with permission from American Sleep Medicine of St. Louis.)

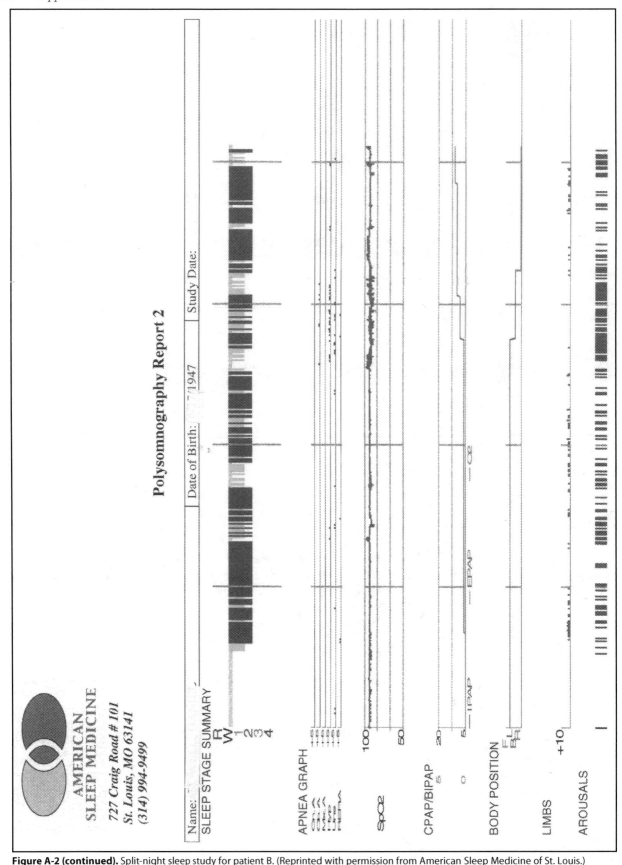

Figure A-2 (continued). Split-night sleep study for patient B. (Reprinted with permission from American Sleep Medicine of St. Louis.)

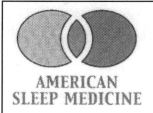

AMERICAN SLEEP MEDICINE

Patient:

Acct :

Physician:

DOS: -12

DOB: -47

CONSULT

REQUESTING PHYSICIAN:

REASON FOR CONSULTATION: I snore something terrible.

History of Present Illness:

He is aware of snoring since he was a teenager. He has frequent sleep interruptions. He has seen an ENT physician. He was advised that fixing his nose will relieve his snoring for the most part. He had fractured his nose, and had surgery, several times. His main concern is sleep interruptions. During the day, he is OK as long as he is physically active. If he is idle he will doze. This last symptom has been present in Grade School. He thinks he slept less than his friends. As a teen, if he stayed up he could not sleep beyond six in the morning. He is a worrier. He is anxious. Currently, he is treated for anxiety with Xanax.If he takes 1 mg, he sleeps or lethargic. At sleep onset, his feet and calves burn. He has neuropathy. There is a sense of crawling in his calves. Cymbalta and a soft pillow to lift his feet relieve this feeling. He is a restless sleeper. There is history of witnessed apnea. He gained 4-5 lbs in the past five years. One year prior to this visit, he was rear ended. He has had a need to stretch his back in the middle of the night since is accident. A typical night is described to fall asleep in a long period. There are two long interruptions. He sleeps but feels, and dreams, of being awake. He has vivid dreams. He does not have visual hallucinations or dream at sleep onset. He wears a wrist brace and has awakened having pulled them off. He took them off while dreaming of pulling a cow. Bedtime is 11 pm and Wake up time is 4: 45 during the week and 7 am on weekends. Epworth Score is 8.

Medical History:

anxiety. CAD. degenerative disc disease. depression. heart attack. disc disease from an accident with nerve root injury from it, CTS. arthritis.

Surgical History:

cardiac surgery - coronary artery bypass graft. repair/pin left ankle 2/2012. lumbar disc surgery x 2.

Family History:

depression - father, brother. *snoring* - father, brother. *anxiety* - brother. *daytime fatigue* - brother.

727 Craig Road   Suite 101   St. Louis, MO 63141
(314) 994-9499   Fax (314) 991-6844   www.americansleepmedicine.com

Figure A-2 (continued). Split-night sleep study for patient B. (Reprinted with permission from American Sleep Medicine of St. Louis.)

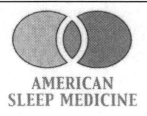

**AMERICAN
SLEEP MEDICINE**

Patient: DOS: -12
Acct :   DOB: -47
Physician:

Social History:
tobacco use - former smoker - length of tobacco use 2 packs/day x 40 years, quit date 2007.
alcohol use - occasional used to drink a lot as a young man. Now he will have 1-2 drinks every
many months - how many/much per day not specified. *caffeine consumption* - coffee 2-3 /day
cups per day. *marital status/living arrangements* - married. *current employment* - unemployed,
disabled on the basis of back injury. *occupation* - Patient's occupation is mechanic-shift work.

Allergies: No known drug allergies

Current Medications:
Cymbalta (duloxetine) 60 mg Capsule, Delayed Release(E.C.) 2 capsule twice a day
Lyrica (pregabalin) 150 mg Capsule Take 1 capsule twice a day
Plaquenil (hydroxychloroquine) 200 mg Tablet Take 1 tablet once a day
Ultram ER (tramadol) 200 mg Tablet Extended Release 24 hr Take 1 tablet twice a day
Vicodin HP (hydrocodone-acetaminophen) 10-660 mg Tablet Take 1 tablet every six hours, as
needed
Xanax (alprazolam) 0.5 mg Tablet Take 1 tablet at bedtime
Zocor (simvastatin) 5 mg Tablet Take 1 tablet once a day

Review of Systems:
Constitutional Symptoms: Denies fatigue, insomnia.
Eyes: wears glasses.
Ears, nose, throat: Denies nasal congestion.
Cardiovascular: Denies shortness of breath.
Pulmonary: Denies cough, productive, dyspnea on exertion.
Gastrointestinal: Complains of altered bowel habits constipation.
Genitourinary: bladder dysfunction, he self catheterizes.
Musculoskeletal: *back* - Denies arthritis of back.
Integumentary: normal, no problems indicated.
Neurological: see HPI.
Psychiatric: *mood* - Denies anxiety, depression.
Endocrine: normal, no problems indicated.
Hematologic, Lymphatic: normal, no problems indicated.
Immunologic: seasonal. Denies hay fever.

727 Craig Road   Suite 101   St. Louis, MO 63141
(314) 994-9499   Fax (314) 991-6844   www.americansleepmedicine.com

Figure A-2 (continued). Split-night sleep study for patient B. (Reprinted with permission from American Sleep Medicine of St. Louis.)

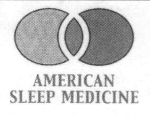

**AMERICAN
SLEEP MEDICINE**

Patient: DOS: -12
Acct :   DOB: -47
Physician:

Vitals: **Height** 72 inches (182.88 cm) **Weight** 189 pounds (85.73 kg) **BMI** 25.63 **Pulse** 74 bpm
Blood Pressure 120 / 83

Exam: **General appearance:** well developed. **ENMT:** *oropharynx, oral mucosa, palates*:
large tongue , tilted palate. **Neck:** *neck*: circumference 17". **Respiratory:** normal.
Cardiovascular: normal. **Musculoskeletal:** normal. **Neurologic:** Snout (No). Glabellar (No).
Romberg: Normal. *Cranial Nerves*: Full visual fields to confrontation, symmetrical facial
expression and sensation. Midline tongue protrusion and palate elevation. No head turning
weakness or difficulty swallowing. *Cognitive Functions*: normal. *Speech*: normal flow, clear to
understand. *Motor System*: Mass, tone and strength is normal. *Sensory System*: Normal
distribution. *Deep Tendon Reflexes*: normal throughout. *Cerebellar System*: Normal bilaterally.
Gait and Balance: bilateral symmetry of length, alignment and position. *Extrapyramidal
System:* Normal.

Problems:
1. ANXIETY STATE UNSPECIFIED (300.00)
2. DEPRESSION (311)
3. LUMBAR DISC DEGENERATION (722.52)
4. OBSTRUCTIVE SLEEP APNEA (327.23)
5. There are two issues with sleep in this gentleman: insomnia secondary to uncontrolled
   anxiety/ depression and age changes. Of course one has to be concerned about obstructive
   sleep apnea in one with CAD.

Plan Note
Patient Education
Sleep Hygiene
Sleep Study scheduled on April 20, 2012

---

727 Craig Road   Suite 101   St. Louis, MO 63141
(314) 994-9499   Fax (314) 991-6844   www.americansleepmedicine.com

Figure A-2 (continued). Split-night sleep study for patient B. (Reprinted with permission from American Sleep Medicine of St. Louis.)

Tech Initials   NB   Chart #___

Patient Satisfaction Survey

American Sleep Medicine, is committed to providing quality sleep medicine services. Please answer this questionnaire to help us improve our service. Your response is confidential.

Communication:

1. Did you have a consultation with ASM sleep specialist physician?   ☒ Yes   ☐ No
2. Were you satisfied with your wait time to see the physician?   ☒ Yes   ☐ No
3. Were you given adequate information in preparation for testing?   ☒ Yes   ☐ No
4. Were questions you had prior to the testing adequately addressed?   ☒ Yes   ☐ No
5. Did you have any difficulty scheduling your testing?   ☐ Yes   ☒ No
   If yes, please explain: _____

Do you have any suggestions or comments for our physician?

_____

Do you have any suggestion as to how we can improve our communication?

_____

Comfort of the sleep center:
Please rate on a scale of 1 to 4 (circle the number)

1. Cleanliness of the room:	4 Excellent	3 Good	2 Average	1 Poor
2. Noise level	4 Excellent	3 Good	2 Average	1 Poor
3. Room temperature:	4 Excellent	3 Good	2 Average	1 Poor

Do you have specific suggestions as to how we could have made your stay in our center more comfortable?
MORE sound proofing of Rooms

Sleep Center Staff:
Please rate our staff on the following 1 to 4 scale (circle the number)

1. Professionalism	4 Excellent	3 Good	2 Average	1 Poor
2. Friendliness/helpfulness	4 Excellent	3 Good	2 Average	1 Poor

Do you have any suggestion as to how our staff can serve you better?

_____

General Questions:

1. Please rate the overall quality of services you received in our sleep disorders laboratory.
      ☐ 4 Excellent   ☒ 3 Good   ☐ 2 Average   ☐ 1 Poor

2. Would you recommend our services to family or friends?   ☒ Yes   ☐ No

3. If you have received similar services at another sleep laboratory/center, how do we compare?

_____

How did you hear about us (circle one)?

Advertisement   Health Fair   Friend   (Physician Referral)   Other

Please feel free to write any additional comments or suggestions:

_____

Patient Signature   Date of Study: 4/20/12

Figure A-2 (continued). Split-night sleep study for patient B. (Reprinted with permission from American Sleep Medicine of St. Louis.)

SLEEP STUDY EXAMPLE THREE

Patient C is a 70-year-old female with a long history of fibromyalgia and pelvic floor dysfunction. She reported nonrestorative sleep and chronic sleep-onset insomnia. She scored high on the FSS, but had a normal score on Epworth. She was noted to have markedly dysfunctional mechanics of respiration. Because of her chronic pain and reports of nonrestorative sleep and insomnia, she was sent for a sleep study. Her study was initially read as essentially normal, but a closer analysis determined that she has extended sleep latency. Review of her stage 2 sleep (N2) revealed that she produced sleep spindles without K-complexes, which are seen in individuals with fibromyalgia. Because of her symptoms, she was referred for neurofeedback. Prior to her sleep study, she took 150-mg trazodone and 2.5 to 5 mg of Ambien at night for sleep and still reported insomnia and nonrestorative sleep. After going through neurofeedback specifically for disordered sleep, at the time of this writing, she reported markedly improved sleep and less fatigue and improved functional capacity during activities of daily living. She has reduced her sleep medication and is now only taking 25 mg of trazodone and has stopped taking Ambien altogether.

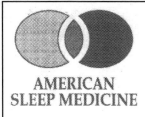

**AMERICAN
SLEEP MEDICINE**

Patient: DOS: -11
MRN: DOB: 40
Account:
Physician:

SOCIAL HISTORY: A 30-pack-year history of tobacco use. She quit 23 years ago. She has one glass of tea per day and denies alcohol use.

REVIEW OF SYSTEMS: Significant for mild shortness of breath, constipation, pain in her back and feet. All other systems were reviewed and are negative.

PHYSICAL EXAMINATION:

VITALS: Blood pressure is 128/75. Pulse is 89. Respiratory rate is 12. Height is 5 feet 6.5 inches. Weight is 120 pounds. BMI is 19. Neck circumference is 11 inches.

GENERAL: She appeared in no acute distress.

HEENT: Normocephalic, atraumatic. Mallampati score was III.

CHEST: Heart had a regular rate and rhythm.

LUNGS: Clear to auscultation bilaterally.

ABDOMEN: Soft, nontender, nondistended.

EXT: Showed no edema.

NEUROLOGIC: Cranial nerves II through XII were grossly intact. Strength was 5/5 bilaterally.

SKIN: Appeared clear.

MENTAL STATUS: Mood was "pretty good." Affect was euthymic. Thought content was negative for suicidal ideation, homicidal ideation, hallucination, or delusion.

ASSESSMENT: This is a 70-year-old female with difficulties with sleep initiation, history of depression, anxiety, and snoring. Diagnostic possibilities include upper airway resistance syndrome, obstructive sleep apnea syndrome, and primary snoring. In addition, her sleep is affected by the depression being treated by Dr. Giuffra. Vicodin and Xanax could cause sleep disruption when withdrawal occurs.

727 Craig Rd.   Suite 101   St. Louis, MO 63141
www.americansleepmedicine.com   (314) 994-9499   Fax (314) 991-6844   *info11@americansleepmedicine.com*

Figure A-3. Sleep study for patient C. (Reprinted with permission from American Sleep Medicine of St. Louis.)

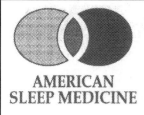

**AMERICAN
SLEEP MEDICINE**

Patient: DOS: ·11
MRN: DOB: 40
Account:
Physician:

PLAN:
1. All-night polysomnography followed by CPAP titration if needed. She was scheduled for January 22, 2011.
2. We discussed sleep related reading material.
3. Follow-up in clinic after sleep studies to decide on treatment.

Many thanks for involving us in the care of this interesting patient. If you have further questions, please feel free to contact us at 314-994-9499.

Figure A-3 (continued). Sleep study for patient C. (Reprinted with permission from American Sleep Medicine of St. Louis.)

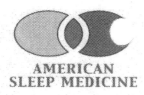

AMERICAN
SLEEP MEDICINE
727 Craig Road # 101
St. Louis, MO 63141
(314) 994-9499

Polysomnography Report

NARRATIVE REPORT

PATIENT'S NAME:
DOB: 1940
DATE OF RECORDING:
REQUESTING M.D.:
ATTENDING M.D.:

Study Performed: Nocturnal Polysomnography

HISTORY: This is a 70 year old female who presented with complaints of difficulties with sleep initiation for many years, she also reports snoring. She has a history of hyperlipidemia, osteoporosis, COPD with planned PFTs, IBS, and mile osteoarthritis. Her Epworth Sleepiness Scale score is 7.

PROCEDURE: This is a nocturnal technician attended polysomnography using the American Sleep Medicine Protocol utilizing continuous digital recording. Recorded channels included: EEG (international 10-20 electrode placement), eye movement, chin EMG, nasal and oral airflow, ECG, respiratory effort, oximetry, body position, snoring sound, pulse rate and limb movement. All events are scored according to the current AASM criteria. Hypopneas (4a) have a 30% reduction in airflow and at least a 4% desaturation and are calculated within the AHI. Alternative Hypopneas (4b) have a 50% reduction in airflow and are accompanied by either a 3% desaturation or an arousal and is calculated within the RDI.

SUMMARY:
1. Sleep Architecture: Lights out occurred at 22:15:22. Lights on occurred at 05:44:23. Total recorded time was 453.6 minutes, with a total sleep time of 408.5 minutes and a sleep efficiency of 91.0 %. The patient's sleep latency was 8.5 minutes. Latency to REM was 215.5 minutes. There was 8.0% of Stage N1 sleep, 36.6% stage N2 sleep, 38.1% stage N3 sleep, and 17.4% REM sleep. Total number of arousals was 105. Arousal index was 15.4.

2. Respiratory Data: During the study the patient had 25 episodes of apneas and (4a) hypopneas (4% oxygen desaturations or greater) making the **Apnea/Hypopnea Index (AHI) 3.7** events per sleep hour. Mean length of the apnea/hypopnea was 22.9 seconds and the longest was 47.8 seconds.

In addition to the above events, there were other hypopneas (4b) and "respiratory arousals" which did not strictly fulfill CMS criteria for desaturation, but were associated with arousals or sleep disruption. When these were considered, the total **Respiratory Disturbance Index (RDI)** was **7.2** events per sleep hour. During non REM sleep there were 6.2 events per sleep hour, and during **REM** sleep there were **11.8** events per sleep hour. Respiratory disturbance index during sleeping in the supine position was **10.0** events per sleep hour and the patient slept **144.5** minutes in the supine position. Respiratory disturbance index while sleeping on both sides was **0.2** events per sleep hour, and the patient slept for 264.0 minutes on both sides. **Mild/Moderate** snoring was noted.

Figure A-3 (continued). Sleep study for patient C. (Reprinted with permission from American Sleep Medicine of St. Louis.)

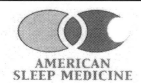

**AMERICAN
SLEEP MEDICINE**

*727 Craig Road # 101
St. Louis, MO 63141
(314) 994-9499*

Polysomnography Report

PATIENT'S NAME:
DOB: ·1940
DATE OF RECORDING:

3. Oxygen Data: The patient spent 99.7 percent of sleep time with oxygen saturation equal to or above 90 percent, the patient spent 0.0 percent of sleep time with oxygen saturation equal to or below 88 percent and the lowest oxygen saturation was 88%.

4. EKG Data: No arrhythmias were noted during the sleep study.

5. Other Data: No leg movements were noted, with a PLM index of 0.0 and a leg movement arousal index of 0.6.

CONCLUSION:

1. The study showed evidence suggestive of underlying upper airway resistance syndrome. This is based on a total AHI of only **3.7** and a total respiratory disturbance index of **7.2** events per sleep hour as compared to a normal of 5 or less.

2. The study showed no prolonged hypoxia, but there were transient desaturations with the lowest saturation of **88%.**

3. Significantly prolonged slow wave sleep was noted along with reduced stage 2 sleepand slightly increased spindle activity. She had delayed REM onset which could be due to medication effect. Her sleep efficiency was within normal limits at 91.0%.

DIAGNOSIS:
    1. Upper Airway Resistance Syndrome (a variant of OSA 327.23)
    2. Mild to Moderate Snoring (786.09)
    3. Idiopathic Insomnia (307.42)

RECOMMENDATION: The patient is scheduled for a follow-up appointment on ███████ to discuss the results of the sleep study and treatment options. If you would like to discuss this case feel free to call me at ██████████ The patient was instructed not to drive or operate heavy machinery if having symptoms of sleepiness.

Figure A-3 (continued). Sleep study for patient C. (Reprinted with permission from American Sleep Medicine of St. Louis.)

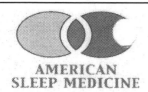

**AMERICAN
SLEEP MEDICINE**

*727 Craig Road # 101
St. Louis, MO 63141
(314) 994-9499*

Polysomnography Report

Summary

Study Information

Name:		Date of Study:	
Date of Birth: .1940		Sex: Female	
Height: 5'6.5"	Wt: 120 lbs.		BMI: 19.1
Requesting Physician:		Diagnosis:	

Staging Summary Information

Recording Start Time:	22:10:53	Recording End Time:	05:44:26
Lights Out:	22:15:22	Lights On:	05:44:23
Total Recording Time (min) :	7:33.5	Total Sleep Time:	6:48.5
Sleep Efficiency (%):	91.0	Number of Awakenings:	8
Sleep Onset Latency (min):	8.5	Stage REM Latency (min):	215.5
(Lights Out to first epoch of 3 consecutive			
sleep epochs, stg. 1, 2, 3, 4, or one epoch of REM)		(Sleep onset to first REM epoch)	
Wake After Sleep Onset (min):	31.0		

Staging Table

Sleep Stage	Duration (min)	% Sleep Time	% Normal
Wake	31.0		
Stage N1 Sleep	32.5	8.0	10%
Stage N2 Sleep	149.5	36.6	50%
Stage N3 Sleep	155.5	38.1	15%
Stage REM	71.0	17.4	25%

SaO2 Summary

SaO2 Awake Average (%)	95
Lowest SaO2 (%)	88

Saturation Levels

Saturation Levels	Hours/Minutes
Time Equal to or Below 95%	6:46:26.0
Time Equal to or Below 90%	0:00:39.0
Time Equal to or Below 85%	0:00:0.0

Figure A-3 (continued). Sleep study for patient C. (Reprinted with permission from American Sleep Medicine of St. Louis.)

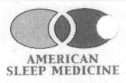

**AMERICAN
SLEEP MEDICINE**
*727 Craig Road # 101
St. Louis, MO 63141
(314) 994-9499*

Polysomnography Report

| Name: | | Date of Birth: | '1940 | Date of Study: | |

Respiratory Events Summary

Parameter	Obstructive	Mixed	Central	Total Apnea	Hypopnea	Alternative Hypopnea	RERA
Number	23	0	0	23	2	8	16
Index (per hour)	3.4	0.0	0.0	3.4	0.3	1.2	2.4
Average Duration (sec)	21.3	0.0	0.0	21.3	42.3	30.0	17.6
Longest Duration (sec)				38.3	47.8		24.8
Number in NREM	15	0	0	15	1	1.2	4
Number in REM	8	0	0	8	1	0.8	12

Respiratory Events – REM/NREM

Parameter	REM	Non-REM	Sleep
Apneas	8	15	23
Hypopneas (4%)	1	1	2
Apneas + Hypopneas	9	16	25
Alternative Hypopneas (3%)	1	7	8
RERA's (Respiratory limitation with arousal and 2% or less desaturation)	4	12	16
Duration in Apnea (min)	3.3	4.8	8.2
Duration in Hypopnea (min)	0.8	0.6	1.4
Duration in Apnea + Hypopnea (min)	4.1	5.4	9.6
AHI (/hr) Apnea/Hypopnea with 4 % oxygen desaturation or greater	7.6	2.8	3.7
RDI (/hr) AHI plus hypopneas with 3% oxygen desaturations and RERAs	11.8	6.2	7.2

Respiratory Events Index (/hr) by Position (sleep time)

Position	Obstructive	Mixed	Central	Hypopnea	Alternative Hypopnea	RERA
Index Supine	9.1	0.0	0.0	0.8	2.9	5.8
Index Non-Supine	0.2	0.0	0.0	0.0	0.2	0.5

Figure A-3 (continued). Sleep study for patient C. (Reprinted with permission from American Sleep Medicine of St. Louis.)

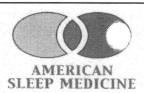

**AMERICAN
SLEEP MEDICINE**

*727 Craig Road # 101
St. Louis, MO 63141
(314) 994-9499*

Polysomnography Report

Name:	Date of Birth:	1940	Date of Study:

Heart Rate Summary

Average Heart Rate	**65**
Slowest Heart Rate	42
Fastest Heart Rate	103
Number of Bradycardic Periods	0
Number of Tachycardic Periods	0

Arousal Summary

Number of	REM	Non-REM	Sleep
Respiratory Arousal	9	28	37
Limb Arousal	0	4	4
Spontaneous Arousal	13	51	64
Total			105
Per Hour			
Respiratory Arousal	7.6	5.0	5.4
Limb Arousal	0.0	0.7	0.6
Spontaneous Arousal	11.0	9.1	9.4
Total			15.4

Leg Movements Summary

	REM	NREM	Total
Number of Limb Movement Associated Arousals	0	4	4
PLM Episodes	0	0	0
Number of Limb Movements per Hour	0.0	5.3	4.4
PLM Index	0.0	0.0	0.0
Limb Movement Arousal Index	0.0	0.7	0.6

A PLM index of less than 5 is considered normal.
  *Ref: THE INTERNATIONAL CLASSIFICATION OF SLEEP DISORDERS Diagnostic and Coding Manual,
1990*

Figure A-3 (continued). Sleep study for patient C. (Reprinted with permission from American Sleep Medicine of St. Louis.)

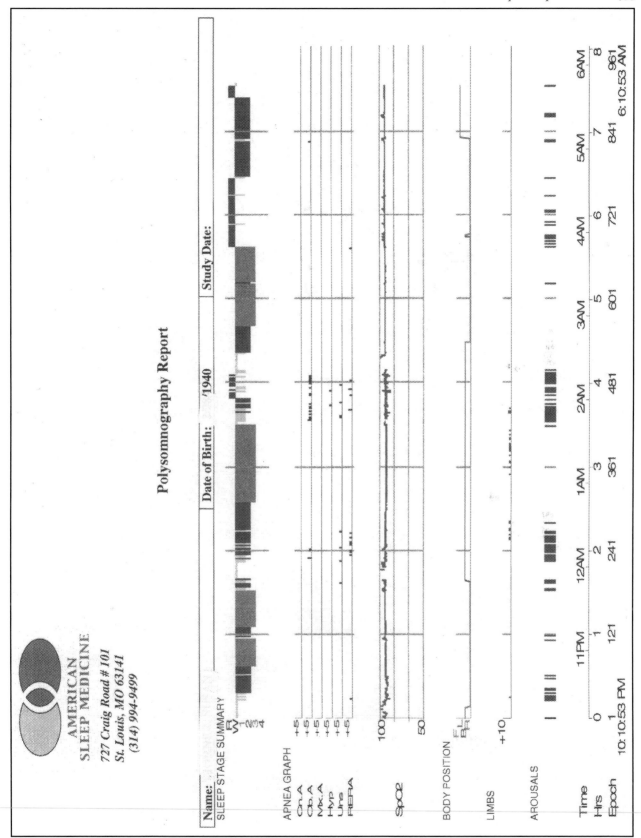

Figure A-3 (continued). Sleep study for patient C. (Reprinted with permission from American Sleep Medicine of St. Louis.)

SUMMARY

These examples show a variety of patient symptoms that lead to referral for sleep study. Each of these patients was being seen by multiple medical professionals, but the impact of disordered sleep was not identified. Perhaps because of the increased patient contact time and understanding of the importance of sleep, the significance of these symptoms was recognized in the rehabilitation setting. The disordered sleep in these patients is likely a contributing factor in the conditions for which these patients were referred for rehabilitation.

A Primer on Brain Waves

Julie M. Hereford, PT, DPT

A. Alpha waves—encephalograph (EEG) oscillations with a frequency of 8 to 13 Hz (slower among children and older adults compared to younger adults) (Figure B-1).

1. Variable amplitude (generally <50 µV among adults).

2. Present when a person is relaxed and drowsy and eyes are closed.

3. Also present during arousals from sleep.

4. Originate in the occipital cortex; more prominent in the occipital leads compared with central leads.

5. Eye opening suppresses alpha activity.

6. Alpha waves are reduced with open eyes and drowsiness and sleep. Historically, they were thought to represent the activity of the visual cortex in an idle state. More recent papers have argued that they inhibit areas of the cortex not in use or, alternatively, that they play an active role in network coordination and communication. Occipital alpha waves during periods of eyes closed are the strongest EEG brain signals.

7. An alpha-like variant called mu (µ) can be found over the motor cortex (central scalp) that is reduced with movement, or the intention to move. Alpha waves do not start to appear until 3 years of age.

8. Alpha wave intrusion occurs when alpha waves appear with non-rapid eye movement (NREM) sleep when delta activity is expected. It is hypothesized to be associated with fibromyalgia, although the study was too small to be conclusive.

B. Alpha-delta—alpha waves occurring during NREM stages 3 and 4 (slow wave or delta) sleep.

C. Beta waves—EEG oscillations with a frequency of 13 to 35 Hz and an amplitude that is usually less than 30 µV (Figure B-2).

1. Present during alert wakefulness.

2. Low-amplitude beta waves with multiple and varying frequencies are often associated with active, busy, or anxious thinking and active concentration.

3. Over the motor cortex, beta waves are associated with the muscle contractions that happen in isotonic movements and are suppressed prior to and during movement changes. Bursts of beta activity are associated with a strengthening of sensory feedback in static motor control and reduced when there is movement change. Beta activity is increased when movement has to be resisted or voluntarily suppressed.

D. Sleep spindles—brief oscillations with a frequency of 12 to 14 Hz lasting 0.5 to 1.5 seconds and an amplitude generally less than 50 µV (Figure B-3).

1. More prominent and which highest voltage over the central leads.

2. May occur during NREM stages 2, 3, and 4 sleep; not seen in NREM stage 1 sleep and REM sleep.

3. Generated in midline thalamic nuclei.

4. Compared to sleep spindles, alpha waves are slower (8–13 Hz).

5. Pseudo-spindles or drug spindles secondary to benzodiazepines have a higher frequency (about 15 Hz).

6. Sometimes referred to as *sigma bands* or *sigma waves*; may represent periods where the brain is

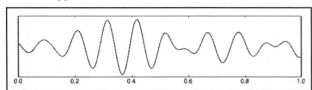

Figure B-1. Alpha waves. (Reprinted with permission from CORE Services, Inc.)

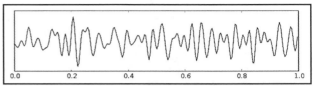

Figure B-2. Beta waves. (Reprinted with permission from CORE Services, Inc.)

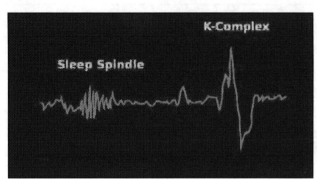

Figure B-3. Sleep spindles and K-complexes characteristic of N2 sleep. (Reprinted with permission from CORE Services, Inc.)

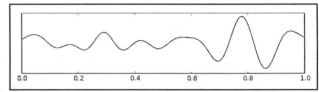

Figure B-4. Theta waves. (Reprinted with permission from CORE Services, Inc.)

inhibiting processing to keep the sleeper in a tranquil state. Along with K-complexes, they are defining characteristics of NREM stage 2 sleep and indicate its onset. They are often tapered at both ends and may or may not be synchronous, but they should be symmetrical and bilateral.

E. K complex—high-amplitude, bi-phasic wave (an initial sharp negative deflection followed by a positive high-voltage slow wave) with a duration of at least 0.5 seconds.

  1. They have 2 proposed functions. First, suppressing cortical arousal in response to stimuli that the sleeping brain evaluates not to signal danger and, second, aiding sleep-based memory consolidation.

  2. Seen maximally over the vertex (central or central-parietal leads).

  3. Believed to represent evoked responses to internal and external stimuli.

F. Sawtooth wave—theta waves with notched waveform.

  1. More prominent over the vertex and frontal leads.

  2. Occur during REM sleep.

G. Theta waves—EEG oscillations with a frequency of 4 to 7 Hz (Figure B-4).

  1. Function is not clear but may be related to memory and learning.

  2. Originate in the hippocampus.

  3. Maximal over the central and temporal leads.

H. Vertex sharp deflections—sharp negative deflections with amplitudes less than 250 μV that are maximal over the vertex.

Glossary of Terms

acetylcholine: A biogenic amine.

action potential: A nerve impulse that is generated by depolarization of the membrane to a threshold (firing) value.

adenosine: An endogenous nucleotide that is a constituent of ribonucleic acid yielding adenine and ribose on hydrolysis; a potent neuromodulator that is distributed at almost all synapses.

ambient temperature: Temperature of the environment.

apnea: Absence of breathing.

atonia: Absence of muscle tone. Tone is the resistance of a muscle to passive elongation or stretch; it is due to the asynchronous, sustained firing of motorneurons.

atropine: A competitive inhibitor of the actions of the neurotransmitter acetylcholine at the musarinic receptors of effector sites, particularly those innervated by cholinergic nerves; parasympatholytic agent that produces relaxation of the smooth muscles in various organs.

basal condition: Basic state essential for maintaining the fundamental vital activities of an organism.

benzodiazepines: A group of drugs used mainly in the treatment of anxiety including, among others, chlordiazepoxide (Librium), diazepam (Valium), and oxazepam (Serax).

biological clock: The brain mechanisms that determine when periods of increased and decreased activity occur in various biological systems.

brainstem: The lower part of the brain; a collective term for the medulla oblongata, pons, and midbrain. The part of the neuraxis, located at the base of the brain, that connects the spinal cord with the rest of the brain; it is thought to contain the mechanisms that regulate sleep and waking behavior, especially rapid eye movement (REM) sleep and wakefulness.

cataplexy: A sudden dramatic decrease in muscle tone and loss of certain reflexes, usually precipitated by strong emotional expression or by the intention of making a sharp movement or by startle; a part of the tetrad of narcolepsy.

cholinergic (nerve): Liberating acetylcholine; a nerve that releases acetylcholine as its neurotransmitter when it is stimulated; for example, all motor nerves of the somatic nervous system.

complex partial seizures: Involve associative areas, notably the limbic system, and there is impaired consciousness, which may be associated with affective changes, automatisms, and amnesia. Partial seizures are seizures in which the first clinical changes indicate activation of an anatomical and/or functional system of neurons limited to a part of a single hemisphere.

depolarization: The reciprocal of hyperpolarization.

desynchronous: (Relative to brain waves) An electroencephalographic (EEG) record that lacks regularity of frequency, thought to indicate a varying and variable pattern of firing of brain cells.

diurnal: Recurring every day.

dopamine: A major neurotransmitter in certain areas of the central nervous system, especially in the nigrostriatal tract; the immediate precursor of norepinephrine in the body; an alpha-adrenergic stimulant.

electroencephalogram: A recording of differences in electrical activity between 2 regions of the brain, ordinarily recorded by means of electrodes applied to the scalp.

eDS: Excessive daytime sleepiness.

entrain: (Synchronize) Zeitgebers; that is, indicators of time, which may be clocks, mealtimes, work periods, position of the sun, etc.

free-running period: A sleep–wake cycle that is internally generated and not responsive to subtle 24-hour time cues associated with the solar day; it can be modified by factors such as the environmental light intensity and hormones .

histamine: An active endogenous substance that functions as a local hormone; acts to modulate local circulation, influence the process of inflammation, and stimulate gastric acid secretions; it is present in the central nervous system and possibly acts as a neurotransmitter.

homeostatic mechanisms: Feedback mechanisms that preserve the stability of the internal environment of a normal organism despite the presence of influences capable of causing profound changes.

hypercapnia: Excess carbon dioxide in the blood that results in overstimulation of the respiratory center.

hyperpolarization: An increase in the relative negativity of the interior of a neuron with respect to the exterior. It may be produced either by an alteration in the charge held by the membrane capacitor or by the movement of ions across the membrane. Hyperpolarization is accompanied by a decrease in excitability.

hypersomnolence: Pathologically excessive drowsiness or sleepiness.

hypoxia: Oxygen deficiency.

insomnia: Dissatisfaction with the quantity or quality of sleep.

internal desynchronization: Occurs when the internal relationships between the numerous daily rhythms that compose the human circadian system are disrupted.

jet lag: Circadian desynchronization and sleeplessness that occurs due to jet aircraft travel to destinations that are several time zones away from the site of origin.

locus coeruleus: A region (bluish in the fresh brain) in the lateral portion of the pons.

metabolic rate: The total quantity of heat that is released per unit of time by the body; this value is expressed in terms of heat energy; that is, calories.

microsleep: Brief intrusions of EEG indications of sleep.

midbrain: (Mesencephalon) Part of the brain stem above the pons and below the diencephalon; forms the upper part and limit of the brain stem.

morpheus: The Greek god of dreams.

myoclonus: A brief and involuntary contraction of one or several muscles that displaces a segment of a limb, a whole limb, or even the entire body in a jerk-like movement.

narcolepsy: A disease in which the afflicted individual periodically finds it impossible to stay awake during the daytime (cataplexy, sleep paralysis, and hypnogogic hallucinations together with narcolepsy complete the tetrad of narcolepsy).

night terrors: A sleep pathology that usually starts with a piercing scream; there is sweating and rapid breathing and an increase in heart rate.

noradrenergic: That is, norepinephrine = noradrenaline not noradrenergic.

ontogenetic: Refers to the complete developmental history of the individual organism.

peptide: A secondary protein derivative characterized by a combination of 2 or more amino acids.

polyneuropathies: The general term denoting functional disturbances and/or pathological changes in the peripheral nervous system.

polysomnography: The simultaneous evaluation of multiple physiological parameters during sleep.

pons: The smallest part of the brain stem lying between the medulla oblongata and the mesencephalon.

Pons tegmentum: The dorsal part of the pons.

postsynaptic inhibition: Inhibition of a cell that is produced by the liberation, from a presynaptic cell, of a neurotransmitter that produces a decrease in excitability.

raphe nuclei: A complex of 9 narrow cellular clusters on the midline that extends through the length of the brain stem (containing serotonin).

reticular formation: A diffuse system of nerve cell bodies and fibers in the brain stem that extends from the medulla oblongata to the thalamus.

sleep cycle: The regular alternation between non-rapid eye movement (NREM) and REM sleep that characterizes any relatively lengthy and undisturbed period of mammalian sleep. An NREM period plus the following REM period equals one sleep cycle.

sleep stages: Subdivisions of the sleep states.

solitary tract: A bundle of nerve fibers consisting of afferent (sensory) input from the vagus, glossopharyngeal, and facial nerves.

somnambulism: Episodes of nocturnal walking during which the subject is asleep or at least incompletely awake.

soporific: Causing or tending to cause sleep; tending to dull awareness or alertness.

spindle: A typical waveform seen in the EEG during NREM sleep; it is characterized by a burst of very regular oscillations at a frequency of from 12 to 14 cycles per second. Sleep spindles are observed most often during NREM stage 2 sleep.

suprachiasmatic nucleus: A group of nerve cells located above the optic chiasm.

Suggested Readings

Chaitow L, Bradley D, Gilbert C. *Multidisciplinary Approaches to Breathing Patter Disorders.* Edinburgh, Scotland: Churchill Livingstone; 2002.

Cohen H. *Neuroscience for Rehabilitation.* Philadelphia, PA: JB Lippincott Company; 1993.

DeMent WC. *The Promise of Sleep.* New York, NY: Random House; 1999.

Goddard S. *Reflexes, Learning and Behavior: A Window Into the Child's Mind.* Eugene, OR: Fern Ridge Press; 2005.

Goodman CC, Boissonnault WG, Fuller KS. *Pathology: Implication for the Physical Therapist.* Philadelphia, PA: Elsevier; 2003.

Kryger H, Roth T, DeMent WC. *Principles and Practice of Sleep Medicine: Expert Consult.* 5th ed. St Louis, MO: Elsevier; 2011.

Lee-Chiong T. *Sleep Medicine: Essentials and Review.* New York, NY: Oxford University Press; 2008.

Leonard CT. *The Neuroscience of Human Movement.* St. Louis, MO: Mosby-Yearbook; 1998.

McNamara P, Barton RA, Nunn CL. *Evolution of Sleep: Phylogenetic and Functional Perspectives.* Cambridge, NY: Cambridge University Press; 2010.

Saunders NA, Sullivan CE. *Sleep and Breathing.* 2nd ed. New York, NY: Marcel Dekker; 1994.

Seuss D. *Sleep Book.* New York, NY: Random House; 1962.

Siegel J. *The Neural Control of Sleep and Waking.* New York, NY: Springer-Verlag; 2002.

Stickgold R, Walker M. *The Neuroscience of Sleep.* London, UK: Academic Press; 2009.

Wiley TS, Fromby B. *Lights Out: Sleep, Sugar and Survival.* New York, NY: Simon & Schuster; 2000.

Financial Disclosures

Dr. Julie M. Hereford has no financial or proprietary interest in the materials presented herein.

Dr. J. Paul Rutledge has no financial or proprietary interest in the materials presented herein.

Dr. Michael D. Hoefs has no financial or proprietary interest in the materials presented herein.

Dr. Duane C. Keller has no financial or proprietary interest in the materials presented herein.

Dr. Bridget E. Lovett has no financial or proprietary interest in the materials presented herein.

Dr. Lauren Milton has no financial or proprietary interest in the materials presented herein.

Dr. Mark Murray has no financial or proprietary interest in the materials presented herein.

Dr. Catherine Siegenskon has no financial or proprietary interest in the materials presented herein.

Index

Printed in the United States
by Baker & Taylor Publisher Services